Dedication

Dedicated to the memory of Michael Wollman, founder and c... Trainers Association (NETA). Michael was a true visionary and believed fitness educa... should be accessible to anyone with a dream and desire to learn.

Michael Wollman
1945 – 2000

In Memoriam

In memory of our dear friend and colleague, Randy Micheau. Randy was a national presenter for the National Exercise Trainers Association (NETA) for many years during which time he inspired countless fitness professionals to expand their knowledge and attain fulfillment in their careers. Randy had an infectious personality allowing him to connect with all and to find a special place in the hearts of many.

Randy Micheau
1960 - 2012

Acknowledgments

NETA would like to thank the countless individuals who have helped us, over the past 40 years, make continual strides toward excellence. Many highly-qualified individuals have been instrumental in writing, illustrating, editing, and designing previous versions of NETA fitness manuals since 1980. The fifth edition is a compilation of these predecessors as well as additional subject matter, and updated recommendations and guidelines.

Graphic Design/Illustrator/Page Layout:
Donna Crespo

Photography:
Glenn Hagen (on-site location courtesy of Gold's Gym)

The NETA Team:

President/Executive Director:
Mario Crespo

Vice President of Operations:
Nicole Miska

Director of Education:
Samantha Protokowicz

Director of Certification:
Michael Iserman

Director of Marketing and Events:
Amara Viaene

Business Development Manager:
Nicole Anderson

Customer Service:
Mou Xe Yang, Jamie McCalley

The web addresses cited in this text were current as of June 2017, unless otherwise noted.

ISBN: 978-0-578-18656-6

©Copyright 2018 National Exercise Trainers Association. All rights reserved. This material may not be reproduced or duplicated in whole or in part, by any means, without permission of:

National Exercise Trainers Association (NETA)
12800 Industrial Park Blvd., Suite 220
Minneapolis, MN 55441
www.NETAfit.org

To order additional copies of this manual, call toll-free 1-800-237-6242, (In Minnesota 763-545-2505)

Vision Statement

NETA's vision is to help our society achieve optimal health facilitated by access to and guidance from a network of well-qualified fitness professionals.

Mission Statement

NETA's mission is to support and inspire the development of well-qualified fitness professionals through the delivery of high-quality educational programs incorporating evidence-based research and practical application. We are committed to guiding fitness professionals throughout their careers by offering affordable, accessible educational opportunities.

Welcome

NETA welcomes you. We are here to help you achieve your personal and professional career goals in the diverse and rapidly-growing fitness industry.

The fifth edition of NETA's *The Fitness Professional's Manual* is an in-depth, user-friendly guide to the foundational theories, concepts, and essential knowledge necessary to support your education and professional development.

In this Manual you will find topics including:

- The role and responsibilities of the fitness professional;
- Effective communication and interpersonal relationship-building skills;
- Techniques to facilitate behavioral change and motivation;
- Introduction to wellness coaching;
- Overview of exercise sciences including anatomy, kinesiology, biomechanics, and exercise physiology;
- Principles of nutrition and weight management;
- Administration and interpretation of health and fitness assessments;
- Guidelines to develop safe and effective exercise programs;
- Fundamentals of leading group exercise classes;
- Exercise-related medical considerations and guidelines for special populations; and
- Administrative and legal considerations for fitness professionals.

It is our sincere hope that this Manual will serve as an invaluable study tool and an ongoing informational resource throughout your fitness career.

For additional resources, such as information regarding our workshops, certification programs, and continuing education offerings, please visit the NETA website at www.netafit.org.

The fitness industry is constantly evolving and advancing. As new research and evidence emerges to expand our understanding of health, fitness, and other dimensions of the exercise profession, changes in programming recommendations, guidelines, and standards are inevitable. The authors and reviewers of this manual have made every effort to verify information contained herein with credible and reliable sources to ensure the content of this manual reflects the up-to-date science and best practices at the time of publication. However, considering the possibility of human error and/or changes in the fitness industry, neither the authors, NETA, or any party who has contributed to this manual warrants that the information provided is accurate or complete, and they are not responsible for errors or omissions, or any outcomes that may result from the use of information contained within this manual.

Reviewers

Ashley Artese, MS, ACE-CPT, ACE-GFI
Florida State University
Tallahassee, FL

Elizabeth Baker, MA, NSCA-CPT, NETA-CGEI
Normandale Community College
Bloomington, MN

Amy Bakken, MA, NSCA-CPT, NETA-CGEI
OptumHealth
Minneapolis, MN

Sarah Cheffy, MS, ACE-CPT
EMPOWER! Mind. Body. Life., LLC
Greensboro, NC

Jon Giese, MEd, NETA-CPT
Rochester Athletic Club
Rochester, MN

Darci Kruse, MS, CSCS, TSAC-F
Marine Corps Community Services, Semper Fit
Marine Corps Base Camp Pendleton, CA

Matt Larson, MS, CSCS
YMCA of Greater Indianapolis
Indianapolis, IN

Michael Lucchino, MEd, CSCS
Loudoun County Public Schools
Sterling, VA

AmberLynn Pappas, MS, ACE-CPT, ACE-GFI
Independent Fitness Professional
Wilmington, NC

Riley Peterson, MA, CSCS
YMCA of the Greater Twin Cities
Burnsville, MN

Samantha Protokowicz, MSEd, ACSM EP-C
National Exercise Trainers Association
Minneapolis, MN

Angie Schroeder, MBA, NETA-CPT, NETA-CGEI
Terra State Community College
Fremont, OH

Jon Staton, MEd, NETA-CPT
Odessa College
Odessa, TX

Jennifer Turpin-Stanfield, MA, ACSM EP-C
Wright State University
Dayton, OH

Table of Contents

Section One: Communication, Interpersonal Relationships, & Behavioral Science

Chapter 1: The Role of Fitness Professionals 3
- Ideal Qualities and Characteristics 3
- Personal Trainer 3
- Group Exercise Instructor 5
- Wellness Coach 5
- Ethics and Professional Standards 5
- NETA's Professional Code of Ethics 5
- Continuing Education 6
- Credible Sources of Information 6

Chapter 2: Relationship-Building & Communication Skills 11
- Rapport 11
- First Impressions 12
- Approaching Members 13
- Impact of a Message 14
- Active Listening Skills 14
- Nonverbal Listening Skills 14
- Understanding Body Language 15
- Verbal Listening Skills 15
- Effective Questions 15
- Reflective Statements 17

Chapter 3: Behavioral Change & Motivation 21
- Transtheoretical Model 21
- Decisional Balance 23
- Self-Efficacy 23
- Social Cognitive Theory 25
- Self-Determination Theory 26
- Health Belief Model 26
- Goal-Setting 26
- SMART Goals 26
- Motivation and Adherence 27

Chapter 4: Introduction to Wellness Coaching 31
- The Art of Wellness Coaching 31
- Motivational Interviewing 32

Appreciative Inquiry 34
The GROW Coaching Model 35

Section Two: Exercise Science

Chapter 5: Human Anatomy 43
Location Terminology 43
Planes of Motion 44
The Skeletal System 44
The Vertebral Column 44
Types of Articulations 46
The Muscular System 49
Structure of Skeletal Muscle 49
Sliding Filament Theory 51
Types of Muscle Action 51
Muscle Functions 52

Chapter 6: Applied Kinesiology & Biomechanics 55
Movement Terminology 55
Kinesiology of the Shoulder Complex and Upper Extremities 55
Kinesiology of the Torso Muscles 59
Kinesiology of the Hips and Lower Extremities 59
Newton's Laws of Motion 67
Biomechanics of Torque 69
Types of Lever Systems 70
Types of Mechanical Stress 71
Deformation Response to Force 72
Posture and the Kinetic Chain 72
Principles of Applied Biomechanics 73

Chapter 7: Exercise Physiology 79
The Cardiorespiratory System 79
The Pathway of Blood Flow 80
Oxygen Consumption 83
Oxygen Deficit and Debt 83
The Bioenergetics Systems 84
The Phosphagen System 84
Anaerobic Glycolysis 85
The Aerobic System 85
Anaerobic Threshold 87

The Neuromuscular System..87
Skeletal Muscle Fiber Types 87
The Motor Unit 89

Section Three: Principles of Nutrition & Weight Management

Chapter 8: Essential Nutrients for Health & Performance 95
The Digestive System 95
Carbohydrates...95
Protein 96
Fat 97
Vitamins 97
Minerals...100
Water 101

Chapter 9: Dietary Guidelines..105
Key Elements of Healthy Eating Patterns 105
Key Recommendations of Healthy Eating Patterns 106
Shifting Toward Healthy Eating Patterns...108
Everyone Has a Role 111
MyPlate 111
Nutrition Facts Label 112
Calculating Macronutrients in Foods... 113
Updates to the Nutrition Facts Label... 114

Chapter 10: Weight Management 119
The Prevalence and Impact of Obesity... 119
Metabolism..120
Calculating Resting Metabolic Rate 122
Guidelines for Safe Weight Loss...122
Motivational Interviewing and Weight Loss...123
National Weight Control Registry..123
Calculation of Goal Body Weight 124

Chapter 11: Eating Disorders 129
Prevalence of Eating Disorders...129
General Risk Factors 129
Anorexia Nervosa..130
Bulimia Nervosa 130
Binge-Eating Disorder 131

Feeding or Eating Disorders Not Elsewhere Classified 132
Female Athlete Triad 132

Section Four: Health & Fitness Assessments

Chapter 12: Initial Intake & Preparticipation Screening 139
Informed Consent 139
Physical Activity Readiness Questionnaire (PAR-Q) 140
Personal Health and Lifestyle Questionnaire 141
ACSM Preparticipation Screening Recommendations 141
Signs and Symptoms of Disease 141
Medical Clearance 142
Risk Factors for CVD 142

Chapter 13: Health Screening Assessments 149
Resting Heart Rate 149
Resting Blood Pressure 149
Body Mass Index 150
Waist-to-Hip Ratio 151
Circumference Measurements 151

Chapter 14: Postural Analysis 155
Posture and the Kinetic Chain 155
Pelvic Alignment 156
Spinal Misalignments 156
Static Postural Screening 157
Dynamic Posture 158
Postural Distortion Patterns 158
Dynamic Postural Screening 159

Chapter 15: Health-Related Physical Fitness Assessments 165
Best Practices 165
Assessment of Body Composition 166
Assessment of Cardiorespiratory Endurance 170
Assessment of Muscular Strength 174
Assessment of Muscular Endurance 175
Assessment of Muscular Flexibility 178

Section Five: Fitness Programming

Chapter 16: Physical Activity & Health 185
Health Benefits of Physical Activity 185
Physical Activity Recommendations for Improved Health 185
Physical Activity Guidelines for Americans 186
Physical Activity Intensity and METs 187
Physical Activity Epidemiology 188
Components of Physical Fitness 189
Principles of Training 190

Chapter 17: Cardiorespiratory Fitness Programming 195
Elements of the Cardiorespiratory Exercise Session 195
Guidelines for Cardiorespiratory Exercise 196
Monitoring Intensity via Heart Rate 197
Monitoring Intensity via Perceived Exertion 198
Strategies for Cardiorespiratory Programming 199

Chapter 18: Muscular Fitness Programming 205
Benefits of Resistance Training 205
Types of Resistance Training 205
General Adaptation Syndrome 207
Resistance Training Guidelines 208
Resistance Training Program Design Models 209
Periodization of Training 211
Common Resistance Training Exercises 212–248

Chapter 19: Flexibility Programming 253
Sensory Receptors 253
Types of Flexibility Exercises 253
Benefits of Stretching 255
Flexibility Training Guidelines 256
Common Flexibility Training Exercises 256–261

Section Six: Fundamentals of Group Exercise

Chapter 20: Introduction to Group Exercise 267
Introduction to Group Exercise 267
Pre-class Leadership 268
Monitoring Cardiorespiratory Intensity 270

Chapter 21: Group Exercise Formats & Components ... 277
Group Exercise Class Formats ... 277
Class Components ... 280
Cardiorespiratory Segment ... 281
Muscular Conditioning Segment ... 281
Cool-down ... 282
Flexibility Segment ... 283

Chapter 22: Leadership, Communication, & Motivation ... 287
Pre-class Leadership ... 287
Communication Skills ... 287
Transtheoretical Model & Readiness to Change ... 289
Motivation ... 289
Type of Learning ... 290

Chapter 23: Teaching a Group Exercise Class ... 293
Class Design ... 293
Fundamental Choreography ... 295
Choreography Delivery Strategies ... 296
Integrating Music ... 297
Music Mastery ... 298
Music Copyright Laws and Licensing ... 299
Cueing ... 300

Section Seven: Injury Management, Emergency Response, Medical Considerations, & Special Populations

Chapter 24: Injury Management & Emergency Response ... 307
Occurrence of Exercise-Related Injuries ... 307
Common Exercise-Related Injuries ... 308
Sprains and Strains ... 308
Chondromalacia Patellae ... 309
Meniscus Tears ... 309
Patellofemoral Pain Syndrome ... 309
Tendonitis ... 310
Shoulder Impingement Syndrome ... 310
Plantar Fasciitis ... 310
Shin Splints ... 311
Bone and Stress Fractures ... 311
Low Back Pain ... 312
Wounds and Lacerations ... 312

Overtraining 312
Care for Exercise-Related Injuries 313
Injury Prevention Strategies 313
Heat-Related Disorders 314
Cardiovascular Events 316
Emergency Response Plan 318

Chapter 25: Medical Conditions & Special Populations 323
Asthma 323
Arthritis 324
Diabetes 325
Hypertension 326
Osteoporosis 327
Pregnancy 328
Youth and Adolescents 330
Older Adults 332

Section Eight: Administrative & Legal Considerations

Chapter 26: Risk Management for Fitness Professionals 339
Standard of Care 339
Negligence 339
Liability Exposures 340
Scope of Practice 340
Risk Management Plan 341
Professional Liability Insurance 342
Case Studies 342

Chapter 27: Documentation & Record Keeping 347
Participant Files 347
Confidentiality and HIPAA 347
Waiver and Release of Liability 347
Informed Consent 348
Preparticipation Screening Questionnaires 348
Progress (SOAP) Notes 349
Additional Forms and Record Keeping 351

Appendices:

PAR-Q & You 357
PAR-Q+ for Everyone 358–361
PARmed-X for Pregnancy 362–365
Health and Lifestyle Questionnaire 366–369
Medical Clearance for Exercise Participation 370
Sample Personal Training/Exercise Log 371–372
Sample Health & Fitness Assessment Data Sheet 373–374

Gloss-a-dex of Terms: 375

Answers to Review Questions 384

Section I

Communication, Interpersonal Relationships, & Behavioral Science

Even the most scientifically-based and artfully-designed exercise program is of little value unless the individual actually adheres to the plan. The physical act of performing exercise, and the ensuing physiological adaptations and fitness outcomes are often stifled by psychological barriers. Fear, lack of confidence, and negative self-beliefs prevent many from taking the first step and still others from adhering to healthy lifestyle behaviors such as physical activity.

Over the years, the role of the fitness professional has evolved and expanded. Likewise, the expectations, needs, and considerations of the typical health seeker and fitness enthusiast have also increased and become more complex. In order to successfully guide clients toward their health and fitness goals, it is essential for fitness professionals to establish positive connections and build meaningful relationships with both potential customers and current participants. In addition, fitness professionals must have strong communication skills as well as an understanding of the theory and best practices related to the facilitation of behavioral change.

Chapter 1 will introduce the role of fitness professionals including the personal trainer, the group exercise instructor, and the wellness coach. In addition, this chapter will present NETA's Professional Code of Ethics.

Chapter 2 provides an introduction to communication skills and strategies used to establish meaningful interpersonal relationships with clients. Topics covered include making a positive first impression, establishing rapport and trust, asking effective questions, and utilizing active listening skills.

Chapter 3 presents the theoretical models related to behavioral change and techniques to enhance motivation for the pursuit and maintenance of healthy lifestyles. To successfully facilitate behavioral change, fitness professionals must understand stages of change, self-efficacy, sources of motivation, and effective goal-setting strategies.

Chapter 4 builds upon the principles of behavioral change with an introduction to the fundamentals of wellness coaching. Fitness professionals will learn the basic principles and processes of coaching through the use of techniques such as motivational interviewing and appreciative inquiry. Coaching skills provide an invaluable asset that enables fitness professionals to empower their clients to make positive change and achieve their desired goals.

1
The Role of Fitness Professionals

Introduction
The fitness industry is still relatively young and the role of the fitness professional is continuously evolving and expanding. Fitness professionals find employment opportunities in a variety of settings including commercial health clubs, community-based wellness centers (e.g., community centers), not-for-profit facilities (e.g., YMCA's, YWCA's, JCC's), corporate fitness centers, university recreation centers, clinical/medical fitness centers, as well as self-employment. In addition, as the health care industry slowly moves toward more preventative strategies, a growing number of opportunities for fitness professionals may arise within the public health and primary care settings (Francis, 2012). Unfortunately, the vast majority of Americans continue to live sedentary lifestyles with only an estimated 21 percent of adults in the United States meeting the recommended levels for aerobic physical activity and for muscle-strengthening exercises in 2010 (Schiller et al., 2012). Subsequently, the prevalence of physical inactivity and the subsequent epidemic of obesity and obesity-related chronic diseases (e.g., type 2 diabetes, cardiovascular disease, metabolic syndrome) have contributed to a growing demand for fitness professionals. According to the U.S. Department of Labor's Bureau of Labor Statistics (2016), employment of fitness trainers and instructors is projected to grow 8 percent from 2014 to 2024, about as fast as the average for all occupations. As businesses, government, and health insurance companies continue to recognize the benefits of health and fitness programs for their employees and subscribers, incentives to join fitness centers or other types of health clubs are expected to drive the continued need for personal trainers and group exercise instructors (BLS, 2016).

Although 'fitness professional' is a commonly-used title, many others are also utilized within the fitness industry to describe the sub-disciplines of fitness occupations. These titles may include: personal trainer, personal fitness trainer, fitness instructor, fitness leader, group exercise instructor, group fitness instructor, fitness coach, wellness coach, and many other derivatives of these labels. Throughout this manual, we will use the title 'fitness professional' or 'exercise professional' when making general references to the larger group and 'personal trainer', 'group exercise instructor', or 'wellness coach' when discussing the respective sub-disciplines.

Roles of the Fitness Professional
Fitness professionals working in various capacities must be prepared to wear a number of different 'hats.' Depending on the environment and the individuals being served, some hats may be worn more often than others. The following list includes some, but not all, of the possible roles a fitness professional may play for their clients and class participants.

- **Instructor**: provides information and explanation
- **Coach**: asks questions, facilitates self-directed change
- **Facilitator**: maintains focus, establishes environment
- **Leader**: provides optimism, sets the course
- **Role Model**: demonstrates habits of healthy living
- **Referral Source**: establishes a multidisciplinary network of health care professionals

Ideal Qualities and Characteristics
The list of ideal qualities and characteristics for a fitness professional is quite extensive and is likely to vary based on the role of the professional (e.g., group exercise instructor, personal trainer, wellness coach), the environment in which he or she works (e.g., club setting, corporate fitness, post-rehabilitation, non-profit facility), and the type of clientele or participants they serve (e.g., health seekers, fitness enthusiasts, special populations, athletes). Nevertheless, some qualities and characteristics seem to be important across all domains. These include:

- **Empathy**: demonstrating the ability to show compassion and understanding for someone's feelings and their situation; to put yourself in their shoes
- **Respectfulness**: honoring the differences of others, treating others as you would expect to be treated
- **Enthusiasm**: being energetic, positive, optimistic, loving what you do
- **Lifelong Learner**: pursuing personal and professional self-development; seeking new knowledge, abilities, and skills
- **Genuineness**: being yourself, keeping it real, having integrity

Personal Trainer
As stated in NETA's Personal Trainer practice analysis (also called role delineation or job task analysis), "Person-

al trainers are fitness professionals who promote health. They accomplish this by developing and implementing exercise programs designed to safely and effectively meet the unique goals of the clients they serve. This practice takes place in the context of their unwavering commitment to client safety and service and their adherence to the highest principles of ethical behavior." Personal trainers offer fee-based services delivered on both a private (one-on-one) and semi-private/small group (typically 2-5 participants) basis. Personal training continues to be one of the most prevalent services in the fitness industry, offered by nearly all health clubs and fitness facilities (Schroeder & Dolan, 2010). According to IHRSA (2013), approximately 6.4 million Americans used personal fitness training services in 2011. One of the many benefits of personal training services is the focus on the individual's goals, needs, and limitations in the design and implementation of the customized fitness program.

The first step toward becoming a personal trainer is attaining the knowledge, skills, and abilities necessary for a successful career. Many obtain this education through colleges and universities that offer programs granting an associate's, a bachelor's, or even a master's degree in a fitness-related discipline (e.g., exercise science, kinesiology, exercise physiology). At the present time, formal education of this nature is not required for employment as a personal trainer. However, career advancement, increasing consumer expectations, and perhaps even state legislation adopted in the future may dictate the need for fitness professionals to complete higher education. Certification provides an assessment of an individuals' minimum competency to safely perform the tasks necessary of a personal trainer. Unfortunately, there are literally hundreds of 'certifications' each having their own prerequisites, standards, and eligibility requirements to earn the distinction of 'certified personal trainer.' The vast menu of certification options makes it difficult for both consumers and individuals wishing to enter the fitness industry to discern the reputable credentials from those less distinguished. In an attempt to facilitate enhanced self-regulation and quality assurance of fitness credentialing, the International Health, Racquet, & Sportsclub Association (IHRSA) issued the following recommendation statement, amended from a previously-released version (IHRSA, 2005):

> "Whereas, given the increasing importance of personal training in health, fitness and sports clubs, IHRSA recommends that, beginning January 1, 2006, member clubs hire personal trainers holding at least one current certification from a certifying organization/agency that has begun third-party accreditation of its certification procedures and protocols from an independent, experienced, and nationally recognized accrediting body."

When the recommendation was first issued, the IHRSA Board of Directors identified the National Commission for Certifying Agencies (NCCA) as being an acceptable accrediting organization. In response to this recommendation statement, many fitness certification providers have earned and maintain NCCA accreditation. NETA's Personal Trainer and Group Exercise Instructor certification programs earned initial NCCA accreditation in 2007 and 2009, respectively.

NCCA accreditation is widely-recognized as a 'gold standard' for certification programs in the fitness industry and for credentialing programs in many adjacent health care professions such as athletic training, dietetics, occupational therapy, recreational therapy, and nursing. NCCA accreditation requires compliance with twenty-four rigorous standards pertaining to areas such as program governance, policies and procedures, candidate information, examination development and administration, and recertification.

Employers and other stakeholders may require fitness professionals to maintain an NCCA-accredited certification, and should verify the validity of these certifications.

The newly-certified personal trainer must now set out to establish the clientele necessary to support their financial and career-oriented goals. The process of identifying, qualifying, and obtaining clients is known as *prospecting*. Changing a prospect into a paying personal training client is largely dependent upon interpersonal communication and relationship-building skills (see chapter 2). In addition, personal trainers must also develop their business acumen, which refers to the understanding of finances, marketing, time management, competitors, and operational

Figure 1-1 Three Dimensions of Success

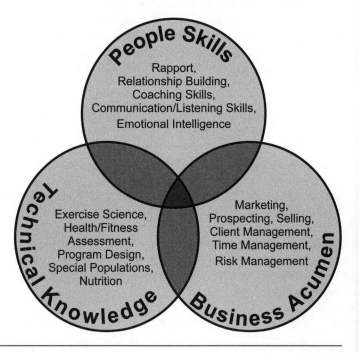

processes necessary to run a successful business. Taken together, technical knowledge, people skills, and business acumen represent the three dimensions of a successful career in personal training. See figure 1-1.

Group Exercise Instructor

Group exercise instructors are fitness professionals who promote enhanced health and increased fitness. They accomplish this by developing and leading group fitness classes designed to safely and effectively meet the unique goals of the individuals they serve. Group exercise instructors apply knowledge and skill to facilitate positive health and fitness outcomes among diverse populations using a variety of class formats and exercise modalities. Group exercise instructors have the opportunity to motivate and inspire numerous individuals simultaneously through various class formats such as group cycle, step aerobics, cardio kickboxing, yoga, boot camp, and group strength training. The wide variety of class offerings provides group exercise instructors with the unique opportunity to reach a wider array of individuals than other fitness professionals. The group dynamics, collective energy, and social support provided by group exercise classes are attractive to many individuals, and facilitates exercise adherence. In addition, instructors who develop an inviting and welcoming class atmosphere for individuals of all ability levels create a positive and enjoyable class experience, which further contributes to successful outcomes and participant retention. Whereas, personal training services typically impact anywhere from 3% to 8% of a club's membership base, group exercise classes achieve participation rates of 20% or more of a club's membership. Subsequently, group exercise instructors have the widest breadth of impact upon the overall health and fitness of those individuals who might not otherwise seek out one-on-one training or coaching.

Wellness Coach

NETA's Wellness Coach role delineation states, "Wellness Coaches are health and fitness professionals who work collaboratively with individuals in a client-centered process to facilitate the achievement of self-determined goals related to balanced healthy living. Successful behavioral change takes place when Wellness Coaches apply clearly defined knowledge and skills, empowering clients to mobilize their internal strengths and external resources for the adoption and maintenance of healthy lifestyle behaviors." Over the past decade, wellness coaching has been an emerging trend within the fitness industry, among health care providers, and in the health insurance industry. Fitness trend reports compiled by the American College of Sports Medicine (ACSM) have ranked wellness coaching among the top 20 worldwide fitness trends every year since 2010 (Thompson, 2015). Wellness coaches utilize techniques such as active listening, thoughtful questioning, and motivational interviewing to facilitate self-directed behavioral change among their clients. The underlying premise of wellness coaching is not to direct clients and 'prescribe' behavioral change strategies, but rather to empower clients to identify their intrinsic motivators and to chart their own pathway for change.

Ethical and Professional Standards

Ethics is a system or code of morals, values, and conduct of a person or within a group of people. This conduct deals with the discipline of good and bad or right and wrong. Good ethical behavior involves bringing the highest values into one's work and aspiring to do the right thing during all interactions and in all situations.

The primary purpose of an accredited fitness certification is to assess the individual's achievement of a minimum level of competency in order to protect the public from harm. Along with the base knowledge required to provide safe and effective exercise programs to the general public, NETA believes fitness professionals must also adhere to an ethical code of conduct. Your professionalism is established through a high level of integrity, positive attitude and image, valid credentials (e.g., fitness/specialty certification, safety certifications), practical skills, and good communication.

In addition, personal trainers, group exercise instructors, and wellness coaches must establish and maintain professional boundaries when working with clients and class participants. A boundary is a limit observed by an individual regarding the nature of a relationship. Friends and family have personal boundaries that may be very different from the boundaries that exists between the fitness professional and a client or participant. These boundaries exist during face-to-face interactions (e.g., 'personal space') as well as within the overall trainer-client relationship. Some examples of inappropriate behavior that crosses outside of generally recognized professional boundaries may include: sending inappropriate messages or images to a client or participant via text message, email, or social media; making sexual advances or entering into an intimate relationship with a client or participant; and acting or speaking in a disrespectful or demeaning manner to a client or participant. It is also very important, both legally and ethically, that fitness professionals maintain client and participant confidentiality. Confidentiality relates to the duty or responsibility to maintain the privacy of clients and class participants. It is likely that fitness professionals will become privy to various types of personal information (e.g., medical history, medications), which must remain confidential at all times.

NETA's Professional Code of Ethics

A Codes of Ethics is a set of guidelines established by professional organizations to direct the conduct and actions related to common business practices within a given profession. The following code of ethics is designed to assist certified fitness professionals of the National Exercise Trainers Association to maintain - both as individuals and as an industry - the highest levels of professional and ethical conduct. This Code of Professional Ethics reflects the level of commitment and integrity necessary to ensure that all NETA Certification Board (NETA-CB) certified health and fitness professionals provide the highest level of service and respect for all colleagues, allied professionals, and the general public.

The NETA-Certified Fitness Professional must be aware of and practice the standards of ethical behavior of his or her profession as follows:

- Respect the rights, welfare, privacy, and dignity of clients, co-workers, and the public at large.
- Provide and maintain a safe and effective training environment and exercise programming.
- Provide equal, fair, and reasonable treatment for all individuals.
- Comply with all applicable laws governing business practices, employment, and property usage.
- Maintain appropriate documentation (e.g., informed consent, PAR-Q, health & lifestyle questionnaire, progress notes, training logs, etc.).
- Respect and maintain the confidentiality of all client information.
- Recognize and abide by the recognized scope of practice consistent with exercise certification(s) held; avoid actions or behaviors restricted to the scope practice for adjacent health care professionals.
- Do not diagnose illness, injury, or medical conditions; refer clients to a more qualified health, fitness, or medical professional when appropriate.
- Strive to remain up-to-date with current practical and theoretical fitness/health research through continuing education, conferences, home studies and networking with other fitness professionals.
- Maintain appropriate safety certifications at all times. A minimum of adult CPR for group exercise instructors, and adult CPR/AED for personal trainers. CPR/AED certification must include a live hands-on practical skills evaluation.
- Establish and practice clear professional boundaries.
- Avoid engaging in any behavior or conduct that could be construed as a conflict of interest or reflects adversely on the fitness profession, NETA, or the NETA-CB.
- Represent credentials and certifications in a honest, accurate, and appropriate manner.
- Strive to protect the public from those who misrepresent the health and fitness professions or are in direct violation of this code of ethics by communicating concerns with the NETA-CB.

Continuing Education

Earning a certification is only the beginning of a fitness professional's educational journey. The fitness industry is very dynamic with new information, understanding, and philosophies emerging and expanding at a breakneck pace. It's imperative for fitness professionals to stay engaged with respected and credible sources of information and research. All NETA certifications are valid for two (2) years from the date of certification. To renew credential(s) and remain a NETA-Certified professional, one must complete twenty (20) continuing education credits (CECs) over the two-year period beginning on the date of certification and ending on the expiration date. Of these 20 CECs, six (6) must be from NETA workshops or NETA home study courses. In addition, group exercise instructors must hold a valid adult CPR certification and personal trainers must hold a valid adult CPR/AED certification. CPR/AED certification must include a live hands-on practical skills evaluation. To complete the renewal process, eligible candidates must submit a completed application, proof of valid CPR (for group exercise instructors) or CPR/AED (for personal trainers), documentation of CECs earned (i.e., certificates of completion), and applicable payment to NETA's office prior to the designated expiration date as indicated on the current certification.

Credible Sources of Information

The volumes of health and fitness information readily available in both print and electronic formats is overwhelming. Unfortunately, much of this information may be inaccurate, tainted by author bias and personal agendas, and/or a misrepresentation of research findings. As such, it is often difficult for fitness professionals and consumers to discern credible and accurate sources of information from the staggering amount of misinformation. The questions and tips provided below can be helpful when evaluating the credibility of health and fitness information (Cottrell et al., 2012).

- Source: What type company or organization (e.g., nonprofit organization, government agency, for-profit business, educational institution) is disseminating the information? Frequently, website addresses ending in ".edu," ".gov," or ".org" are known and typically reputable organizations or institutions. Be cautious of sites that have an internet address ending in ".com" as they are commercial sites and may be selling a product or service.
- Review: Has the content or information been verified or undergone an expert panel or peer review process? Reputable publications, such as articles printed in professional journals, must receive approval from an editorial or a peer review panel prior to acceptance for publication. These review panels consist of well-recognized experts in the field.
- Author(s): Are the author's credentials clearly pro-

vided? Are the author's education, background, and expertise consistent with the subject matter being presented? Does the author provide contact information? Does the author have any obvious conflicts of interest? Readers should be leery of authors who claim to be health or fitness 'experts' yet lack the requisite credentials consistent with such a designation.

- References: Does the author provide appropriate references? Is the underlying source of information considered credible? Have other reputable authors or organizations referenced this information? If the author proclaims information is based on research, facts, or evidence, then the appropriate source of the information should be cited. Dig deeper to verify the legitimacy of the information.

- Facts: Are the facts consistent with information obtained from other reputable sources? Is the author providing the information in a biased manner or presenting facts out of context? Does the information seem plausible? Although new discoveries do occur and innovative thinking may challenge conventional wisdom, readers should always maintain some skepticism when new ideas deviate radically from accepted scientific principles and widely-recognized best practices.

- Date: When was the information published or last updated? Is the information current or perhaps outdated? Although some seminal publications and articles have stood the test of time, information published years ago may not be relevant or accurate today. Readers should always seek the most recent edition of textbooks or the most up-to-date version of standards, guidelines, and/or position/consensus statements.

Chapter Summary

The fitness industry is very young and dynamic. Both the role and the opportunity for fitness professionals continues to grow at a rapid, yet steady pace. Successful fitness professionals will be those who possess the ideal characteristics as well as knowledge, skills, and abilities with regard to technical subject matter, communication skills, and business acumen. It's imperative that fitness professionals conduct themselves with integrity and in accordance with ethical standards. In addition, fitness professionals must continue to expand their knowledge and skill in order to deliver their services in a safe and effective manner.

Chapter References

Bureau of Labor Statistics, U.S. Department of Labor, Occupational Outlook Handbook, 2016-17 Edition, Fitness Trainers and Instructors, on the Internet at http://www.bls.gov/ooh/personal-care-and-service/fitness-trainers-and-instructors.htm (retrieved July 19, 2016).

Cottrell, R.R., Girvan, J.T., & McKenzie, J.F. (2012). *Principles and Foundations of Health Promotion and Education,* 5th edition. San Francisco, CA: Benjamin Cummings Publishing.

Francis, P.N. (2012). Is there a public health role for fitness professionals? *IDEA Fitness Journal,* 9(1).

International Health, Racquet, & Sportsclub Association (2005). On the Internet at http://www.ihrsa.org/blog/2014/8/15/personal-trainer-accreditation.html. Accessed March 22, 2017.

International Health, Racquet, & Sportsclub Association (2013). *The IHRSA Health Club Consumer Report: 2012 Health Club Activity, Usage, Trends & Analysis.*

Schiller, J.S., Lucas, J.W., Ward, B.W., & Peregoy, J.A. (2012). Summary health statistics for U.S. adults: National health interview survey, 2010. National Center for Health Statistics. *Vital and Health Statistics.* Series 10 (252).

Schroeder, J., & Dolan, S. (2010). 2010 IDEA fitness programs & equipment trends. *IDEA Fitness Journal,* 7(7).

Thompson, W.R. (2015). Worldwide survey of fitness trends for 2016: 10th anniversary edition. *ACSM's Health & Fitness Journal,* 19(6), 9-18.

Chapter 1 Review Questions

1. The NETA Group Exercise and Personal Trainer certifications are valid for _____ years from the date of certification. NETA-certified professionals must complete a minimum of _____ continued education credits (CECs) prior to the certification expiration date in order to be eligible for renew?
    A. 3, 15
    B. 2, 20
    C. 5, 20
    D. 4, 26

2. Which of the following is considered to be a violation of NETA's Professional Code of Ethics?
    A. Store personal training client files in a locked file cabinet in a secure office space within your health club.
    B. Refer clients with special medical needs to a qualified health care provider.
    C. Enter into an intimate sexual relationship with an emotionally-vulnerable personal training client.
    D. Inspect all fitness equipment on a regular basis to ensure proper function and safety.

3. Which of the following roles or 'hats' of a fitness professional is BEST represented by asking thoughtful questions to facilitate self-directed behavioral change?
    A. Instructor
    B. Role Model
    C. Leader
    D. Coach

4. According to the U.S. Department of Labor's Bureau of Labor Statistics, employment opportunities for fitness professionals are expected to _____ over the current decade ending in 2014.
    A. remain unchanged
    B. decrease
    C. increase
    D. be eliminated

5. Which of the following is a set of guidelines established by professional organizations to direct the conduct and actions related to common business practices within a given profession?
    A. Code of Ethics
    B. Accreditation
    C. Certification
    D. Articles of Order

6. Successfully obtaining a/an _____ indicates that an individual has passed a written assessment, demonstrating a minimum level of knowledge and competency to safely perform the basic duties of a personal trainer or group exercise instructor.
    A. accreditation
    B. certification
    C. job
    D. certificate of completion

Answers to Review Questions on Page 384
Note: Review questions are intended to reinforce learning and comprehension of subject matter presented in the corresponding chapter. The review questions are not intended to be representative of actual certification exam questions in terms of style, content, or difficulty.

2
Relationship-Building & Communication Skills

Introduction

The ability to effectively communicate and build meaningful relationships with other people is among the most important skill-sets for fitness professionals. Certainly fitness professionals must possess the 'technical' knowledge related to exercise science, nutrition, assessment of health and fitness, and program design; however, this knowledge will do little by way of assisting others to achieve their healthy living goals if the fitness professional is unable to establish personal connections with their prospective clients and class participants. This chapter will review concepts and strategies related to relationship-building and communication skills such as questioning and active listening. The acquisition of these skills will provide the foundation from which fitness professionals will be able to enhance the individual's overall experience, facilitate positive behavioral change, and guide their clients and participants toward their health and fitness goals.

Building Relationships

Rapport

The first step toward building a meaningful relationship with another person is to establish rapport. Rapport may be simply defined as a positive interaction or connection experienced between two or more people. It has been proposed that rapport is created through the interrelation of three components including mutual attentiveness, positivity, and coordination (Tickle-Degnen & Rosenthal, 1990). Mutual attentiveness is displayed through a shared expression of interest with one another. Positivity is seen as the reciprocation of friendliness and caring during an interaction. Coordination can also be thought of as harmony or balance between two individuals. Although some people may be particularly skilled at developing rapport, it is not an inherent personality trait, but rather an experience that results from the combination of qualities that emerge from each individual during an interaction (Tickle-Degnen & Rosenthal, 1990). This positive connection or experience may be expressed when people say they 'hit it off,' 'clicked,' 'had good chemistry,' were 'on the same page' or 'in sync.' Rapport is essential to the establishment of trust, honest open communication, and understanding. The presence of rapport between two individuals is believed to facilitate influence and responsiveness, which is essential for fitness professionals attempting to guide behavioral change among their clients and participants. Certainly, if rapport is established with another person, then that individual is more inclined to like, trust, and respect the fitness professional, which increases the probability that they may want to utilize your fitness services.

An invaluable set of principles that are very effective to establish rapport have been identified by Dale Carnegie in his best-selling book, *How to Win Friends and Influence People* (1981). These principles are referred to as the "six ways to make people like you" (Carnegie, 1981). The first principle is to become genuinely interested in other people. Showing interest in other people not only demonstrates respect, but also allows the trainer to learn more about that person, their interests, goals, and underlying motivations. Many fitness professionals have gained a significant amount of knowledge and have a passion to share this knowledge with anyone willing to listen. Unfortunately, this information may not be relevant, interesting, or even important to the other person. Those who are just beginning their journey toward healthy living may be intimidated by the fitness professional and the fitness setting. Becoming overloaded with too much information may increase their feelings of anxiety. Focus your energy on taking interest in others rather than trying to get others to take interest in you. Remember, 'no one cares how much you know until they know how much you care.'

Perhaps the most simple of these principles is to smile. A warm, authentic smile is very likely to elicit a smile in response. A simple smile can brighten someone's day, makes you more approachable, and indicates a positive disposition.

The third principle is to remember peoples' names. Many people claim to be 'bad with names' and that may be true, but remembering peoples' names is a skill that can be learned and improved. A person's name is to that person the sweetest-sounding and most important word in any language (Carnegie, 1981). By remembering a person's name, you are showing respect for that individual and giving them a sense of importance. During the initial introduction, concentrate on the person's name, repeat it out loud in the conversation and in your mind. When meeting many

> **Good to Know**
>
> **"Six Ways to Make People Like You"**
> - Become genuinely interested in other people.
> - Smile
> - Remember people's names.
> - Be a good listener. Encourage others to talk about themselves.
> - Talk in terms of the other person's interests.
> - Make the other person feel important and do it sincerely.

new people, as in a fitness center setting or group exercise class, it can be particularly challenging to remember names and important details about each person. Take a moment after each initial interaction and write the person's name down in a small pocket notebook. Include a brief physical description, distinguishing characteristics, and noteworthy points from the conversation. Use this name book as a reference before engaging the person in a future conversation, allowing you greet them by name and feel confident in doing so.

Principle number four is essential to building rapport and effective communication; be a good listener and encourage others to talk about themselves. The art of listening is also a learnable skill. Listening attentively not only demonstrates that you are taking genuine interest in the other person, but it is also one of the highest compliments and displays of respect you can show toward another person. In addition, by listening closely you are able to learn and understand more about that person and the topics of importance to them. As you learn more about their interests, ask questions they will enjoy answering and encourage them to talk more about themselves. By listening intently, it will appear as though you are a great conversationalist. Resist the temptation to dominate the conversation by talking endlessly about your qualifications, services, and the benefits of working with you in an attempt to convince them that you are worthy of hire. Ask thoughtful questions, listen, and learn about the other person as you gain insight into their goals, motivations, and challenges. In doing so, you will be in a much better position to present solutions that best fit their uniqueness.

Many people get excited when others take interest in their hobbies and passions. Although you cannot be an expert on all topics, make a point to learn a little more about the other person's interests. They will appreciate your efforts to gain knowledge about their interests and to have an intelligent conversation on subjects that matter most to them. The road to a person's heart is to talk about topics of greatest importance to them. Principle number five – talk in terms of the other person's interests.

The final principle touches upon one of the deepest needs of human nature, the need to feel important. According to Maslow's Hierarchy of Needs (see figure 2-1), our most basic needs are physiological, such as the need for oxygen, food, water, warmth, sleep, and even physical activity. Next in this hierarchy is the need for safety. This includes shelter, security, financial stability, and freedom from fear. Above these needs is the need for relationships and social connections including family, friends, loved ones, and significant others. The need for esteem relates to internal feelings of self-efficacy, respect, confidence, and of course importance. In addition, the need for esteem is also satisfied through the respect, recognition, and acceptance received from others. The highest-order need in this model is self-actualization. This represents the achievement of one's full potential, expressions of creativity, the pursuit of knowledge, spiritual fulfillment, and a sense of being a part of something larger than one's self.

Figure 2-1 Hierarchy of Needs

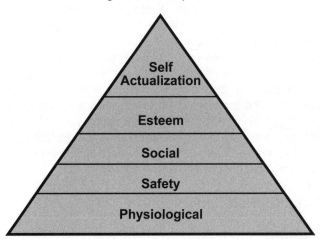

Making others feel important supports the need for esteem and in doing so also contributes to our own needs in this area. You can make people feel important in a variety of ways. In fact, many of the preceding principles contribute to the feeling of importance you create for others. In addition, you may also deliver a meaningful compliment, remember a birthday or special occasion by sending a card, or praise their skills and accomplishments. Regardless of what you say or do to make others feel important, you must be sincere in your efforts, without the expectation for something in return. Through a conscious effort to make others feel important as well as adherence to the other principles described above, you will establish good rapport and meaningful relationships with many people.

First Impressions

The initial reaction and first impressions formed during an encounter with another person have a lasting effect on the development of a relationship, or lack thereof, between two people (Sunnafrank & Ramirez, 2004). These first impressions are made quickly, often during the initial moments of a conversation or even through observations made prior to any verbal communication (Sunnafrank & Ramirez, 2004). The so-called *7-11 rule of first impressions* suggests that people make eleven decisions about you within the first seven seconds of an interaction (Coffman, 2006). These eleven decisions include: are you friendly, attractive, knowledgeable, professional, empathetic, credible, confident, clean, helpful, courteous, and responsive. Researchers have also suggested that within 10 milliseconds of seeing a stranger's face, people make five trait judgments regarding an individual's attractiveness, likability, trustworthiness, competence, and aggressiveness (Willis & Todorov, 2006). According to the Predicted Outcome Value Theory, we analyze our first impressions of another person in an effort to predict the likelihood that future contact with this person will bring us personal rewards and positive outcomes (Sunnafrank & Ramirez, 2004). Based on these first impressions, we proceed to develop relationships with those we expect to be most rewarding and we limit or restrict interaction with those who appear to have fewer benefits to offer (Sunnafrank & Ramirez, 2004).

Whether you realize it or not, you are being watched. Potential clients, class participants, and club members make countless decisions and judgments about you, often even before an actual interaction. People are casually assessing your attitude, demeanor, professionalism, and competence, among many other attributes. Their assessment will often determine whether or not they will initiate or reciprocate a conversation with you. The following strategies may help to establish a positive impression, facilitate interactions, and lead to new relationships and opportunities:

- **Attire**: Dress like a professional. Wear appropriately-fitted and clean clothes (e.g., club-logoed apparel, shirt tucked in, looking sharp).
- **Personal Hygiene**: Make sure you are well-groomed, with fresh breath, and minimize the use of heavy fragrances.
- **Attentiveness**: When working with a client or club member, stay engaged. Keep your focus on the individual with whom you are working.
- **Body Language**: Be aware of the messages you send, both positive and negative, through your posture, body position, facial expressions, and use of physical cues.
- **Professional Greeting**: When meeting someone remember to smile, make eye contact, shake hands with confidence and respect, introduce yourself first, and engage the other person in conversation.
- **Listen**: Listening is among the best conversational strategies to make a positive first impression and to establish rapport with others. (See previous section)
- **Speech**: Use non-technical language when possible. Communicate with confidence, clearly articulate words, and ask thoughtful questions.
- **Courteous**: Remember the 'golden rule', treat others as you would like to be treated.

Approaching Members

It is important for fitness professionals to be approachable, but also to proactively approach club members. For personal trainers, creating visibility and connecting with 'new' members (i.e., any club member the fitness professional has not met) is an important strategy when building their clientele. However, the manner in which the fitness professional approaches members will have a significant influence on the trajectory of their relationships. The first interaction with a member must be professional, pleasant, and most important, non-threatening. Begin with genuine praise and honest appreciation. Compliment the member on something specific. Avoid approaching members with questions that they may perceive as challenging to their beliefs, judgments, and competency. For example, the personal trainer may have observed a member incorrectly performing an exercise and felt inclined to approach the member to offer assistance. The personal trainer might initiate the conversation with one of the following questions:

- "Can I make a suggestion?"
- "May I show you the correct way to perform that exercise?"
- "May I show you a better way to do that?"
- "Can I help you with that exercise?"
- "Can I show you a safer technique for that exercise?"

Although the intentions may be good, this approach may not be received positively by the member. Each of these questions either directly or indirectly suggests that the member does not know how to correctly perform the exercise. Although this is likely to be true, they may be nonetheless offended or embarrassed to have their competency challenged. The experienced exerciser may believe that they already know what they are doing. The novice exerciser may have fear, insecurity, and anxiety about their abilities, which you have just exacerbated with your approach validating their low self-efficacy. In addition, this type of approach may elicit a conditioned response to any perceived solicitation. As is often heard by the department store clerk in response to their offer of assistance, "No thanks, I am just looking."

Certainly, fitness professionals have an obligation and a duty to correct a member who is performing an exercise incorrectly. Intervention is particularly important when the member is in immediate danger or risk of serious injury. However, in most cases, improper technique is not likely to present such an imminent risk. Although it is still prudent and recommended for the fitness professional to provide proper instruction, this information and assistance is more likely to be well-received once rapport and trust have been established. Therefore, the objective of the initial interaction with a club member is to simply make a positive connection and to learn their name. This can be accomplished through a technique called the 'greet-and-go.' The 'greet-and-go' is a brief interaction during which the fitness professional compliments the member, makes an introduction, learns the member's name, and then leaves them to continue their workout. During this conversation, the fitness professional should avoid asking questions that could result in a 'no' response. An example of a 'greet-and-go' statement is provided below.

> "Hello, I can see you are in the middle of your workout and I don't want to take up too much of your time. My name is Michael and I am a Certified Personal Trainer here at the ABC Fitness Center. I just wanted to compliment you on your great effort today. If there is anything at all I can do to assist you, please don't hesitate to ask…. By the way, what is your name? …. It is very nice to meet you, Susan. Enjoy the rest of your workout."

Having made a non-threating positive connection, future interactions may be initiated on a first-name basis allowing the personal trainer to continue building a meaningful relationship with the member while gaining their trust and acceptance. The personal trainer is well-positioned to learn more about the member's health and fitness goals, and to offer guidance when appropriate.

Communication Skills

Impact of a Message

The word communication originates from the Latin word '*communis*', meaning to share or to make common. Communication is the act of conveying and receiving information through the exchange of messages delivered by speech, visual aids, signals, writing, body language, or behavior. The information you deliver to and receive from another individual is represented by both verbal and nonverbal messages. The relative impact of these components has been estimated by early researchers (Archer & Akert, 1977; Mehrabian & Ferris, 1967). The verbal messages include both the words you speak and how you express these words. It is has been estimated that only 7% of the message you send or receive is communicated by what you say. An additional 38% of the message is conveyed by how you say the words. This includes elements such as your tone of voice, pronunciation, speaking rate, and vocal projection. The final 55% of the message is derived from nonverbal communication which includes body language, facial expressions, gestures, posture, and movements of the head. See figure 2-2. Although these percentages are commonly referenced, it is likely that the relative importance of words, tonality, and body language is dependent on the context of the communication (e.g., phone conversations).

Active Listening Skills

As noted earlier in this chapter, listening is a key strategy to establish rapport with another person. In addition, listening is an essential communication skill necessary to ensure information is correctly interpreted and understood. Although nonverbal cues represent over half of a communicated message, information transmitted verbally, through both words and tonality, is also of obvious importance. Anecdotally, it has been said that since we have two ears and one mouth, we should listen twice as often as we speak. In addition, we also use our eyes both to communicate and interpret messages.

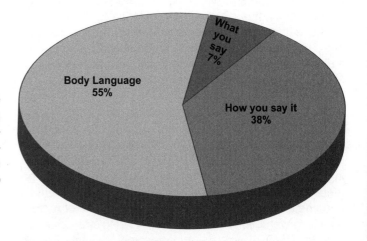

Figure 2-2 Impact of a Message

Nonverbal Listening Skills

Nonverbal listening skills require an individual to hear what is being communicated through both words and tone of voice. The listener must comprehend the words being used, but also interpret the manner in which those words are spoken. It is possible and common to passively listen to someone speak, meaning you hear the sound of their voice, but are not truly paying attention to what they are saying. True listening is an active process, which requires concentration and focus. It is also a skill that can be learned and improved.

In order to develop the ability to actively listen, you must increase your awareness of and attempt to eliminate listening barriers. First and foremost, give the other person your full attention. Do not attempt to multi-task during meaningful conversations and make every effort to eliminate potential distractions (e.g., cell phone, television, background noise). Don't talk too much. If you are trying to learn about the other person, then you must allow them to speak. During meetings such as a consultation, the fitness professional should speak about 30% of the time, whereas the remaining 70% of the 'talk time' is reserved for the other person. Ask questions and then be quiet, allowing the other person to respond. In addition, try to stop yourself from thinking you know what the other person is going to say, thinking that you already have all the answers, or thinking about what you are going to say next. After the other person concludes a statement, it's okay to allow for a brief pause in the conversation as you process the information and then formulate your response or follow-up question. Certainly don't cut the other person off in the middle of a statement or attempt to finish sentences on their behalf.

Understanding Body Language

Another nonverbal 'listening' skill is actually performed with your eyes as you observe the body language of the other person. Body language may include any number of conscious or unconscious movements of the body used to communicate a message to another person (Sielski, 1979). These methods of communication may include facial expressions, eye contact, head and body position, posture, and gestures. These often hidden messages delivered through nonverbal cues both compliment and at times contradict the spoken word. In addition to delivering a message, these cues may also reflect attitudes and feelings (Sielski, 1979). Since the messages delivered through body language play such a crucial role in communication, it's important for the fitness professional to recognize, interpret, and understand these nonverbal signals. Table 2-1 provides examples of some common nonverbal cues and their possible meanings.

Verbal Listening Skills

Another component of active listening is to verbally communicate back with the other person. This serves several purposes which include indicating that you are in fact paying attention, seeking clarification, and confirming understanding. The verbal active listening skills are summarized in table 2-2.

Effective Questions

In addition to listening, the use of meaningful questions is among the most important communication skills. Asking questions allows the fitness professional to gather the information necessary to design an appropriate exercise program and to facilitate behavioral change. As noted above, questioning is an active listening skill used to ensure understanding of objective information as well as thoughts and feelings communicated by another person. There are two general categories of questions: closed-ended and open-ended.

Closed-Ended Questions

Closed-ended questions are those that generally require a very brief response such as 'yes' or 'no.' This type of question is often used when seeking factual or objective information. Some examples of closed-ended questions include:

- "Do you smoke?"
- "Do you have high blood pressure?"
- "How much do you currently weigh?"
- "Are you currently taking any prescription medications?"
- "How often do you exercise?"
- "What is your health or fitness-related goal?"

Although closed-ended questions may occasionally elicit a more elaborate reply, the nature of the question is such that we typically anticipate a short, objective response. Closed-ended questions are appropriate when gathering factual information; however, this type of question rarely provides much insight into an individual's beliefs, feelings, or emotions.

Open-Ended Questions

Open-ended questions are constructed and asked with the intention of uncovering more subjective and emotionally-based information such as personal opinions, feelings, and beliefs. The purpose of an open-ended question is not to limit the possible responses, but rather to encourage the respondent to provide a more elaborate reply. Open-ended questions often begin with 'How', 'What', or 'Why', but may also be delivered as statements such as "Tell me more about…" Questions that ask 'why' should be used with caution since these questions may evoke resistance or defensiveness due to the judgmental tone that can often accompany 'why.' However, when asked thoughtfully and at the correct time during a conversation, questions beginning with 'why' may be very effective at uncovering thoughts and feelings. Examples of open-ended questions include:

- "What is most important to you in achieving this goal?"
- "How will you feel if your current situation does not change?"
- "Tell me about the obstacles preventing you from attaining this goal."
- "What do you enjoy most about exercise and physical activity?"
- "What do you believe will be the most challenging aspects of adopting a healthier diet?"

Try to utilize a variety of questioning techniques and sentence structures. Avoid asking too many consecutive questions of the same type, which may make the other person feel as though they are being interrogated. The exchange of information should feel free-flowing and conversational using a variety of questions and active verbal listening skills. Always ask questions in a non-judgmental and positive manner. Ask thoughtful questions that reflect your genuine curiosity in the other person. Open-ended questions which dig deeper into a person's thoughts and feelings will be more appropriate once rapport and trust has been established with the individual.

Table 2-1 Body Language

Cue: Description	Possible Interpretation
Open Position: arms relaxed to sides of body, palms of hands exposed, eye-contact	Indicates openness and willingness to communicate
Closed Position: arms crossed, legs crossed, head tilted slightly down, scowling expression	A defensive posture, not interested in communicating, not listening, does not accept what is being said
Covering Mouth: fingers or entire hand over mouth	Attempting to hide their words, not being truthful, sharing embarrassing information
Rubbing Nose: lightly rubbing or touching side of nose with index finger	Expression of doubt, puzzlement, or may imply deception
Finger Tapping: lightly and repetitively tapping fingers on a table top or flat surface	Indicates impatience or boredom
Hand on Chin: hand resting on or under chin, stroking the chin, often with head tilted to side	Processing information or thoughts, making a decision
Leaning Back: leaning torso backwards, retracting head, perhaps even stepping back	Attempting to regain personal space, feeling smothered, keeping the other at arms-length
Fidgeting: frequently making minor adjustments to posture, jingling change in pocket, picking at finger nails, picking lint off clothes, playing with hair, toe tapping	Signs of nervousness or lack of interest, also used as self-comforting techniques

Table 2-2 Active Listening Skills

Active Listening Skill	Example
Paraphrasing: re-stating *using similar words and similar phrase arrangement* to those used by the speaker. (Also called a simple reflection).	*Client*: "I am finding it hard to workout due to my kids' busy schedules." *Trainer*: "So, it has been difficult for you to exercise because your kids are involved in a lot of activities."
Reflecting: stating what you heard the speaker say using your own words and sentence structure, often making an assumption with regard to the underlying meaning of the statement. See page 29 for types of reflective statements.	*Client*: "Last summer, we were just as busy as we always seem to be, but I made a point to pencil in some time for exercise on my calendar." *Trainer*: "So exercise retained importance in your busy schedule and you were more deliberate to set aside time for yourself last summer."
Repeating *(Parroting)*: re-stating the message using exactly the same words used by the speaker.	*Client*: "I just can't seem to stop having fast food for lunch every day." *Trainer*: "You can't seem to stop having fast food for lunch every day?"
Summarizing: stating the key points of a long thought or conversation. Also used to close conversation or transition to a new topic of discussion.	*Client*: "I have good intentions of doing it, but we have been so busy lately and other things always seem to get in the way. Last Thursday I had a doctor's appointment. On Friday we had friends over for dinner. Yesterday, we went to a play. On top of that, we have also been trying to make arrangements for our trip this summer." *Trainer*: "It sounds like you have been very busy with doctor's appointments, social events, and planning for your big trip."
Minimal Encouragers: words or short phrases used to encourage the speaker to continue. Also may be nonverbal movements.	*Client*: "I think I finally discovered an effective way to add more vegetables to my diet." *Trainer*: "Really?"
Questioning: gathering information using both open- and closed-ended questions.	*Trainer*: "On a scale of 1 to 10, how important is it to you to improve your diet at this time?" (Closed) *Trainer*: "How do you feel about your eating habits at the present time?" (Open)

Reflective Statements

Active listening includes the thoughtful and strategic use of reflective statements. The objective of reflective statements may include a demonstration of understanding, clarification of a client's statement, confirmation of the client's thoughts or feelings, and facilitation of the process of self-discovery (Resnicow & McMaster, 2012). In addition, a fitness professional may also use reflections to test an assumption about what a client means or feels, or to make a guess regarding the direction of the client's 'story' (Resnicow & McMaster, 2012). Many reflective statements will begin with the phrases, "It sounds like…", "If I understood you correctly…", or "So, if I heard you correctly..." (Resnicow & McMaster, 2012). Examples of various types of reflective statements are provided below.

A *simple reflection* paraphrases and restates what the client has said utilizing their own words without exaggeration, interpretation, or distortion.
Client: "I have been so busy with work and family that I just don't have time to exercise."
Trainer: "I hear you saying that you don't have time to exercise due to your busy schedule of work and family obligations."

Complex reflections add some meaning or emphasis to what the client has said, making a guess about the unspoken message or what might be coming next.
Client: "I have been so busy with work and family that I just don't have time to exercise."
Trainer: "So you would like to take time to exercise, but you are just too busy and overwhelmed with work and family obligations."

Amplified reflections maximize or minimize what the client has said, in an exaggerated form, but without sarcasm.
Client: "I have been so busy with work and family that I just don't have time to exercise."
Trainer: "So I hear you saying that it's absolutely impossible for you to fit time for exercise into your schedule."

A *double-sided reflection* acknowledges what the client has just said, but also incorporates reference to a contradictory or inconsistent statement they have made in the past.
Client: "I have been so busy with work and family that I just don't have time to exercise."
Trainer: "It sounds like you are just too busy to fit exercise into your schedule. However, I remember you have also mentioned that exercise makes you feel better and helps to manage the stress of your demanding schedule."

Feeling reflections involve expressing in one's own words the emotions stated or implied by the client. Feelings can be reflected from both verbal and nonverbal responses of the client.
Client: "I have been so busy with work and family that I just don't have time to exercise."
Trainer: "So you are feeling overwhelmed by all of your commitments and frustrated that exercise has not fit into your schedule."

A *reframing reflection* offers a alternate meaning or different perspective from that which the client has expressed. A reflection of this nature suggests a new and positive interpretation of a statement having negative inferences made by the client.
Client: "Lately, my husband has really been bothering me to begin an exercise program."
Trainer: "Your husband must really care about you and would like to see you remain healthy."

Chapter Summary

This chapter introduced the essential relationship-building and communication skills for fitness professionals. First impressions may positively or negatively influence the likelihood and direction of a relationship with another person. During the initial interaction, it is crucial to make a positive first impression and to establish rapport, which leads to trust and open communication. Effective communication includes the interpretation and understanding of both verbal and nonverbal messages as well as self-awareness of messages sent to others. Active listening skills, such as paraphrasing, summarizing, and questioning, are used to communicate understanding and to gather additional information.

Chapter References

Archer, D., & Akert, R.M. (1977). Words and everything else: Verbal and nonverbal cues in social interpretation. *Journal of Personality and Social Psychology, 35*(6), 443-449.

Carnegie, D. (1981). *How to Win Friends and Influence People*. New York: Simon and Schuster.

Coffman, S. (2006). *Tools to Grow and Retain Your Client Base*. WebEdu home study course: Desert Southwest Fitness.

Mehrabian, A., & Ferris, S.R. (1967). Inference of attitudes from nonverbal communication in two channels. *Journal of Consulting Psychology, 31*(3), 248-252.

Pease, B., & Pease, A. (2006). *The Definitive Book of Body Language*. New York, NY: Bantam Books.

Resnicow, K., & McMaster, F. (2012). Motivational interviewing: Moving from why to how with autonomy support. *International Journal of Behavioral Nutrition and Physical Activity, 9*(19), 1-9.

Sielski, L.M. (1979). Understanding body language. *The Personnel and Guidance Journal, 57*(5), 238-242.

Sunnafrank, M., & Ramirez, A. (2004). At first sight: Persistent relational effects of get-acquainted conversations. *Journal of Social and Personal Relationships, 21*(3), 361-379.

Tickle-Degnen, L., & Rosenthal, R. (1990). The nature of rapport and its nonverbal correlates. *Psychological Inquiry, 1*(4), 285-293.

Willis, J., & Todorov, A. (2006). First impressions making up your mind after a 100-ms exposure to a face. *Psychological Science, 17*(7), 592-598.

Chapter 2 Review Questions

1. Which of the following is considered to be an open-ended question?
    - A. How many days per week do you perform resistance training?
    - B. Do you enjoy exercise?
    - C. How do you imagine you will feel when you achieve this goal?
    - D. What was your average heart rate during today's workout?

2. Which of the following may indicate a defensive position suggesting that an individual is not interested in communicating or interacting?
    - A. Hand placed over mouth.
    - B. Arms crossed over front of chest.
    - C. Leaning backward.
    - D. Arms held to the sides of the body with palms open.

3. You observe a member that you do not know performing the lat pulldown exercise incorrectly. You decide to approach the member. Which of the following is likely to be the most effective statement to initiate the conversation?
    - A. "Hi, do you mind if I show you the correct way to perform that exercise?"
    - B. "Hello, why are you performing the exercise that way?
    - C. "Hi, can I show you a more safe and effective way to perform that exercise?"
    - D. "Hello, I don't think we have met before. I just wanted to say 'hi.' My name is…"

4. Your new client states, "I just don't seem to have enough time to work exercise into my busy schedule. I really want to exercise more often, but I just have so many other things to do." Which of the following active listening skills is an example of paraphrasing this statement?
    - A. "Tell me more about your busy schedule?"
    - B. "So, although you would like to exercise more often, your busy schedule makes it difficult for you to find the time."
    - C. "If you want to achieve your goal, then you are going to need to adjust your busy schedule to find more time for exercise."
    - D. "What are some of the commitments that keep your schedule so busy and preventing you from finding the time to exercise?

5. Which of the following nonverbal aspects is likely to have the MOST significant impact on the meaning of a message?
    - A. The selection and use of words being communicated.
    - B. The body position and facial expressions of the speaker.
    - C. The projection and volume of the speaker's voice.
    - D. The education and experience of the speaker.

6. Which of the following is an appropriate and effective strategy to establish rapport with a potential client?
    - A. Smile and make a point of remembering the person's name.
    - B. Make sure the prospect is aware of your education, certification, and experience.
    - C. Tell the potential client about the success stories of other clients.
    - D. Give the person your business card and a brochure including your rates.

Answers to Review Questions on Page 384

Note: Review questions are intended to reinforce learning and comprehension of subject matter presented in the corresponding chapter. The review questions are not intended to be representative of actual certification exam questions in terms of style, content, or difficulty.

3
Behavioral Change & Motivation

Introduction
When performed regularly, physical activity and exercise result in countless physical and physiological adaptations. These adaptations facilitate improved health, increased fitness, and enhanced performance. Although the act of exercising is a physical process, the adoption and maintenance of healthy lifestyle behaviors, such as regular physical activity, is largely mediated by psychological factors. A well-constructed and scientifically-based exercise program is of little benefit if the client is not willing or motivated to perform the activities.

Fitness and wellness professionals work with a wide variety of individuals, each having unique goals, sources of motivation, personal beliefs, values, and barriers to change. In order to facilitate and guide behavioral change, the fitness professional must discover, understand, and appreciate the uniqueness of each individual. Chapter 3 reviews the widely-accepted theories associated with behavior change as well as effective approaches to goal-setting and strategies to increase motivation and adherence. As the fitness industry slowly undergoes a paradigm shift from an approach focused largely on telling and directing, toward a philosophy of facilitating and guiding, knowledge of these behavioral sciences will help today's fitness professional to be a catalyst for change in the lives of their clients and participants.

Behavioral Change

Repeating a pattern, over time, forms specific behaviors. Behaviors are complex and have many determinants. They are influenced by social, environmental, psychological and/or biological factors. Each of these factors plays a significant role in the acquisition, maintenance, and cessation of behavioral patterns. Awareness of the need for changing a behavior, its origins, and consequences, is important in beginning the path to change.

Behavior change starts in the mind with a change in thoughts and thought processes. Studies show that the brain can make actual physical and neurological changes through a process called *neuroplasticity*. This process involves changing neurons within the brain through new experiences. The new experiences may be as subtle as repeating a positive statement to oneself regularly, such as an affirmation. The brain 're-wires' itself based on pathways that are developed by this new consistent pattern of thinking.

If your clients or class participants think positively or have positive thoughts about change, their brain may begin to 're-wire' itself to accept the changes. Maintaining a positive outlook toward behavior change will help clients and class participants make the beneficial changes they need to achieve their goals. The following sections summarize several of the models and theories regarding behavioral change including the transtheoretical model, the social cognitive theory, the self-determination theory, and the health belief model.

Transtheoretical Model
The **transtheoretical model (TTM)** originally emerged in the late 1970s as the result of studies and observations regarding individuals involved in smoking cessation (Lox et al., 2010; Prochaska & DiClemente, 1983). Since that time, the TTM has been applied to other types of behavioral change including the adoption of regular physical activity (Barkley, 2012; Hutchinson et al., 2009; Marshall & Biddle, 2001). In fact, among all models and theories of behavioral change, the TTM is perhaps the most commonly adopted with regard to increasing physical activity behavior (Hutchison et al., 2009). According to the transtheoretical model, also known as the "stages of change model," individuals move through five stages of change including precontemplation, contemplation, preparation, action, and maintenance (Barkley, 2012; Lox et al., 2010; Moore & Tschannan-Moran, 2010). A brief description of each of these stages, as they pertain to physical activity, is provided in table 3-1.

Individuals in pursuit of behavior change may take an undesirable, yet foreseeable detour into a lapse or relapse from the desired behavior. A *lapse* may describe a very brief and temporary departure from the desired behavior or a return to an undesirable behavior. For example, a client may miss two or three exercise sessions due to a particularly busy work schedule, yet then successfully return to their normal exercise routine the following week. A lapse may occur among those in either the action or main-

Table 3-1 Transtheoretical Model

TTM Stages of Change	
Precontemplation	The individual is not thinking about adopting physical activity or an exercise program and has no intention of beginning in the foreseeable future (e.g., the next 6 months). At this stage, the individual does not perceive any problems with their present lifestyle. They consider the disadvantages of exercise to outweigh the advantages and may even fail to recognize the benefits of regular physical activity entirely. Individuals in precontemplation may be defensive when others suggest or attempt to convince them to be more active. However, without intervention, individuals will stay in this stage for a long period of time. Individuals in precontemplation often have the attitude that "I won't" or "I can't" with regard to exercise.
Contemplation	The individual has intentions of becoming more physically active and/or beginning an exercise program within the next 6 months. There is a growing awareness of the advantages and benefits of exercise; however, this is off-set by perceived disadvantages and barriers. As such, the individual is weighing the pros and cons (i.e., decisional balance). There is a feeling of ambivalence in that the individual may simultaneously feel or express desires to become active and remain inactive at the same time. In the contemplation stage, the general attitude toward physical activity is "I may."
Preparation	The preparation phase is characterized by intentions to become physically active or start exercising within the next month. Individuals are preparing for exercise by joining a health club, purchasing new fitness apparel or exercise equipment, or scheduling a consultation with a fitness professional. At this stage, the individual may be performing some sporadic leisure-time physical activity or exercise, but not to the minimum threshold to be considered physically active. Individuals in the preparation stage are thinking, "I will."
Action	The individual is performing regular physical activity and/or exercise up to the minimum level, defined as the equivalent of at least 150 minutes of moderate-intensity leisure-time physical activity per week. Among all the stages of change, action is the most unstable as people attempt to maintain this new behavior while navigating the inevitable obstacles to their success. Individuals in the action stage can report, "I am" physically active.
Maintenance	Individuals move into the maintenance stage once they have sustained regular physical activity at or above the minimum levels for 6 consecutive months. The physical and psychological benefits they have attained, along with the belief in their own ability to live a physically-active lifestyle, continues to fuel their motivation and adherence to exercise. Although effort is still required to avoid set-backs, the individual's self-confidence regarding exercise is strong. Individuals in the maintenance stage say, "I still am."

Lox et al. (2010); Moore & Tschannan-Moran (2010)

Table 3-2 Identifying the Stage of Change

Identifying The Stage of Change		
	No	Yes
1. I am currently Physically active.		
2. I intend to become more physically active in the next 6 months.		
For activity to be regular, it must add up to a total of 30 minutes or more per day and be done at least 5 days per week. For example, you could take one 30-minute walk or take three 10-minute walks for a daily total of 30 minutes.		
	No	Yes
3. I currently engage in regular physical activity.		
4. I have been regularly physically active for the past 6 months.		

Scoring Algorithm
    If question 1 and 2 = 'No', then client is at in precontemplation stage
    If question 1 = 'No' and 2 = 'Yes', then client is in contemplation stage
    If question 1 = 'Yes' and 3 = 'No', then client is in preparation stage
    If question 1 and 3 = 'Yes', and 4 = 'No', then client is in action stage
    If question 1, 3, and 4 = 'Yes', then client is in maintenance stage		

Marcus & Forsyth (2009)

tenance stage of change with a quick recovery back to either of those stages. A *relapse* represents a longer-term departure from behavioral change often accompanied by decreased desire and motivation to resume the targeted behavior. For example, this same individual may be overwhelmed by a busy work schedule, travel, and family obligations, which lead to several months away from their exercise routine. A relapse may occur for those in the maintenance stage, but more often strikes those still in the inherently unstable action stage. In this situation, the individual may be able to move themselves directly back into the action stage, but is more likely to revert back to an earlier stage such as preparation or even contemplation. In some cases, an individual may relapse due to negative coping strategies, which are characterized by unhealthy psychological or emotional responses to a lapse in behavior. The individual may experience feelings of failure, loss of control, guilt, or shame. The initial lapse may cause the individual to believe that all hope for positive behavior change is lost and that attempts to adopt the desired behavior are futile. This is known as the *abstinence violation effect* (Lox et al., 2010). Figure 3-1 provides a schematic representation of the transtheoretical model's stages of change.

Decisional balance refers to an individual's perceptions, beliefs, and interpretation of the pros and cons related to changing their behavior (ACSM, 2018; Janis & Mann, 1977; Lox et al., 2010; Moore & Tschannan-Moran, 2010). In the precontemplation stage, individuals perceive there to be more cons or barriers to adopting a physically active lifestyle (Lox et al., 2010; Marcus & Forsyth, 2009). Individuals in the contemplation stage are seeing a fairly equal balance between the pros and cons to physical activity (Lox et al., 2010; Marcus & Forsyth, 2009). The relative balance between their perception of the pros and cons at this stage contributes to their feelings of ambivalence toward engaging in physical activity. As individuals move into the preparation stage, the decisional balance scale begins to tip in favor of the advantages and benefits of physical activity, which fuels their motivation for change. See figure 3-2. As the individual moves forward into action and maintenance, their belief in the advantages and the value they place in the pros of being physically active continues to strengthen (Lox et al., 2010; Marcus & Forsyth, 2009). Table 3-3 provides a sample 2 x 2 decision-making matrix as it may look for an individual contemplating the adoption of physical activity.

Figure 3-1 TTM Stages of Change

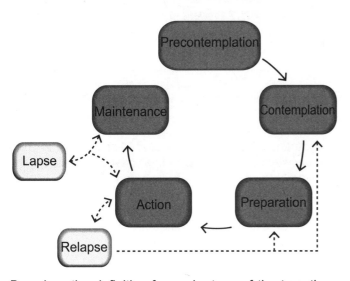

Figure 3-2 Decisional Balance

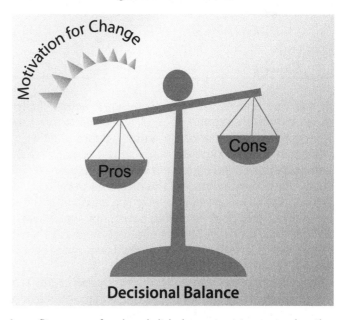

Based on the definition for each stage of the transtheoretical model, Marcus & Forsyth (2009) have presented a series of brief statements that may be used by fitness professionals to identify an individual's stage of change. The statements and interpretation algorithm are provided in table 3-2.

Decisional Balance and Self-Efficacy

Among the many factors that influence an individual's position and movement through the stages of change, two variables are of particular importance, especially during the earlier stages. These variables include decisional balance and self-efficacy.

As a fitness professional, it is important to recognize the pros and cons perceived by potential clients and class participants. In the early stages of behavioral change, it is important to emphasize the benefits of regular physical activity and to help individuals to identify effective strategies to overcome perceived barriers.

Another important factor that influences an individual's adoption or avoidance of physical activity is self-efficacy. **Self-efficacy** refers to situational or task-specific self-confidence. In this situation, self-efficacy is an individual's belief that they are capable of performing physical activity

Table 3-3 Sample Decisional Balance Worksheet

Pros of Physical Activity	Pros of Remaining Inactive
• I will be more fit and strong. • I will have more energy. • I may lose some weight and reduce my belly fat. • I will look better in my summer clothes. • My blood pressure and cholesterol may be lower. • I will feel more confident and will get more positive attention from people.	• I will have time to go out with my friends and watch my favorite TV shows. • I can sleep in a little longer in the morning. • I won't feel tired and sore like I used to after a workout. • I won't have to do laundry all the time washing those sweaty clothes. • I don't have to face the embarrassment of walking into a health club.
Cons of Physical Activity	**Cons of Remaining Inactive**
• I don't have enough time in my busy schedule. • I am too tired after a long day of work. • It costs too much to join a health club. • I don't feel safe walking alone in my neighborhood. • I may have to miss some of my favorite TV shows. • I will have to get up earlier in the morning. • I will be sore and may get hurt.	• I will probably continue to gain weight which will make me feel horrible. • My blood pressure and cholesterol will only get worse and I may get heart disease. • I won't be ready for the beach during our summer vacation. • My spouse will keep making me feel guilty for not exercising. • I won't have the energy or fitness to play with my kids.

or exercise and adhering to a physically-active lifestyle or an exercise program. Lack of self-efficacy can have a very powerful influence on an individual's inaction toward change. Unfortunately, many people do not have the self-awareness to recognize the influential role low self-efficacy plays in their personal situation. The belief that one is incapable of successfully performing a task (e.g., physical activity, exercise) can be so strong that the individual will not even make an attempt to adopt the new behavior due to fear of failure or thinking it would be a waste of time.

The **self-efficacy theory (SET)**, introduced in 1977 by Albert Bandura, is central to many models of behavioral change and describes how individuals form perceptions regarding their own ability to engage in a certain behavior (Lox et al., 2010). There are several factors that may either increase or decrease an individual's self-efficacy. Having knowledge of these factors, the fitness professional may utilize various strategies to help the individual overcome the internal barrier of low self-efficacy regarding physical activity and exercise.

Past performance accomplishments refers to the individual's perception of success related to previously performed activities similar to, or the same as, the current target behavior (Lox et al., 2010). For example, looking back in time and recalling instances when the individual was able to successfully maintain an active lifestyle, participate in an exercise program, or perform athletic endeavors, may strengthen self-efficacy with regard to activity in the present day. With the reminder of their past performance, the individual may begin to think, "I've done it before so I can do it again."

Mastery experiences are somewhat similar, but related to small achievements made in very recent past or at the present time, which contribute to building self-efficacy for the targeted behavior or task. Challenging a sedentary individual to train for and run a marathon would be perceived as an overwhelming and obviously infeasible task. The individual's present situation is too far removed from the seemingly unbelievable feat of running a marathon. However, the individual may simply begin by walking a mile, running their first continuous mile, successfully completing a 5-kilometer run, then a 10-kilometer run, eventually followed by a half-marathon. Each smaller accomplishment represents a mastery experience that gradually builds the individual's self-efficacy not only for running, but also with regard to crossing the finish line of a marathon. What once appeared to be unfathomable to the individual is now within their realm of possibility.

Another source of self-efficacy may be found through vicarious experiences, also known as social modeling. Vicarious experience refers to the observation of the behaviors or accomplishments of other individuals, which are similar to those desired by the observer (Lox et al., 2010). The greater the similarity between the individual and the social model, the greater the influence may be on that person's self-efficacy. These vicarious experiences may be represented by client testimonials and success stories, other class participants achieving similar goals, someone who has overcome an illness or injury to return to health and physical activity, or even the distant influence of a celebrity having achieved a fitness goal. Seeing others adopt physical activity and successfully achieve exercise-related goals provides inspiration and builds self-efficacy. The individual may begin to think, "If he or she can do it, then so can I."

Social persuasion is also a factor that may contribute to the development of self-efficacy. Social persuasion typically involves verbal statements of encouragement, affirmation, or positive-reinforcement. Of course, to be most effective, this social persuasion must be genuine, sincere, and without ulterior motive. In addition, the most impactful persuasion is that which comes from a significant other (e.g., friend, spouse, family member) or a respected figure (e.g., physician, fitness professional). In its simplest form, social persuasion may be statements like, "I know you can do it!", "Keep up the great work, you are doing awesome!", or "I believe in you!".

> **Good to Know**
>
> **Factors that influence self-efficacy:**
> - Past performance accomplishments
> - Mastery experiences
> - Vicarious experiences/social modeling
> - Social persuasion
> - Physiological states
> - Affective states

Two final sources of self-efficacy involve both physiological and affective states. Physiological states may include physical sensations that accompany physical activity such as rapid heart rate, respiration, soreness, and fatigue. These sensations may impact self-efficacy both negatively or positively depending upon the individual's expectation and interpretation of these sensations. Initially, these physical sensations may be perceived as a warning sign or as an indication of an inability to perform exercise. However, as the body adapts to the stress of physical activity and exercise, the individual may feel increased self-efficacy resulting from their enhanced ability to tolerate the demands of the activity. They may even begin to interpret the physiological state associated with exercise as a good sensation and one that they enjoy experiencing.

Affective or emotional states can also influence self-efficacy either positively or negatively. An individual who is experiencing positive emotions such as happiness, excitement, or pride would be expected to view the anticipated bout of physical activity with high self-efficacy (Lox et al., 2010). On the other hand, an individual holding negative emotions such as anxiety, fear, or disappointment is likely to approach physical activity with low self-efficacy (Lox et al., 2010). Increased stress response can negatively affect self-efficacy if it is above the 'zone,' the ideal state of arousal for optimal performance. For example, a person with test anxiety will not perform as well as a person who is calm and thinking "I got this!".

Other Models of Behavioral Change

In addition to the transtheoretical model, several other theories have also been proposed to interpret and explain the psychological processes involved in behavioral change. Many of these theories have been applied to the adoption and maintenance of regular physical activity. A brief summary of each of these models is also provided in the following paragraphs. Readers are encouraged to pursue additional knowledge and understanding of these behavioral change models through a review of the references corresponding to this chapter.

Social Cognitive Theory

The **social cognitive theory (SCT)**, proposed by psychologist Albert Bandura, suggests that behavior change and learning is affected by three variables including personal characteristics, environmental factors, and behavioral attributes (ACSM, 2018; Barkley, 2012; Marcus & Forsyth, 2009). The three-way interaction between these dynamic variables is known as 'reciprocal determinism' (Barkley, 2012; Marcus & Forsyth, 2009). Personal characteristics may include emotions, thoughts and perceptions, values and beliefs, personality traits, and biological factors (ACSM, 2018; Barkley, 2012). Environmental factors include social influences such as friends, family, co-workers, media, public policy, and cultural norms; and aspects related to physical space such as home, neighborhood, and workplace (ACSM, 2018; Barkley, 2012). Behavioral attributes refer to past and present behaviors and experiences. Two central concepts in the social cognitive theory are self-efficacy and outcome expectations. The concept of outcome expectations suggests that in order for an individual to adopt a new behavior (e.g., physical activity) there must be a strong belief that the behavior will provide positive outcomes (e.g., more energy, improved health, enhanced mental function, better appearance), which are valued by the individual and perceived to outweigh any potential negative outcomes (e.g., physical discomfort, fatigue, less time for other activities) associated with the new behavior (ACSM, 2018; Marcus & Forsyth, 2009).

Self-Determination Theory

The **self-determination theory (SDT)** suggests that individuals seek to satisfy three primary psychosocial needs including a need for autonomy (i.e., self-determined behavior), a need to demonstrate competence (i.e., experience mastery), and a need for meaningful social interactions (ACSM, 2018; Lox et al., 2010). Subsequently, an individual's actions and behaviors seek to satisfy one or more of these needs (Lox et al., 2010). The SDT also suggests that an individual's level of motivation for a particular behavior lies somewhere along a continuum from amotivation to various forms of extrinsic motivation to intrinsic motivation (ACSM, 2018; Lox et al., 2010). *Motivation* is the degree of determination, drive, or desire with which an individual approaches (or avoids) a behavior. *Amotivation* refers to a complete lack of motivation or desire to engage in a certain behavior or activity. *Extrinsic motivation* is motivation driven by factors external to or outside of the individual such as financial incentives, awards, competition with others, or approval from others. *Intrinsic motivation* originates internally and refers to the motivation to perform a task (e.g., physical activity) for the inherent pleasure, satisfaction, or the personal challenge. Individuals with amotivation have no desire or intention to exercise and therefore low self-determination for physical activity (ACSM, 2018; Lox et al., 2010). Those who are intrinsically motivated also have high self-determination and subsequently the strongest commitment to exercise, even when challenged by barriers and obstacles (ACSM, 2018, Lox et al., 2010).

Health Belief Model

The **health belief model (HBM)** suggests that individuals will modify their behavior (e.g., become physically active) to prevent or manage a disease or undesirable health condition if they believe they are susceptible to the disease or condition (ACSM, 2018; Barkley, 2012; Champion & Skinner, 2008). The HBM is based on the premise that individuals will take action to become physically active if six constructs are satisfied including: (1) perceived susceptibility to the disease or medical condition; (2) the disease or condition is perceived to be of a serious nature; (3) adopting physical activity is perceived to provide benefits to reduce susceptibility to the disease or condition; (4) the perceived barriers to physical activity are outweighed by the benefits; (5) the individual has self-efficacy regarding their ability to adopt and maintain physical activity; and (6) the individual is exposed to cues or prompts to action (e.g., recognition of risk factors, signs or symptoms, a doctor's recommendation to exercise) (ACSM, 2018; Barkley, 2012; Champion & Skinner, 2008). Advocates of the health belief model suggest that all six of these constructs combine to influence an individual's motivation to begin regular physical activity as a means to reduce the risk of the disease or health condition of concern (Barkley, 2012).

Goal-Setting

An important element to facilitate the adoption of physical activity is effective goal-setting. In addition, setting well-designed goals can also increase motivation and improve adherence to physical activity and exercise. Generally speaking, there are two broad categories of goals including action-oriented goals and outcome-oriented goals.

Action-oriented goals are also often referred to as process goals or performance goals. An action-oriented goal is short-term and focuses on the steps or actions to be taken toward achieving the desired outcome. A new client may express a desired outcome of weight loss; however, the individual may quickly become discouraged, or even discontinue their efforts, if progress toward the desired outcome (i.e., weight loss) is not achieved within what they perceive to be a realistic timeframe. Their lack of immediate control over this targeted outcome creates frustration, discouragement, and may demotivate the client. By refocusing the individual's attention toward action-oriented goals, a sense of control and achievement will be created, which maintains the individual's motivation and efforts toward the desired outcome. In this scenario, rather than focusing on weight loss, action-oriented goals may be established that focus on performing a targeted amount of physical activity or specific modifications to dietary habits. For example, an action-oriented goal related to physical activity may be, "Perform 150 minutes of moderate-intensity physical activity each week." The preceding goal statement is focused on an action (i.e., performing a designated amount of physical activity) and is short-term (i.e., within one week). By achieving this goal each week, it will contribute toward progress to the desired outcome. In addition, this goal places responsibility back in the hands of the client providing a sense of control and accountability.

Outcome-oriented goals are long-term in nature and relate to the outcome or result of consistent actions and behaviors. An example of an outcome-oriented goal may be, "I will lose 20 pounds within the next 6 months." Certainly to achieve this goal, specific behaviors will require modification such as physical activity and dietary habits. The outcome is contingent upon successful performance of the actions.

Often times, individuals will frame their goals around desired outcomes and unfortunately will state them in very vague terms. For example, a client may say, "I want to lose weight", "I want to tone up", or "I want to get in better shape." To provide better clarity and focus, the fitness professional should collaborate with the client to restate these goals with less ambiguity. To accomplish this, an effective goal-setting strategy is to establish SMART goals. **SMART** is an acronym that stands for specific, measurable, attainable, relevant, and time-bound (YMCA, 2006). This approach to goal-setting should be applied to both the establishment of action-oriented and outcome-oriented goals. Table 3-4 provides a brief explanation regarding each component of a SMART goal.

Several additional derivatives of the SMART acronym have also been suggested including: SMARTS - specific, measurable, action-oriented, realistic, timely, and self-determined (ACSM, 2018); SMART – specific, measurable, agreed, realistic, time-phased (Whitmore, 2009); SMART- specific, measurable, actionable, realistic, and time-lined (Moore & Tschannen-Moran, 2010); SMART – specific, measurable, assignable, realistic, time-related (Doran, 1981); SMART- specific, measurable, achievable, realistic/relevant, timed (Bovend'Eerdt et al., 2009).

Motivation and Adherence

In many ways, designing an exercise program is the 'easy' part in the delivery of personal training and fitness services. The real challenge for the fitness professional is presented when attempting to motivate a client or class participant to actually perform and adhere to the exercise program. The following section provides a list of best practices that may be used by fitness professionals to facilitate increased motivation and adherence to regular physical activity and structured exercise programs.

Enjoyable Activities: It may seem obvious, but it's worth stating. If the activities incorporated into the exercise program and the experience created by the fitness professional are enjoyable, then the individual is much more likely to be motivated, perhaps intrinsically, to participate in the program or class. Provide activities that appeal to a specific client.

Availability and Convenience: Among the many environmental factors that influence exercise participation is accessibility to fitness facilities. As might be expected, those who reside in close proximity to convenient and accessible facilities (e.g., community centers, health clubs, YMCAs) demonstrate higher levels of physical activity participation (Humpel et al., 2002). Offering flexibility in scheduling and a wide variety of class offerings can also increase participation. The convenience of offering onsite child care also favorably influences participation.

Effective Goal-Setting: As noted earlier, setting appropriate goals, using the SMART approach, can facilitate increased motivation and program adherence. For most individuals, accountability and successful behavior modification will be most effective when the emphasis is placed on action-oriented goals.

Emphasize Health Benefits Versus Appearance: Research has demonstrated that exercise for the purpose of improving physical appearance as a primary outcome measure may negatively affect self-esteem, reduce positive affect, increase negative perceptions of body image, increase social physique anxiety, and increase depression (Lox et al., 2010). On the other hand, when individuals (women in particular) exercise primarily to improve physical function (e.g., strength, endurance) they are more likely to experience satisfaction and more positive feelings toward one's body (Lox et al., 2010). Similarly, participants in a health-oriented class reported greater enjoyment and intention to join the class in the future than those participating in an appearance-oriented class (Lox et al., 2010).

Social Support: Clients who do not have friends, relatives, or significant others who are willing to support them during a lifestyle change find the process much more difficult, if not impossible. In many cases, the fitness professional may serve as an individual's only source of social support. One of the many important elements of both small group personal training and group exercise classes is the social support offered by these programs and services. With regard to overall member retention, it has been suggested that member-to-member connections and the social environment created within a health club setting may actually be more important than staff-to-member conections

Table 3-4 Setting SMART Goals

Setting SMART Goals	
Specific	Establish clear, well-defined goals. The goal must specifically indicate exactly what is to be accomplished. The goal must be easily understood and unambiguous.
Measurable	The goal should include an objective method of measuring the progress toward and attainment of the goal. The measurement and tracking will help evaluate whether an individual is on track to attain a specific goal and will also indicate whether modifications are needed for the goal to be reached.
Attainable	The goal should be realistically attainable by the individual. If an individual believes that a goal is possible, it helps provide the motivation and perseverance to attain the goal. It is important to stretch for a goal, but the actual goal must be within reason. Setting goals that are obviously too high may cause frustration, discouragement, and demotivation.
Relevant	The goal should be pertinent to the unique needs, interests, and abilities of the individual. Action-oriented goals should have a correlation to the achievement of the desired outcome. If a goal is relevant, the individual will be motivated to strive toward its achievement. Goal-setting must be a collaborative process to ensure the participant is 'buying-in' to the goal.
Time-bound	Identify the specific timeframe within which the goal is to be achieved. A schedule of steps to achieve the goal should be developed to provide a specific plan of action with a predetermined deadline for completion of the individual steps (actions) and the desired outcome.

YMCA (2006)

(McCarthy, 2007). Fitness professionals should make an effort to help individuals to expand their network of connections within classes, programs, and the overall health club setting.

Develop a Plan: Fitness professionals should collaborate with their clients, as well as club members seeking their guidance, to develop a clear plan toward desired outcomes. The plan should include appropriate short- and long-term goal setting as well as the specific step-by-step processes to be followed in pursuit of these goals. In addition, the plan may outline strategies to deal with foreseeable barriers and potential lapses. Although the plan may have structure, it should also provide flexibility to accommodate other commitments and obligations. It is important that the client or club member plays an active role to create this personalized plan; therefore, creating a sense of ownership and self-accountability to the plan.

Behavioral Contracts: Behavioral contracts are written non-legal agreements specifying target behaviors, exercise frequency, rewards and consequences, and a timeline for specific achievements or outcomes. Behavioral contracts may be effective to create a sense of commitment to both self and others, and may serve as a reminder and an extrinsic motivator to exercise.

Acknowledge and Reward Progress: Affirmations, positive reinforcement, and tangible awards can be powerful tools to support a client's efforts to implement behavioral change. As a type of social persuasion, these strategies may help to increase self-efficacy and can serve as effective sources of extrinsic motivation during the early stages of behavioral change. The use of positive reinforcement is a key element of B.F. Skinner's stimulus-response theory (SRT), which suggests an explanation regarding how people learn new behaviors through classic conditioning (Lox et al., 2010).

Self-Monitoring and Tracking: It has been said that "if you don't measure it, you can't manage it." Self-monitoring and tracking either through written journals or the use of technology-based tracking tools (e.g., heart rate monitors, pedometers, accelerometers, mobile device applications) may be an effective motivator and an antecedent to physical activity and exercise adherence. In addition, these tools are also effective for dietary tracking, awareness, and accountability.

Chapter Summary
This chapter provided an overview of the transtheoretical model as well as several other theories and models proposed to explain the psychosocial factors that influence behavioral change such as the adoption and maintenance of physical activity. In addition, several strategies were suggested to increase motivation and adherence to physical activity including the use of effective goal-setting. Since many Americans struggle to successfully adopt favorable lifestyle behaviors such as regular physical activity and healthy dietary habits, fitness professionals must have knowledge and skill in helping individuals to successfully achieve behavioral change.

Chapter References
American College of Sports Medicine (2018). *ACSM's Guidelines for Exercise Testing and Prescription*, 10th edition. Philadelphia, PA: Wolters Kluwer.

Barkley, S. (2012). Behavioral theory and counseling techniques for increasing physical activity participation. *ACSM's Certified News, 22*(4), 4-5,12.

Bovend'Eerdt, T.J., Botell, R.E., & Wade, D.T. (2009). Writing SMART rehabilitation goals and achieving goal attainment scaling: A practical guide. *Clinical Rehabilitation, 23*(4), 352-361.

Champion, V.L., & Skinner, C.S. (2008). The health belief model. In: K. Glanz, B.K. Rimer, and K. Viswanath (Eds.), *Health Behavior and Health Education: Theory, Research, and Practice*, 4th edition (pp. 45-65). San Francisco, CA: Jossey-Bass.

Doran, G.T. (1981). There's a S.M.A.R.T. way to write management's goals and objectives. *Management Review, 70*(11), 35-36.

Humpel, N., Owen, N., & Leslie, E. (2002). Environmental factors associated with adults' participation in physical activity: A review. *American Journal of Preventive Medicine, 22*(3), 188-199.

Hutchison, A.J., Breckon, J.D., & Johnston, L.H. (2009). Physical activity behavior change interventions based on the transtheoretical model: A systematic review. *Health Education & Behavior, 36*(5), 829-845.

Janis, I.L., & Mann, L. (1977). *Decision Making: A Psychological Analysis of Conflict, Choice, and Commitment*. New York, NY: Collier Macmillan.

Lox, L.L., Martin-Ginis, K.A., & Petruzzello, S.J. (2010). *The Psychology of Exercise: Integrating Theory and Practice*, 3rd edition. Scottsdale, AZ: Holcomb Hathaway.

Marcus, B., & Forsyth, L. (2009). *Motivating People to be Physically Active*, 2nd edition. Champaign, IL: Human Kinetics.

Marshall, S.J., & Biddle, S.J. (2001). The transtheoretical model of behavior change: A meta-analysis of applications to physical activity and exercise. *Annals of Behavioral Medicine, 23*(4), 229-246.

McCarthy, J. (2007). *IHRSA's Guide Go Member Retention: Industry Lessons On What, And What Not, To Do.* 2nd edition. International Health Racquet and Sportsclub Association.

Moore, M., & Tschannan-Moran, B. (2010). *Coaching Psychology Manual*. Baltimore, MD: Lippincott, Williams & Wilkins.

Prochaska, J.O., & DiClemente, C.C. (1982). Transtheoretical theory: Toward a more integrative model of change. *Psychotherapy Theory Research and Practice, 19*(3), 276-288.

Prochaska, J.O., & DiClemente, C.C. (1983). Stages and processes of self-change of smoking: Toward an integrative model of change. *Journal of Consulting and Clinical Psychology, 51*(3), 390-395.

Whitmore, J. (2009). *Coaching for Performance: GROWing Human Potential and Purpose*, 4th edition. Boston, MA: Nicolas Brealey Publishing.

YMCA of the USA (2006). *YMCA Personal Training Manual*, 2nd edition. Champaign, IL: Human Kinetics.

Recommended Reading
American College of Sports Medicine (2018). Chapter 12: Behavioral Theories and Strategies for Promoting Exercise. In, *ACSM's Guidelines to Exercise Testing and Prescription*, 10th edition. Philadelphia, PA: Wolters Kluwer.

Chapter 3 Review Questions

1. You are meeting with a new member of the health club who has scheduled an initial fitness consultation. This member indicates that he has been active on an inconsistent basis for the past five weeks and would like to begin a structured exercise program to improve his cardiorespiratory fitness and to lose some weight. Based on this information, you conclude that he is in which stage of the transtheoretical model?
   A. Precontemplation
   B. Preparation
   C. Contemplation
   D. Action

2. A friend indicates that she would like to begin an exercise program, but at the same time enjoys spending her limited free time in sedentary activities such as watching TV and checking out social media updates. She recognizes the benefits of being physically active, but also perceives an equal number of disadvantages and sacrifices she would have to make in order to become active. Based on this information, what is this individual's current stage of behavioral change in the transtheoretical model?
   A. Precontemplation
   B. Preparation
   C. Contemplation
   D. Maintenance

3. Which of the following goal statements is an example of a SMART action-oriented goal?
   A. "I will lose 10 pounds over the next 10 weeks through increased exercise and decreased caloric intake."
   B. "I will increase my maximal oxygen consumption by 5 mL/kg/min over the next 3 months."
   C. "I will reduce my abdominal fat by doing more core exercises."
   D. "I will complete a minimum of two full-body resistance training sessions each week."

4. Which of the following is an example of an intrinsic source of motivation?
   A. Giving a class participant a T-shirt for perfect attendance in a series of classes.
   B. Earning a partial reimbursement of membership dues for visiting the club a minimum number of times each month.
   C. Feelings of satisfaction and accomplishment after running a marathon (26.2 miles).
   D. Receiving compliments from others regarding your recent weight loss.

5. You have just started working with a 52-year-old male client. When asked what prompted him to begin an exercise program, your client indicates that a close friend of his had recently suffered a heart attack. The client is overweight and has high blood pressure. He is worried that he too may be at risk for a heart attack if he does not start taking better care of himself by exercising regularly and improving his diet. Which of the following theoretical models of behavioral change may best explain this scenario?
   A. Self-Determination Theory
   B. Health Belief Model
   C. Transtheoretical Model
   D. Social-Cognitive Theory

6. Which of the following is most likely to increase a client's self-efficacy related to exercise?
   A. Sharing success stories of other individuals who have achieved fitness goals similar the client's.
   B. Educating the client with regard to the risks of a sedentary lifestyle
   C. Highlighting the many health benefits that can be obtained from regular physical activity.
   D. Setting aggressive long-term goals using the SMART approach to goal-setting.

Answers to Review Questions on Page 384
Note: Review questions are intended to reinforce learning and comprehension of subject matter presented in the corresponding chapter. The review questions are not intended to be representative of actual certification exam questions in terms of style, content, or difficulty.

4
Introduction to Wellness Coaching

Introduction
Similar to many health care providers (e.g., physicians, dietitians, physical therapists), fitness professionals have largely been trained in an 'expert' approach, which places focus on a problem, deficit, or weakness and a corresponding solution or treatment. To a large extent, moving individuals toward their health and fitness goals has relied on the technical knowledge and skills of a fitness professional to conduct an initial assessment and develop an exercise program designed to achieve the desired goal. Although some individuals may adhere to a program derived from expert advice, the majority do not. Generally speaking, people desire autonomy and resist being told what to do even when the advice serves their best interest (Frates et al., 2011). Even the most scientifically-based exercise program is ineffective when the individual lacks the desire and intrinsic motivation to follow through with the plan. On the other hand, a wellness coach relies on the inherent knowledge possessed by the client, helping them to help themselves through the process of behavioral change.

As noted in chapter one, wellness coaching has been an emerging trend in the health and fitness industries over the past decade. Preparing for and earning a wellness coach certification may serve as an important step in the career progression of a fitness professional. At the very minimum, fitness professionals must have a general understanding of fundamental coaching skills necessary to effectively guide their clients and class participants toward behavioral change and desired goals. Building upon the topics of effective communication skills and principles of behavioral change presented in the previous two chapters, this chapter will introduce fundamental skills and concepts related to coaching.

The Art of Wellness Coaching
It is not too surprising that the term 'coach' conjures up thoughts and images of a sports coach with a whistle draped around their neck during a practice or pacing the sidelines during the game. A sport coach's tactics may include barking commands at their players, providing instruction, drafting up strategic plays, or delivering inspirational speeches with the hope of motivating their players for competition. However, in the context of health, wellness, and behavioral change a coach plays a much more subtle role. Wellness coaches ask thoughtful questions, provide gentle guidance, and work collaboratively with their clients to develop client-centered plans for change. A wellness coach acts like a co-pilot, always mindful to keep the client positioned in the driver's seat, charting the course toward their personal goals.

The following quotes nicely capture the essence of coaching as it pertains to behavioral change to attain improved health and well-being.

> "Coaching is the art of creating an environment, through conversation and a way of being, that facilitates the process by which a person can move toward desired goals in a fulfilling manner" (Gallwey, 2000).
>
> "Coaching is more about asking the right questions than providing answers – a coach engages in a collaborative alliance with the individual to establish and clarify purpose and goals and to develop a plan of action to achieve these goals" (Zeus & Skiffington, 2000).
>
> "Coaching is chiefly about discovery, awareness, and choice. It is a way of effectively empowering people to find their own answers, encouraging and supporting them on the path as they continue to make important choices. Coaching is a form of conversation with unspoken ground rules regarding certain qualities that must be present: respect, openness, compassion, empathy, and a rigorous commitment to speaking the truth" (Whitworth et al., 2007).
>
> "Coaching is unlocking people's potential to maximize their own performance. It is helping them to learn rather than teaching them…The underlying intent of every coaching interaction is to build the coachee's self-belief" (Whitmore, 2009).

Taken together, these quotes capture many of the essential characteristics required of effective wellness coaches including empathy, compassion, and acceptance. In addition, these quotations represent fundamental coaching skills such as questioning, listening, collaborating, and facilitating. Although a wellness coach may have extensive knowledge or even expertise in disciplines such as exercise science, fitness programming, nutrition, or psychology, having this knowledge is not necessarily requisite to successfully coach a client toward behavioral change and desired outcomes. At the heart of coaching is the assumption, "people have the inherent creativity, intelligence, and tacit knowledge they need to succeed but may need help in gaining access to it" (Hargrove, 1995). As such, wellness coaching is not about directing individuals, disseminating endless information, providing unsolicited advice, or telling people what to do. Table 4-1 outlines the differences between the expert- and the coach-approach.

Motivational Interviewing

Motivational interviewing has been shown to be an effective approach to facilitate the adoption and maintenance of healthy lifestyle behaviors including physical activity (Britt et al., 2004; Lundahl & Burke, 2009; Martins & McNeil, 2009). **Motivational interviewing (MI)** was originally introduced in the early 1980s by psychologist, William R. Miller, PhD, and further developed and described with his colleague Stephen Rollnick, PhD. In the most recent edition of their popular book *Motivational Interviewing*, Miller and Rollnick (2012) offer several definitions of motivational interviewing. The layperson's definition of motivational interviewing states, "Motivational interviewing is a collaborative conversation style for strengthening a person's own motivation and commitment to change" (Miller & Rollnick, 2012). Miller and Rollnick (2012) also provide a more technical definition which states, "Motivational interviewing is a collaborative, goal-oriented style of communication with particular attention to the language of change. It is designed to strengthen personal motivation for, and commitment to, a specific goal by eliciting and exploring the person's own reasons for change within an atmosphere of acceptance and compassion." MI has become central to the strategies used by wellness coaches to guide their clients through the process of behavioral change.

The Spirit of Motivational Interviewing

The technical definition of MI also represents the four elements that create the underlying 'spirit' of motivational interviewing, which include partnership, acceptance, compassion, and evocation (Miller & Rollnick, 2012). MI is always performed in partnership with the client, such that it is a collaborative effort, with the client clearly being the indisputable expert about themselves (Miller & Rollnick, 2012). In the spirit of MI, the coach maintains an attitude of acceptance toward the client, honoring the uniqueness and potential of the individual (Miller & Rollnick, 2012). Acceptance is also reflected in the respectful, empathetic, and nonjudgmental approach characteristic of MI conversations. Motivational interviewing is also performed with compassion and a deliberate commitment to the personal goals, desires, and interests of the client (Miller & Rollnick, 2012). MI is not a technique to manipulate people's behavior, to trick them into changing, or to coerce them to act in a manner that serves the needs of the coach or a hidden agenda. Lastly, motivational interviewing focuses on the strengths of the individual under the assumption that they already possess the knowledge to develop their own solutions. As such, the coach evokes this inherent knowledge and elicits 'change talk' (i.e., statements that favor or support change) expressed by the client (Barkley, 2013; Miller & Rollnick, 2012).

The Process of MI

Motivational interviewing involves four key processes that include engaging, focusing, evoking, and planning (Miller & Rollnick, 2012). *Engaging* is the first of these processes, which is to establish rapport, mutual trust, and a respectful helping relationship (Miller & Rollnick, 2012). *Focusing* is the process by which the coach identifies and maintains a specific direction in the MI conversation regarding change (Miller & Rollnick, 2012). *Evoking* is the process of discovering the client's own motivation for change, assisting clients to overcome their ambivalence to change, guiding clients to recognize discrepancies between their current behavior and their broader life goals or values, and to elicit client statements in favor change (i.e., change talk) (Barkley, 2013; Miller & Rollnick, 2012; Resnicow & McMaster, 2012). The final step in MI is the process of *planning*, which encompasses developing commitment to change and formulating a specific action plan (Miller & Rollnick, 2012).

Core Communication Skills of MI

Communication skills are essential to effective motivational interviewing. Throughout the process of motivational

Table 4-1 Expert vs. Coach

Expert vs. Coach	
Expert	**Coach**
• Instructs individuals • Provides education and information • Relies on knowledge and skills of the expert • Strives to have all the answers • Focuses on problems, deficits, and weaknesses • Advises and directs	• Helps individuals to help themselves • Builds motivation, self-efficacy, and engagement • Relies on inherent knowledge, self-awareness, and insights of the individual • Strives to help individuals to find their own answers and solutions • Focuses on strengths • Collaborates

Adapted from Frates et al. (2011)

interviewing and in accordance with its guiding principles, there are four core communication skills that are used by coaches during MI conversations. These communication skills create the acronym **OARS**: open-ended questioning, affirming, reflective listening, and summarizing.

As discussed in chapter 2, *open-ended questions* do not limit an individual's response and invite elaboration and conversation. Some examples of open-ended questions used during MI include:

- "How do you hope I might be able to help you?"
- "Where do you think your current lifestyle will lead you?"
- "In what ways do you think it is important for you to become more physically active?"

Affirming is the second core skill used during motivational interviewing. Affirming is to highlight the positive or to recognize and acknowledge the strengths of the client, their good actions, and their inherent value as a person (Miller & Rollnick, 2012). For example, affirmation statements may include:

- "Thank you for taking time out of your busy schedule to meet with me today."
- "You did a really great job with your exercise program last week."
- "I can see that you are very committed to making this change."

Perhaps one of the most frequently used communication skills in MI is *reflective listening*. Reflective listening actually involves many different types of reflection statements which can vary in complexity and purpose (Miller & Rollnick, 2012; Resnicow et al., 2002; Resnicow & McMaster, 2012). The goals of reflective statements may include a demonstration of understanding, clarification of a client's statement, confirmation of the client's thoughts or feelings, and facilitation of the process of self-discovery (Resnicow & McMaster, 2012). In addition, a coach may also use reflections to test an assumption about what a client means or feels, or to make a guess regarding the direction of the client's 'story' (Resnicow & McMaster, 2012). Many reflective statements will begin with the phrases, "It sounds like…", "If I understood you correctly…", or "So, if I heard you correctly..." (Resnicow & McMaster, 2012). Some sample reflective statements include:

Client: "I have been so busy over the last week that I have not had time to breathe let alone exercise."
Coach: "You are feeling overwhelmed by your schedule and frustrated that you have not been able to exercise." (feeling reflection)

Client: "I know I should exercise more often, but when I get home from work I just like to sit down and relax while I watch my favorite shows."
Coach: "So on the one hand you would like to exercise more, but on the other hand doing so may mean giving up some of the time you spend watching TV." (double-sided reflection)

Client: "My wife has really been bothering me to start an exercise program."
Coach: "It sounds like she must really care about you." (reframing reflection)

The last of the four core motivational interviewing skills is summarizing. *Summarizing* is a type of reflection used to pull together a series of interrelated items (i.e., collecting summary); a reflection used to connect something the client has just said to an earlier or past statement (i.e., linking summary); or to reflect on a series of thoughts or statements in preparation for a shift to a new topic (i.e., transitional summary) (Miller & Rollnick, 2012). For example, the coach may present an open-ended question such as, "What are some of the of reasons you have considered becoming more physically active?" The client will respond by sharing a list of reasons they have considered. The coach will then reflect with a collecting summary to restate these reasons, which may be followed by the simple question, "Anything else?" or "Do any of those really stick out in your mind as having greater importance to you?" In these scenarios, the coach may be attempting to evoke more information or to focus the direction of the MI conversation.

Rating Rulers
Another important strategy often used in motivational interviewing, particularly to elicit change talk, is a rating ruler or 'change ruler' (Barkley, 2013; Miller & Rollnick, 2012; Resnicow et al., 2002; Resnicow & McMaster, 2012). Rating rulers are used to assess the level of importance behavioral change has to the client and their confidence (i.e., self-efficacy) in making this change. The question of importance is, "On a scale of 0 to 10, with 10 being the highest, how important is it to you to become more physically active?" The question of confidence is, "Again, on the same scale from 0 to 10, with 10 being the highest, assuming you want to be more physically active, how confident are you that you could do it?" After the client provides their response to either question, the coach follows up with the question "What makes you rate it as a 6 instead of a lower number like a 2 or 3?" This may be followed by another question such as, "What might it take to get you to a higher number like an 8?" The use of rating rulers may help the coach to understand the client's readiness for change and their self-efficacy for change. In addition, these questions may facilitate the client's self-awareness and elicit client statements in favor of making the change.

The Four Principles of MI

Using the previously discussed communication skills, the processes of MI are guided by four general principles. Using these principles, the coach can assist the client to gain self-awareness of their thoughts and enable clients to resolve ambivalence to behavioral change (Moore & Tschannan-Moran, 2010). The first of these four principles is to "express empathy." Empathy is an understanding and acceptance of another person's experiences, thoughts, and feelings. Expressions of empathy help to establish rapport. When the client feels heard and understood, they are more likely to communicate openly, which in turn facilitates the process of change. Coaches maintain a non-judgmental disposition and accept that ambivalence is a normal part of the change process. The skillful use of reflective listening is fundamental to expressions of empathy.

The second principle of MI is to "develop discrepancy." Behavioral change is often motivated by a perceived discrepancy between an individual's current behavior and their personal goals or values (Moore & Tschannan-Moran, 2010). To develop discrepancy, the coach may begin with an exploration of the client's goals, values, and beliefs. Open-ended questions, reflective listening, and rating rulers are often utilized to identify and develop discrepancy between behavior and these values. Using these strategies, the coach guides the client to notice these discrepancies and moves them to make their own arguments for change.

It is natural for individuals to resist change, particularly if they feel that the change is being imposed or pushed upon them. Direct persuasion, confrontation, and argumentation are to be avoided during motivational interviewing. Nevertheless, the coach is likely to encounter occasional resistance, sometimes referred to as *resistance talk* or *sustain talk*. The third principle of MI is to "roll with resistance." If a client expresses resistance the coach should not oppose or challenge this resistance, but instead should acknowledge and explore the client's thoughts, feelings, and concerns. Resistance talk should also serve as a signal for the coach to change their approach or strategy. A commonly-used metaphor describes the MI conversation more like a dance than a wrestling match (Resnicow et al., 2002). The conversation may be guided by either the coach or the client, but the pair should always move in the same direction rather than struggling against each other. To minimize chances of resistance talk, the coach must resist the temptation to respond to their 'righting reflex', which is the desire to correct what appears to be wrong with people and their situations, and to point them in the right direction, which often relies on a directive style (Miller & Rollnick, 2012).

The last guiding principle of motivational interviewing is to "support self-efficacy." As noted in chapter 3, self-efficacy is an individual's task-specific or situation-specific confidence. The coach supports the development of self-efficacy by helping the client to look back on past successes, recognizing and affirming the client's strengths and skills, and expressing optimism in the client's ability to change.

To learn more about motivational interviewing please see Miller & Rollnick (2012) and Clifford & Curtis (2016).

Good to Know	
Framework of Motivational Interviewing	
The 'Spirit' of MI	*The Key Processes of MI*
Partnership	Engaging
Acceptance	Focusing
Compassion	Evoking
Evocation	Planning
Guiding Principles of MI	*Core Skills of MI*
Express Empathy	Open-ended questioning
Develop Discrepancy	Affirming
Roll with Resistance	Reflective listening
Support Self-Efficacy	Summarizing

Appreciative Inquiry

Appreciative inquiry was originally developed by Dr. David Cooperrider and his colleagues at the Case Western Reserve University School of Management in the 1980s (Moore & Charvat, 2006; Moore & Tschannan-Moran, 2010; Watkins & Cooperrider, 2000). Originally, appreciative inquiry was developed as an affirmation process for creating change within organizations by focusing on the positive or what was 'right' in an organization (Moore & Charvat, 2006; Watkins & Cooperrider, 2000). The philosophy of appreciative inquiry has since been adopted as an approach to facilitate health behavior change. In this context, **appreciative inquiry (AI)** is a coaching mindset and an approach that focuses on exploring and amplifying an individual's strengths in order to motivate behavioral change (Moore & Tschannan-Moran, 2010). There are five underlying principles of appreciative inquiry which are listed and briefly described in table 4-2.

The principles of appreciative inquiry have been applied toward behavioral change in various ways among which the *5-D Model of AI* has become the most common (Bushe, 2011; Moore & Tschannan-Moran, 2010). The 5-D Model of AI includes define, discover, dream, design, and destiny (Bushe, 2011; Moore & Tschannan-Moran, 2010). See figure 4-1.

The first step of the 5-D model is to define the desired outcome and the focus of the inquiry. This allows the coach and the client to establish clarity and focus with regard to the coaching conversations and the targeted behavioral change.

Table 4-2 Principles of Appreciative Inquiry

Principles of Appreciative Inquiry	
Positive Principle	The positive principle asserts that positive energy, thoughts, and emotions build the aspiration and motivation to move an individual toward behavioral change. Positivity expands awareness, increases resiliency, enhances creativity, and facilitates growth.
Constructionist Principle	The constructionist principle indicates that positivity stems from the conversations and interactions we have with other people. This principle stresses the importance of social and physical environments. Constructionism suggests that we create the reality in which we live.
Simultaneity Principle	The simultaneity principle suggests that positive questions and positive reflections simultaneously create positive conversations and interactions. The questions we ask and the manner in which we ask them are at the root of change.
Anticipatory Principle	The anticipatory principle proposes that when we anticipate a positive future, it becomes so. Likewise, it is the image of a positive future that guides positive behavior in the present. If we can see and believe in the change, then we can do it.
Poetic Principle	The poetic principle contends that "when we focus on problems, we get more problems. When we focus on possibilities, we get more possibilities." We will get more of what we focus on.

Moore & Tschannan-Moran (2010)

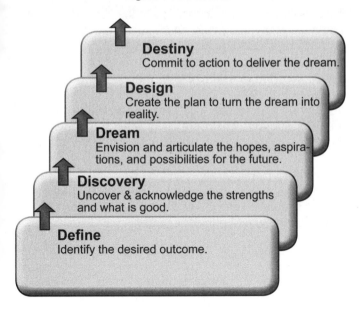

Figure 4-1 5-D Model of AI

The next step is the discovery phase during which the coach utilizes open-ended questions and reflections to uncover the client's strengths, past and present successes, and core values. The focus of the discovery phase is to identify and emphasize the positive and what is working or has worked well. This phase of the 5-D model may be the most important in terms of developing self-efficacy and creating positive energy for the upcoming phases.

The dream phase of the 5-D model is used to look into the future at what might be. The client is encouraged to visualize and articulate their hopes, aspirations, and the possibilities that could be. The client describes how things would be and how they will feel when they successfully execute the desired behavioral change. The coach may also ask the client to share their 'three wishes' for the future. The design phase creates the structure necessary to turn the dream into reality. Recalling the observations and insights from the discovery phase, the coach and the client collaborate to develop a specific plan to attain the desired behavioral change and ultimately the dream.

The final phase of the 5-D model is destiny (formerly referred to as the delivery phase). This phase of the model is arguably the most difficult since it represents implementation of the plan. Successful behavioral change requires commitment to action and personal responsibility. The coach offers support by keeping the spotlight on what is working and by checking in with the client regularly to ensure accountability to the plan.

The GROW Coaching Model

According to Whitmore (2009), the two key principles of effective coaching are building awareness and responsibility within the client. Building self-awareness enables the client to recognize and understand how their thoughts, emotions, and desires distort their own perception of reality (Whitmore, 2009). Raising self-awareness is essential since it facilitates self-discovery and improvement (Whitmore, 2009). Creating a sense of responsibility empowers the client to be accountable for their own thoughts and actions (Whitmore, 2009). This returns to the concept of autonomy previously noted. Individuals will demonstrate greater commitment to actions and behaviors that they have chosen, rather than those that they were advised or ordered to perform. Effective coaching always keeps the client in the driver's seat establishing their own pathway to success.

To guide the coaching conversation while building awareness and responsibility, Whitmore (2009) has developed the GROW model. **GROW** is an acronym that stands for goal, reality, options, and what will you do (Whitmore, 2009). Similar to other approaches to coaching, the GROW model is guided by effective questions and reflections.

The first step is to establish the goal. This stage is used to clarify the focus and direction for a coaching session as well as the short-term (action-oriented) and long-term (outcome-oriented) goals to be achieved. The coach may establish the focus of an interaction by asking questions such as:

- "What would be the most helpful topic of conversation for you during today's session?
- "What do you hope to accomplish during our meeting today?"

In addition, the coach will collaborate with the client to create SMART goals focused on desired outcomes. Later in the process (i.e., during the 'what will you do' phase) the client and the coach will work together to establish specific action-oriented goals.

Once the desired outcome has been identified, the next step is to explore the client's current reality, which is their perception of the current situation. A primary objective in this stage of the GROW model is to build a client's self-awareness of their thoughts and feelings, and how these cognitions impact their perception and behavior. The coach utilizes nonjudgmental, open-ended questions and reflective statements to create a picture of the client's situation, while expressing empathy and understanding. Questions asked during the reality stage may include:

- "What actions have you taken so far?"
- "What is currently going well for you?"
- "What has worked best in the past?"
- "What obstacles or barriers have you encountered?"
- "How do you feel about the present situation?"
- "If you were able to change anything in the present time, what might it be?"

Having established the direction and thoroughly explored the client's reality, the next step is to guide the client to generate a list of options. The options do not need to be the 'right' solutions, but they should originate from the client. As noted previously, a fundamental belief in coaching is that the individual inherently possesses the knowledge and ability to create their own pathway to change. The coach facilitates a brain-storming of options by tapping into the internal knowledge and creativity of the client. The coach may ask:

- "What options do you currently see?"
- "What steps have you considered taking toward this goal?"
- "What advice would you give to a friend in a similar situation?"
- "What else could you do?"

The final step in the GROW model is to create the plan for change. In other words, what will you do? In essence, the list of options generated by the client provides the foundation from which specific action-oriented goals may be created. To assist the client in developing their own plan for change, the coach may use questions such as:

- "Of the options you have shared with me, which sounds like the best place to start?"
- "Considering all of the options you have identified, where would you like to begin?"
- "Of these options, which do you feel most confident you can carry out?"

As the action plan is developed, it is also an opportunity for the coach to strengthen commitment and reinforce the client's personal responsibility to the desired outcome. The coach may use rating rulers such as, "On a scale of 0 to 10, rate your degree of certainty that you will carry out the actions you have identified?". The coach may follow-up with the question, "What makes your rating an 8 versus a 9 or 10?". In addition, the coach should discuss a follow-up plan to check progress as well as explore the need for support, which the client feels will ensure their success.

In conjunction with other strategies (e.g., motivational interviewing, appreciative inquiry), the GROW model provides a simple yet effective approach for coaches to guide their clients toward behavioral change.

Good to Know

The GROW Coaching Model

Goal - What is the desired outcome?
Reality - What is the current situation?
Options - What could you do?
What - What will you do?

Chapter Summary

As the prevalence of chronic disease continues to rise, countless individuals seek behavioral change to adopt and maintain healthy lifestyle behaviors such as regular physical activity and proper nutrition. Unfortunately, the expert-approach providing education, advice, and direction has been shown to be largely ineffective. A coach-approach offers an appealing alternative which has shown positive outcomes with regard to lasting behavioral change. This chapter has merely provided an introduction to the theoretical basis, philosophy, and selected models for coaching. Fitness professionals are encouraged to expand their knowledge through a review of the recommended readings provided at the end of this chapter. In addition, the artful skill of coaching must be developed through hands-on practice gained under the guidance of an experienced wellness coach.

Chapter References

Barkley, S. (2013). Counseling techniques for increasing physical activity participation. *ACSM's Certified News, 23*(1), 4-5,13.

Britt, E., Hudson, S.M., & Blampied, N.M. (2004). Motivational interviewing in health settings: A review. *Patient Education and Counseling, 53*(2), 147-155.

Bushe, G.R. (2011) Appreciative inquiry: Theory and critique. In Boje, D., Burnes, B. and Hassard, J. (eds.) *The Routledge Companion To Organizational Change* (pp. 87-103).Oxford, UK: Routledge.

Clifford, D., & Curtis, L. (2016). *Motivational Interviewing in Nutrition and Fitness.* New York, NY: The Guilford Press.

Frates, E.P., Moore, M.A., Lopez, C.N., & McMahon, G.T. (2011). Coaching for behavior change in physiatry. *American Journal of Physical Medicine & Rehabilitation, 90*(12), 1074-1082.

Gallwey, W.T. (2000). *The Inner Game of Work.* New York, NY: Random House.

Hargrove, R. (1995). *Masterful Coaching.* San Francisco, CA: Jossey-Bass.

Lundahl, B., & Burke, B.L. (2009). The effectiveness and applicability of motivational interviewing: A practice-friendly review of four meta-analyses. *Journal of Clinical Psychology, 65*(11), 1232-1245.

Martins, R.K., & McNeil, D.W. (2009). Review of motivational interviewing in promoting health behaviors. *Clinical Psychology Review, 29*(4), 283-293.

Miller, W.R., & Rollnick, S. (2012). *Motivational Interviewing: Helping People Change.* 3rd edition. New York: Guilford Press.

Moore, M., & Tschannan-Moran, B. (2010). *Coaching Psychology Manual.* Baltimore, MD: Lippincott, Williams & Wilkins.

Moore, S.M., & Charvat, J. (2007). Promoting health behavior change using appreciative inquiry: Moving from deficit models to affirmation models of care. *Family & Community Health, 30*(15), S64-S74.

Resnicow, K., DiIorio, C., Soet, J.E., Borrelli, B., Hecht, J., & Ernst, D. (2002). Motivational interviewing in health promotion: It sounds like something is changing. *Health Psychology, 21*(5), 444-451.

Resnicow, K., & McMaster, F. (2012). Motivational interviewing: Moving from why to how with autonomy support. *International Journal of Behavioral Nutrition and Physical Activity, 9*(19), 1-9.

Watkins, J.M., & Cooperrider, D. (2000). Appreciative inquiry: A transformative paradigm. *OD Practitioner, 32*(1), 6-12.

Whitmore, J. (2009). *Coaching for Performance: GROWing Human Potential and Purpose,* 4th edition. Boston, MA: Nicolas Brealey Publishing.

Whitworth, L., Kimsey-House, K., Kimsey-House, H., & Sandahl, P. (2007). *Co-Active Coaching: New Skills for Coaching People Toward Success in Work and Life,* 2nd edition. Boston, MA: Davies-Black.

Zeus, P., & Skiffington, S. (2000). *The Complete Guide to Coaching at Work.* Roseville, NSW, Australia: McGraw-Hill.

Recommended Reading

Arloski, M. (2009). *Wellness Coaching for Lasting Lifestyle Change,* 2nd edition. Duluth, MN: Whole Person Associates.

Clifford, D., & Curtis, L. (2016). *Motivational Interviewing in Nutrition and Fitness.* New York, NY: The Guilford Press.

Gavin, J., & Mcbrearty, M. (2013). *Lifestyle Wellness Coaching,* 2nd edition. Champaign, IL: Human Kinetics.

Miller, W.R., & Rollnick, S. (2012). *Motivational Interviewing: Helping People Change.* 3rd edition. New York: Guilford Press.

Moore, M., & Tschannan-Moran, B. (2010). *Coaching Psychology Manual.* Baltimore, MD: Lippincott, Williams & Wilkins.

Tice, L. (1997). *Personal Coaching for Results: How to Mentor and Inspire Others to Amazing Growth.* Nashville, TN: Thomas Nelson Publishers.

Whitmore, J. (2009). *Coaching for Performance: GROWing Human Potential and Purpose,* 4th edition. Boston, MA: Nicolas Brealey Publishing.

Chapter 4 Review Questions

1. Which of the following processes of motivational interviewing is characterized by discovering the client's motivation for change and eliciting change talk?
   A. Engaging
   B. Focusing
   C. Evoking
   D. Planning

2. The principle of appreciative inquiry that suggests positive questions and positive reflections directly result in positive conversations and interactions is known as the _____ Principle.
   A. Constructionist
   B. Simultaneity
   C. Positivity
   D. Anticipatory

3. Which of the following is the best example of an affirming statement?
   A. "Lately, you have really persevered over your busy schedule to keep up with your exercise program."
   B. "You are feeling overwhelmed by your busy schedule and frustrated that you have not been able to exercise."
   C. "If I hear you correctly, on one hand you would like to be exercising more frequently, but on the other hand you don't have the energy after a busy day at work."
   D. "I have been so busy lately that I have not had any time to exercise."

4. In which stage of the 5-D model of appreciative inquiry is a coach most likely to ask the question, "Looking into the future, what would your ideal state of health look like?"
   A. Define
   B. Discover
   C. Design
   D. Dream

5. Which of the following is representative of a coach-approach to behavioral change?
   A. Providing education and information to an individual
   B. Relying on the inherent knowledge and creativity of an individual
   C. Providing advice and direction to an individual
   D. Attempting to have all the answers to an individual's problem

6. Which of the following questions is a coach most likely to ask during the "R" stage of the GROW model?
   A. "How do you feel about your current level of physical activity?"
   B. "What would you tell a friend who was struggling to achieve a similar goal?"
   C. "On a scale of 0 to 10, how confident are you that you will complete that task next week?"
   D. "What alternatives are you considering?"

Answers to Review Questions on Page 384

Note: Review questions are intended to reinforce learning and comprehension of subject matter presented in the corresponding chapter. The review questions are not intended to be representative of actual certification exam questions in terms of style, content, or difficulty.

Section II

Exercise Science

The various subdisciplines of exercise science include human anatomy, kinesiology, biomechanics, and exercise physiology. Collectively, these areas provide the foundation for all fitness programming. A comprehensive understanding of the exercise sciences is necessary for the fitness professional to design scientifically-based, safe, and effective programs.

Chapter 5 provides an overview of human anatomy. Two major systems will be covered including the skeletal system and the muscular system. In addition, important terms and definitions will be introduced, enabling the fitness professional to easily locate and identify anatomic structures throughout the body.

Chapter 6 builds upon this knowledge of the musculoskeletal system by exploring the movement sciences of kinesiology and biomechanics. The information presented in this chapter will provide the fitness professional with a comprehensive understanding of human movement, which is necessary for the selection and implementation of appropriate exercises.

Chapter 7 presents the topics of exercise physiology, which include neuromuscular physiology, the bioenergetic systems, and cardiorespiratory physiology. In this chapter, the fitness professional gains insight of the complex biological processes that support exercise, the immediate physiologic responses to exercise, and the long-term adaptations to various types of activity.

5
Human Anatomy

Introduction
Anatomy is a biological science which studies the structure of the body. There are many interrelated systems that comprise the human body. This chapter will focus primarily on the skeletal and muscular systems. The anatomical structures of other systems such as the circulatory and respiratory systems will be included within chapter 7 – Exercise Physiology. Understanding the 'language' of anatomy will allow the fitness professional to understand, locate, and identify structures throughout the human body. Important terms and definitions will be introduced that will soon become a natural part of the fitness professional's vocabulary.

Location Terminology
The study of human anatomy begins with the **anatomical position**. In the anatomical position, the body is standing erect, the feet are positioned hip-width apart with the toes pointing forward, the arms are hanging to the sides of the body with palms of the hands facing forward, and the head and eyes are looking directly forward. Figure 5-1 illustrates the anatomical position. This position serves as the reference point from which structures of the body are named and located in relation to each other. With some exceptions, movements of the human body are also referenced using the anatomical position as the starting point.

The **median**, also known as the *midline*, divides the body into the right and left halves. Horizontally, a body part located closer to the midline of the body is said to be **medial**, whereas body parts located further away from the midline are referred to as **lateral**. Vertically, a body part located closer to the head is **superior** and a body part located away from the head (closer to the feet) is called **inferior**. When identifying the relative location of points on the extremities (arms and legs), the term **proximal** ('in close proximity to') refers to a point located closer to the attached end of a limb or the center of the body. **Distal** ('a greater distance from') refers to a point located further away from the attached end of a limb or the center of the body. For example, the wrist is located distal to the elbow; whereas, the elbow is located proximal to the wrist. The term **anterior** is used in reference to a body part on or toward the front of the body. **Posterior** refers to a body part on or toward the back of the body. For example, the quadriceps muscle group is on the anterior side of the leg and the hamstrings muscle group is located on the posterior aspect. Finally, **superficial** refers to a point or a body part located closer to (external) or on the surface of the body and **deep** refers to a point or a body part located further beneath (internal) another point or away from the surface of the body. For example, the rectus abdominis muscle is superficial in relation to the transverse abdominis muscle, which is deep. Table 5-1 provides a summary of anatomical location terminology.

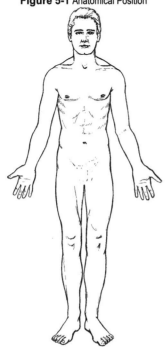

Figure 5-1 Anatomical Position

Table 5-1 Anatomical Location Terminology

Term	Definition
Medial	Closer to the midline or the middle of the body
Lateral	Away from the midline or the middle of the body
Superior	Closer to the head (away from the feet)
Inferior	Away from the head (closer to the feet)
Proximal	Closer to the attached end of a limb or the center of the body
Distal	Away from the attached end of a limb or the center of the body
Anterior	On or toward the front of the body
Posterior	On or toward the back of the body
Superficial	Closer to or on the surface of the body
Deep	Further beneath or away from the surface of the body

Planes of Motion

Human movement is often performed in three dimensions, each of which is identified in relation to a specific plane. A **plane** is a flat, level surface extending into space. Movement of the body is classified as occurring in three planes including sagittal, frontal, and transverse. The **sagittal plane** extends from the median dividing the body into the right and left sides. The **frontal plane** divides the body into the anterior (front) and posterior (back). The **transverse plane** (sometimes referred to as the horizontal plane) separates the body into the upper and lower segments. Figure 5-2 illustrates the three anatomical planes of motion. When a movement occurs in a specific plane of motion, it will "draw the plane" or run parallel to the plane of motion. For example, from the anatomical position, the movements of elbow flexion and extension occur in the sagittal plane in that the arm moves parallel to the designated plane, but does not cross it. Movements of the body and the corresponding planes of motion will be covered in greater detail in chapter 6.

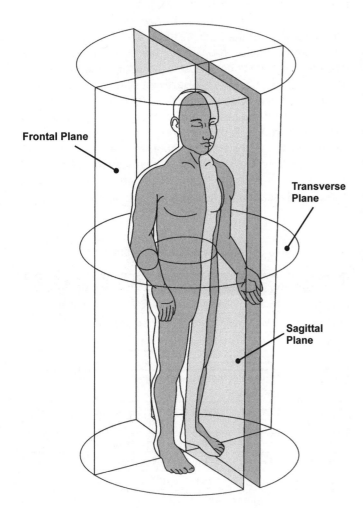

Figure 5-2 Planes of Motion

The Skeletal System

The skeletal system consists of 206 bones. Figures 5-3 (anterior) and 5-4 (posterior) illustrates the major bones of the human body. The skeletal system provides the supportive framework for the maintenance of posture. The bones and the corresponding joints also provide the lever system, which works in collaboration with the muscles to produce movement. In addition, the skeletal system also protects the vital organs (e.g., brain, heart, lungs), serves as a storage site for essential minerals (e.g., calcium, phosphorous), and within the bone marrow, produces blood cells (e.g., red blood cells, white blood cells, platelets).

The 206 bones of the human body are categorized into the axial skeleton and the appendicular skeleton. The **axial skeleton**, consisting of 80 bones, includes the skull, spinal column, sternum, and ribs. The axial skeleton provides the supportive axis for the body and protects the central nervous system (brain and spinal cord) and the organs within the ribcage. The **appendicular skeleton**, which consists of the remaining 126 bones, includes the upper and lower extremities (i.e., arms, legs) as well as the shoulder and pelvic girdles. The appendicular skeleton is largely responsible for movement and locomotion of the body.

> **Good to Know**
>
> Many terms are utilized to name and identify bony structures, many of which serve as muscle attachment points. Some of these include:
> **Fossa:** a broad shallow area of a bone
> **Tubercle:** a relatively small projection or bump on a bone
> **Process:** a relatively large or prominent bump on a bone
> **Foramen:** an opening or a hole in a bone through which nerves, blood vessels, and other structures may pass

The Vertebral Column

The **vertebral column** (also called the spinal column) consists of as many as 33 of the bones within the axial skeleton. Figure 5-5 illustrates the vertebral column. The individual bones of the vertebral column are called **vertebra**. The vertebral column is separated into three primary regions including the cervical, thoracic, and lumbar vertebrae. The **cervical** region of the spine consists of 7 vertebrae, which support the skull and neck. The first two cervical vertebrae, called the *atlas* (C1) and *axis* (C2), create a *pivotal joint,* which allows the head to rotate from side to side. The **thoracic** region, consisting of 12 vertebrae, articulates (connects) to the ribs providing support to the thorax. The 5 vertebrae of the **lumbar** region are the largest of the vertebral column. The size and strength of the lumbar vertebrae is necessary to

Figure 5-3 Anterior Skeletal Anatomy

Figure 5-4 Posterior Skeletal Anatomy

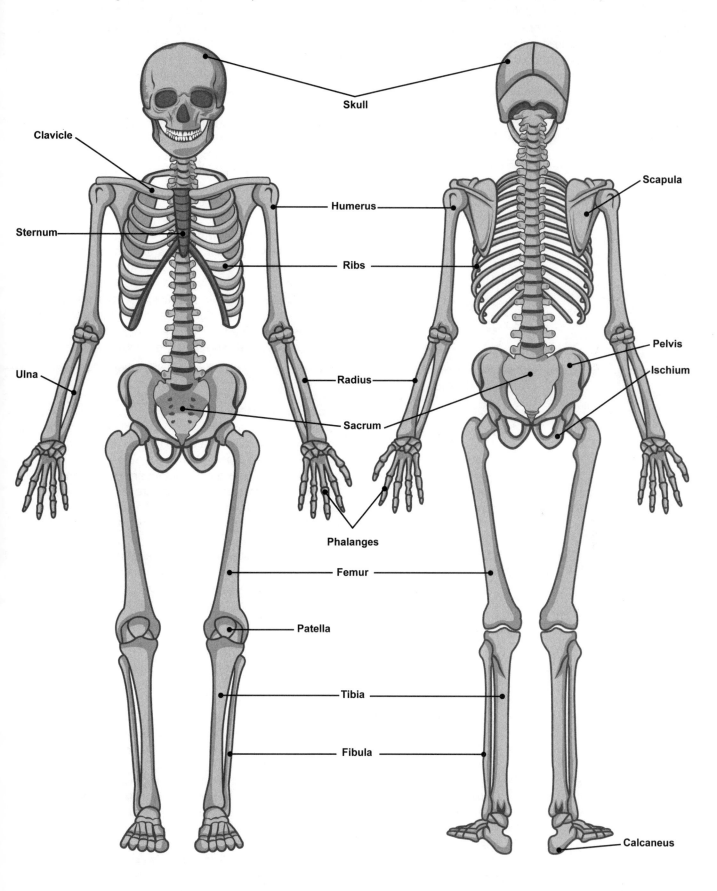

support a significant portion of the body's weight as well as sustain various forces applied to the body. The most inferior portion of the vertebral column includes the **sacrum**, a single bone consisting of 5 fused vertebrae, and the **coccyx** consisting of up to 4 fused vertebrae. The sacrum transmits body weight to the hip joints through articulations with the pelvic girdle. The coccyx is considered to be functionally insignificant.

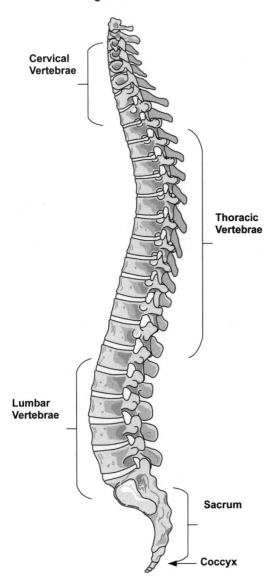

Figure 5-5 Vertebral Column

Bone Tissue
Skeletal tissue is comprised of a collagen matrix, which gives bone flexible properties, and mineral content (i.e., calcium and phosphates), which provides the stiffness. There are two types of bones: cortical bone and trabecular bone. *Cortical* or compact bone is found mainly in the long shafts of bones and accounts for about 80% of all bone tissue. *Trabecular* bone is a spongy tissue having a lattice or honeycomb structure, and is found in the vertebrae, pelvis, flat bones, and ends of long bones. Bone is a dynamic tissue with the ability to grow and self-repair.

The bone matrix consists of three types of bone cells including osteoclasts, osteoblasts, and osteocytes. *Osteoclasts* are bone-destroying cells that cause resorption of the bone tissue. *Osteoblasts* are bone-building cells that stimulate the formation of new bone tissue. *Osteocytes* are mature bone cells that help to regulate bone remodeling. Bone remodeling is a continuous process involving the coupled action of osteoclasts and osteoblasts, in which osteoclasts first resorb (i.e., breakdown) older bone and osteoblasts subsequently form and mineralize new bone.

During periods of growth and maturation, the activity of osteoblasts exceeds osteoclasts, so bones grow, increase mineral density, and gain strength. After peak bone mass is attained, typically in the mid-to-late twenties, the activity of osteoclasts gradually outpaces osteoblasts leading to loss of bone mineral density and strength. The rate of bone loss is influenced by genetics, hormonal factors, dietary habits, and other lifestyle behaviors. If the loss of bone mineral density becomes significant, it may result in osteopenia or osteoporosis.

Types of Bones
Bones may be classified as long, short, flat, and irregular. The bones of the limbs such as the humerus, radius, ulna, femur, tibia, fibula and phalanges (fingers and toes) are long bones, which provide rigid levers for movement. The carpals (wrist) and tarsals (ankle) are short bones having a relatively similar length and width. The short bones provide greater strength, but decreased movement capability. The flat bones, such as the ribs, sternum, scapula, and ilium, serve as broad sites for muscle attachment. The irregular bones come in a variety of shapes and generally do not fall in any of the other three categories. These bones include the ischium, pubis, the vertebrae, certain bones of the skull, and many others.

Types of Articulations
The junction between two adjacent bones is called an **articulation** or a *joint*. There are three major types of articulations in the body. These joint classifications include synarthrodial (also called *fibrous*), amphiarthrodial (also called *cartilaginous*), and diarthrodial (also called *synovial*) joints. The **synarthrodial joints** are held together by tough, fibrous connective tissue making them an *immovable joint* such as those found between suture joints of the skull. The **amphiarthrodial joints** are often connected by fibrocartilaginous tissue such as a pad or a disc like that found between two adjacent vertebrae. Amphiarthrodial articulations are often *slightly moveable* joints. **Diarthrodial joints** are *freely movable* joints and are the most common in the body. As noted above, these joints are also called *synovial joints* arising from their

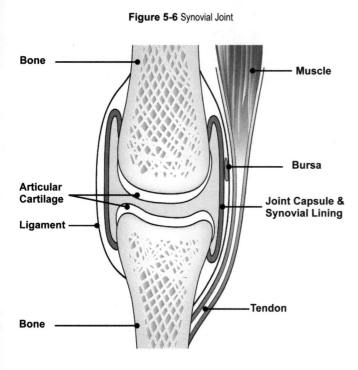

Figure 5-6 Synovial Joint

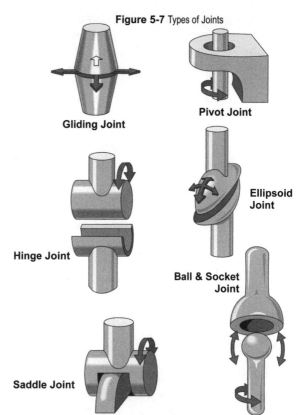

Figure 5-7 Types of Joints

characteristic synovial membrane and the synovial fluid which lubricates the joint. In addition, synovial joints also contain articular cartilage and a joint capsule. Examples of synovial joints within the human body include the shoulder, elbow, hip, and knee. Many joints also obtain passive support from **ligaments**, which connect bone to bone. Figure 5-6 illustrations the components of a synovial joint.

Joints can be further classified according to their structure and pattern of movement. Figure 5-7 provides illustrations of these various joint classifications. The shoulder and the hip are examples of **ball-and-socket** joints in which the ball-like head of one bone fits into the cup-shaped socket of another. This type of joint is the most freely moveable allowing for movement in all three planes of motion. A **hinge** joint consists of the c-shaped surface of one bone rotating or 'swinging' around the rounded surface of another. Hinge joints typically allow for movement in only one plane of motion (e.g., sagittal) such as that seen at the elbow and knee. A **saddle** joint consists of the convex surface of one bone sitting in the concave surface of another. Although this type of joint is limited in its ability to rotate, it does allow for movement in the remaining two planes of motion. The carpal-metacarpal joint of the thumb is one of the few examples of a saddle joint in the body. **Ellipsoid** joints are also referred to as *condyloid* joints. This joint configuration is best described as a reduced ball-and-socket-like joint in which the oval-shaped surface of one bone fits into the elongated or elliptical-shaped cavity of another. Examples of ellipsoid joints include the wrist as well as the metacarpophalangeal (finger) and metatarsophalangeal (toe) joints. A **pivot** joint allows for rotation and is characterized by the 'ring' of one bone fitting into or around the process of another. As noted earlier, the first two cervical vertebrae create a pivot joint under the base of the skull. The radius and ulna (radioulnar joint) at the elbow also create a pivot joint allowing supination and pronation of the forearm. Finally, the flat surfaces of two adjacent bones create a **gliding** joint allowing the bones to glide in all directions over each other. The joints between the carpals of the hands and the tarsals of the feet are gliding joints.

Vertebral Articulations

The vertebral column is extremely complex and subsequently has earned its own dedicated field of medicine (i.e., chiropractic). The vertebral column is a series of interconnected joints including numerous muscles, ligaments, and nerves. The vertebrae are bonded together by two long, thick ligaments (posterior longitudinal and anterior longitudinal ligaments), which span the length of the spinal column, as well as smaller ligaments that connect the multiple joints between adjacent vertebrae.

As noted earlier, the primary joint between two vertebrae is created by the fibrocartilaginous tissue called the **intervertebral disc** located between the bodies of the vertebrae. The outer portion of the disc is made of a several layers of tough connective tissue with obliquely-oriented fibers called the **annulus fibrosus**. The center of the disc contains a jelly-like substance called the **nucleus pulposus**. The intervertebral discs serve an important function to absorb shock and dissipate *ground reaction forces* that arise from movements such as walking, running, and jumping. The tough fibrous tissue of the discs is quite resilient to these forces; however, it is not uncommon for acute and chronic injuries to occur. The cumulative effects of chronic poor posture and/or faulty lifting techniques may contribute to premature degeneration and weakening of the disc, eventually resulting in injury (e.g., bulge or herniation).

Additional intervertebral joints are formed at the superior and inferior facets (also called articular processes) located on the two transverse processes of each vertebra. These *facet joints* function to limit motion and protect the spine from excessive rotation, lateral flexion, and *shearing* forces. These joints may also become injured as the result of spinal instability, poor body mechanics or lifting techniques, and unsafe exercises. An illustration of vertebrae and the significant structures can be seen in figure 5-8.

The Shoulder Complex

The shoulder complex is comprised of three bones including the humerus, scapula, and clavicle. These bones articulate to create several joints throughout the shoulder complex. The ball-and-socket joint between the head of the humerus and the glenoid fossa of the scapula is called the *glenohumeral joint*. The articulation between the acromion process of the scapula and the distal end of the clavicle is called the *acromioclavicular joint*. A musculotendinous joint, called the *scapulothoracic joint*, is also created between the anterior surface of the scapula and the posterior rib cage. The shoulder joint requires a balance of both mobility (i.e., ability to move through a normal and functional range of motion) and stability. Movements of the shoulder complex will be discussed in greater detail in chapter 6. Figures 5-9 (anterior view) and 5-10 (posterior view) illustrate the major anatomical structures of the shoulder complex.

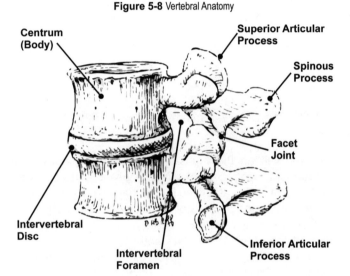

Figure 5-8 Vertebral Anatomy

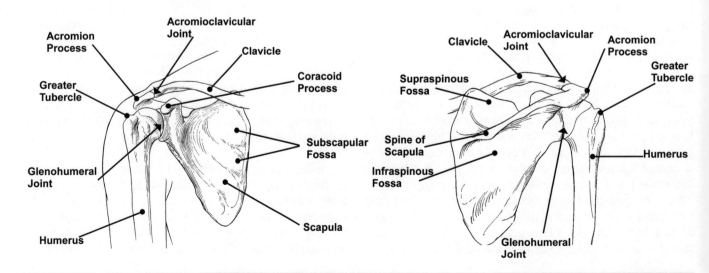

Figure 5-9 Shoulder Complex (Anterior View)

Figure 5-10 Shoulder Complex (Posterior View)

The Knee Joint

The knee, which functions as a hinge joint, is comprised primarily of the femur, tibia, and patella. The articulations of these bones create two joints. The joint between the tibia and the femur is called the *tibiofemoral joint*. The articulation between the patella and the femur is called the *patellofemoral joint*. The patella is the largest *sesamoid bone* in the body and functions to increase the biomechanical efficiency of the quadriceps to extend the knee and provides a protective shield for the tibiofemoral joint (Tecklenburg et al., 2006). Like the shoulder, the knee is a very complex joint and therefore vulnerable to dysfunction as well as injuries such as patellofemoral syndrome and anterior cruciate ligament (ACL) tears (see chapter 24). Figure 5-11 indicates the major structures of the knee joint.

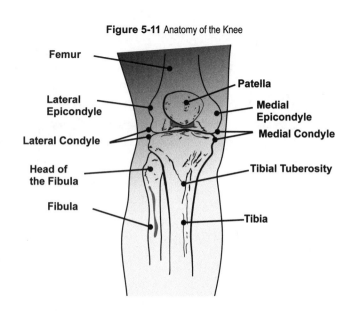

Figure 5-11 Anatomy of the Knee

The Muscular System

Muscles of various types throughout the body serve different purposes. There are three general classifications of muscle tissue: cardiac, smooth, and skeletal. The **cardiac muscle tissue**, comprising the walls of the heart, is extremely efficient, fatigue resistant, and well-adapted to maintain the ongoing pumping action of the heart. Cardiac muscle is involuntary since we do not maintain conscious control of this muscle action. Another type of involuntary muscle is **smooth muscle tissue**, which lines the internal organs (e.g., stomach, intestines) and blood vessel walls. Smooth muscle serves to move food through the digestive system and blood through the arteries and veins. The most abundant type of muscle in the human body is **skeletal muscle tissue**. Skeletal muscle is a voluntary muscle since it is largely under our conscious control to accelerate (create movement), decelerate (slow movement), and stabilize (prevent movement). Skeletal muscle is primarily comprised of water (~75%). Another approximately 20% of the muscle composition is contractile proteins and the remaining approximately 5% includes high-energy phosphates, key minerals, and energy sources needed for the production of force. The human body includes well over 600 different skeletal muscles. Figure 5-13 (anterior view) and figure 5-14 (posterior view) indicate the major muscles of the body. A more comprehensive review of skeletal muscle anatomy will be covered in conjunction with applied kinesiology in chapter 6.

Structure of Skeletal Muscle

Skeletal muscle consists of long, cylindrical cells called **muscle fibers**. Each muscle fiber is comprised of hundreds to thousands of smaller, threadlike structures called **myofibrils**. Myofibrils are arranged parallel to each other and span the length of the muscle fiber. A gelatin-like substance called the *sarcoplasm* surrounds the myofibrils. The *mitochondria*, known as the 'powerhouse' of a muscle fiber, are found within the sarcoplasm. The energy needed to support aerobic activity is produced in the mitochondria. The myofibrils are comprised of even smaller contractile proteins called **myofilaments**. The two myofilaments include **actin**, the thin filament, and **myosin**, the thick filament. Each myosin filament is surrounded by six actin filaments. These myofilaments overlap lengthwise to form a series of interconnected segments called sarcomeres. A **sarcomere** is often referred to as the smallest functional unit of the skeletal muscle fiber. The ends of each sarcomere are designated by a dense *Z-line*. When examined under magnification, the overlapping of actin and myosin creates light and dark bands which, along with the Z-lines, give the skeletal muscle a striped or striated appearance. For this reason, skeletal muscle is also referred to as *striated muscle*. Figure 5-12 depicts the structure of skeletal muscle.

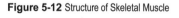

Figure 5-12 Structure of Skeletal Muscle

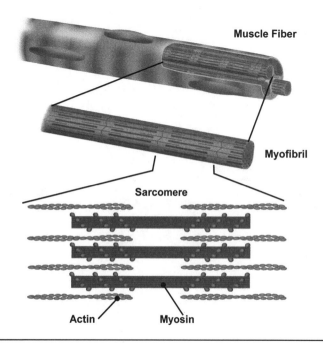

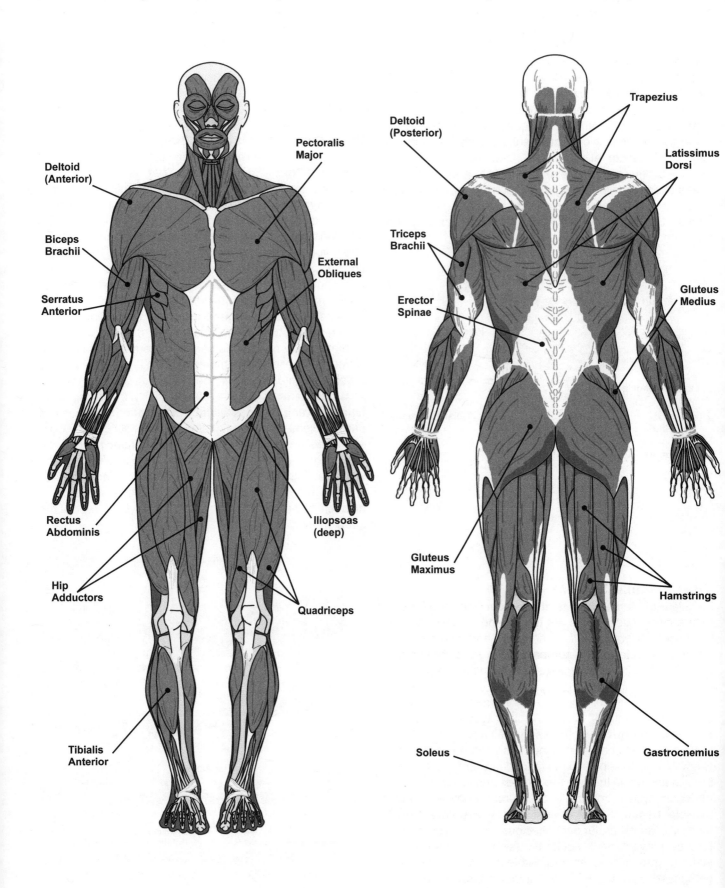

Figure 5-13 Anterior Muscle Anatomy

Figure 5-14 Posterior Muscle Anatomy

Sliding Filament Theory

The widely-accepted **sliding filament theory** has been suggested as an explanation regarding the process of skeletal muscle contraction (Huxley & Niedergerke, 1954; Huxley & Hanson, 1954; Huxley, 1974). The sliding filament theory states that when sufficiently stimulated (known as an *action potential*) by the central nervous system, the small heads extending from the myosin filaments bind with the actin filaments creating cross-bridges. The actin filaments are then pulled (called a *power stroke*), in a sliding fashion, across the myosin filament. This sliding action brings the Z-lines closer together, shortening the sarcomere without the myofilaments themselves changing length. As this sliding action occurs throughout the entire series of adjacent sarcomeres, the end result is a muscular contraction (shortening of the muscle). See figure 5-15 for a depiction of the sliding filament theory. Once the stimulus from the nervous system is removed, the cross-bridges between actin and myosin will release and the muscle will relax to its normal resting length. In order for this contraction to occur, the muscle must first receive an action potential from the central nervous system and an adequate supply of energy must be available within the muscle. Both of these topics will be discussed further in chapter 7.

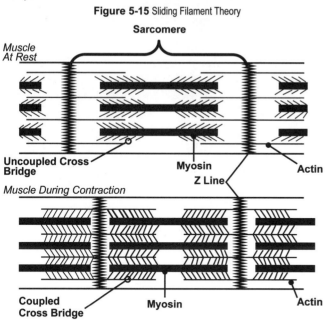

Figure 5-15 Sliding Filament Theory

Connective Tissue of Skeletal Muscle

The overall architecture of skeletal muscle resembles that of a telecommunications cable made up of bundles of wires. The outer most covering on the muscle itself is called the *fascia* which covers the next immediate layer surrounding the whole muscle called the *epimysium*. Within the muscle, groups of muscle fibers are bundled together into *fascicles* which are covered by a connective tissue called *perimysium*. The individual muscle fibers within the fascicle are surrounded by *endomysium*. Not only does each of the connective tissues play an important role in maintaining the structure of skeletal muscle, but they are also vital to the transmission of forces from the muscle to the bone causing movement. Each layer of connective tissue spans the length of the muscle, merging to from the **tendon** which attaches the muscle to the bone. Figure 5-16 illustrates the connective tissues within skeletal muscle. The musculotendinous attachment that is located at the more stable end of the body segment, which tends to be located *proximally*, is called the **origin**. The musculotendinous attachment that is located at the moving end of the body segment, which tends to be located *distally*, is called the **insertion**.

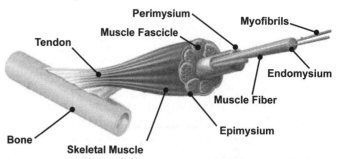

Figure 5-16 Muscle Structure and Connective Tissue

Types of Muscle Action

The skeletal muscles produce the force necessary to move the skeleton as well as external objects. There are two main types of muscle actions during which force is produced. During an **isometric** action, the muscle produces force, but there is no resulting movement and no change in the muscle length. This is also sometimes referred to as a *static contraction*. Using the arms to push outward against the frame of a doorway is an example of an isometric action. Although muscular force is exerted against the door frame, no movement occurs. The other type of muscle action is called **isotonic**. During isotonic actions, the muscle shortens and lengthens as force is generated against an external load. The shortening phase of an isotonic muscle action is called the **concentric phase**, during which the external load is lifted. The lengthening phase is known as the **eccentric phase**, during which the load is lowered. For example, when performing a dumbbell biceps curl (see figure 5-17), the concentric phase occurs as the dumbbell is lifted (i.e., elbow flexion) toward the shoulder and the eccentric phase occurs as the dumbbell is lowered (i.e., elbow extension) in a controlled manner back to the starting position. In this example, the biceps provides the muscular force during each phase of the exercise, to both lift the dumbbell and to control the descent as the dumbbell is lowered with each repetition. When identifying the concentric and eccentric phases of a resistance training exercise, a good rule of thumb is that the concentric phase always occurs as the weight is lifted away from the ground. During resistance training, the concentric and eccentric phases are sometimes referred to as the positive and negative phases, respectively.

Muscle Functions

Muscles may be called upon to play a variety of roles during resistance training, which is determined by the objective of the exercise. The muscle or group of muscles that are primarily responsible for a specific movement is called the **agonist**, also known as the *prime mover*. Other muscles that assist the agonist to perform a certain movement are known as the **synergists**. For example, when performing the seated leg curl exercise, the hamstrings muscle group acts as the agonist and the gastrocnemius muscle functions as a synergist, to collectively create flexion of the knee. The muscle or group of muscles that work in direct opposition to the agonist is called the **antagonist**. In the example above, the quadriceps muscle group functions as the antagonist since these muscles are responsible for the opposite joint movement (i.e., knee extension). Muscles can also function as **stabilizers**. In this role muscles support and stabilize a body segment or position, which enables the agonist muscles to effectively perform the desired movement. For example, during a dumbbell biceps curl, several muscles (e.g., rhomboids, trapezius, deltoid, rotator cuff) function to stabilize the shoulder complex and other muscles (rectus abdominis, obliques, erector spinae) function to stabilize the core and posture. Most muscles can take on any of the previously mentioned functions depending upon the desired movement. However, some muscles are used inherently more for stabilization such as the core muscles to stabilize the lumbo-pelvic-hip complex and the rotator cuff muscles to stabilize the shoulder (glenohumeral) joint.

Chapter Summary

The study of human anatomy includes a vast and complicated language of scientific terminology. This chapter has barely skimmed the surface of general anatomical concepts and the major structures of both the muscular and skeletal systems. It is crucial for fitness professionals to have practical knowledge of basic human anatomy in order to better understand the related exercise sciences and to safely implement effective exercise programs for their clients and participants.

Chapter References

Huxley, A.F., & Niedergerke, R. (1954). Structural changes in muscle during contraction: Interference microscopy of living muscle fibres. *Nature*, 173(4412), 971–973.

Huxley, A.F. (1974). Muscular contraction. *The Journal of Physiology*, 243(1), 1-43.

Huxley, H., & Hanson, J. (1954). Changes in the cross-striations of muscle during contraction and stretch and their structural interpretation. *Nature*, 173(4412), 973–976.

Tecklenburg, K., Dejour, D., Hoser, C., & Fink, C. (2006). Bony and cartilaginous anatomy of the patellofemoral joint. *Knee Surgery, Sports Traumatology, Arthroscopy*, 14(3), 235-240.

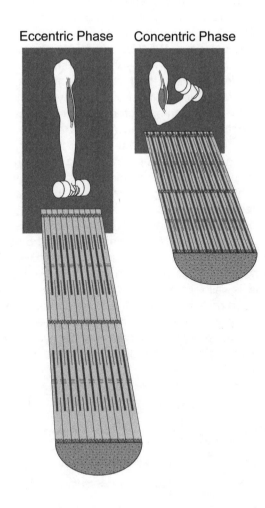

Figure 5-17 Isotonic Muscle Actions

Eccentric Phase   Concentric Phase

Chapter 5 Review Questions

1. The anatomical plane which divides the body into the anterior and posterior sides is called the
    A. sagittal plane.
    B. transverse plane.
    C. frontal plane.
    D. horizontal plane.

2. Which of the following anatomical structures is located distal to the elbow joint?
    A. Metacarpals
    B. Glenohumeral joint
    C. Acromion process
    D. Humerus

3. Which of the following bones is included within the axial skeleton?
    A. Scapula
    B. Tibia
    C. Sternum
    D. Ulna

4. The major muscle located on the posterior aspect of the tibia is called the _____.
    A. hamstrings
    B. triceps
    C. tibialis anterior
    D. gastrocnemius

5. According to the sliding filament theory, which of the following events occurs first during a muscular contraction?
    A. The actin filaments are pulled across the myosin filaments.
    B. An action potential is delivered by the central nervous system to the muscle.
    C. The actin and myosin filaments bind to create cross-bridges.
    D. The Z-lines move closer together causing the sarcomere to shorten.

6. Which of the following is considered to be a diarthrodial joint?
    A. The suture joints between the bones of the skull.
    B. The joint between the bodies of two adjacent vertebrae.
    C. The joint between the glenoid fossa of the scapula and the humerus.
    D. The joint between the sternum and a rib.

Answers to Review Questions on Page 384

Note: Review questions are intended to reinforce learning and comprehension of subject matter presented in the corresponding chapter. The review questions are not intended to be representative of actual certification exam questions in terms of style, content, or difficulty.

6
Applied Kinesiology & Biomechanics

Introduction
Kinesiology is derived from two Greek words, *kinēsis*, meaning movement or motion, and *ology*, meaning knowledge. Kinesiology is the study of human movement. **Biomechanics** is the study and the application of the principles of mechanics to the biological systems of the human body. This chapter will build upon the knowledge of human anatomy previously gained in chapter 5, to ensure the fitness professional has a practical understanding of the movement sciences. Collectively, this knowledge will prepare the fitness professional to select and implement appropriate exercises for their clients and participants.

Applied Kinesiology

Movement Terminology
The study of kinesiology begins with a review of fundamental movement terminology. Although there may be some exceptions, the *anatomical position* serves as the starting point from which movements are identified. The anatomical position also marks the 'neutral' point or zero degrees (0°) for joint *range of motion*.

A movement that decreases the relative joint angle or brings two body parts closer together is called **flexion**. The opposite movement is called **extension** during which the relative joint angle increases or two body segments move further apart and back toward the anatomical position. The term **hyperextension** is used to describe the continuation of extension that goes beyond the anatomical position. However, in fitness vocabulary, extension is often used when the movement occurs within the individual's normal and safe range of motion; whereas, hyperextension is reserved to define extension that continues beyond normal range of motion and is likely to cause injury. Flexion and extension movements typically occur in the sagittal plane of motion. At the ankle joint, the movements equivalent to flexion and extension are specially named, dorsiflexion and plantar flexion, respectively. **Dorsiflexion** refers to the movement which brings the top (dorsal surface) of the foot toward the anterior aspect of the lower leg. **Plantar flexion** refers to the movement of the bottom (plantar surface) of the foot toward the ground (e.g., pointing the toes away from the body).

The side-to-side movements that occur in the frontal plane are called abduction and adduction. Movement away from the midline of the body is called **abduction**. Movement toward the midline of the body is called **adduction**. However, when the arms move in this manner through the transverse plane, then **horizontal abduction** is used to describe movement parallel to the ground, away from the midline of the body, and **horizontal adduction** refers to movement parallel to the ground, toward the midline of the body. In this case, it is also acceptable to use the terms *horizontal extension* and *horizontal flexion*, respectively. At the ankle joint, specialized terms are used to describe the side-to-side motion of the foot in the frontal plane. **Inversion** refers to the movement of the bottom of the foot inward, toward the midline of the body. **Eversion** refers to the movement of the bottom of the foot outward, away from the midline of the body.

Movement around the long axis of a bone (e.g., humerus, femur) or a body segment (e.g., vertebral column) is called **rotation**. In the upper and lower extremities, a movement away from the body (outward) is called **external rotation** and a movement toward the body (inward) is called **internal rotation**. Rotational movements of the head and torso are simply called right rotation and left rotation, accordingly. The terms supination and pronation are used to specifically describe the rotational movements of the forearm (radioulnar joint). **Pronation** refers to the rotational movement turning the palms of the hands down or posteriorly and **supination** refers to the rotational movement turning the palms of the hands up or anteriorly, returning to the anatomical position. At the ankle and foot, supination is also used to describe the combined motions of inversion and dorsiflexion; whereas, pronation describes the combined motions of eversion and plantar flexion. Table 6-1 provides a summary of the movement terminology. Figures 6-1 to 6-9 provide illustrations of movements occurring at the major joints throughout the body.

Kinesiology of the Shoulder Complex and Upper Extremities
The shoulder complex, including the glenohumeral and scapulothoracic joints, requires a balance of stability and mobility for proper function. The stability of the glenohumeral joint is largely provided by the four rotator cuff muscles. This group of muscles can be remembered by the acronym **SITS**: *supraspinatus*, *infraspinatus*, *teres minor*, and *subscapularis*. All four of the rotator cuff muscles originate from various aspects of the scapula and insert on the proximal aspect of the humerus. The

Table 6-1 Movement Terminology

Term	Definition
Flexion	Decreasing the joint angle or bringing two body segments closer together
Extension	Returning from flexion to the anatomical position, increasing the joint angle, or moving two body segments further apart
Hyperextension	A continuation of extension beyond the anatomical position
Dorsiflexion	Movement bringing the top of the foot toward the anterior aspect of the lower leg
Plantar Flexion	Movement of the bottom of the foot away from the body or toward the ground
Abduction	Movement of a body part (e.g., arm or leg) away from the midline of the body.
Adduction	Movement of a body part (e.g., arm or leg) toward the midline of the body
Horizontal Abduction	Movement of a body part (i.e., arm) parallel to the ground away from the midline of the body
Horizontal Adduction	Movement of a body part (i.e., arm) parallel to the ground toward the midline of the body
Inversion	Movement of the bottom of the foot inward, toward the midline of the body
Eversion	Movement of the bottom of the foot outward, away from the midline of the body
Rotation	A movement (inward or outward) around the long axis of a bone or body segment
Pronation	Rotational movement turning the palms of the hand down or posteriorly
Supination	Rotational movement turning the palms of the hands up or anteriorly

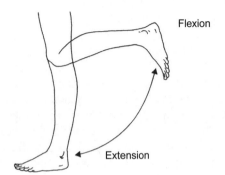

Figure 6-1 Movements of the Knee

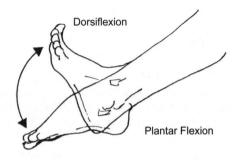

Figure 6-2 Movements of the Ankle

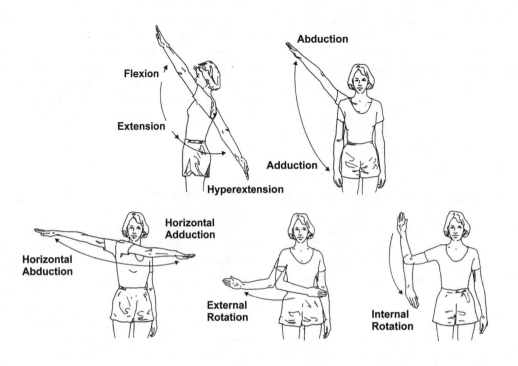

Figure 6-3 Movements of the Shoulder

56   Section II, Chapter 6 — Applied Kinesiology and Biomechanics

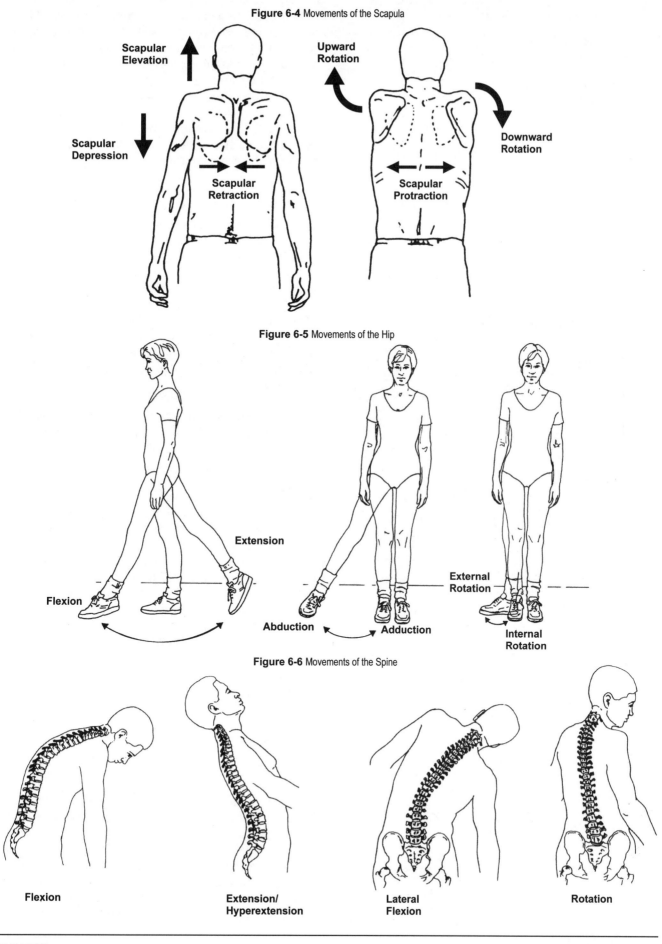

Figure 6-4 Movements of the Scapula

Figure 6-5 Movements of the Hip

Figure 6-6 Movements of the Spine

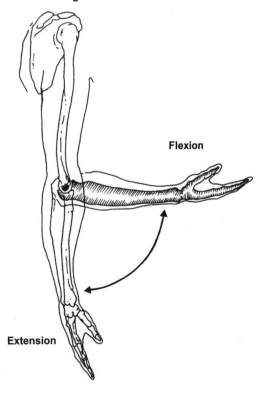

Figure 6-7 Movements of the Elbow

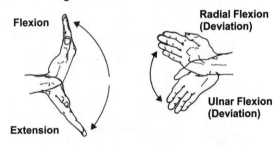

Figure 6-8 Movements of the Wrist

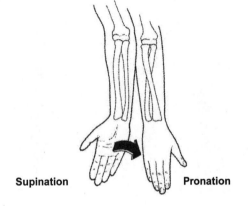

Figure 6-9 Movements of the Forearm

rotator cuff muscles provide stability to the shoulder joint and function as *force couples* to maintain congruency within the joint during rotation and other movements of the shoulder. In addition to providing glenohumeral stability, the rotator cuff muscles also produce various movements of the shoulder. The **supraspinatus** functions to assist with shoulder abduction, primarily during the first 30 degrees of movement. The **infraspinatus** and **teres minor** function as external rotators, and the **subscapularis** is an internal rotator of the shoulder (humerus).

The larger, superficial **deltoid** muscle produces several movements of the shoulder, corresponding to the three directions in which these muscle fibers are oriented. The **anterior deltoid** produces shoulder flexion, the **middle deltoid** produces shoulder abduction, and the **posterior deltoid** is responsible for shoulder horizontal abduction and to a lesser extent contributes to shoulder extension. The primary mover for both shoulder extension and shoulder adduction is the **latissimus dorsi,** which is assisted by the **teres major** acting as a synergist during both of these movements. Located on the anterior side of the upper body, the **pectoralis major** is primarily responsible for shoulder horizontal adduction.

The stability of the shoulder complex is also related to the scapulothoracic joint between the scapula and the posterior rib cage. Several muscles interact on this joint to ensure both stability as well as proper movement mechanics of the shoulder. The **serratus anterior** originates from the anterior and posterior ribs and inserts on the anterior surface of the scapula acting to stabilize, protract, and upwardly rotate the scapula. The **pectoralis minor** also attaches to the anterior ribs (3-5) and the coracoid process of the scapula. It acts to protract and also to depress the scapula. The **trapezius** is the large kite-shaped muscle of the upper back. Like the deltoid it has three components based on the directional orientation of the muscle fibers. The **upper trapezius** functions to elevate and upwardly rotate the scapula. The **lower trapezius** downwardly rotates and depresses the scapula. The **middle trapezius** retracts the scapula. Deep to the middle trapezius lies the **rhomboids**, which originates from the spinous processes of vertebrae C7-T5 and inserts on the medial (vertebral) border of the scapula. The rhomboids are responsible for scapular retraction as well as downward rotation. The **levator scapula** lies deep to the upper trapezius and, as the name implies, is responsible for scapular elevation.

The major muscles of the upper arm include the biceps brachii and the triceps brachii. The **biceps** is located on the anterior side of the humerus. The biceps has two heads, the long head, which originates from the glenoid fossa of the scapula, and the short head, which originates from the coracoid process of the scapula. The two heads of the biceps share a common insertion point on the proximal aspect of the radius (radial tuberosity). The primary function of the biceps is elbow flexion; however, given the attachment points on the scapula, the biceps can also assist the anterior deltoid during shoulder flexion. The **triceps** is located on the posterior aspect of the upper arm. As the name implies, the triceps has three heads including the long head, which originates from the inferior edge of the glenoid fossa of the scapula, and the medial (short) and lateral heads originating from posterior aspects of the humerus. The triceps inserts on the olecranon process of the ulna. The primary function of the triceps is elbow extension.

Tables 6-2 to 6-5 summarize the attachment points, functions and recommended exercises for the upper extremity muscles. Figures 6-10 to 6-19 provide illustrations of the muscles acting on the upper extremities.

Scapulohumeral Rhythm

The combined motion of shoulder abduction and upward rotation of the scapula, (occurring at the glenohumeral and scapulorthoracic joints, respectively) is known as *scapulohumeral rhythm* (Crosbie et al., 2008; Inman & Abbott, 1944; Kibler et al., 2012). After the initial 30 degrees of abduction, every 2 degrees of humeral movement (abduction) is matched by 1 degree of scapular movement (upward rotation) (Crosbie et al., 2008). Maintenance of normal scapulohumeral rhythm and appropriate shoulder function is the combined effort of many muscles providing both stability and mobility to the shoulder complex. Disruption of normal shoulder mechanics due to poor posture, muscle imbalance, and joint dysfunction can lead to chronic shoulder injuries such as *shoulder impingement syndrome* (DePalma & Johnson, 2003). Shoulder impingement syndrome will be addressed in greater detail in chapter 24.

Kinesiology of the Torso Muscles

The muscles of the torso are responsible for stabilization, support, and movement of the spine. Collectively, these muscles are often referred to as the 'core.' Since the torso has minimal skeletal support, it must rely on the strength and stability provided by the multiple layers of abdominal wall musculature. The deepest of these muscles is the transverse abdominis. The **transverse abdominis** is comprised of horizontally-oriented fibers and functions primarily to stabilize the pelvis and lumbar spine. The transverse abdominis also compresses the abdomen and assists during forced exhalation. The next layers of abdominal muscles include the **internal obliques** and **external obliques**. The internal and external obliques function synergistically to stabilize, rotate, and flex the spine. The fibers of the obliques are oriented diagonally with the internal oblique fibers running upward and medially; whereas, the external oblique fibers run downward and medially (similar to the direction of your fingers when reaching into your front pockets). The most superficial muscle of the anterior torso is the **rectus abdominis**. The fibers of the rectus abdominis run vertically from the pubic bone to the xiphoid process and the costal cartilage of the 5th through 7th ribs. The rectus abdominis is separated vertically by a midline band of connective tissue called the *linea alba* and horizontally by 3-4 fibrous bands called *tendinous inscriptions*. These bands of connective tissue create several bilateral muscle sections, which give rise to the slang term 'six-pack' in reference to the rectus abdominis. In addition to assisting with spinal stability, the rectus abdominis also functions to flex the spine and control the tilt of the pelvis.

The large muscle group on the posterior aspect of the torso, running vertically from the sacrum to the cervical spine is called the **erector spinae**. The erector spinae is comprised of three muscle subdivisions called the *longissimus*, *spinalis*, and the *iliocostalis*. These subdivisions are further divided into groups deriving their names from the respective attachment points along the spine. These groups include the *lumborum*, *thoracis*, *cervicis*, and *capitis* sections of the erector spinae muscle groups. Collectively, the erector spinae muscles are responsible for spinal extension. Deeper muscles, such as the *multifidi*, provide intrinsic support and stability to the spine. From the origin to the insertion, the multifidi muscles span between 1-3 vertebrae throughout the spinal column.

Table 6-6 summarizes the attachment points, functions and recommended exercises for the muscles of the torso. Figures 6-20 to 6-24 provide illustrations of the muscles acting on the torso.

Kinesiology of the Hips and Lower Extremities

The pelvic girdle is comprised of three paired bones called the *ilium*, *ischium*, and *pubis*. As the skeleton matures, these three bones unite to form a triangular suture joint within a cup-shaped socket called the *acetabulum*. The ball-shaped head of the femur articulates with the acetabulum to form the ball-and-socket joint of the hip. The vast majority of muscles acting on the hip originate from the pelvic girdle. One exception to this is the psoas muscles (major and minor), which originate from the transverse processes of T12-L5. The **psoas major** and **psoas minor** merge with the **iliacus** to insert on the lesser trochanter of the femur. Together, these three muscles are called the **iliopsoas** and are primarily responsible for flexion of the hip. Therefore, the iliopsoas muscle is also commonly referred to as the 'hip flexors.' Given the origin of the psoas, tightness or over-activity of these muscles can cause increased lordosis (arching) of the lumbar spine, particularly in the absence of adequate core strength to stabilize the spine and pelvis.

On the posterior aspect of the hip is the large **gluteus maximus** muscle, which works in opposition (antagonist) to the iliopsoas to perform hip extension. During hip

Table 6-2 Muscles of the Shoulder

Muscle	Origin	Insertion	Action (Primary in Bold)	Recommended Exercises
Deltoid	Lateral third of the clavicle, the acromion process, and the spine of scapula	Deltoid tuberosity of the humerus	Anterior: **Flexion** Middle: **Abduction** Posterior: **Horizontal abduction** and extension	Shoulder Press Lateral Raise (Scaption) Reverse Fly
Supraspinatus	Supraspinous fossa of the scapula	Greater tubercle of the humerus	**Shoulder abduction** and glenohumeral stabilization	First 30 degrees of lateral raise and scaption
Infraspinatus	Infraspinous fossa of the scapula	Greater tubercle of the humerus	**Shoulder external rotation**, glenohumeral stabilization	External rotation with cable or tubing, side-lying with dumbbell
Teres Minor	Axillary border of the scapula	Greater tubercle of the humerus	**Shoulder external rotation**, glenohumeral stabilization	External rotation with cable or tubing, side-lying with dumbbell
Subscapularis	Subscapular fossa of the scapula	Lesser tubercle of the humerus	**Shoulder internal rotation**, glenohumeral stabilization	Internal rotation with cable or tubing, side-lying with dumbbell
Teres Major	Dorsal surface of the inferior angle of scapula	Lesser tubercle of the humerus	**Shoulder adduction and extension**	Exercises similar to latissimus dorsi

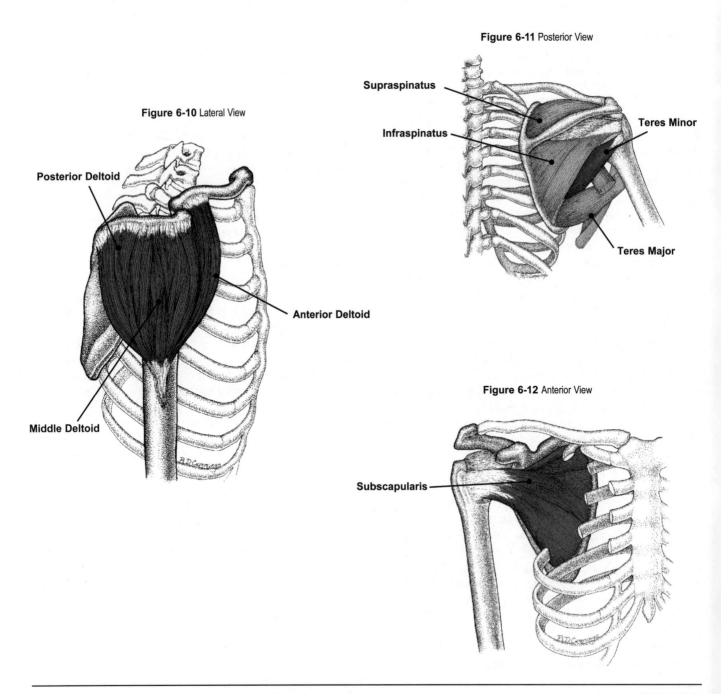

Figure 6-10 Lateral View

Figure 6-11 Posterior View

Figure 6-12 Anterior View

Table 6-3 Muscles of the Anterior Upper Body

Muscle	Origin	Insertion	Action (Primary in Bold)	Recommended Exercises
Pectoralis Major	Sternum, clavicle, costal cartilage of upper 6 ribs	Greater tubercle of the humerus lateral lip of intertubercular groove of the humerus	**Arm horizontal adduction**, shoulder flexion, shoulder internal rotation	Bench Press, Chest Press Machine, Chest Fly, Dumbbell Chest Press, Push-up
Pectoralis Minor	3rd through 5th ribs	Coracoid process of scapula	**Protracts scapula**, depresses scapula	"Push-up plus" Supine Scapular Protraction with Dumbbell
Serratus Anterior	Muscular digitations from the anterior and posterior aspect of the first 8-9 ribs	Length of the anterior surface of the vertebral border of the scapula	Protracts, stabilizes, and upwardly rotates the scapula	Any exercise involving movement or stabilization of the scapula

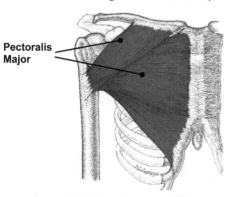

Figure 6-13 Pectoralis Major

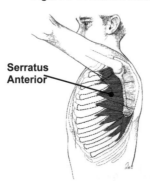

Figure 6-14 Serratus Anterior

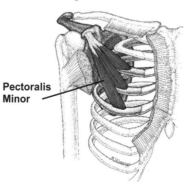

Figure 6-15 Pectoralis Minor

Table 6-4 Muscles of the Posterior Upper Body

Muscle	Origin	Insertion	Action (Primary in Bold)	Recommended Exercises
Trapezius	Occipital bone, ligamentum nuchae, and the spinous processes of C7 - T12	Acromion process and spine of scapula	Upper: Scapular elevation and upward rotation Middle: Scapular retraction Lower: Scapular depression and downward rotation	Seated Narrow Row, Seated Wide Row, Shrugs, Lat Pulldown, Assisted Pull-up, Shoulder Press
Levator Scapulae	Transverse processes of C1 – C4	Vertebral border of scapula superior to spine of scapula	**Scapular elevation**, neck lateral flexion	Shrugs
Rhomboids	Spinous processes of C7 – T5	Vertebral border of scapula	**Retraction** and downward rotation of the scapula	Seated Narrow Row, Seated Wide Row, Lat Pulldown, Assisted Pull-up
Latissimus Dorsi	Spinous processes of T7 - L5 and sacrum via the thoracolumbar fascia	Medial intertubercular groove of the humerus	**Shoulder extension**, **arm adduction**, arm internal rotation	Lat Pulldown, Assisted Pull-up, Straight Arm Pulldown, Dumbbell Row

Figure 6-16 Upper Back 1

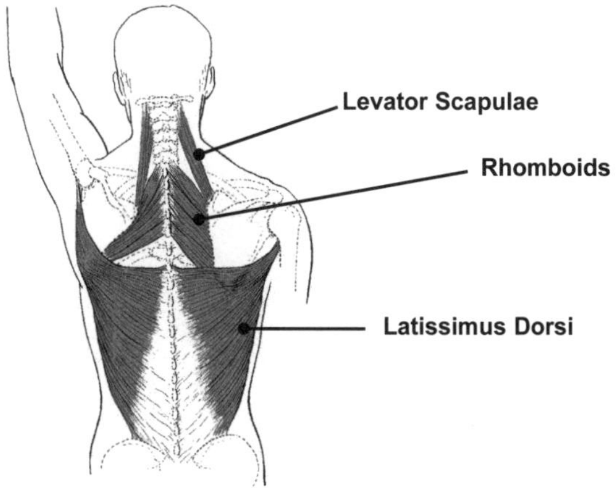

Figure 6-17 Upper Back 2

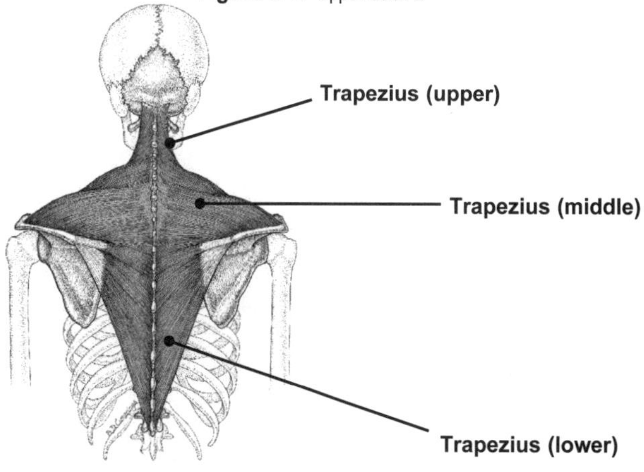

Figure 6-5 Muscles of the Upper Arm

Muscle	Origin	Insertion	Action (Primary in Bold)	Recommended Exercises
Biceps Brachii	Long Head: glenoid fossa of scapula Short Head: coracoid process of scapula	Radius	**Elbow Flexion**, shoulder flexion, forearm supination	Dumbbell Biceps Curl Preacher Curl Biceps Curl Machine Barbell Curl
Triceps Brachii	Medial and Lateral Heads: proximal humerus Long Head: infraglenoid tubercle of scapula	Olecranon process of the ulna	**Elbow Extension**, shoulder extension	Cable Triceps Pushdown Supine Dumbbell Extension French Press Dumbbell Triceps Kickback

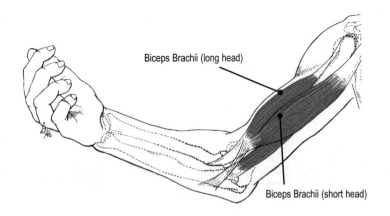

Figure 6-18 Biceps

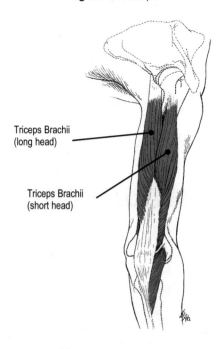

Figure 6-19 Triceps

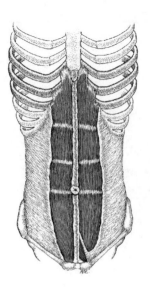

Figure 6-20 Rectus Abdominis

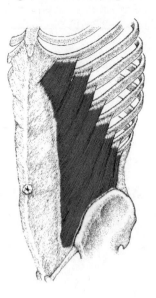

Figure 6-21 External Obliques

Table 6-6 Muscles of the Torso

Muscle	Origin	Insertion	Action (Primary in Bold)	Recommended Exercises
Rectus Abdominis	Pubis	Xiphoid process and the cartilage of the 5th through 7th ribs	Spinal Stabilization, **spinal flexion**	Abdominal Crunches, Stability Ball Crunches, Reverse Crunches, Abdominal Machine
External Obliques	Lower 8 ribs	Linea alba, pubis and iliac crest	**Spinal Stabilization**, spinal rotation, flexion, and lateral flexion	Oblique Crunches, Trunk Rotation, Stability Ball Crunches, Side-Lying Planks
Internal Obliques	Inguinal ligament, iliac crest and part of the thoracolumbar fascia	Lower 3 ribs, linea alba and Xiphoid process	**Spinal Stabilization**, spinal rotation, flexion, and lateral flexion	Oblique Crunches, Trunk Rotation, Stability Ball Crunches, Side-Lying Planks
Transverse Abdominis	Inguinal ligament, iliac crest, thoracolumbar fascia and cartilages of the lower 6 ribs	Xiphoid process, linea alba, inguinal ligament and pubis	**Spinal Stabilization**, abdominal compression	Any exercise involving stabilization or movement of the torso
Erector Spinae	At various sites along the spine, ribs, and iliac crest	At various sites on the skull, spine and ribs	**Spinal Extension**	Back Extension Machine, Prone Cobra, Roman Chair

Figure 6-22 Internal Obliques

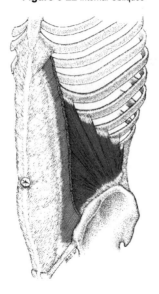

Figure 6-23 Transverse Abdominis

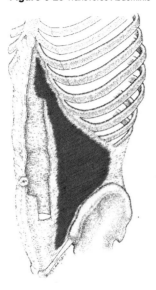

Figure 6-24 Erector Spinae

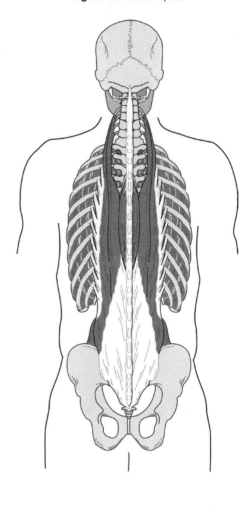

Table 6-7 Muscles of the Hip

Muscle	Origin	Insertion	Action (Primary in Bold)	Recommended Exercises
Tensor Fascia Latae	Anterior iliac crest and anterior superior iliac spine (ASIS)	Iliotibial band	Assists with hip flexion, abduction, and internal rotation	Standing Hip Abduction, Seated Hip Abduction, Side Leg Lift
Gluteus Maximus	Posterior pelvis along lower part of ilium, sacrum, and coccyx	Gluteal tuberosity of femur and iliotibial band	**Hip extension** and external rotation	Squat, Leg Press, Glute Kick-Back, Rotary Hip Machine
Gluteus Medius	Outer surface of the Ilium	Greater trochanter of femur	**Hip abduction**, internal rotation and pelvic stabilization in single leg stance	Standing Hip Abduction, Seated Hip Abduction, Side Leg Lift
Gluteus Minimus	Outer surface of the Ilium	Greater trochanter of femur	**Hip abduction** and internal rotation	Standing Hip Abduction, Seated Hip Abduction, Side Leg Lift
Iliopsoas: Psoas Major, Psoas Minor, Iliacus	Transverse processes of T12 – L5, and iliac crest	Lesser trochanter of the femur	**Hip flexion**, Trunk flexion	Supine Leg Lift, Rotary Hip Machine

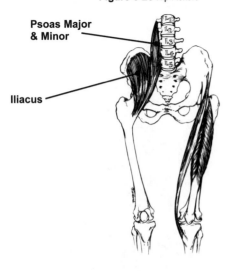

Figure 6-25 Hip Flexors

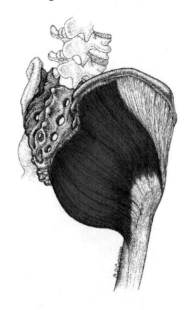

Figure 6-26 Gluteus Maximus

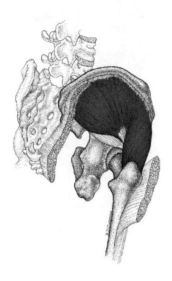

Figure 6-27 Gluteus Medius

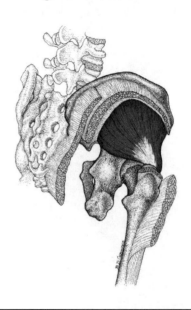

Figure 6-28 Gluetus Minimus

Table 6-8 Muscles of the Hip Adductors

Muscle	Origin	Insertion	Action (Primary in Bold)	Recommended Exercises
Adductor Magnus	Inferior ramus of the pubis and the ischium, and the ischial tuberosity	Most of the length of the linea aspera and the adductor tubercle of femur	**Hip adduction**, hip external rotation, and assists with hip extension	Seated Hip Adduction, Standing Hip Adduction, Squat, Leg Press
Adductor Longus	Crest of the symphysis pubis	Middle third of the linea aspera of the femur	**Hip adduction**, hip external rotation, and assists with hip flexion	Seated Hip Adduction, Standing Hip Adduction
Adductor Brevis	Inferior ramus of the pubis	Upper part of the linea aspera of the femur	**Hip adduction**, hip external rotation	Seated Hip Adduction, Standing Hip Adduction
Pectineus (not pictured)	Superior ramus of the pubis	Posterior surface of the femur inferior to the lesser trochanter	**Hip adduction**, hip flexion and external rotation	Seated Hip Adduction, Standing Hip Adduction
Gracilis (not pictured)	Symphysis pubis and the pubic arch	Medial surface of the tibia inferior to the condyle	**Hip adduction**, and assists with knee flexion	Seated Hip Adduction, Standing Hip Adduction

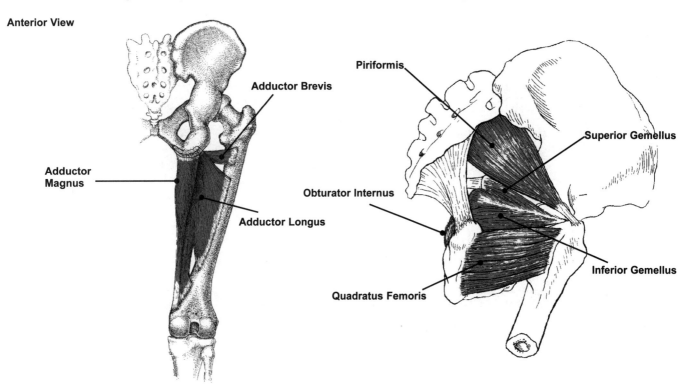

Figure 6-29 Hip Abductors

Anterior View

Figure 6-30 Deep Hip Rotators

Table 6-9 Muscles of the Deep Hip Rotators

Muscle	Origin	Insertion	Action (Primary in Bold)	Recommended Exercises
Piriformis	Anterior surface of sacrum	Superior border of the greater trochanter of femur	**Hip external rotation**, assists with hip extension and abduction	Seated Hip Abduction, Hip External Rotation with resistance tubing
Obturator Internus	Inner surface of obturator foramen and obturator membrane	Greater trochanter of femur	**Hip external rotation**	Hip External Rotation with resistance tubing
Superior Gemellus	Ischial spine	Greater trochanter of femur	**Hip external rotation**	Hip External Rotation with resistance tubing
Inferior Gemellus	Ischial tuberosity	Greater trochanter of femur	**Hip external rotation**	Hip External Rotation with resistance tubing
Obturator Externus (not pictured)	Outer surface of obturator foramen and obturator membrane	Trochanteric fossa of femur	**Hip external rotation**	Hip External Rotation with resistance tubing
Quadratus Femoris	Ischial tuberosity	Shaft of femur inferior to greater trochanter	**Hip external rotation**	Hip External Rotation with resistance tubing

Table 6-10 Muscles of the Upper Leg

Muscle	Origin	Insertion	Action (Primary in Bold)	Recommended Exercises
Quadriceps: Rectus Femoris Vatus Lateralis Vastus Intermedius Vastus Medialis	Rectus femoris originates on the anterior inferior iliac spine. Vastus muscles originate on the greater trochanter and proximal femur	Tibial tuberosity via the patellar tendon	**Knee extension**, (hip flexion – rectus femoris)	Squat, Smith Squat, Leg Press, Leg Extension, Stability Ball Squat, Lunge
Hamstrings: Biceps Femoris Semimebranosus Semitendonosus	Ischial tuberosity	Biceps femoris: lateral head of fibula and lateral condyle of tibia Semi's: Medial surface of proximal tibia	**Knee flexion, hip extension**	Seated Leg Curl, Prone Leg Curl, Stability Ball Leg Curl

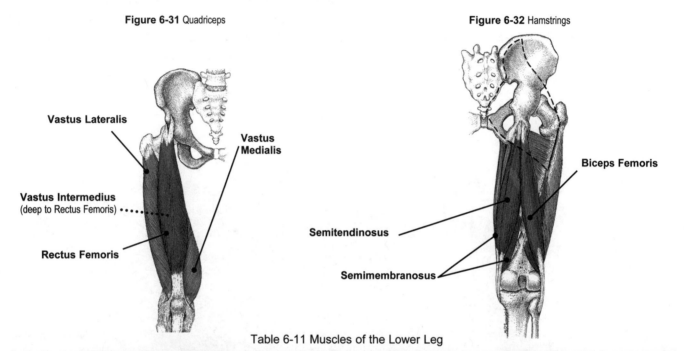

Figure 6-31 Quadriceps

Figure 6-32 Hamstrings

Table 6-11 Muscles of the Lower Leg

Muscle	Origin	Insertion	Action (Primary in Bold)	Recommended Exercises
Gastrocnemius	Lateral and medial (posterior) condyles of the femur	Calcaneus (via the Achilles tendon)	**Plantar flexion** and knee flexion	Standing Heel Raise, Calf Raise Machine
Soleus	Head of the fibula and inner border of the tibia	Calcaneus (via the Achilles tendon)	**Plantar flexion**	Seated Heel Raise, Standing Heel Raise
Tibialis Anterior	Shaft of the tibia and posterior surfaces of the interosseous membrane	First cuneiform (small bones in the feet) and base of the first metatarsal	**Dorsiflexion** and inversion of the foot	Standing Toe Raise, Dorsiflexion against tubing

Figure 6-33 Lower Leg - Posterior View

Figure 6-34 Lower Leg - Lateral View

Figure 6-35 Lower Leg - Anterior View

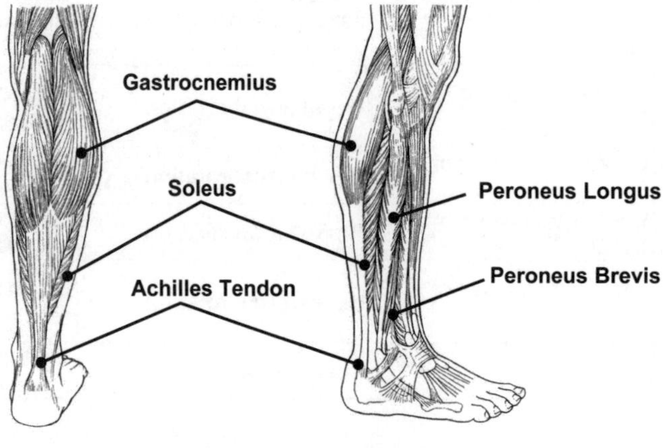

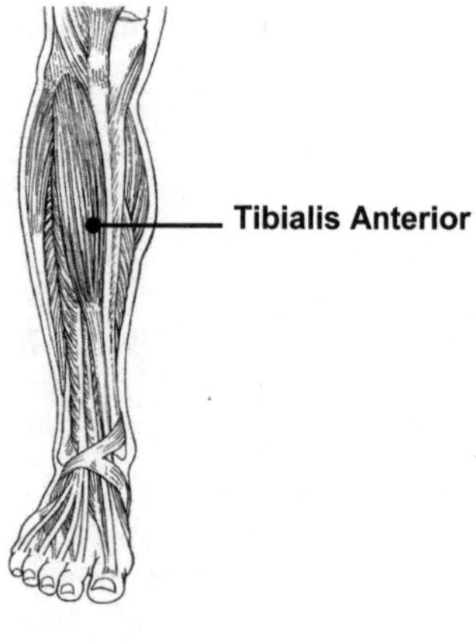

extension, the gluteus maximus is assisted by another large muscle group called the **hamstrings**. The hamstrings muscle group, which is comprised of three muscles including the **biceps femoris**, **semitendinosus**, and the **semimembranosus**, collectively inserts on the ischial tuberosity. As a two-joint muscle, the hamstrings insert on various aspects of the proximal tibia and fibula allowing them to also function as a primary knee flexor.

The antagonist muscle group to the hamstrings is the **quadriceps**, located on the anterior side of the femur. The primary function of the quadriceps is knee extension. The quadriceps is comprised of four muscles including the **rectus femoris**, **vastus lateralis**, **vastus intermedius**, and **vastus medialis**. One of these muscles, the rectus femoris, also crosses the hip joint, allowing it to act as a synergist to the iliopsoas during hip flexion.

The **gluteus medius** and **gluteus minimus** are located on the lateral aspect of the hip. Both muscles originate from the outer (lateral) surface of the ilium and insert on the greater trochanter of the femur. The gluteus medius and minimus are primarily responsible for hip abduction and can also assist with hip internal rotation. In addition, the gluteus medius is also an important muscle providing pelvic stabilization (i.e., prevent hip adduction and pelvic drop) during single leg stance. Also located on the lateral side of the hip, the **tensor fascia latae** assists with hip abduction, hip flexion and hip internal rotation.

The hip abductors are opposed by a large group of five muscles known as the hip adductors. The *hip adductors* include the **adductor magnus**, **adductor longus**, **adductor brevis**, **pectineus**, and **gracilis**. These muscles originate from various aspects of the pubic bone and the ischial tuberosity. Most of the hip adductor muscles insert at various points along the femur; however, the gracilis also spans the knee joint inserting on the medial tibia. Collectively, this large group of muscles functions as powerful hip adductors as the name implies.

Deep within the hip joint is a group of muscles known as the 'six deep lateral rotators.' This group of relatively small muscles is the primary mover for hip external rotation. The six deep lateral rotators include the *obturator internus, obturator externus, superior gemellus, inferior gemellus, quadratus femoris*, and perhaps the best known of the group, the **piriformis**.

Table 6-7 to 6-10 summarizes the attachment points, functions and recommended exercises for the muscles of the hip and upper leg. Figures 6-25 to 6-32 provide illustrations of the muscles acting on the hip and knee.

There are several muscles of the lower leg that act primarily on the ankle and foot. The ankle joint is comprised of the articulation between three bones: the distal end of both the tibia and fibula, and the proximal aspect of the talus. The ankle joint, also called the *talocrural joint*, functions like a hinge joint allowing the movements of plantar flexion and dorsiflexion. Two muscles are primarily responsible for ankle plantar flexion, the **gastrocnemius** and the **soleus**. These muscles merge together into a common insertion point on the calcaneus via the *Achilles tendon*. Since the gastrocnemius muscle spans the posterior aspect of the knee, attaching to the medial and lateral condyles of the femur, it can also function to assist the hamstrings during knee flexion. The primary muscle performing ankle dorsiflexion is the **tibialis anterior**, located on the anterior aspect of the lower leg. Another important joint of the ankle is the *subtalar joint* formed by the articulation between the talus and the calcaneus. The subtalar joint allows for inversion and eversion of the foot. The tibialis anterior also performs inversion of the foot along with the *tibialis posterior*. Two key muscles that contribute to foot eversion include the *peroneus longus* and *peroneus brevis*.

Table 6-11 summarizes the attachment points, functions and recommended exercises for the muscles of the lower leg. Figures 6-33 to 6-35 provide illustrations of the muscles acting on the ankle and foot.

Biomechanics

Newton's Laws of Motion

Sir Isaac Newton (1642-1727), was a physicist, mathematician, astronomer, and philosopher. He wrote the *Mathematical Principles of Natural Philosophy* first published in 1687. This body of work includes Newton's three laws of motion as well as the laws of universal gravitation. These laws explain how objects move on earth and describe the relationship between forces acting upon the body and the body's resulting motion. The three physical laws of motion have formed the basis for biomechanics.

Figure 6-36 Sir Isaac Newton

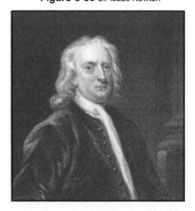

Newton's first law, **the law of inertia**, states that an object at rest will stay at rest and an object in motion will stay in motion (in the same direction and velocity) unless an external force acts upon the object. In other words, an object that is not in motion (i.e., velocity = zero) will remain stationary until a force causes it to move. The magnitude of this inertia is proportional to the mass of the object such that a heavier object (i.e., greater mass) will possess more inertia or reluctance to move. Likewise, an object in motion will continue moving at its current speed and in its current direction until a force (e.g., gravity) causes its velocity (e.g., speed and/or direction of movement) to change. **Inertia** is the reluctance of an object to change its current state of motion. When the forces acting upon an object are equal, the object is said to be in a state of **equilibrium**. An object that is not moving is in a state of *static equilibrium*. If an object is in motion without any change in velocity (i.e., no acceleration, deceleration, or change in direction), then the object is in a state of *dynamic equilibrium*.

Since many synovial joints rotate around an axis of rotation, many movements of the body are rotational in nature. Closely related to the law of inertia is the concept of rotational inertia. **Rotational inertia (RI)** refers to the reluctance of a body segment or object to rotate around an axis of rotation (e.g., joint). It is proportional to the mass of the object and the distance of the object's center of mass from the axis of rotation or joint. A heavier object located a greater distance from the axis of rotation possesses more rotational inertia (i.e., 'reluctance to rotate'). For example, a baseball bat has less rotational inertia when held by the barrel of the bat (thick end) rather than by the handle since the bat's center of mass is moved closer to the axis of rotation in this position. Likewise, when a little league coach instructs a player to "choke up on the bat," the strategy is to shift the bat's center of gravity closer to the body creating less rotational inertial and allowing the player to more easily swing the bat.

The **law of acceleration**, Newton's second law, states that a force applied to an object causes acceleration of the object in the direction of the force that is proportional to the force and inversely proportional to the mass of the object. The greater the external force acting upon an object, the more acceleration the force will generate. Similarly, a lighter object subjected to the same magnitude of force will experience greater acceleration. For example, when a soccer ball is kicked it will accelerate at a velocity proportional to the force of the kick and in the same direction as the net force vector at the time the foot strikes the ball. If a more powerful kick (i.e., greater force) is applied to the ball, then the ball will accelerate at a greater velocity. Conversely, kicking a medicine ball (not advised) with an identical force will result in less acceleration in comparison to the soccer ball. The law of acceleration can be expressed mathematically by the following equations:

Acceleration (a) = Force (f) / Mass (m)
or
Force (f) = Mass (m) x Acceleration (a)

Once an object has been set in motion by an external force it is said to have momentum. **Momentum (p)** is equal to the mass of the object multiplied by its velocity. (Note: in physics, momentum is abbreviated by the lower case "p" to avoid confusion with the abbreviation "m" used for mass.) Momentum can be simply stated as 'mass in motion'. A heavier object will possess more momentum than a lighter object when both are traveling at the same velocity. If two moving objects are of equal mass, the one traveling at the greater velocity will possess more momentum. An object at rest does not have momentum. Since momentum is the product of the object's mass and velocity, it is expressed by the equation:

Momentum (p) = Mass (m) x Velocity (v)

Again, since many joints in the human body move around an axis, this rotational motion creates angular momentum. **Angular momentum** is generated by the mass of the object, the distance of the object from the axis of rotation, and the speed (velocity) at which the object is moving. In other words, angular momentum is the product of the object's mass, the distance of the object from the axis of rotation, and the velocity of the object. For example, when performing a kettlebell swing, more angular momentum is generated by: (1) using a heavier kettlebell, (2) having longer arms, and/or (3) swinging the kettlebell faster. Subsequently, when a weight has more angular momentum it will require less muscular force (concentric) to keep the weight in motion; whereas, a weight moving more slowly (i.e., less angular momentum) requires additional muscular force to keep it in motion. Conversely, a weight possessing more angular momentum will actually require greater muscular forces (eccentric) of the antagonist muscles to decelerate the movement of the object as the end-range of motion is approached.

The third law of motion, the **law of action-reaction**, states that when an object applies a force to another object, there is an equal and opposite force applied back to the original object. In other words, for every action, there is an equal and opposite reaction. While swimming, the individual pushes/pulls the water backward resulting in an opposite reaction force which propels the body forward through the water. In another example, when walking, running, or jumping, the foot exerts force against the ground. The ground exerts an equal and opposite force back against the foot, which is subsequently dispersed throughout the body's kinetic chain (ankle, knee, hip, spine). This is referred to as ground reaction force. **Ground reaction forces (GRF)** may be a concern with regard to exercise and physical activity due to the potential for increased stress on the musculoskeletal system and increased risk for cumulative injuries. Ground reaction forces while walking can be 1–2 times body weight, 2–4+ times body weight when running or sprinting, and can reach 6–8 times body weight when jumping or landing from a jump (Kohrt et al., 2004; McNitt, 1993; Mero et al., 1992; Nilsson & Thorstensson, 1989). Ground reaction forces when running (or walking) will change according to several factors such as the velocity of locomotion, the weight of the individual, and the type of surface. Running at a higher velocity, an individual with greater body mass, and hard surfaces (e.g., concrete, asphalt) will all produce greater ground reaction forces and thus increase the risk of injury. Similarly, variables such as participant mass, height of jump, number of foot contacts, rate of progression, and type of surface should be carefully considered when incorporating *plyometric exercises* into clients' programs.

Biomechanics of Torque

Human movement occurs when a muscle contracts and pulls upon the bone by way of the musculotendinous attachment. Although during some exercises it appears as though muscles are pushing (e.g., chest press, shoulder press, leg press), technically these movements are the result of various muscle groups shortening (i.e., concentric contractions) to pull upon bones and body segments. The affected joint acts as the axis of rotation to allow movement in designated planes and ranges of motion. There are three types of lever systems which will be described below. Each lever system within the human body includes the following three components:

Fulcrum: the pivot point of the lever (i.e., axis of rotation).
Force: the action upon an object causing acceleration or deceleration.
Moment Arm: the perpendicular distance from the fulcrum to the applied force.

When a **force (f)** is applied to a point on a lever away from the axis of rotation, a rotational movement occurs. As defined above, the perpendicular distance from the axis of rotation at which the force is applied is called the **moment arm (MA)**. The degree to which this force causes the lever to rotate is called **torque (T)**. Defined quantitatively, torque is the magnitude of the force multiplied by the length of the moment arm.

Torque (T) = Force (f) x Moment Arm (MA)

In human movement science, we must consider both the external torque applied to the body and the internal torque generated by the musculoskeletal system. Subsequently, the internal force generated by the muscle(s) is termed the **muscle force**. The perpendicular distance from the axis of rotation to the application of the muscle force on the bone (i.e., muscle insertion) is called the **force arm**. The external force applied to the body (e.g., dumbbell, barbell, kettlebell, etc.) is called the **resistance force** and the perpendicular distance from the axis of rotation to the center mass of the resistance force is called the **resistance arm**. Figure 6-37 illustrates the components of the lever system that operate around the elbow joint during a dumbbell biceps curl.

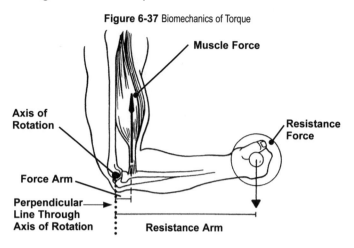

Figure 6-37 Biomechanics of Torque

The most obvious option to alter the magnitude of the external torque applied to a body segment is to change the resistance force. For example, selecting a heavier dumbbell will increase the external torque; whereas, a lighter dumbbell applies less torque. In some cases, the length of the resistance arm may also be adjusted. During a dumbbell lateral raise, bending the elbows slightly moves the dumbbell closer to the axis of rotation, decreasing the torque, and in effect making the same dumbbell feel as though it is lighter. Likewise, during standing hip abduction the leg strap may be repositioned closer to the knee than the ankle, making the resistance feel lighter. As the resistance force is applied more proximally on the lower leg, the length of the resistance arm is shortened, and the magnitude of the external torque applied through the hip joint is reduced.

The resistance force during free weight (e.g., dumbbell, barbell) exercises is the result of gravity pulling downward on the mass of the object. The line of this gravitational pull is always downward, toward the ground. Therefore, when moving a free weight through a full *range of motion*, as seen with the biceps curl in figure 6-37, the length of the resistance arm changes as the resistance force moves toward and away from the perpendicular line through the axis of rotation. In the position illustrated (~90° of elbow flexion) the dumbbell is at its greatest distance from this perpendicular line. Subsequently, the length of the resistance arm is greatest in this position creating the maximal external torque that will be experienced throughout the range of motion. In this position, often called the 'sticking point', the dumbbell feels the heaviest. At the upper and lower positions of this movement, the resistance arm is relatively shorter, the external torque is decreased, and the dumbbell feels lighter, although the actual mass of the dumbbell has not changed.

Types of Lever Systems

In a **first class lever**, the muscle force and the resistance force act on opposite sides of the fulcrum, similar to a see-saw. See figures 6-38 and 6-39. If the fulcrum is closer to the resistance force, then the muscle will be at a *mechanical advantage* (able to overcome the resistance force by generating less muscular force than the resistance force acting against it). However, if the fulcrum is closer to the muscle force, then the muscle will be at a *mechanical disadvantage* (requires greater muscular force in comparison to the resistance force).

Figure 6-38 First Class Lever

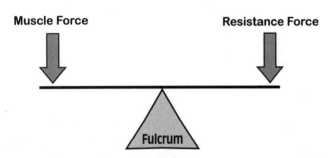

Figure 6-39 See-Saw

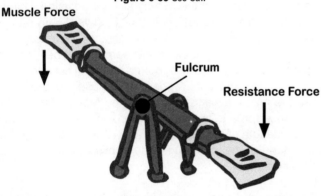

Figure 6-40 First Class Lever

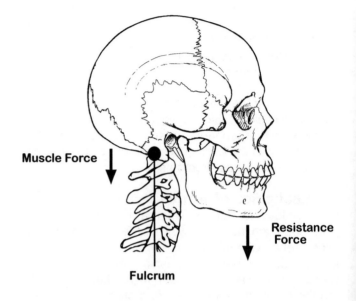

An example of a first class lever system in the body is the skull moving forward and backward (flexion/extension) on the first cervical vertebra (called the atlas). In this example, the atlas is the fulcrum, the weight of the head is the resistance force (being pulled by gravity into a position of cervical flexion) and the muscle force is applied at the base of the skull by cervical extensor muscles (semispinalis capitus, splenius capitus, upper trapezius) in order to prevent the head from falling forward. See figure 6-40.

In a **second class lever**, the muscle force and the resistance force act on the same side of the fulcrum so that the muscular force is applied through a longer arm than the opposing resistance force. See figure 6-41. Second class levers create a significant mechanical advantage allowing the muscle force to overcome substantial resistance forces as in the case of a wheelbarrow. See figure 6-42.

Figure 6-41 Second Class Lever

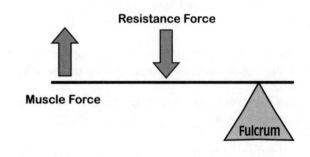

Figure 6-42 Wheelbarrow

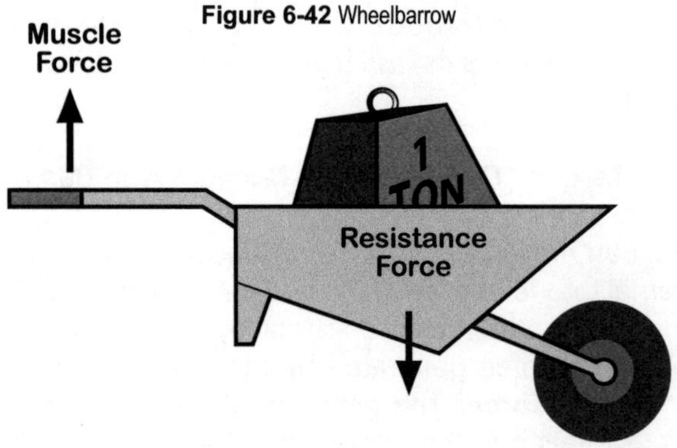

An example of a second class lever in the body is seen when elevating up on the balls of the feet (plantar flexion) where the ball of the foot (distal end of first metatarsal) is the axis of rotation, the weight of the body is the resistance force, and the gastrocnemius and soleus provide the muscular force. See figure 6-43. With the mechanical advantage offered by this lever system, the calf muscles are able to lift a significant amount of weight during plantar flexion of the ankle.

Figure 6-43 Second Class Lever Lower Leg

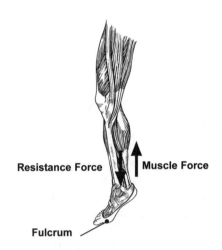

A **third class lever** system is characterized by the application of a muscle force and a resistance force on the same side of the axis of rotation, with the muscle force acting through a moment arm shorter than that of the resistance force. See figure 6-44. The majority of movements around synovial joints in the human body (e.g., shoulder, elbow, hip, knee) function as third class levers. The third class lever system creates a significant mechanical disadvantage that requires the muscle force to be substantially greater than the resistance force acting upon the body. Although not ideal for maximal force production to overcome external loads, third class levers do allow for a significant of range of motion (ROM) as well as speed of movement. As illustrated earlier, the biceps muscle acts through a third class lever system to overcome the resistance of a dumbbell during elbow flexion. Another example of a third class lever can be seen during the dumbbell lateral raise exercise. As the arm is abducted, the glenohumeral joint establishes the axis of rotation, the deltoid muscle provides the muscle force, and the pull of gravity against the dumbbell applies the resistance force. See figure 6-45.

Figure 6-44 Third Class Lever

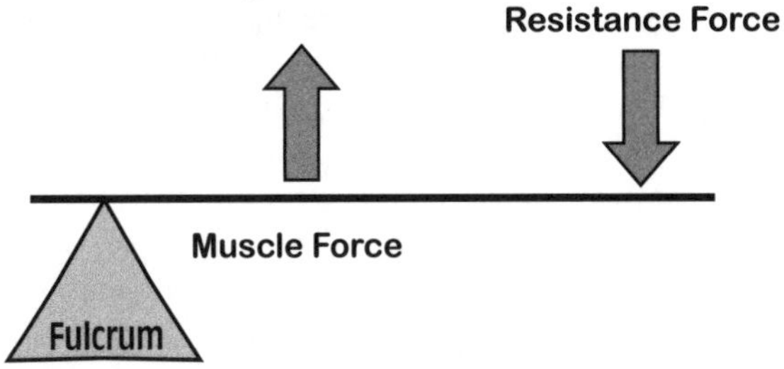

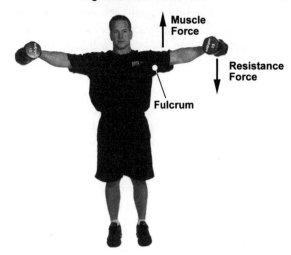

Figure 6-45 Third Class Lever

Types of Mechanical Stress

Various external forces acting against the body create loads upon the muscle, skeletal, and connective tissues. The direction and degree to which these loads change the shape of the tissue determines the type of mechanical stress (Knudson, 2007). **Normal stress** is applied by forces that are perpendicular to the object's cross-section. In other words, when a normal stress is applied through a bone, the load travels parallel to the long axis of the bone. Normal stress can be further classified according to the transformation in shape it tends to create. A **tensile stress** is the result of loading forces that act to pull apart, elongate, or stretch the tissue. An obvious example of this can be seen during a static stretch when force is applied to a body segment to lengthen the muscle tissue. **Compressive stress** has the opposite effect in that it causes the tissue to shorten, or as the name implies, to be compressed. For example, when running or jumping, as the foot contacts the ground, the load of the body weight and the counteracting ground reaction forces create a compressive stress on the tissue of the foot (and throughout the *kinetic chain*). Figures 6-46, 6-47, and 6-48 illustrate normal, tensile, and compressive stress, respectively.

Another type of mechanical stress is called **shear stress**, sometimes referred to a *shearing force*. This stress is characterized by forces and subsequent loads that are applied in opposite directions across the cross-section of

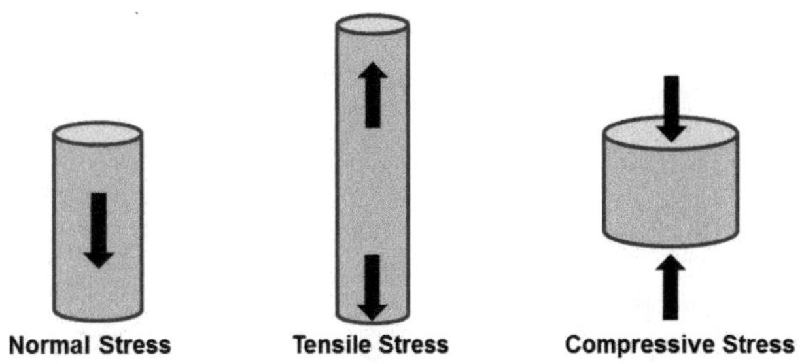

Figure 6-46 Normal   **Figure 6-47** Tensile   **Figure 6-48** Compressive

a bone, tissue, or a joint. See figure 6-49. Shear stress applied across a bone or joint may cause serious injury such as fractures or dislocations. For example, a football player receiving a hit to the lateral aspect of the lower leg may suffer a ligament (anterior cruciate and/or medial collateral) injury due to the shearing stress that is applied across the knee joint (between the femur and tibia). Shearing forces are also experienced across joints during many resistance training exercises. For example, it has been suggested that when performing the leg extension machine, potentially damaging shear forces are applied across the knee joint (tibiofemoral joint) during the last 10-30° of extension, approaching maximum shear force at full extension of the knee (Graham et al., 1993; Nisell et al., 1986; Reeves et al., 1998; Tagesson et al., 2009).

When several forces are acting upon a body segment, they may create a combined load such as torsion or bending (Knudson, 2007). **Torsion** occurs when two spiral forces act on a body segment in opposite directions. See figure 6-50. When performing a rotary torso machine, as one end of the spinal column is stabilized in the machine and the distant end of the trunk rotates in the opposite direction, torsion forces are placed upon the intervertebral discs. **Bending** occurs when forces create a compressive stress on one side of a body segment and a simultaneous tensile stress on the opposite side. See figure 6-51.

Figure 6-49 Shear Stress

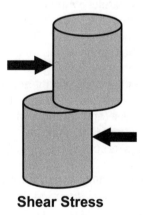

Shear Stress

Figure 6-50 Torsion

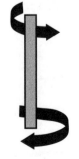

Figure 6-51 Bending

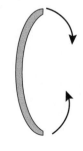

Deformation Responses to Force

When an object, or in this case a tissue of the body, changes shape in response to the loading of external forces, then the material is said to have the property of deformation. The property of *deformation* allows material to change shape in response to the applied loads instead of or in addition to changes in direction or velocity. All objects undergo some degree of deformation in response to applied forces; however, in some cases the degree of deformation may be so small that it cannot be detected or even measured. In these cases, the material or object is said to be *rigid*.

If an object or material remains permanently deformed after the external force is removed, then it is said to have the characteristic of **plastic deformation**. This can be observed when manipulating the shape of Play-doh® or a cooling piece of wax. If an object or material quickly returns to its original shape once the external force(s) are removed, such as a piece of resistance tubing, then it is said to have the characteristic of **elastic deformation**. Most soft tissues, such as muscle, tendons, and ligaments in the human body possess **viscoelastic** properties. This refers to the ability of soft tissues to exhibit properties of both solids and fluids, allowing them to deform in response to an external force and then to gradually return to the original form once the force is removed. For example, when a muscle is subjected to a passive static stretch, it gradually lengthens in response to the forces being applied to the musculotendinous unit. In a review article by Magnusson (1998), it was noted that a single static stretch held for 90 seconds produced viscoelastic stress relaxation in the muscle of approximately 30%, returning to baseline stiffness within 45-60 minutes from the termination of the stretch. Although less dramatic than these results, the viscoelastic properties of muscle can also be seen in a typical static stretch held for 15-30 seconds, returning to baseline stiffness a short period of time later.

Posture and the Kinetic Chain

Posture may be defined as the position of all body parts at any given time. Ideal posture aligns the body segments to minimize the muscular effort necessary to maintain the biomechanical efficiency of the neuromuscular and musculoskeletal systems. Although some individual variation exists, proper posture in the static standing position is typically defined with regard to the *plumb line*. See figure 6-52. Observed from a lateral view, the plumb line (sometimes referred to as the line of gravity) is the imaginary vertical line that drops from the ear through the center of the shoulder joint, along the lateral midline of the trunk, through the bodies of the lumbar vertebrae, slightly anterior to the sacroiliac joint, through the greater trochanter of the femur, anterior to the midline of the knee (posterior to the patella), and slightly anterior to the lateral malleolus of the ankle. This interconnected series of body segments and joints spanning from the feet superiorly to

Figure 6-52 Plumb Line

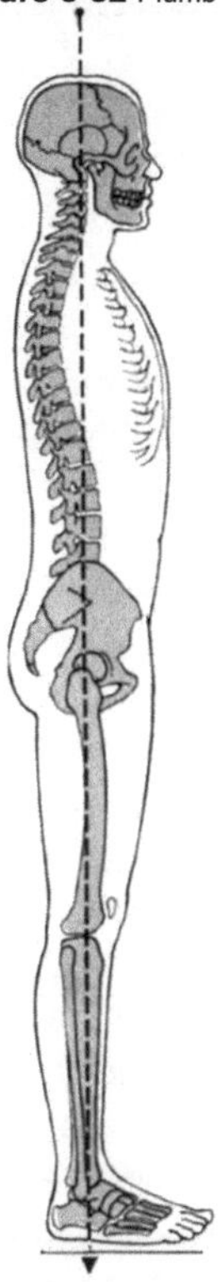

the head is often referred to as the **kinetic chain**. Although typically identified through skeletal landmarks and joints, the kinetic chain is actually an interrelated network that includes the skeletal system, the muscular system, and the nervous system.

Proper postural alignment is crucial for the maintenance of the structural integrity necessary to overcome the various forces and loads applied to the body. When in proper alignment, the muscles are able to maintain their ideal *length-tension relationship* allowing for optimal force production (Clark et al., 2008). In this position, the joints are also able to effectively absorb and distribute external forces thus reducing stress on the joints (Clark et al., 2008). When an individual is chronically placing their body in a position of misalignment, they are likely to develop muscle imbalances, inefficient or restricted movement patterns, and cumulative musculoskeletal injury.

Therefore, it is both important to screen and educate clients with regard to proper postural alignment. Fitness professionals should screen both static (stationary) and dynamic (moving) postural alignment to identify possible muscle weakness and tightness that may need to be addressed as a component of their overall fitness program. Although attempts have been made to place objective criteria in the postural screening protocol, there remains a high level of subjectivity in the fitness professional's ability to observe, interpret, and qualify postural alignment. Static and dynamic postural screening will be reviewed in greater detail in chapter 14.

Principles of Applied Biomechanics

Normal daily activities involve countless **functional** movements including squatting, bending, lifting, pushing, pulling, and rotating. Functional movements are often characterized by the integration of multiple joints performing in a multi-planar (sagittal, frontal, transverse), three-dimensional manner. Subsequently, additional principles of applied biomechanics must be considered and understood. Among these are the concepts of balance, stability, and coordination.

Balance refers to an individual's ability to control the position of his or her body against external forces. Balance is controlled and maintained by a number of sensory systems in the body including the eyes (visual system), inner ears (vestibular system), and the awareness of the body's position in relation to space and the external environment (proprioceptive system). The sensory information gathered by receptors within these various systems is communicated through the *afferent neurons* to the brain ensuring appropriate information and messages are sent back, via the *efferent neurons*, to the muscles controlling movement and maintaining balance.

Stability refers to the ease with which balance can be maintained. In most static positions and dynamic movements, stability is achieved by keeping the body's center of gravity within the base of support. The **center of gravity (COG)** is the theoretical point at which the body's mass is concentrated and balanced between all three planes of motion. Although the exact location varies among individuals based on their somatotype (i.e., ectomorph, endomorph, mesomorph) and stature (i.e., height), the center of gravity is generally located at the level of the sacrum. The **base of support** is established by the body's contact point(s) with the ground or other stable surface. When in the *anatomical position*, the base of support is created by the feet – generally positioned hip-width apart (in line with the anterior superior iliac spine of the pelvis) and the feet pointing directly forward. In the anatomical position, the most stable state is achieved when the center of gravity is directly in the center of the base of support. See figure 6-53.

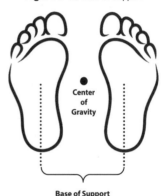

Figure 6-53 Base of Support

Stability is directly proportional to the distance of the center of gravity from the outer limits of the base of support; indirectly proportional to the height of the center of gravity from the ground or contact surface, and directly proportional to the weight of the body. Referring to figure 6-53, if the center of gravity is shifted to either the left or right or to the front or back (anterior/posterior), then the body becomes less stable. If the center of gravity is moved outside the limits of the base of support, then the loss of stability will result in the individual falling. A taller individual is also going to be inherently less stable since their center of gravity is located higher from the ground. In this situation it would be easier for a given external force to disrupt their stability as compared to a person of shorter stature. However, if the center of gravity is lowered by slightly bending the knees and hips, more stability will be created by lowering the center of gravity. An individual with greater body mass will also be inherently more stable since it would require a greater external force to disrupt the position of the body.

During some exercises and activities, the location of the center of gravity is changing relative to the base of support. For example, during a standing biceps curl, as the weight is lifted forward (via elbow flexion) the combined center of mass shifts forward in the sagittal plane to follow the movement of the dumbbell. If the weight of the dumbbell exceeds the individual's ability to stabilize the core muscles, then they may be tempted to compensate by leaning backward (extending the spine) in an effort to bring the center of gravity back toward the center of the base of support. In this exercise, many individuals may benefit from standing in a stride stance with one foot slightly in front of the other. Doing so will allow the exerciser to more easily maintain the forward-moving center of gravity within the base of support thus increasing stability.

Depending upon the goal of the participant and the exercise program, many exercises can be progressed or regressed to either decrease or increase stability, respectively. Figure 6-54 illustrates a sample pyramid of progressions that may be used for exercises performed in a standing position.

In some activities, the center of gravity is intentionally shifted outside the base of support. For example, when walking or running the center of gravity is shifted slightly anterior to the base causing forward momentum (controlled falling) that is caught by moving a foot forward to reestablish a new base of support.

The ability to integrate several movements of the body simultaneously and/or sequentially to achieve a complex task is called **coordination**. Examples of coordination include a player dribbling a basketball across a court while changing direction to avoid an opponent, or swinging a golf club to drive a ball down the fairway. Many fundamental movements and skills are learned early in life such as walking, jumping, and throwing. The field of *motor learning* is dedicated to the study of this subdiscipline of exercise science. When introduced to a new skill or movement, many individuals will benefit from having the activity broken down into small components (i.e., task analysis) to facilitate learning. As these new skills are learned, the movements will become more fluid and synchronized requiring less thought and in many cases less effort (e.g., muscle recruitment, energy expenditure). In resistance training, this effect is often called *neuromuscular education*, where the nervous system and muscular system are 'learning' how to coordinate the activation of appropriate muscles to produce smooth synchronized movement. Most of the early strength gains achieved through resistance training maybe be attributed to neuromuscular education.

Chapter Summary

This chapter introduced the fundamental concepts and principles related to the human movement sciences of kinesiology and biomechanics. The physical laws that govern movement are universal in nature, since they apply to all objects and bodies in the universe. Newton's laws, including inertia, acceleration, and action-reaction, cannot be broken as they are natural laws of motion. The lever systems established by the musculoskeletal system allow for movement and generation of force against external loads. Of these lever systems, the third class lever is the most common in the human body. In addition to creating movement, external forces may also result in deformation of tissue. The principles of applied biomechanics include balance, stability, and coordination, each of which is essential to functional movement and activities of daily living. Fitness professionals must develop a practical understanding of the kinesiological movement terminology as well as biomechanics in order to safely select and implement exercises for their clients.

Figure 6-54 Pyramid of Stability Progressions

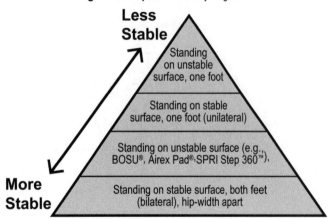

Chapter References

Clark, M.A., Lucett, S., & Corn, R.J. (2008). *NASM Essentials of Personal Fitness Training*, 3rd edition. Philadelphia, PA: Lippincott Williams & Wilkins.

Crosbie, J., Kilbreath, S.L., Hollmann, L., & York, S. (2008). Scapulohumeral rhythm and associated spinal motion. *Clinical Biomechanics*, 23(2), 184-192.

DePalma, M.J., & Johnson, E.W. (2003). Detecting and treating shoulder impingement syndrome. *The Physician and Sportsmedicine*, 31(7), 180-189.

Graham, V.L., Gehlsen, G.M., & Edwards, J.A. (1993). Electromyographic evaluation of closed and open kinetic chain knee rehabilitation exercises. *Journal of Athletic Training*, 28(1), 23-30.

Inman, V.T., & Abbott, L.C. (1944). Observations on the function of the shoulder joint. *The Journal of Bone and Joint Surgery (American)*, 26(1), 1-30.

Kibler, W.B., Sciascia, A., & Wilkes, T. (2012). Scapular dyskinesis and Its relation to shoulder injury. *Journal of the American Academy of Orthopaedic Surgeons*, 20(6), 364-372.

Kohrt, W.M., Bloomfield, S.A., Little, K.D., Nelson, M.E., and Yingling, V.R. (2004). American College of Sports Medicine Position Stand: Physical activity and bone health. *Medicine and Science in Sports and Exercise*, 36, 1985–1996.

Knudson, D. *Fundamentals of Biomechanics*, 2nd edition. (2007). New York, NY: Springer Publishing.

Magnusson, S.P. (1998). Passive properties of human skeletal muscles during stretch maneuvers. *Scandinavian Journal of Medicine & Science in Sports*, 8(2), 65-77.

McNitt-Gray, J.L.(1993). Kinetics of the lower extremities during drop landings from three heights. *Journal of Biomechanics*, 26(9), 1037–1046.

Mero, A., Komi, P.V., & Gregor, R.J. (1992). Biomechanics of sprint running: A review. *Sports Medicine*, 13(6), 376-392.

Nilsson J. & Thorstensson, A. (1989). Ground reaction forces at different speeds of human walking and running. *Acta Physiologica Scandinavica*, 136(2), 217-227.

Nisell, R., Németh, G., & Ohlsén, H. (1986). Joint forces in extension of the knee: Analysis of a mechanical model. *Acta Orthopaedica*, 57(1), 41-46.

Reeves, R.K., Laskowski, E.R., & Smith J. (1998). Weight training injuries: Part 1: Diagnosing and managing acute conditions. *The Physician and Sportsmedicine*, 26(2),67-83.

Tagesson, S., Öberg, B., & Kvist, J. (2009). Tibial translation and muscle activation during rehabilitation exercises 5 weeks after anterior cruciate ligament reconstruction. *Scandinavian Journal of Medicine & Science in Sports*, 20(1), 154-164.

Chapter 6 Review Questions

1. Which of the following joint actions occurs during the concentric phase of a dumbbell chest press?
    A. Elbow flexion
    B. Shoulder horizontal abduction
    C. Shoulder extension
    D. Elbow extension

2. The primary muscle during shoulder adduction is the _____.
    A. pectoralis major
    B. latissimus dorsi
    C. middle deltoid
    D. levator scapula

3. The joint action created by a concentric contraction of the iliopsoas muscle group is
    A. hip flexion.
    B. hip abduction.
    C. ankle dorsiflexion.
    D. hip extension.

4. In a third class lever system, the muscle force and the resistance force are located on the _____ side of the fulcrum with the muscle force _____ to/from the axis of rotation then the resistance force.
    A. same, further
    B. opposite, further
    C. opposite, closer
    D. same, closer

5. During the seated leg extension exercise, moving the leg pad closer to the ankle will _____ the external torque around the knee joint.
    A. decrease
    B. not affect
    C. increase
    D. eliminate

6. Your client is able to perform a body weight squat while maintaining appropriate postural and joint alignment. Which of the following is considered the next logical progression to increase the instability challenge for this client?
    A. Single leg squat on an inflatable balance disc
    B. Single leg squat on stable floor.
    C. Bilateral squat performed on a BOSU®
    D. Squat performed using Smith machine

Answers to Review Questions on Page 384
Note: Review questions are intended to reinforce learning and comprehension of subject matter presented in the corresponding chapter. The review questions are not intended to be representative of actual certification exam questions in terms of style, content, or difficulty.

7
Exercise Physiology

Introduction

Exercise physiology is the study of the physical, biological, and chemical responses that occur within the body's cells, tissues, organs, and systems in response to exercise. This chapter will provide an overview of three interrelated systems of the body including the cardiorespiratory system, the energy systems (bioenergetics), and the neuromuscular system. Fitness professionals must understand the acute responses and chronic adaptations experienced within each of these systems in response to exercise and physical activity.

The Cardiorespiratory System

The **cardiorespiratory system** is comprised of two interdependent systems including the *circulatory* (often called the *cardiovascular*) and the *respiratory* systems. The circulatory system consists of the heart, blood vessels, and the blood. The respiratory system is comprised of the upper respiratory tract including the nose, mouth, trachea (wind pipe), and bronchi; and the lower respiratory tract consisting of the lungs and its components including the bronchioles, alveolar ducts, and alveoli. See figure 7-1 illustrating the respiratory system. The primary function of the cardiorespiratory system is to deliver oxygen and nutrients to the tissues and cells of the body and to remove carbon dioxide and other waste products.

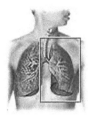
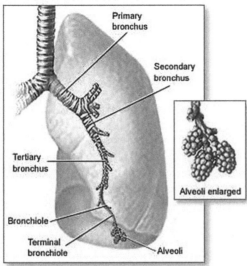

Figure 7-1 Respiratory System

The Heart

The **heart** is a four-chambered organ comprised of highly specialized cardiac muscle. The heart functions as a pump to move the blood through the network of blood vessels. The right side of the heart, known as the *pulmonary side*, is responsible for collecting and circulating deoxygenated (oxygen-depleted) blood to the lungs. The left side of the heart is known as the *systemic side* and is responsible for circulating oxygenated (oxygen-rich) blood to the organs, tissues, and cells of the body. The four chambers of the heart include two atria and two ventricles. The atria are smaller chambers which lie superior to the ventricles and collect blood. The ventricles are larger chambers which pump blood away from the heart. See figure 7-2 for an illustration of the heart anatomy.

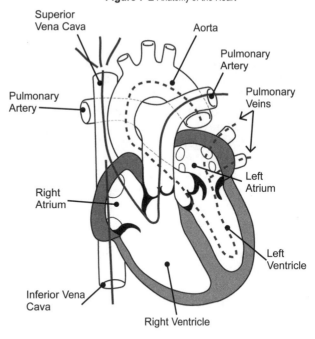

Figure 7-2 Anatomy of the Heart

Blood Vessels

Blood is transported throughout the body in a network of blood vessels. A blood vessel that carries oxygenated blood away from the heart and to the targeted tissue (e.g., organs, muscles, tissues, cells) is called an **artery**. The largest artery is the *aorta,* which transports blood pumped from the left ventricle. The oxygen-rich blood travels through the aorta to the thick-walled arteries and then to the smaller **arterioles**. Arterioles play a significant role during exercise to regulate blood flow to the appropriate tissues through *vasoconstriction* and *vasodilation*. During exercise, blood is diverted to the working skeletal muscles to deliver the oxygen necessary to support the activity, and to the skin to dissipate heat. The arterioles branch into an extensive network of microscopic blood vessels called the **capillaries**. The capillaries are so tiny that some of the blood cells are forced to flow through the vessel single file. The thinness of the capillary walls and the slow speed of the blood flow through these tiny vessels make them excellent for gas, nutrient, and waste exchange to and from the surrounding tissues. From the capillaries, the blood is collected by a network of **venules,** which move blood to the larger veins. The venules and veins return the deoxygenated blood back to the heart. The walls of many veins contain one-way valves that help to maintain venous blood return to the heart by preventing back flow under the relatively low pressures found in the venous blood vessels. The large veins returning blood to the heart from the upper and lower body are called the *superior vena cava* and the *inferior vena cava*, respectively.

The Pathway of Blood Flow

The pathway of blood flow through the heart begins with venous (deoxygenated) blood returning from the peripheral aspects of the body, which enters the right artrium by way of the superior and inferior vena cava. The deoxygenated blood moves from the right atrium into the right ventricle (via the right atrioventricular valve, also called the tricuspid valve). From the right ventricle, the blood is pumped to the lungs via the pulmonary arteries. In the lungs, the blood is re-oxygenated as it picks up oxygen from the ambient air and releases carbon dioxide (via capillaries surrounding the alveoli in the lungs). The now oxygenated blood returns to the heart via the pulmonary veins and enters the left atrium of the heart. Oxygenated blood moves from the left atrium to the left ventricle (via the left atrioventricular valve, also called the bicuspid or mitral valve). The blood is then pumped from the left ventricle through the aorta and the arterial network of blood vessels to the targeted tissues (e.g., skeletal muscles) and organs in the body. Oxygen and nutrients are delivered to the targeted tissue, carbon dioxide and waste products are removed, the blood returns to the heart via the venous blood vessels, and the process starts over.

Heart Rate

Familiar to most, **heart rate (HR)** is the number of beats or cardiac cycles of the heart per minute. The number of heart beats at rest is called the **resting heart rate (HR$_{rest}$ or RHR)**. The normal resting heart rate range for an adult is between 60 and 90 beats per minute. Generally speaking, those with a well-conditioned cardiorespiratory system will have a lower resting heart rate, even below this normal range. The decrease in resting heart rate seen with regular cardiorespiratory exercise is the result of increased *parasympathetic nervous system* tone (i.e., 'rest and digest' response) as well as the increased stroke volume to more efficiently fulfill the needed cardiac output and oxygen demands at rest (discussed in more detail later). In other cases, a low resting heart rate may be indicative of those taking prescription medications, which slow the heart rate (e.g., blood pressure medication such as β-blockers), or individuals with certain types of heart disease. A resting heart rate less than 60 beats per minute is called *bradycardia*. A resting heart rate greater than 100 beats per minute is called *tachycardia,* which may suggest a serious illness or disease.

During exercise, heart rate increases in proportion to the exercise intensity. The increase in heart rate is modulated by the sympathetic nervous system (i.e., 'fight or flight' response), which adjusts to meet the increasing metabolic and oxidative demands placed on the body during exercise. The relatively constant heart rate sustained at a given exercise intensity is called the *steady state heart rate*. As regular cardiorespiratory exercise is performed, the *submaximal heart rate* at any given level of exercise will be lower in comparison to pre-training levels. This decreased submaximal heart rate response is an expected adaptation, which reflects improving cardiorespiratory efficiency during exercise.

The highest attainable heart rate during exhaustive exercise is called the **maximum heart rate (HR$_{max}$ or MHR)**. Many factors, such as age and genetics, will influence maximum heart rate; however, it generally is not sensitive to cardiorespiratory exercise and should not be expected to change with training. There are some obvious safety concerns associated with pushing an individual to maximal exertion in order to determine their maximum heart rate. Therefore, several equations have been developed to predict HR$_{max}$, most of which are based on age. These equations will be discussed further in chapter 17.

Stroke Volume

The amount of blood pumped by the left ventricle of the heart with each beat is called the **stroke volume (SV)**. A typical stroke volume for an adult at rest is 60-100 milliliters per beat (mL/b). During cardiorespiratory exercise, stroke volume increases in response to the increasing need for oxygen. Whereas heart rate increases linearly up to maximum values in response to exercise intensity, in low-to-moderately trained individuals, stroke volume increases up to approximately 40-50% of their maximal capacity and then plateaus. However, it has been suggested that the stroke volume of highly trained endurance athletes continues to increase up to maximum effort (Zhou et al., 2001). One of the primary adaptations to regular cardiorespiratory exercise is an increase in left ventricular stroke volume at rest, during submaximal exercise, and at maximal exertion. The increase in stroke volume allows the heart to beat less frequently (reduced heart rate), yet still supply the necessary volume of blood to the body and the muscles.

Cardiac Output

The product of the heart rate and the stroke volume represents the **cardiac output (Q)**, the volume of blood pumped by the heart per minute.

Cardiac Output (Q) = Heart Rate (HR) x Stroke Volume (SV)

At rest, an adult's cardiac output is approximately 5 liters of blood per minute (L/min). Since heart rate and stroke volume both increase in response to exercise intensity, cardiac output also rises in proportion to exercise. At maximal exercise, the average cardiac output may increase to 20-25 L/min. For highly conditioned endurance athletes, the maximum attainable cardiac output may be up to 30-40 L/min. Greatly influenced by stroke volume, cardiac output also increases at maximal levels in response to regular cardiorespiratory exercise. In addition, after a period of training, an individual is also able to attain a higher absolute workload, which requires more oxygen when exercising at maximal capacity. However, cardiac output at rest and during any given submaximal intensity, may be unchanged after training since improvements in stroke volume and reductions in heart rate largely off-set each other to obtain a similar cardiac output compared to baseline. Furthermore, peripheral adaptations occurring within the skeletal muscles (i.e., adaptations influencing oxygen extraction, see page 82) allow more oxygen to be removed from the circulating blood, thereby reducing the need for a greater volume of blood to be delivered to the muscles.

Blood Pressure

The measurement of pressure exerted by the circulating blood against the walls of the arterial blood vessels is called **blood pressure (BP)**. The unit of measurement for blood pressure is millimeters of mercury (mmHg). Blood pressure is the product of the cardiac output and the *total peripheral vascular resistance (TPVR)*.

Blood Pressure (BP) = Cardiac Output (Q) x Total Peripheral Vascular Resistance (TPVR)

As noted earlier, cardiac output represents the total volume of blood pumped by the heart per minute. The total peripheral vascular resistance represents systemic resistance to blood flow encountered or created within the arterial blood vessels. A major factor that influences vascular resistance is the inner diameter of the blood vessels. A blood vessel that is *vasoconstricted* will have a smaller inner diameter resulting in greater resistance to blood flow. The inner diameter of a blood vessel may also be reduced by *atherosclerosis* characterized by thickening of the arterial walls and the accumulation of plaque (e.g., fatty acids and cholesterol) within the arterial blood vessels. On the other hand, *vasodilation* results in an increase of the inner diameter of the blood vessel and a reduced resistance to blood flow. *Baroreceptors* located within the aorta and the carotid arteries sense changes in blood pressure through stretching of the arterial wall. The baroreceptors signal the brain to adjust cardiac output and alter the diameter of the blood vessels via vasoconstriction or vasodilation in an effort to maintain appropriate blood pressure.

Blood pressure is expressed in terms of both the systolic blood pressure and the diastolic blood pressure. The **systolic blood pressure** represents the pressure exerted against the arterial vessel walls during a left ventricular contraction of the heart. The systolic pressure is the top number of a blood pressure measurement. A healthy systolic blood pressure is less than 120 mmHg. The **diastolic blood pressure** represents the pressure in the arterial vascular system during the relaxation phase of the cardiac cycle. The diastolic pressure is the bottom number of a blood pressure measurement. A healthy diastolic blood pressure is less than 80 mmHg.

During cardiorespiratory exercise, the systolic blood pressure will normally respond by progressively increasing in proportion to the exercise intensity. This is the result of increasing cardiac output, which is greater than the corresponding decrease in peripheral vascular resistance (due to vasodilation) experienced during a bout of exercise. The vasodilation that occurs within the arterioles during cardiorespiratory exercise causes the diastolic pressure to remain unchanged or to decrease slightly.

As the result of regular cardiorespiratory exercise, systolic and diastolic blood pressures have been shown to decrease at rest and during submaximal intensities comparable to the pre-training levels (Chobanian et al., 2003; Cornelissen & Fagard, 2005). This adaptation to cardiorespiratory exercise is more pronounced in hypertensive and prehypertensive populations and serves as an effective strategy to prevent and or manage hypertension (high blood pressure). Generally speaking, blood pressure at rest and during submaximal exercise is lower in trained versus untrained individuals. Although regular aerobic exercise is likely to provide the most substantial improvements in blood pressure (Whelton et al., 2002), resistance training programs have also been demonstrated to be an effective strategy to reduce resting blood pressure (Kelley & Kelley, 2000). Blood pressure screening and classification will be reviewed in chapter 13.

Oxygen Extraction

The arterial blood transports oxygen to the skeletal muscles during exercise. Within the blood, oxygen is bound to an iron-containing protein called *hemoglobin*, which acts as the oxygen transportation vehicle. In a resting state, every 100 mL of atrial blood contains approximately 20 mL of oxygen. As the atrial blood circulates through the capillaries in the skeletal muscle, some of the oxygen is removed. This is referred to as **oxygen extraction**. At rest, the venous blood returning to the heart from the skeletal muscles contains approximately 15 mL of oxygen per 100 mL of blood. During exercise, to fulfill the increasing demands for oxygen, the oxygen content of venous blood may be as low as 5 mL of oxygen per 100 mL of blood, representing an acute increase in oxygen extraction. Since the oxygen extraction represents the difference between the oxygen content of the arterial and the venous blood, it is also referred to as the *arterial-venous oxygen difference (a-vO$_2$ diff)*.

Just as oxygen extraction increases during exercise to accommodate the increasing demand, it will also increase at rest as well as during submaximal and maximal exercise as the result of regular cardiorespiratory training. The increased capacity of the skeletal muscle to extract and utilize oxygen is the result of adaptations including increased capillary density, increased size and number of *mitochondria*, increased aerobic enzymes, and increased myoglobin. The increased number of capillaries allows for more oxygen-rich blood to be delivered to the muscles, and also provides more surface area for the exchange of both oxygen and carbon dioxide between the blood and the muscles. The exchange of gases (i.e., oxygen and carbon dioxide) between the blood and the cells (e.g., muscle fibers) is referred to as *internal respiration*. Mitochondria are structures in the muscle fiber within which oxygen is utilized to produce energy needed for muscular contractions. Mitochondria are often referred to as the 'powerhouse' of the cell. A greater number of mitochondria allows for more oxygen to be 'burned' for energy production. Just as hemoglobin transports oxygen in the blood, *myoglobin* is an iron-rich protein found in the muscle serving to shuttle oxygen from the blood to the mitochondria. Higher levels of myoglobin allow for greater transport of oxygen from the blood and into the mitochondria within the skeletal muscle.

Although small increases may be seen with regard to oxygen extraction at rest and during submaximal exercise, more pronounced improvements are observed at maximal intensity. In conjunction with increased maximal cardiac output, the adaptations influencing oxygen extraction play a significant role to improve cardiorespiratory capacity.

Ventilation

The lungs are responsible for the exchange of oxygen and carbon dioxide between the ambient air and the blood, known as *external respiration*. In the lungs, the *bronchi* branch into smaller *bronchioles* which divide into an extensive network of *alveoli*. The alveoli are small sacs, clustered together like grapes, and surrounded by a web of capillaries. See figure 7-3. It is across the alveolar-capillary membrane that the exchange of oxygen and carbon dioxide occurs between the air and the blood, a process known as *diffusion*. The ambient air inhaled into the lungs contains approximately 21% oxygen as well as approximately 78% nitrogen and lesser amounts of other gases.

Figure 7-3 Alveoli

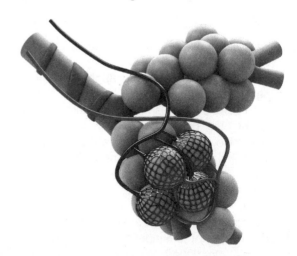

The amount of air inhaled and exhaled with each breath is called the **tidal volume (V_T)**, named because it goes in and out like the tides of the ocean (Morehouse & Miller, 1976). An adult has a resting tidal volume of approximately 500 mL per breath, which varies slightly based on the size of the individual's body. During exercise, tidal volume increases in response to the greater demand for oxygen. As the exercise intensity increases to higher levels, exhalation becomes more forceful in an effort to expel additional carbon dioxide. As an adaptation to regular cardiorespiratory exercise, tidal volume at rest and during submaximal exercise increases minimally as the result of trained respiratory muscles. The improvements in tidal volume seen with conditioning are more pronounced at maximal levels of exercise.

The number of breaths taken per minute is called the **respiratory rate (f_B)** or frequency of breaths. A normal respiratory rate at rest is approximately 12 breaths per minute. During exercise, the respiratory rate increases in response to the demands of the exercise. As the result of regular cardiorespiratory exercise, respiratory rate decreases at rest and during submaximal exertion. However, maximal respiratory rate increases due to higher attainable workloads post-training and the subsequently greater oxygen demands and carbon dioxide production.

The product of the tidal volume and the respiratory rate is the **pulmonary ventilation (V_E)**. This represents the total amount of air inhaled and exhaled by the lungs per minute; therefore, pulmonary ventilation is also called *minute ventilation*.

Pulmonary Ventilation (V_E) = Respiratory Rate (f_B) x Tidal Volume (V_T)

An adult at rest will have a pulmonary ventilation of approximately 6 liters of air per minute (12 breaths per minute x 500 mL air per breath = 6 L/min). Since tidal volume and respiratory rate both increase in response to increasing exercise intensity, pulmonary ventilation also rises during exercise. During submaximal exercise, the increase seen in pulmonary ventilation occurs linearly with the exercise intensity; however, as exercise approaches near-maximal and maximal levels, respiratory rate becomes more pronounced and pulmonary ventilation rises more rapidly. During maximal exercise, a well-trained individual may achieve gender-dependent maximal pulmonary ventilation between 150 L/min to 200 L/min. Although individuals do have conscious control over ventilation, during exercise the ventilatory responses are modulated to a large extent by sensory receptors within joints and chemical receptors in the circulatory system, which signal the central nervous system to increase ventilation in response to the demands of exercise.

In response to cardiorespiratory training, pulmonary ventilation at rest and during submaximal exercise is unchanged or perhaps minimally decreased; whereas maximal pulmonary ventilation will increase.

Oxygen Consumption

As noted earlier in this section, one of the primary functions of the cardiorespiratory system is to deliver oxygen to the skeletal muscles. Nearly all of the components of the cardiorespiratory system discussed thus far play an important role in fulfilling this function. The combined and interrelated contribution of each component supports the utilization of oxygen to produce energy for the working muscles. The amount of oxygen that is utilized by the body (e.g., muscles) at rest or during a specific level of exercise is called **oxygen consumption (VO_2)**. The rate at which oxygen is consumed is determined by the product of the cardiac output and the oxygen extraction. This is known as the Fick Equation.

Oxygen Consumption (VO_2) = Cardiac Output (Q) x Oxygen Extraction (a-vO_2 diff)

Oxygen consumption may be expressed in absolute terms as liters of oxygen consumed per minute (L/min) or in relative terms as milliliters of oxygen consumed per kilogram of body weight per minute (mL/kg/min). Oxygen consumption may also be expressed in terms of *metabolic equivalents (METs)*. One (1) MET represents the amount of oxygen consumed at rest, which is equivalent to 3.5 mL/kg/min. In response to regular cardiorespiratory training, resting oxygen consumption remains unchanged.

During exercise, oxygen consumption increases linearly in response to the exercise intensity. Submaximal oxygen consumption remains unchanged or may decrease slightly (due to increased biomechanical efficiency of movement) in response to regular training. The highest amount of oxygen that is utilized or consumed during maximal, exhaustive exercise is called **maximal oxygen consumption (VO_2max)**. Maximal oxygen consumption is influenced by uncontrollable factors such as genetics, age, and gender. In addition, VO_2max is also related to exercise habits. Maximal oxygen consumption is expected to increase as an adaptation to a well-designed cardiorespiratory program and is also considered by most to be the best indicator of cardiorespiratory fitness. Several researchers investigating healthy subjects have demonstrated increases of 10% to 30% in VO_2max following exercise training, with the greatest improvements occurring among the least fit individuals at baseline (Pate et al., 1995). Maximal oxygen consumption values among the most well-conditioned endurance athletes may be as high as approximately 75 mL/kg/min in women and approximately 85 mL/kg/min in men (Ehrman, 2010).

Oxygen Deficit and Debt

At the onset of exercise, the demand for oxygen increases instantaneously from the resting level to that required to support the specific level of exercise. However, the ability of the cardiorespiratory system to supply the needed oxygen lags behind this demand. The difference between the supply and the demand for oxygen during the initial minutes of exercise is called the **oxygen deficit**. Since an inadequate supply of oxygen is present during these initial minutes of exercise, the body must rely on the anaerobic metabolic pathways (discussed later in this chapter) to provide the energy necessary for muscular work. When the transition from a resting state to a level of high-intensity exercise is very rapid, a larger supply and demand disparity will occur. This scenario produces a greater oxygen deficit. On the other hand, if the transition from rest to exercise is more gradual and progresses from low-, to moderate-, to high-intensity activity, then the oxygen deficit is minimized since the cardiorespiratory system is able to keep pace with the rising yet gradual demand for oxygen.

The point at which the supply of oxygen meets the demand is called **steady state**. During steady state exercise, the cardiorespiratory system is able to fulfill the demand for oxygen and can rely predominately on the aerobic metabolic pathways to produce the required energy. Steady state can often be attained within 2 to 4 minutes, but is dependent upon the exercise intensity and the cardiorespiratory conditioning of the exerciser. Higher-intensity exercise will prolong the time needed to attain steady state. Aerobically-trained individuals will achieve steady state more quickly than the untrained. Steady state exercise may be sustained for an extended period of time (e.g., 10–60+ minutes), again dependent upon the relative intensity and individual level of conditioning, and is characteristic of most traditional endurance training programs.

Upon the conclusion of exercise, the demand for oxygen will quickly return to the baseline resting level. However, the amount of oxygen that is actually consumed remains elevated for several minutes following exercise. The additional oxygen consumed above resting requirements following exercise is called the **oxygen debt** or the **excess post-exercise oxygen consumption (EPOC)**. The magnitude of the EPOC is related to both the intensity of the exercise and the duration, with higher levels of each contributing to a greater EPOC. Many factors have been suggested to play a role in the physiologic necessity of EPOC including: dissipation of heat, replenishment of muscular phosphagen and glycogen stores, removal of lactate and other metabolic byproducts, clearance of blood catecholamines ('fight or flight' hormones), and restoration of blood and muscle oxygen (Farinatti et al., 2012; Gaesser & Brooks, 1984). Figure 7-4 illustrates the dynamics of oxygen consumption at the onset and conclusion of exercise.

Table 7-1 summarizes the variables of the cardiorespiratory system, including the acute responses and chronic adaptations to aerobic training.

The Bioenergetic Systems

All biological work performed by the body's cells (e.g., muscles) requires energy. The foods we eat including carbohydrates, fats, and to a lesser extent protein, are the major substrates for energy production. These substrates are broken down into their simplest components (i.e., glucose and fatty acids) through a process called *metabolism*. Ultimately these components are synthesized into the usable form of energy called **adenosine triphosphate (ATP)**, the energy currency of the cell. A very small amount of ATP is stored within the skeletal muscle, only enough to fulfill the demands of 1 to 2 seconds of maximal exertion. Catalyzed by an enzyme called *myosin ATPase*, the high-energy bond may be broken between the second and third phosphate groups within the ATP molecule. This releases the energy needed for cellular function (e.g., muscular contractions) and results in ADP and an inorganic phosphate (P_i).

$$Adenosine\text{\textasciitilde}P_i\text{\textasciitilde}P_i\text{\textasciitilde}P_i + H_2O \xrightarrow{myosine\,ATPase} Adenosine\text{\textasciitilde}P_i\text{\textasciitilde}P_i + P_i + Energy$$

$$ATP + H_2O \xrightarrow{myosine\,ATPase} ADP + P_i + Energy$$

Upon depletion of this stored ATP, the muscles must turn to other metabolic pathways to obtain the energy necessary to support ongoing activity. There are three metabolic pathways that provide the needed ATP including the phosphagen system, anaerobic glycolysis, and the aerobic system.

The Phosphagen System

Since the supply of stored ATP is very limited and only able to support the demands of just a couple seconds of maximal exercise, the body must rely on other metabolic pathways to resynthesize additional ATP to provide the energy for ongoing muscular effort. The most immediate source of additional ATP is the phosphagen system. The **phosphagen system** utilizes another high-energy phosphate compound found within the skeletal muscles

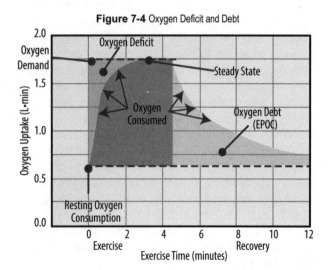

Figure 7-4 Oxygen Deficit and Debt

Table 7-1 Cardiorespiratory Responses to Exercise

Variable	Acute Response	Long Term Adaptations		
		Rest	Submax	Max
Heart Rate (HR): The number of beats per minute.	↑	↓	↓	↔
Stroke Volume (SV): Amount of blood pumped per beat.	↑	↑	↑	↑
Cardiac Output (Q): Volume of blood pumped per minute.	↑	↓	↔ or ↓	↑
Systolic Blood Pressure: Pressure against the arterial walls during a left ventricular contraction of the heart.	↑	↓	↓	↑
Diastolic Blood Pressure: Pressure against the arterial walls during the relaxation phase of cardiac cycle.	↔ or ↓	↓	↓	↑ or ↓
Respiratory Rate (f_B): Number of breaths per minute	↑	↓	↓	↑
Tidal Volume (V_T): Amount of air moved through lungs per breath	↑	↑	↑	↑
Pulmonary Ventilation (V_E): The volume of air exchanged in lungs per minute	↑	↔	↔ or ↓	↑
Oxygen Extraction (a-vO_2 diff): Amount of oxygen removed from circulating blood into the skeletal muscles.	↑	↑	↑	↑
Oxygen Consumption (VO_2): Amount of oxygen utilized by the skeletal muscles.	↑	↔	↔ or ↓	↑

called *creatine phosphate (CP)*. After the stored supply of ATP is broken down, creatine phosphate is used to quickly resynthesize additional ATP, a chemical reaction catalyzed by the enzyme *creatine kinase*.

$$ADP + CP \xrightarrow{(creatine\ kinase)} 1\ ATP + Creatine$$

Since this chemical reaction does not require oxygen, it is considered to be an *anaerobic* metabolic pathway. Although this reaction occurs very rapidly and is able to maintain the supply of ATP necessary for high-intensity exercise, the amount of creatine phosphate stored within the muscles is extremely small. There is likely to be enough creatine phosphate to support up to 10 seconds of maximal exertion during which time the supply of creatine phosphate is quickly depleted. Subsequently, the phosphagen system is the dominant metabolic pathway for the production of ATP during high-intensity, very short duration activities such as short sprints (e.g., < 100 meters), a set of heavy resistance training (e.g. 1–5 RM), most field events in track and field, or a spike in volleyball. Fortunately, approximately 70% of the creatine phosphate is restored in the skeletal muscles within 30 seconds, and 100% after 3 to 5 minutes of recovery (Tomlin & Wegner, 2001). Generally, adequate recovery can be attained within 2 to 3 minutes, preparing the muscles for the next bout of high-intensity activity.

Anaerobic Glycolysis

If the body is to continue performing high-intensity activity, then the relative intensity level must be reduced slightly and the muscles must transition to a different metabolic pathway for a source of ATP. The metabolic pathway responsible for short-term ATP production during high-intensity exercise is called **anaerobic glycolysis**. As noted earlier, anaerobic means in the absence of oxygen, and glycolysis is the breakdown (i.e., metabolism) of glucose. Carbohydrates ingested as part of an individual's diet are broken down into their simplest form, glucose, which can then be stored in both the skeletal muscle and the liver as glycogen (a long chain of glucose molecules). The breakdown of a glucose molecule through anaerobic glycolysis yields 2-3 ATPs.

$$Glucose \xrightarrow{(via\ anaerobic\ glycolysis)} 2\text{-}3\ ATPs + Lactate + H_2O + Heat$$

Like the phosphagen system, anaerobic glycolysis is able to provide a fairly rapid, although limited, source of ATP to support high-intensity exercise over a relatively short-period of time, typically up to 2-3 minutes. The process of anaerobic glycolysis occurs in the sarcoplasm of the muscle fibers resulting in the incomplete breakdown of glucose into a substance called pyruvate. In the absence of sufficient oxygen, the mitochondria in the muscle fibers are unable to oxidize all of the available pyruvate, leading to the conversion of some pyruvate to lactate. Lactate accumulates when production exceeds the body's ability to clear or utilize lactate. Although lactate was long believed to be a dead end metabolic by-product responsible for the onset of fatigue, it is now understood that lactate serves as an important intermediate of carbohydrate metabolism and additional energy production (Hall et al., 2016; Mann, 2007).

During high-intensity exercise supported by anaerobic glycolysis, a concomitant accumulation of hydrogen ions (protons) within the muscle causes acidosis (i.e., decreased pH). The production and accumulation of hydrogen ions has been attributed to non-mitochondrial hydrolysis of ATP (breakdown of ATP to ADP) (Hall et al., 2016; Mann, 2007; Robergs et al., 2004). This metabolic acidosis, not the accumulation of lactate, slows the process of glycolysis, disrupts muscular contraction, creates the 'burning' sensation in the muscle, and ultimately causes muscle fatigue resulting in the slowing or cessation of exercise. Although lactic acid and lactate have been mistakenly blamed for the acidosis and ensuing muscle fatigue, it is now believed that lactate actually resists acidosis since the formation of lactate from muscle glycogen consumes two hydrogen ions (Mall, 2007; Robergs et al., 2004).

Anaerobic glycolysis is the primary metabolic pathway during high-intensity, short-duration activities lasting up to 2 to 3 minutes such as middle-distance sprints (e.g., 200–800 meters), moderate-intensity resistance training (e.g., 6–15 RM), a rally during racquetball, or a short uphill climb on a bike. The clearance of lactate following a bout of high-intensity exercise occurs rapidly; however, the concentration of lactate in the muscle and blood is not restored to pre-exercise levels for 30 to 60 minutes after the conclusion of exercise (Gollnick et al., 1986; Tomlin & Wegner, 2001). An active recovery (e.g., continued low-intensity activity at 50–60% of VO_2max) has been shown to facilitate more rapid lactate clearance (Donne, 2000), and more aerobically conditioned individuals tend to recover more quickly from repeated bouts of high-intensity exercise (Gollnick et al., 1986).

The Aerobic System

As the intensity of exercise decreases and the duration increases, the body is able to transition into the more plentiful sources of ATP derived from the aerobic systems. Aerobic means 'in the presence of oxygen.' The aerobic system is comprised of two interrelated subsystems including *aerobic glycolysis* and *fatty acid oxidation*, which collectively supply the long-term source of energy. The aerobic system relies on the cardiorespiratory system to supply the oxygen needed at rest and during exercise to create ATP.

Aerobic Glycolysis

When an adequate supply of oxygen is available within the muscle, the pyruvate produced through glycolysis is shuttled into the mitochondria of the muscle fiber. The mitochondria contain oxidative enzymes that catalyze the steps involved in **aerobic glycolysis**. In the mitochondria, the pyruvate is converted to *acetyl-CoA*, which then enters the *Kreb's cycle*, a complex series of chemical reactions resulting in the production of ATP. Carbohydrates, in the form of glycogen and glucose, serve as the substrate for aerobic glycolysis. When metabolized aerobically, one molecule of glucose provides 32-38 ATPs. As noted earlier in this chapter, regular cardiorespiratory exercise increases the size and number of mitochondria as well as the concentration of oxidative enzymes, leading to an increased capacity to produce energy through the aerobic system.

$$\text{Glucose} + O_2 \xrightarrow{\text{via aerobic glycolysis}} \text{ATPs} + CO_2 + H_2O + \text{Heat}$$

Fatty Acid Oxidation

The muscles are also able to utilize fats (stored as fatty acids) to aerobically produce ATP through a process called **fatty acid oxidation (FAO)**. Like aerobic glycolysis, FAO also occurs in the mitochondria of the muscle fibers. Although fatty acid oxidation plays a role in energy production across the continuum of exercise intensities, its relative contribution increases substantially during prolonged, low-intensity exercise. At rest, the majority of the energy needs are fulfilled by fatty acid oxidation. During moderate- to high-intensity exercise, carbohydrates (i.e., glucose) are the preferred substrate. As the exercise intensity decreases, the body is able to transition into the more abundant source of potential energy found in fatty acids. The metabolism of fatty acids requires more oxygen than the metabolism of glucose. Therefore, fat becomes a readily accessible source of energy during low-intensity activity when the cardiorespiratory system is more capable of fulfilling the needed oxygen demand. Fat is also a very dense source of energy. The breakdown of a fatty acid molecule provides 129 ATPs, or more depending on the type o fat utilized. A 16-carbon fatty acid yields 129 ATPs and an 18-carbon fatty acid yields 147 ATPs.

$$\text{Fatty Acid} + O_2 \xrightarrow{\text{via fatty acid oxidation}} \text{ATPs} + CO_2 + H_2O + \text{Heat}$$

The aerobic system supplies the energy needed during moderate- to low-intensity activities that last for a prolonged period of time (i.e., >2–3 minutes). These activities include those that utilize the large muscle groups of the body, in a continuous and rhythmic fashion such as walking, running, cycling, swimming, aerobic dancing, and cross-country skiing.

Figure 7-5 depicts a summary of the metabolic pathways involved in glycolysis and fatty acid oxidation.

During exercise, the ability to produce ATP through the aerobic system is limited initially by the supply of oxygen. During very long periods of cardiorespiratory exercise (e.g., >3 hours) the ability to produce ATP aerobically is limited by the availability of muscle glycogen and blood

Figure 7-5 Metabolic Pathways

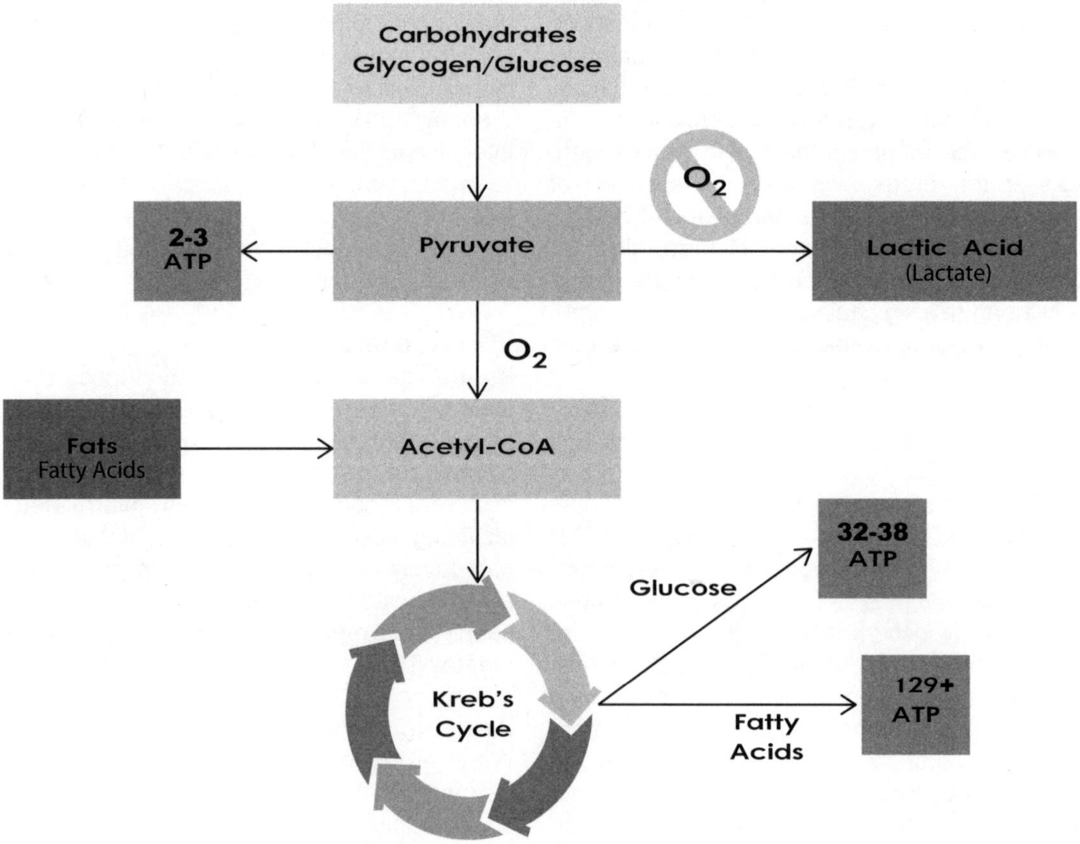

Table 7-2 Energy Systems

Energy System	Intensity	Duration	Type of Activity	Rate of ATP Production	Amount of ATP
Phosphagen System	Very High to Maximal	1-10 seconds	Power & Speed	Fast	1
Anaerobic Glycolysis	High	Up to 2-3 minutes	Speed & Strength	Intermediate	2-3
Aerobic Systems	Moderate to Low	> 3 minutes	Endurance	Slow	32-129+

glucose. During endurance events such as a marathon (26.2 miles) the point at which muscle glycogen stores are depleted is commonly referred to as 'hitting the wall.' It is very unlikely that depletion of fatty acids will limit exercise; however, fatty acid oxidation may be inhibited by a lack of muscle glycogen, since aerobic glycolysis is necessary to 'ignite' fatty acid oxidation. For this reason, it is often said that 'fat burns in a carbohydrate flame.' Other factors that contribute to the onset of fatigue during endurance exercise may include: dehydration, electrolyte imbalance, elevated core body temperature, central nervous system inhibition, muscular fatigue, mental fatigue, and environmental conditions (e.g., heat, humidity, altitude) (Bassett & Howely, 2000; Marcora et al., 2009).

Recovery from endurance activities typically occurs within 2 to 24 hours depending on the intensity and duration of exercise as well as the magnitude of musculoskeletal stress applied to the body. Replenishment of depleted glycogen stores occurs optimally within 45 to 60 minutes after exercise. Likewise, rehydration should occur immediately following activity. Remodeling of damaged musculoskeletal tissue may require 24 hours or more. Recovery from ultra-endurance events such as marathons, ultra-marathons, and triathlons may require several days to weeks before normal training intensities and volumes are resumed. Table 7-2 provides a summary of the metabolic systems.

Anaerobic Threshold

Upon initiation of exercise, the immediate demand for ATP outpaces the cardiorespiratory system's ability to mobilize sufficient oxygen for aerobic energy production. Therefore, ATP is derived from anaerobic pathways and there is a corresponding slight increase of blood lactate above resting values (Hall et al., 2016). As the cardiorespiratory system responds to the exercise stimulus by supplying more oxygen to the working muscles, blood lactate levels decrease and stabilize (Hall et al., 2016). When exercise intensity remains at a comfortable low-to-moderate level (e.g., steady state), lactate production and clearance are in equilibrium and lactate does not accumulate substantially.

As exercise intensity increases substantially, there is a point at which the aerobic energy pathways can no longer efficiently provide energy. This point also marks a disproportionate and unavoidable rise in lactate accumulation called the **anaerobic threshold** (AT). At intensities above the anaerobic threshold, the muscles derive energy primarily through the anaerobic metabolic pathways. As the body relies more heavily on anaerobic metabolism, a discrepancy once again arises between the oxygen supply and demand. This results in an oxygen deficit similar to that seen at the onset of exercise.

The anaerobic threshold may be increased through proper training strategies such as interval training, which alternates short periods of high-intensity exercise with low-intensity active recovery. A conditioned individual will be able to tolerate higher levels of lactate and will hit their anaerobic threshold at a higher exercise intensity or workload in comparison to their pre-training levels. See figure 7-6. Increasing anaerobic threshold allows the participant to sustain a relatively higher intensity of exercise supported by aerobic metabolism; therefore, increasing performance and maximizing caloric expenditure.

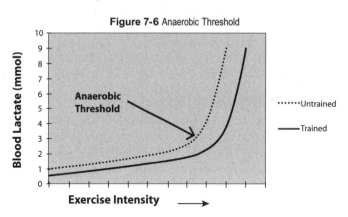

Figure 7-6 Anaerobic Threshold

The Neuromuscular System

Skeletal Muscle Fiber Types

Although each skeletal muscle fiber is unique, each may be placed into two general categories based largely on their speed of contraction and their metabolic characteristics. The two muscle fiber categories include **slow twitch** and **fast twitch** muscle fibers. Although there is general agreement regarding the classification of muscle fiber types among fitness professionals, the scientific community has yet to arrive at a full consensus on the appropriate classifications.

Table 7-3 Muscle Fiber Types

Type I slow twitch slow oxidative	Type IIa fast twitch fast oxidative glycolytic	Type IIb or IIx fast twitch fast glycolytic
• Slow speed of contraction • Low force production • High resistance to fatigue • High capillary density & large number of mitochondria • High concentration of aerobic enzymes & myoglobin • Produces energy through aerobic metabolism	• Fast speed of contraction • Moderate force production • Moderate resistance to fatigue • Produces energy through both aerobic and anaerobic metabolism	• Fast speed of contraction • High force production • Low resistance to fatigue • Produces energy through anaerobic metabolism • Greatest potential for hypertrophy

Slow Twitch Muscle Fibers

Slow twitch muscle fibers are also known as **type I** or more descriptively, **slow oxidative muscle fibers**. Type I muscle fibers are characterized by a slower speed of contraction. This does not imply that movements controlled by type I muscle fibers are slow, but rather it reflects the relatively slower speed of contraction, in terms of milliseconds, compared to fast twitch muscle fibers. As the naming of type I fibers suggests, they also derive the majority of their energy from the oxidative or aerobic metabolic pathways. Subsequently, type I muscle fibers are well-suited for low- to moderate-intensity endurance activities such as walking, jogging, and cycling. Type I muscle fibers produce a relatively low amount of force, yet are highly resistant to fatigue. In light of their dependence on aerobic metabolism, type I fibers are also characterized by a large number of mitochondria, a high capillary density, and a greater concentration of oxidative enzymes and myoglobin. Due to the high amounts of myoglobin and the greater capillary density, type I fibers appear reddish in color (Scott et al., 2001).

Fast Twitch Muscle Fibers

In comparison to slow twitch muscle fibers, fast twitch fibers have a fast speed of contraction, again a difference measured in milliseconds. Fast twitch fibers are further divided into two subtypes: **type IIa** and **type IIb**. Previously, the fastest muscle fibers were known as type IIb fibers; however, more recent research discoveries regarding the histological properties of the fast twitch fibers led exercise scientists to the identification of a third fast twitch fiber called **type IIx** (Greising, 2012; Schiaffino & Reggiani, 2011). The type IIx fiber classification is now used interchangeably with or in place of type IIb.

The type IIx muscle fibers are also known as **fast glycolytic fibers**. The type IIx fibers contain a higher concentration of glycolytic enzymes allowing them to supply the majority of their energy needs from anaerobic metabolism. As the largest of the muscle fibers, the type IIx fibers are able to produce a very high amount of force, yet also fatigue rapidly. The type IIx fibers are well-adapted for activities that require power, speed, and strength. These muscle fibers also possess the greatest capacity for muscle *hypertrophy* – the increased cross-sectional size of a muscle fiber in response to resistance training.

The second subclassification of fast twitch fibers is the type IIa fiber. This fiber functions as an intermediate fiber and is called a **fast oxidative glycolytic** muscle fiber. Although type IIa fibers are still considered fast twitch, they do possess greater endurance capacities and resistance to fatigue in comparison to the type IIx fibers. These muscle fibers are very adaptable to both strength and endurance activities. Type IIa fibers are largely involved in speed and strength activities, but are able to sustain effort longer than the type IIx fibers. Since both subtypes of fast twitch fibers have a smaller concentration of myoglobin and a lower capillary density compared to slow twitch fibers, they appear with a white coloration. Table 7-3 summarizes the major characteristics of the three muscle fiber types.

Muscle Fiber Distribution

The distribution of muscle fibers varies among individuals as well as muscles throughout the body. An individual's relative proportion of slow twitch and fast twitch muscle fibers is determined largely by genetics and to a lesser extent by environmental factors and physical activity habits (Simoneau & Bouchard, 1995). The average individual is estimated to have approximately 52% type I, 33% type IIa, and 13% type IIx muscle fibers (Howley & Franks, 1992). The distribution of muscle fiber types is likely to influence the selection of and success with certain types of sport or activities. Endurance athletes such as distance runners have been found to have a higher percentage of type I fibers; whereas, sprinters and weightlifters have been found to have a higher percentage of type II fibers. It is generally accepted that exercise training elicits a conversion between type IIa and type IIx muscle fibers; however, the possibility of conversion between type I and type II fibers remains in question (Scott et al., 2001).

Skeletal muscles throughout the body are comprised of different proportions of muscle fiber types based upon their primary function (Jennekens et al., 1971; Rantanen et al., 1994). For example, postural and stabilization-oriented muscles have a high proportion of type I (slow twitch) muscle fibers given their role to maintain alignment, which requires low force production and high resilience to fatigue. On the other hand, dynamic muscles are predominately comprised of type II (fast twitch) fibers, given their role to move the skeletal system often against external resistance. Subsequently, exercise programs should be planned accordingly to provide a training stimulus specific to the muscle fiber content and function of each muscle group.

The Motor Unit

The functional component of the neuromuscular system is the **motor unit**. A motor unit is comprised of the *motor neuron* (i.e., nerve cell), the branches of the neuron (i.e., *dentrites* and *axons*), and the muscle fibers that are innervated by the nerve. Figures 7-7 and 7-8 provide illustrations of the motor neuron and a motor unit. As indicated in chapter 5, in order for a muscle to contract (see sliding filament theory), an electrical impulse (i.e., action potential) must be delivered via the motor unit to the muscle fibers. A single electrical impulse causing excitation of the muscle fibers followed by complete relaxation is called a **twitch**. A series of electrical stimuli delivered in rapid succession create an additive effect called **summation**. This prevents the muscle fibers from achieving complete relaxation between stimuli and causes the muscle to contract with greater force. The peak force production of a motor unit is achieved when the frequency of stimulation achieves the point of full summation, called **tetanus**. When the electrical stimulation delivered by the central nervous system reaches the threshold necessary to activate the motor unit, then all of the muscle fibers innervated by the motor unit will contract. This is referred to as the **all-or-none principle.** As greater external loads are applied against a muscle, the nervous system will activate additional motor units and subsequently additional muscle fibers to increase the magnitude of force production. The simultaneous activation of additional muscle fibers is called **recruitment**. According to the **size principle**, muscle fibers are recruited in order of size with the smaller type I muscle fibers recruited first, followed by the larger type IIa fibers, and finally the largest type IIx fibers (Henneman, 1957; Mendell, 2005).

The motor units found in the smaller muscles, such as the muscles that control the eyes, innervate a very small number of muscle fibers. This allows for the neuromuscular control required to perform precise movements and fine motor skills. Larger muscles, such as the major muscle groups of the body (e.g., quadriceps, hamstrings, gluteals, pectorals) contain hundreds of motor units each responsible for controlling thousands of muscle fibers. These muscles are better equipped for gross motor skills and greater force production.

Whereas the longer-term (e.g., >6 weeks) gains in strength may be attributed to muscle hypertrophy, the immediate and short-term (e.g., <4 weeks) strength gains seen in response to resistance training are due largely to neuromuscular adaptations. These changes occur without any significant gains in muscle size. The expected neuromuscular changes include an increase in motor unit recruitment and synchronization, increase in motor unit activation rate, increase in coactivation of agonist muscles, inhibition of antagonist muscle activation, and enhanced recruitment of higher threshold type II fibers. In conjunction with the neuromuscular adaptations, individuals will also experience the 'learning effect' in which the coordination and biomechanical efficiency in movement will improve.

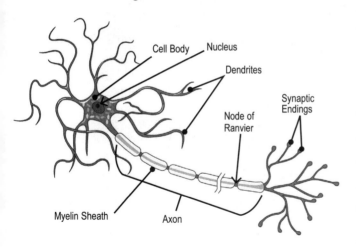

Figure 7-7 Motor Neuron

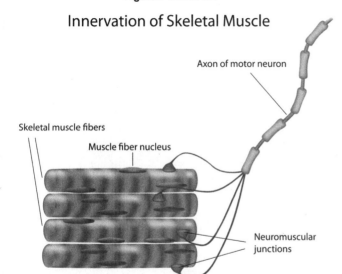

Figure 7-8 Motor Unit

Innervation of Skeletal Muscle

Chapter Summary
This chapter reviewed the physiological systems that support exercise. The cardiorespiratory system supplies the oxygen needed by the cells throughout the body. The skeletal muscle contractions are supported by the bioenergetic systems which supply the energy, in the form of ATP, necessary for all muscular work. Muscular contractions and human movement are controlled by the neuromuscular system. In response to regular physical activity and exercise, the various systems of the body undergo numerous adaptations allowing for more efficient and effective performance of both exercise and activities of daily living.

Chapter References
Bassett, D.R., & Howley, E.T. (2000). Limiting factors for maximum oxygen uptake and determinants of endurance performance. *Medicine and Science in Sports and Exercise*, 32(1), 70-84.

Chobanian, A.V., Bakris, G.L., Black, H.R., Cushman, W.C., Green, L.A., Izzo Jr, J.L., ... & Roccella, E.J. (2003). Seventh report of the joint national committee on prevention, detection, evaluation, and treatment of high blood pressure. *Hypertension*, 42(6), 1206-1252.

Cornelissen, V.A., & Fagard, R.H. (2005). Effects of endurance training on blood pressure, blood pressure–regulating mechanisms, and cardiovascular risk factors. *Hypertension*, 46(4), 667-675.

Ehrman, J.K. (Ed.). (2010). *ACSM's Resource Manual for Guidelines for Exercise Testing and Prescription*, 6th edition. Baltimore, MD: Lippincott Williams & Wilkins.

Farinatti, P., Castinheiras Neto, A.G., & da Silva, N.L. (2012). Influence of resistance training variables on excess postexercise oxygen consumption: A systematic review. *ISRN Physiology*, 2013, Article ID 825026.

Gaesser, G.A., & Brooks, G.A. (1984). Metabolic bases of excess post-exercise oxygen consumption: A review. *Medicine and Science in Sports and Exercise*, 16(1), 29-43.

Gollnick, P.D., Bayly, W.M., & Hodgson, D.R. (1986). Exercise intensity, training, diet, and lactate concentration in muscle and blood. *Medicine and Science in Sports and Exercise*, 18(3), 334-340.

Greising, S.M., Gransee, H.M., Mantilla, C.B., & Sieck, G.C. (2012). Systems biology of skeletal muscle: Fiber type as an organizing principle. *Wiley Interdisciplinary Reviews: Systems Biology and Medicine*, 4, 457-473.

Hall, M.M., Rajasekaran, S., Thomsen, T.W., & Peterson, A.R. (2016). Lactate: Friend or foe. *Physical Medicine and Rehabilitation Journal*, 8(3), S8-S15.

Henneman, E. (1957). Relation between size of neurons and their susceptibility to discharge. *Science*, 126, 1345–1347.

Howley, E.T., & Franks, B.D. (1992). *Health Fitness Instructor's Manual*, 2nd edition. Champaign, IL: Human Kinetics.

Jennekens, F.G., Tomlinson, B.E., & Walton, J.N. (1971). Data on the distribution of fibre types in five human limb muscles. An autopsy study. *Journal of the Neurological Sciences*, 14(3), 245-257.

Kelley, G.A., & Kelley, K.S. (2000). Progressive resistance exercise and resting blood pressure: A meta-analysis of randomized controlled trials. *Hypertension*, 35(3), 838-843.

Mann, T. (2007). Sporting myths: The REAL role of lactate during exercise. *South African Journal of Sports Medicine*, 19(5), 114-116.

Marcora, S.M., Staiano, W., & Manning, V. (2009). Mental fatigue impairs physical performance in humans. *Journal of Applied Physiology*, 106(3), 857-864.

Mendell, L.M. (2005). The size principle: A rule describing the recruitment. *Journal of Neurophysiology*, 93(6), 3024-3026.

Monedero, J., & Donne, B. (2000). Effect of recovery interventions on lactate removal and subsequent performance. *International Journal of Sports Medicine*, 21(8), 593-597.

Morehouse, L.E., & Miller, A.T. (1976). *Physiology of Exercise*, 7th edition. St. Louis, MO: The C.V. Mosby Company.

Pate, R.R., Pratt, M., Blair, S.N., Haskell, W.L., Macera, C.A., Bouchard, C., ... & Wilmore, J.H. (1995). Physical activity and public health. *The Journal of the American Medical Association*, 273(5), 402-407.

Rantanen, J., Rissanen, A., & Kalimo, H. (1994). Lumbar muscle fiber size and type distribution in normal subjects. *European Spine Journal*, 3(6), 331-335.

Robergs, R.A., Ghiasvand, F., & Parker, D. (2004). Biochemistry of exercise-induced metabolic acidosis. *American Journal of Physiology-Regulatory, Integrative and Comparative Physiology*, 287(3), R502-R516.

Schiaffino, S., & Reggiani, C. (2011). Fiber types in mammalian skeletal muscles. *Physiological Reviews*, 91(4), 1447-1531.

Scott, W., Stevens, J., & Binder–Macleod, S.A. (2001). Human skeletal muscle fiber type classifications. *Physical Therapy*, 81(11), 1810-1816.

Simoneau, J.A., & Bouchard, C. (1995). Genetic determinism of fiber type proportion in human skeletal muscle. *FASEB Journal*, 9(11), 1091-1095.

Tomlin, D.L., & Wenger, H.A. (2001). The relationship between aerobic fitness and recovery from high intensity intermittent exercise. *Sports Medicine*, 31(1), 1-11.

Whelton, S.P., Chin, A., Xin, X., & He, J. (2002). Effect of aerobic exercise on blood pressure: A meta-analysis of randomized, controlled trials. *Annals of Internal Medicine*, 136(7), 493.

Zhou, B., Conlee, R.K., Jensen, R., Fellingham, G.W., George, J.D., & Fisher, A.G. (2001). Stroke volume does not plateau during graded exercise in elite male distance runners. *Medicine and Science in Sports and Exercise*, 33(11), 1849-1854.

Recommended Reading
McArdle, WD., Katch, F.I., & Katch, V.L. (2015). *Exercise Physiology: Nutrition, Energy, and Human Performance*, 8th edition. Philadelphia, PA: Wolters Kluwer.

Chapter 7 Review Questions

1. Which of the following is an expected adaptation in response to regular cardiorespiratory exercise?
    A. Decrease in capillary density of type I muscle fibers
    B. Decreased parasympathetic nervous system tone
    C. Increased submaximal left ventricular stroke volume
    D. Increased resting diastolic blood pressure

2. Which of the following activities is most appropriately associated with the anaerobic glycolysis energy system?
    A. Jogging one mile at a half marathon race pace
    B. Running one lap (400 meters) around an Olympic size track
    C. Sprinting three-quarters of the length of a football field
    D. Walking three miles in less than an hour

3. Which of the following adaptations is likely to have the most significant impact on increased maximal oxygen consumption seen with regular endurance exercise training?
    A. Decreased submaximal heart rate
    B. Increased stroke volume
    C. Decreased mitochondrial size and density
    D. Increased maximal heart rate

4. Long chains of glucose are stored as glycogen in the _____ and _____.
    A. tendons, ligaments
    B. stomach, blood
    C. skeletal muscle, liver
    D. lungs, smooth muscle

5. Which of the following metabolic pathways is primarily responsible for the energy supplied during power and speed activities?
    A. Fatty acid oxidation
    B. Phosphagen system
    C. Anaerobic glycolysis
    D. Aerobic glycolysis

6. Which of the following are characteristic of type IIb or IIx muscle fibers?
    A. High resistance to fatigue
    B. Slow speed of contraction
    C. Large number of mitochondria
    D. High force production

Answers to Review Questions on Page 384

Note: Review questions are intended to reinforce learning and comprehension of subject matter presented in the corresponding chapter. The review questions are not intended to be representative of actual certification exam questions in terms of style, content, or difficulty.

Section III

Principles of Nutrition & Weight Management

The achievement and maintenance of optimal health, physical fitness, and athletic performance is contingent upon proper nutrition. Fitness professionals must have practical knowledge of basic principles of nutrition as well as evidence-based dietary recommendations in order to educate and guide their clients.

Chapter 8 provides an overview of the digestive system as well as the six nutrients essential for optimal health and peak performance. These nutrients include carbohydrates, fat, protein, vitamins, minerals, and water.

Chapter 9 provides a summary of the current Dietary Guidelines for Americans. These Guidelines are jointly published by the U.S. Department of Agriculture and the U.S. Department of Health and Human Services. In addition, this chapter will introduce the MyPlate icon, provide an interpretation of a Nutrition Facts label, and review the calculation of macronutrient content in food.

Chapter 10 reviews metabolism and basic guidelines pertaining to safe and effective weight management. In addition, this chapter will summarize some of the key findings of the National Weight Control Registry.

Chapter 11 addresses disordered eating patterns and diseases such as anorexia nervosa, bulimia nervosa, binge-eating disorder, and feeding or eating disorders not elsewhere classified. This chapter includes information to help the fitness professional recognize signs and symptoms of disordered eating and provides resources to address these challenging situations.

8
Essential Nutrients for Health & Performance

Introduction
The cells making up the tissues of the body require a constant source of energy and nutrients. The foods we eat provide the nutrients required for the body to function, which otherwise may not be obtained. These essential nutrients include carbohydrates, protein, fat, vitamins, minerals, and water. The digestive system is responsible for the break-down and absorption of these essential nutrients.

The Digestive System
The overall function of the digestive system is to break up the foods we ingest into smaller molecules, which are then absorbed into the body to support the nutrient and energy needs of the cells. The digestive system is comprised of the mouth, pharynx, esophagus, stomach, small intestine, large intestine, and rectum. See figure 8-1. Food is ingested through the mouth where it is chewed into smaller pieces and blends with saliva, which dissolves some of the food particles and aids in swallowing. Once swallowed, the food passes through the pharynx and into the esophagus. The food is moved through the esophagus through a series of alternating contractions and relaxations of the smooth muscle, a process called peristalsis. Having passed through the esophagus, the food empties into the stomach where digestion of the food continues through both the chemical actions of digestive enzymes and muscular churning processes to break the food into smaller particles. The food (now a liquid mixture known as chyme) moves into the small intestine. The small intestine is the primary site for the digestion of food into smaller molecules and for absorption of the nutrients (carbohydrates, fat, protein, vitamins, minerals, and water) into the bloodstream and lymphatic system. The food (i.e., chyme) is moved through the small intestine through a process similar to peristalsis called segmentation. From the small intestine the food moves into the large intestine (i.e., colon). At this stage of the digestive tract, most digestion and absorption is completed, with only final absorption of water and salts left to occur. The fecal material consisting of fiber, indigestible substances, bacteria and other waste products is expelled from the body through the anus.

The Six Essential Nutrients

Carbohydrates
Carbohydrates are the preferred source of energy for the body. One gram of carbohydrate provides approximately 4 Calories of energy. The simplest forms of carbohydrates are known as *monosaccharides* which include glucose, galactose, and fructose. Glucose is a structural component of most carbohydrates and is the only form of carbohydrate the body can use as a fuel source. See figure 8-2. Therefore, all carbohydrates must be converted into

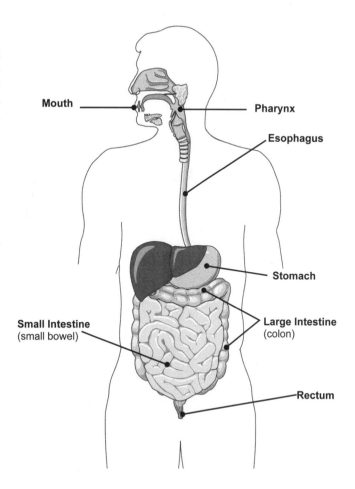

Figure 8-1 Digestive System

Figure 8-2 Glucose

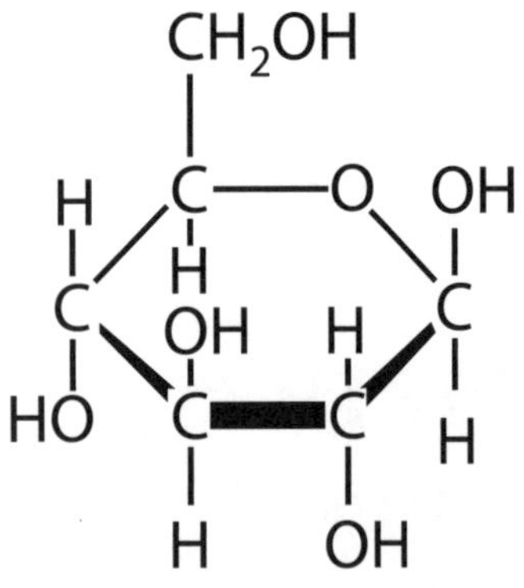

[Chemical structure of glucose]

glucose in order to produce ATP via anaerobic or aerobic glycolysis. Any glucose not immediately used is stored in the skeletal muscle and liver in the form of glycogen (a long chain of glucose molecules). If carbohydrates are ingested at a level greater than the body can utilize or store in the form of glycogen, then the excess will be converted to fatty acids and stored in the adipose (fat) tissue.

Two monosaccharides linked together form a *disaccharide*, which include the milk sugar lactose (glucose + galactose), the common table sugar sucrose (glucose + fructose), and the malt sugar maltose (glucose + glucose). Both monosaccharides and disaccharides are considered to be *simple carbohydrates* (sometimes called simple sugars) and are commonly found in honey, corn syrup, and refined sugars. Many food sources of simple carbohydrates have a low nutrient density meaning they contain a high number of calories, but very few essential nutrients.

A long chain of monosaccharides is referred to as a *polysaccharide*. Glycogen is a polysaccharide found in meats and seafood. Polysaccharides also include starches and cellulose found in vegetables and grains. The food sources containing polysaccharides are often called *complex carbohydrates*. The complex carbohydrates have a higher nutrient density including essential vitamins and minerals as well as dietary fiber – an indigestible form of carbohydrate. Complex carbohydrate foods include whole grains (e.g., cereals, breads, pasta, rice), vegetables, and fruits. In comparison to the simple sugars, complex carbohydrates require more energy to digest and allow glucose to enter the bloodstream more gradually.

It is currently recommended that Americans consume 45% to 65% of their total daily calories from carbohydrates (DGAC, 2015). In consideration of the higher nutrient density, complex carbohydrate food sources are preferred. Ideally, no more than 10% of the total daily calories consumed should be in the form of simple carbohydrates. The carbohydrate recommendations for athletes and highly active individuals range from 6 to 10 grams per kilogram of body weight per day (Rodriguez et al., 2009; Thomas et al., 2016).

Dietary fiber is the nondigestible form of carbohydrates found naturally in plant-based foods. Among the best sources of dietary fiber are legumes, vegetables, fruit, and whole grains. Although bran is not a whole grain, it is also a great source of dietary fiber. There are many health benefits associated with increased dietary fiber consumption including an improved blood cholesterol profile, lower prevalence of obesity, and reduced risk of cardiovascular disease, certain types of cancer, and type 2 diabetes. Unfortunately, most Americans significantly under-consume dietary fiber with an average intake estimated to be just 15 grams per day. The recommended AI for dietary fiber is 14 grams per 1,000 calories, or 25 grams per day for women and 38 grams per day for men (DGAC, 2015).

Understanding Calories

A calorie is a unit commonly used to measure or express the energy content of foods and beverages as well as the energy expended by the body. A calorie (i.e., small calorie) is a unit of heat energy required to raise the temperature of 1 gram of water 1 degree Celsius (°C). One calorie is equivalent to 4.184 joules in the International System of Units. In the popular use of the term and in the labeling of food products in the U.S., a 'calorie' actually refers to a kilocalorie (i.e., large calorie, kilogram calorie, food calorie), or 1,000 calories (Buchholz & Schoeller, 2004). A kilocalorie is the amount of heat energy needed to raise the temperature of 1 kilogram of water from 14.5° to 15.5° Celsius. When fitness professionals and dietitians refer to calories, they are actually referring to kilocalories (kcal), which is most appropriately written as Calorie (with a capital C) and abbreviated as Cal. Throughout this manual, 'calorie' actually represents a kilocalorie or Calorie.

Protein

Protein is the 'building block' for many structures in the body including muscle, skin, hair, connective tissue, nerve tissue, and blood. In addition to its role in the building, maintenance, and repair of tissue, protein also acts as a transportation vehicle for iron, fats, and oxygen. In addition, protein plays a key role in acid-base balance, the formation of enzymes to catalyze chemical reactions in the body, and formation of antibodies to combat infections. In certain circumstances (e.g., energy deprivation), protein can also function as a back-up source of energy. Each gram of protein contains approximately 4 Calories.

Good to Know

1 gram of carbohydrate = 4 kilocalories
1 gram of protein = 4 kilocalories
1 gram of fat = 9 kilocalories
1 gram of alcohol = 7 kilocalories

The structural components of protein are known as **amino acids**. There are approximately 20 amino acids used by the human body to construct various proteins. Different combinations and sequences of amino acids create different types of protein. The **essential amino acids** include the eight to ten amino acids that cannot be manufactured by the body and therefore must be consumed as part of a regular diet. The remaining amino acids are referred to as **nonessential amino acids**. The body is able to manufacture these using nitrogen and components of carbohydrates and fat. Foods that contain all of the essential amino acids are called *complete proteins*. Some complete protein sources include lean meat, fish, poultry, eggs, and dairy products. Plant-based *incomplete protein* sources, such as vegetables, fruit, legumes, and grains, do not contain all or a sufficient amount of the essential amino acids. Consuming incomplete proteins in combination may provide all of the essential amino acids in which case the foods are referred to as *complementary proteins*. Examples include beans + brown rice, peanut butter + whole wheat bread, and peas + pasta. In addition, hummus (chickpeas and tahini) and tofu (coagulated soy milk) provide complete protein sources. Tofu, which is low in saturated fat, low in calories, and cholesterol-free, serves as a high-quality alternative to many animal proteins.

The current Recommended Dietary Allowance (RDA) for protein is 0.8 grams per kilogram of body weight and the Acceptable Macronutrient Distribution Range (AMDR) for protein intake among adults is 10% to 35% of total daily calories (DGAC, 2015; Otten et al., 2006). However, the RDA for protein does not recognize the increased protein needs seen among regularly active individuals and competitive athletes. It has been recommended that endurance-trained athletes consume 1.2 to 1.4 grams of protein per body weight per day and that strength-trained athletes consume 1.2 to 1.7 g/kg/day (Rodriguez et al., 2009). Table 8-1 summarizes the protein intake recommendations.

Table 8-1 Protein

Recommended Protein Intake	
Adult General Population	0.8 g/kg/day
Endurance-Trained Athletes	1.2 – 1.4 g/kg/day
Strength-Trained Athletes	1.2 – 1.7 g/kg/day

More recently, a general daily protein intake range of 1.2 to 2.0 g/kg/day has been recommended for athletes, regardless of a strength or endurance classification of the athlete (Thomas et al., 2016). Although active individuals generally have higher protein requirements, research has not conclusively demonstrated that mega-doses and supplementation of protein (amino acids) beyond the recommended levels will further enhance muscle hypertrophy, improve athletic performance, or contribute significantly to energy needs. When protein intake regularly exceeds the body's needs, the unused amino acids are stored as fat. The waste products (e.g., urea) from fat conversion must be excreted in the urine, which places an additional burden on the kidneys. A diet high in animal proteins may also be associated with elevated intake of saturated fat, triglycerides, and cholesterol, which increases the risk of cardiovascular disease and certain types of cancer.

Fat

Fats serve many important functions throughout the human body including insulation for temperature regulation, cell membrane structure, protection of vital organs, transmission of nerve impulses, vitamin absorption, and hormone production. In addition, fat also serves as a very dense source of energy, providing approximately 9 Calories per gram. Fat provides more than twice the calories per gram than either carbohydrates or protein.

Since fat plays so many vitally important roles throughout the body, it would be unwise to restrict fat intake below the level necessary to maintain proper physiological function. However, too much dietary fat also presents significant health concerns such as overweight and obesity, and elevated risk of many chronic illnesses such as cardiovascular disease, type 2 diabetes, hypertension, and certain types of cancer. It is recommended that Americans consume 20% to 35% of total daily calories from fat, with less than 10% coming from saturated fatty acids and keeping *trans* fatty acids as low as possible (DGAC, 2015; Kris-Etherton et al., 2007). It is recommended that emphasis is placed on the consumption of foods providing polyunsaturated and omega-3 fatty acids (DGAC, 2015; Kris-Etherton et al., 2007).

The major forms of dietary fat are fatty acids or triglycerides (one glycerol molecule with three fatty acids). Fatty acids are categorized based upon the absence or presence of double bonds within the chain of carbon atoms making up the 'backbone' of the fat. A *saturated fatty acid (SFA)* does not contain any double bonds between the carbon atoms and many are found in a solid form (called 'solid fats') at room temperature. Saturated fatty acids are found in relatively high amounts in animal products such as meat and full-fat dairy products. These food sources account for approximately 60% of the saturated fatty acids found in the typical American diet (Kris-Etherton et al., 2007). The high consumption of these animal-based fats is also associated with elevated blood cholesterol, atherosclerosis (plaque and clogging within the arteries), and risk of cardiovascular disease. Saturated fatty acids are also present in tropical vegetable oils such as palm kernel, coconut, and cocoa oils.

Fatty acids that contain one or more double bonds are called *unsaturated fatty acids*. These are further classified as *monounsaturated fatty acids (MUFA)*, containing one double bond, and *polyunsaturated fatty acids (PUFA)*,

Table 8-2 DRIs

Dietary Reference Intakes – Definition of Terms	
Estimated Average Requirement (EAR)	The EAR represents the average daily intake that is likely to meet the nutritional requirements of approximately half of the healthy population. It is not used as an individual nutrient recommendation or a goal, but rather is used for statistical analysis when setting the RDAs.
Acceptable Macronutrient Distribution Range (AMDR)	The AMDR is the range of intake for a particular energy source (e.g., carbohydrate, fat, protein) that is associated with reduced risk of chronic disease while providing intakes of essential nutrients.
Recommended Dietary Allowance (RDA)	The RDA is established at a level which meets the nutrient requirements of nearly all healthy individuals (95% or two standard deviations from the EAR). As such, the RDA will exceed the nutrient needs for most healthy people in the population and intakes below the RDA do not necessarily indicate a deficiency.
Adequate Intake (AI)	When there is insufficient scientific evidence to establish an RDA, an AI is set based on the levels of nutrients consumed by apparently healthy individuals. Although the AI is a less exact measure than an RDA, it is believed to be adequate for nearly all healthy individuals within the population.
Tolerable Upper Intake Level (UL)	The UL represents the highest average level of nutrient intake that does not pose any risk of adverse health effects. Intakes above the UL increase the risk of nutrient toxicity.

Adopted from Francis & Klitzke (2010)

Table 8-3 Vitamins

Nutrient	Recommended Intake* Men	Recommended Intake* Women	Functions	Sources
Vitamin A	900 µg	700 µg	Vision, healthy skin and hair, immune function, growth of bones and teeth	Yellow/orange fruits and vegetables, dark green leafy vegetables, dairy products, liver
Vitamin B1 (Thiamine)	1.2 mg	1.1 mg	Carbohydrate oxidation, growth and function of nerve tissue	Fortified cereals, oatmeal, and whole grain breads, poultry, fish, pork, liver
Vitamin B2 (Riboflavin)	1.3 mg	1.1 mg	Metabolism/energy production from carbohydrates, fats, and protein, vision, healthy skin	Milk, whole grains, green leafy vegetables, broccoli, organ meats, eggs
Vitamin B3 (Niacin)	16 mg	14 mg	Metabolism/energy production from carbohydrates, fats, and protein	Meat, poultry, fish, whole grains, enriched cereals, legumes, dairy products, eggs
Vitamin B5 (Pantothenic Acid)	5 mg	5 mg	Metabolism/energy production from carbohydrates, fats, and protein, fatty acid synthesis	Whole grains, lean meats, legumes, vegetables, fruits
Vitamin B6 (Pyridoxine)	1.3 mg 1.7 mg > 50 yrs	1.3 mg 1.5 mg > 50 yrs	Metabolism and synthesis of protein, neurotransmitter synthesis	Meat, fish, poultry, whole grains, dried beans, bananas, prunes, avocados, potatoes
Vitamin B9 (Folic Acid)	400 µg	400 µg	DNA synthesis, red blood cell production, cell division	Green leafy vegetables, organ meats, dried peas, beans, lentils, whole grains
Vitamin B12	2.4 µg	2.4 µg	Red blood cell formation, nervous system function, folate utilization, metabolism of protein and fat	Meat, dairy products, seafood
Vitamin C (Ascorbic Acid)	90 mg	75 mg	Antioxidant, collagen formation in bone, muscles, and cartilage, iron absorption, maintain blood vessels and gum tissue	Citrus fruits, berries, tomatoes, peppers, potatoes
Vitamin D	15 µg 20 µg > 71 yrs	15 µg 20 µg > 71 yrs	Bone mineralization, calcium and phosphorus absorption, heart and nervous system function	Sunlight, fortified milk, fish, eggs, butter, fortified margarine
Vitamin E	15 mg	15 mg	Antioxidant to protect against cellular damage, immune function	Wheat germ, dark green leafy vegetables, nuts, fortified and multigrain cereals
Vitamin K	*120 µg*	*90 µg*	Blood clotting	Green leafy vegetables, fruit, cabbage, alfalfa, broccoli, synthesized by intestinal bacteria
Choline	*550 mg*	*425 mg*	Precursor of acetylcholine, liver function	Milk, liver, eggs, peanuts

*values provided represent the RDAs (regular font) and AIs (italic font) for adults aged 19 and older unless otherwise noted. µg = micrograms; mg = milligrams

Dietary Reference Intakes

In 1995, the United States (Institute of Medicine) and Canada (Office of Nutrition Policy and Promotion of Health Canada) began collaboration to establish a uniform set of nutrient-based Dietary Reference Intakes (DRIs) (Atkinson, 2011). The purpose of the DRIs is to identify the nutrient intake levels that will promote health, prevent or delay diet-related chronic disease, and avoidance of nutrient overconsumption (Francis & Klitzke, 2010). The DRIs create the scientific basis for public policy such as nutritional labeling, fortification of foods, and menu-planning for school meal programs (Francis & Klitzke, 2010). In addition, the DRIs were used in the creation of The Dietary Guidelines for Americans (see chapter 9) and the MyPlate graphic.

The DRIs include four nutrient reference values to be used for assessing and planning the dietary needs of individuals and groups (Francis & Klitzke, 2010). These values include: *Estimated Average Requirement (EAR)*, *Recommended Dietary Allowance (RDA)*, *Adequate Intake (AI)*, and *Tolerable Upper Intake Level (UL)*. Table 8-2 provides a definition for each of these nutrient reference values. Since no single food contains all of the vitamins and minerals, it is important to consume a variety of nutrient-dense foods to maintain the intake necessary for optimal health. Tables 8-3 and 8-4 provide a summary of essential vitamins and minerals including the common food sources, key functions, and RDAs or AIs for each micronutrient.

Table 8-4 Minerals

Nutrient	Recommended Intake* Men	Recommended Intake* Women	Functions	Sources
Calcium	1,000 mg 1,200 mg >50 yrs	1,000 mg 1,200 mg >50 yrs	Structure of bones and teeth, muscular contraction, heart rhythm, nerve conduction, vasodilation/vasoconstriction.	Milk and dairy products, dark green leafy vegetables, broccoli, canned fish (with bones), whole almonds
Chromium	35 µg	25 µg	Glucose metabolism, insulin function	Corn oil, whole grains, clams, brewer's yeast, dried peas and beans
Copper	900 µg	900 µg	Red blood cell formation, skeletal and collagen health, nerve coverings	Oysters, shellfish, nuts, organ meats, legumes
Fluoride	4 mg	3 mg	Stimulates bone formation, strengthens of tooth enamel	Fluorinated water, teas, marine fish
Iodine	150 µg	150 µg	Control of metabolism as a component of thyroxine, a hormone found in the thyroid gland	Iodized salt, seafood
Iron	8 mg	18 mg	Hemoglobin formation, transportation of oxygen in blood, immune function	Red Meats, organ meats, legumes, green leafy vegetables, enriched grain products
Magnesium	420 mg 400 mg 19-30 yrs	320 mg 310 mg 19-30 yrs	Acid-base balance, energy production, protein synthesis, muscular contraction	Meats, nuts, whole grains, seeds, legumes, vegetables, fruits
Phosphorus	700 mg	700 mg	Skeletal tissue formation, metabolism of protein, fat and carbohydrates, component of many B-vitamin coenzymes	Meats, fish, poultry, eggs, dairy products, grains
Potassium	*4,700 mg*	*4,700 mg*	Fluid/electrolyte balance, contractions of the heart, nervous system and kidney function	Fruits (bananas, melons), potatoes, vegetables, lean meat
Sodium	2,300 mg (UL)	2,300 mg (UL)	Fluid balance, acid-base balance, contraction of the heart, nerve conduction	Table salt, soy sauce, processed/preserved foods
Selenium	55 µg	55 µg	Antioxidant to protect tissue from radiation damage, pollution, and normal metabolic byproducts	Seafood, meat, liver, whole grains
Zinc	11 mg	8 mg	Essential for DNA and RNA, protein synthesis, digestion, aids in healing wounds, immune function	Lean meats, seafood, liver, whole grains, eggs, poultry, nuts legumes

*values provided represent the RDAs (regular font) and AIs (italic font) for adults aged 19 and older unless otherwise noted. µg = micrograms; mg = milligrams

containing two or more double bonds. Fats that contain a higher percentage of unsaturated fatty acids are usually liquid (called 'oils') at room temperature. Unsaturated fatty acids are found in vegetable oils, nuts, olive oils, and seed oils. Many fish and seafoods are heart-healthy sources of polyunsaturated fats called omega-3 fatty acids.

Trans **fatty acids (TFA)** are another type of fat which are found naturally in some foods from ruminant animals (e.g., cattle and sheep) such as beef, lamb, and dairy products. They are also produced during the hydrogenation process used by food manufacturers to convert vegetable oils into semi-solid fats having a longer self-life. Sources of *trans* fatty acids may include commercially prepared baked goods, fried foods, margarine, and snack foods. A number of research studies have demonstrated an association between *trans* fatty acid intake and increased risk of heart disease. Therefore, Americans are encouraged to keep their intake of *trans* fatty acids 'as low as possible' (USDA & HHS, 2015). In 2006, it was federally-mandated that food manufacturers include the amount of *trans* fatty acid on Nutrition Facts labels for foods containing more than 0.5 grams per serving. As the result, consumer awareness of *trans* fatty acids has increased while consumption has slowly decreased. In addition, some food manufacturers have taken action to voluntarily reduce or eliminate the use of partially hydrogenated vegetable oils containing *trans* fatty acids (Mozaffarian et al., 2006).

Vitamins

Vitamins are organic, carbon-based micronutrients essential for the maintenance of normal physiological processes. There are 13 different vitamins essential to the human body, most of which can only be obtained through the foods we ingest. Vitamins are placed into two categories: water-soluble and fat-soluble. The *water-soluble vitamins* include the vitamin B complex and vitamin C. Most water-soluble vitamins cannot be stored in the body and any amounts in excess of those needed to maintain physiological functions are excreted in the urine. Subsequently, overconsumption of water-soluble vitamins is unlikely and regular intake is necessary. The *fat-soluble vitamins* include vitamin A, D, E, and K. The fat-soluble vitamins may be stored in the body for extended periods, which increases the risk of toxicity associated with overconsumption.

Vitamin D is a unique nutrient in that it is produced by the body through sunlight on the skin. However, in the U.S., particularly in more northern locations, most vitamin D is obtained from dietary sources such as fortified foods including milk and yogurt. Adequate vitamin D is necessary for skeletal health. Although vitamin D has been the topic of much scientific research over the recent years, evidence is inconclusive with regard to the many non-skeletal health benefits suggested to arise from increased vitamin D intake (Ross et al., 2011). Although the average dietary intake of vitamin D is estimated to be less than the recommended level, the majority of the U.S. population is meeting their requirements for vitamin D through a combination of dietary sources and sunlight exposure (Ross et al., 2011). Nevertheless, most Americans are likely to benefit from modest increases to vitamin D intake. The RDA for vitamin D is 15 µg/day (600 IU/day) for youth and most adults, and 20 µg/day (800 IU/day) for adults over 71 years.

Minerals

Minerals are inorganic (do not contain carbon) elements that are obtained from the foods we eat and are stored throughout the body. Minerals are critical for many functions such as the regulation of enzyme activity, fluid and acid-base balance, transmission of nerve impulses, and skeletal structure. However, similar to vitamins, minerals do not have any caloric value. Although both vitamins and minerals are essential for energy-producing reactions, they do not supply a direct source of energy. Minerals are classified based largely on the amounts needed by the body. The **major minerals** (also called macrominerals) are those having an RDA in amounts greater than 20 milligrams; whereas, the **trace minerals** (also called microminerals) are needed in amounts less than 20 milligrams. Some major minerals include calcium, magnesium, phosphorus, potassium, and sodium. Trace minerals include copper, iron, iodine, manganese, selenium, zinc, and others.

Calcium is a macromineral responsible for functions such as nerve transmission, skeletal muscle contraction, vasoconstriction and vasodilation of blood vessels, and heart rhythm. In addition, adequate intake of calcium is critical for optimal skeletal health. A significant proportion of the U.S. population is at risk for osteoporosis due to low bone density. Low calcium intake is of particular concern among youth ages 9 and older, adolescent girls, adult women, as well as all adults over the age of 51. All age groups are encouraged to meet their RDA for calcium by increasing consumption of fat-free or low-fat dairy products and/or alternative calcium sources (e.g., calcium-fortified orange juice, dark green vegetables, whole almonds).

Sodium is an essential macromineral needed by the body for fluid balance, acid-base balance, contraction of the heart, and conduction of nerve impulses. However, excessive sodium intake causes a proportional increase in blood pressure and subsequent risk for the development of hypertension. Nearly all Americans are estimated to over-consume sodium with the average estimated intake of 3,400 mg per day among those 2 years and older (NCI, 2010). Although a small proportion of the sodium consumed by Americans comes from salt added to foods at the table or during preparation, most sodium comes from processed foods such as yeast breads, chicken mixed dishes, pizza, pasta dishes, and luncheon meats. Americans should strive to reduce daily sodium intake to less than 2,300 milligrams (mg) and further reduce intake to 1,500 mg among persons who are 51 and older and those of any age who are African American or have hypertension, diabetes, or chronic kidney disease (USDA & HHS, 2015).

Whereas dietary intake of sodium is known to be excessively high in the American diet, intake of **potassium** is generally low. Dietary potassium can counteract the negative effects of sodium on blood pressure. In light of the health benefits of adequate dietary potassium, many would benefit from increased consumption of potassium-rich foods such as baked potatoes, carrots, tomatoes, prunes, oranges, and bananas. The AI for potassium for adults is 4,700 mg per day.

Water

Water and proper hydration are critical for life as well as for optimal performance during exercise and athletic activities. Water is among the most abundant molecule in the body, representing more than 70% of lean tissue (e.g., skeletal muscle) and approximately 60% of the total body weight. Water is crucial for many physiological functions within the body including regulation of body temperature, absorption and transportation of nutrients, digestion and elimination of waste products, protection of vital organs, and maintenance of blood volume. Water also serves as the medium for all biochemical reactions and metabolic processes throughout the body.

Proper hydration is maintained through the balance of water ingested with beverages and foods, and fluids lost through sweat, urine, feces, and water vapor in exhaled air. Fluid losses are accelerated during exercise, especially in hot and humid environments, as sweat production increases substantially to dissipate the heat produced through metabolic reactions. Sweat evaporating from the skin provides the cooling effect to assist the body in regulating unsafe elevations of core body temperature. When fluid losses significantly exceed fluid intake, the body is in a state of **dehydration**. Dehydration of 1% to 2% of body weight will begin to compromise physiological functions of the body and will negatively affect exercise and athletic performance (Casa et al., 2000). Physiological functions are further disrupted with dehydration of greater than 3% of body weight and the risk of developing exertional heat illness increases (see chapter 24) (Casa et al., 2000). Although thirst signals the need for fluid intake, the body may already be dehydrated before the sensation of thirst is experienced. Other signs and symptoms of dehydration may include dizziness, fainting, nausea, hypotension (reduced blood pressure), dark-colored urine, and reduced blood flow to the brain. On the other hand, when excessive amounts of water are ingested, overcompensating for fluid loss through sweat, a dangerous condition known as **hyponatremia** may develop. *Exercise-associated hyponatremia (EAH)* is a condition in which the blood's water-to-sodium ratio is severely elevated causing a decrease in plasma sodium concentration (i.e., dilution of salt in the blood) (Hew-Butler et al., 2005). The signs and symptoms of hyponatremia include bloating, (e.g., "puffiness" in face, hands, and feet), acute weight gain, nausea, vomiting and headache (Hew-Butler et al., 2005). In severe cases, more serious signs and symptoms may develop such as swelling of the brain, confusion, disorientation, seizures, respiratory distress, coma, and death (Hew-Butler et al., 2005). Women are particularly susceptible to hyponatremia, especially those with low body weight, slower running

Table 8-5 Fluid Intake

	Fluid Intake Recommendations	
	National Athletic Trainers Association (Casa et al., 2000)	American College of Sports Medicine (Sawka et al., 2007)
Before Exercise	• Drink adequate fluids the day before training. • Drink at least 16-20 oz. (~500 mL) of fluid 2-3 hours before exercise.	• Drink 5-7 mL per kilogram of body weight at least 4 hours before exercise. • Consume beverages with sodium and/or salted snacks to stimulate thirst and to retain needed fluids.
During Exercise	• Replace sweat losses with equivalent volume of fluid. • Drink 8-10 fl. oz. (~200 mL) every 15-20 minutes of exercise. • During exercise > 50-60 minutes, fluids containing electrolytes and carbohydrates (4%-8% concentration) may maintain performance.	• The amount and rate of fluid replacement depends upon the individual sweating rate, exercise duration, and environment. • Individuals should monitor body weight changes during exercise and competition to estimate sweat losses with respect to environmental conditions. • As a general rule, drink ad libitum (freely) from 14-27 fl. oz./hr. (~400-800 mL/hr.) based on body size, pace/intensity, and environment. • For prolonged exercise, "sports beverages" are recommended containing electrolytes (sodium, potassium) and carbohydrates (~5-10% concentration).
After Exercise	• Drink 24 oz. (~700 mL) for every 1 pound of weight lost through sweat. This represents a fluid replacement of 1.5 times weight loss. • Rehydrate within 2-6 hours post-exercise. • Include beverages containing sodium and carbohydrates (for glycogen replenishment).	• Drink ~1.5 L of fluid for each kilogram of body weight lost (24 oz. fluid per pound lost). • Consume beverages and snacks with sodium to stimulate thirst and fluid retention for rapid and complete recovery.

or performance pace, inexperience with endurance racing, excessive fluid consumption behavior, and exercise duration greater than 4 hours (Hew-Butler et al., 2005).

Under normal conditions, most adults need at least 8 to 10, eight ounce glasses (64-80 fl. oz/day) of water per day. Fluid intake must be increased in conjunction with exercise and athletic activities, especially when performed in hot and humid environments. Table 8-5 summarizes fluid intake recommendations before, during, and after exercise.

Chapter Summary

This chapter provided an overview of the digestive system as well as an introduction to the six essential nutrients. The macronutirents including carbohydrates and fats serve many functions including as a substrate for energy production during physical activity and exercise. Protein provides the building blocks for repair and maintenance of tissue. The micronutrients, including vitamins and minerals, serve a variety of functions to maintain the normal physiologic processes of the body. Water is essential for both life and appropriate hydration is necessary to optimize exercise performance.

Chapter References

Atkinson, S.A. (2011). Defining the process of Dietary Reference Intakes: Framework for the United States and Canada. *The American Journal of Clinical Nutrition*, 94(2), 655S-657S.

Buchholz, A.C., & Schoeller, D.A. (2004). Is a calorie a calorie?. *The American Journal of Clinical Nutrition*, 79(5), 899S-906S.

Casa, D.J., Armstrong, L.E., Hillman, S.K., Montain, S.J., Reiff, R.V., Rich, B.S., ... & Stone, J.A. (2000). National Athletic Trainers Association position statement: Fluid replacement for athletes. *Journal of Athletic Training*, 35(2), 212-224.

Dietary Guidelines Advisory Committee. (2015). *Scientific Report of the 2015 Dietary Guidelines Advisory Committee*. Washington (DC): USDA and US Department of Health and Human Services.

Francis, J.J., & Klitzke, C.J. (2010). Dietary reference intakes: Cutting through the confusion. *Nutrition Guide for Physicians*, 65-70.

Hew-Butler, T., Almond, C., Ayus, J.C., Dugas, J., Meeuwisse, W., Noakes, T., ... & Panel, E.A.H.E.C. (2005). Consensus statement of the 1st international exercise-associated hyponatremia consensus development conference, Cape Town, South Africa 2005. *Clinical Journal of Sport Medicine*, 15(4), 208.

Kris-Etherton, P.M., Innis, S., & Ammerican, D.A. (2007). Position of the American Dietetic Association and Dietitians of Canada: Dietary fatty acids. *Journal of the American Dietetic Association*, 107(9), 1599-1611.

Montain, S.J. (2008). Hydration recommendations for sport 2008. *Current Sports Medicine Reports*, 7(4), 187-192.

Mozaffarian, D., Katan, M.B., Ascherio, A., Stampfer, M.J., & Willett, W.C. (2006). *Trans* fatty acids and cardiovascular disease. *New England Journal of Medicine*, 354(15), 1601-1613.

National Cancer Institute (2010). Mean Intake of Sodium, Mean Intake of Energy, and Percentage Sodium Contribution of Various Foods Among US Population, by Age, NHANES 2005–06. http://riskfactor.cancer.gov/diet/foodsources/sodium/table1a.html. Updated December 21, 2010. Accessed March 7, 2013.

Otten, J.J., Hellwig, J.P., & Meyers, L.D. (2006). *Dietary reference intakes (DRI's): The essential guide to nutrient requirements*. Washington, DC: National Academy Press.

Rodriguez, N.R., DiMarco, N.M., & Langley, S. (2009). Position of the American Dietetic Association, Dietitians of Canada, and the American College of Sports Medicine: Nutrition and athletic performance. *Journal of the American Dietetic Association*, 109(3), 509-527.

Ross, A.C., Manson, J.E., Abrams, S.A., Aloia, J.F., Brannon, P.M., Clinton, S.K., ... & Shapses, S.A. (2011). The 2011 dietary reference intakes for calcium and vitamin D: What dietetics practitioners need to know. *Journal of the American Dietetic Association*, 111(4), 524-527.

Sawka, M.N., Burke, L.M., Eichner, E.R., Maughan, R.J., Montain, S.J., & Stachenfeld, N.S. (2007). American College of Sports Medicine, Position stand: Exercise and fluid replacement. *Medicine & Science in Sports & Exercise*, 39(2), 377-390.

Thomas, D.T., Erdman, K.A., & Burke, L.M. (2016). Position of the Academy of Nutrition and Dietetics, Dietitians of Canada, and the American College of Sports Medicine: Nutrition and athletic performance. *Journal of the Academy of Nutrition and Dietetics*, 116(3), 501-528.

U.S. Department of Agriculture and U.S. Department of Health and Human Services (2010). *Dietary Guidelines for Americans, 2010*. 7th edition, Washington, DC: U.S. Government Printing Office.

U.S. Department of Agriculture and U.S. Department of Health and Human Services (2015). *2015-2020 Dietary Guidelines for Americans*, 8th edition. Available at https://health.gov/dietaryguidelines/

Chapter 8 Review Questions

1. According to the recommended macronutrient proportions for adults, what is the maximum amount of fat per day for a 2,200 calorie diet?
    A. 73 grams
    B. 49 grams
    C. 86 grams
    D. 193 grams

2. Which of the following refers to the established nutrient level, based on scientific evidence, to meet the requirements of nearly all healthy individuals?
    A. Estimated Average Requirement (EAR)
    B. Recommended Dietary Allowance (RDA)
    C. Adequate Intake (AI)
    D. Tolerable Upper Intake Level (UL)

3. Which of the following minerals is considered a major mineral (macromineral)?
    A. Iodine
    B. Calcium
    C. Iron
    D. Zinc

4. The dangerous condition in which the blood's water-to-sodium ratio is severely elevated causing a decrease in plasma sodium concentration is known as:
    A. Dehydration
    B. Hypertension
    C. Hyponatremia
    D. Hyperlipidemia

5. Based on pre- and post-weight measurements, it was determined that your client lost 2 pounds of body weight during a 5-kilometer (3.1 miles) run on a hot summer morning. What is the minimum amount of fluid that should be ingested after the race to rehydrate the athlete?
    A. 24 fluid oz.
    B. 36 fluid oz.
    C. 48 fluid oz.
    D. 72 fluid oz.

6. Which of the following is the BEST example of complementary proteins?
    A. Peanut butter and white bread
    B. Black beans and brown rice
    C. Peanut butter and strawberry jelly
    D. Broccoli and ranch veggie dip

Answers to Review Questions on Page 384

Note: Review questions are intended to reinforce learning and comprehension of subject matter presented in the corresponding chapter. The review questions are not intended to be representative of actual certification exam questions in terms of style, content, or difficulty.

9
Dietary Guidelines

Introduction

The U.S. Department of Agriculture (USDA) and the U.S. Department of Health and Human Services (HHS) have jointly published the *Dietary Guidelines for Americans* (DGA) every five years since 1980. Although the early editions were published voluntarily, federal law was passed in 1990 requiring the DGA to be reviewed, updated, and republished every five years (Watts et al., 2011; USDA & HHS, 2015). Although many of the DGA recommendations have remained relatively consistent over time, the Dietary Guidelines has evolved as research has grown and scientific knowledge has advanced (USDA & HHS, 2015). The first several editions of the DGA were relatively simple consumer-oriented brochures. However, in recent years the DGA has expanded and shifted toward more specific recommendations supported by an extensive evidence-based review process conducted by the Dietary Guidelines Advisory Committee (DGAC).

The main purpose of the Dietary Guidelines is to inform the development of Federal food, nutrition, and health policies and programs. It is written for policymakers, as well as nutrition, exercise, and health professionals, not the general public. The Dietary Guidelines is a critical tool for professionals to help Americans make healthy choices in their daily lives, to help prevent chronic disease, and enjoy a healthy diet. Its recommendations are ultimately intended to help individuals improve and maintain overall health and reduce the risk of chronic disease - its focus is disease prevention. The Dietary Guidelines is not intended to be used to treat disease. Regardless of an individual's current health status, almost all people in the United States could benefit from shifting choices to better support healthy eating patterns. Thus, the Dietary Guidelines may be used by fitness professionals to encourage healthy eating patterns for clients, club members, and class participants.

The eighth edition of the Dietary Guidelines provides five overarching Guidelines that encourage healthy eating patterns, recognize that individuals will need to make shifts in their food and beverage choices to achieve a healthy pattern, and acknowledge that all segments of our society have a role to play in supporting healthy choices (USDA & HHS, 2015). Figure 9-2 lists the five Guidelines. In addition, Key Recommendations provide further guidance regarding how individuals can follow the five Guidelines (USDA & HHS, 2015). Figure 9-3 provides the Key Recommendations. This chapter will review the 2015-2020 Dietary Guidelines and the MyPlate graphic, as well as interpretation of the Nutrition Facts label and calculation of macronutrient content of food. Readers are strongly encouraged to review the entire *2015-2020 Dietary Guidelines for Americans* policy document available at https://health.gov/dietaryguidelines/.

Key Elements of Healthy Eating Patterns

About half of all American adults have one or more preventable chronic diseases, many of which are related to poor quality eating patterns and physical inactivity. These include cardiovascular disease, high blood pressure, type 2 diabetes, certain types of cancer, and poor bone health (i.e., osteopenia, osteoporosis). Concurrent with these lifestyle-related health problems persisting at high levels, trends in food intake over time show that, at the population level, Americans are not consuming healthy eating patterns. For example, the prevalence of overweight and obesity has risen and remained high for the past 25 years, while Healthy Eating Index (HEI) scores, a measure of how food choices align with the Dietary Guidelines, have remained low (USDA & HHS, 2015).

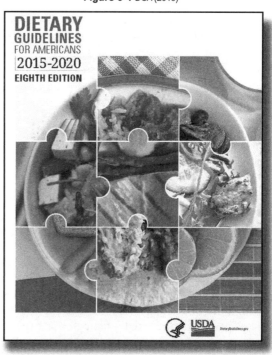

Figure 9-1 DGA (2015)

People do not eat foods and nutrients in isolation but in combination, and this combination forms an overall eating pattern. A growing body of research has examined the relationship between overall eating patterns, health, and risk of chronic disease, and findings on these relationships are sufficiently well established to support dietary guidance. As a result, eating patterns and their food and nutrient characteristics are a primary emphasis of the recommendations in the 2015-2020 edition of the Dietary Guidelines.

An **eating pattern** represents the combination of foods and beverages that constitute an individual's complete dietary intake over time. Often referred to as a 'dietary pattern,' an eating pattern may describe a customary way of eating or a combination of foods recommended for consumption. Throughout the 2015-2020 Dietary Guidelines, the Healthy U.S.-Style Eating Pattern is used to illustrate the specific amounts and limits for food groups and other dietary components that make up healthy eating patterns. Other examples of healthy eating patterns include the Healthy Mediterranean-Style Eating Pattern, the Healthy Vegetarian Eating Pattern, and the Dietary Approaches to Stop Hypertension (DASH) Eating Plan. To learn more about these healthy eating patterns, please refer to the 2015-2020 Dietary Guidelines policy document.

The 2015-2020 Dietary Guidelines for Americans reflects for the first time a robust body of scientific evidence on overall eating patterns and chronic disease. Healthy eating patterns support a healthy body weight and can help prevent and reduce the risk of chronic disease throughout periods of growth, development, and aging as well as during pregnancy. The following principles of healthy eating patterns (also see figure 9-4) apply to meeting the Key Recommendations:

- An **eating pattern** represents the totality of all foods and beverages consumed. All foods consumed as part of a healthy eating pattern fit together like a puzzle to meet nutritional needs without exceeding limits, such as those for saturated fats, added sugars, sodium, and total calories. All forms of foods, including fresh, canned, dried, and frozen, can be included in healthy eating patterns. Eating patterns are more than the sum of their parts and may be more predictive of overall health and disease risk than individual foods or nutrients.

- Nutritional needs should be met primarily from foods. Individuals should aim to meet their nutrient needs through healthy eating patterns that include **nutrient-dense foods**. Foods in nutrient-dense forms contain essential vitamins and minerals and also dietary fiber and other naturally occurring substances that may have positive health effects. In some cases, fortified foods and dietary supplements may be useful in providing one or more nutrients that otherwise may be consumed in less than recommended amounts.

- Healthy eating patterns are adaptable. Individuals have more than one way to achieve a healthy eating pattern. Any eating pattern can be tailored to the individual's socio-cultural and personal preferences

There is more than one type of healthy eating pattern. The Dietary Guidelines embodies the idea that a healthy eating pattern is not a rigid prescription, but rather, an adaptable framework in which individuals can enjoy foods that meet their personal, cultural, and traditional preferences and fit within their budget. Chapter 1 of the *2015-2020 Dietary Guidelines for Americans* policy document focuses on the first three of the five Guidelines listed in figure 9-2.

Key Recommendations of Healthy Eating Patterns

The Dietary Guidelines are supplemented with a number of Key Recommendations that provide more specific guidance on healthy eating patterns. The Dietary Guidelines' Key Recommendations for healthy eating patterns should be applied in their entirety, given the interconnected relationship that each dietary component can have with others. The first Key Recommendation is to *consume a healthy eating pattern that accounts for all foods and beverages within an appropriate calorie level.*

A healthy eating pattern includes:

- *A variety of vegetables from all of the subgroups.* Healthy eating patterns include a variety of vegetables from all five vegetable subgroups including dark green, red and orange, legumes (beans and peas), starchy, and other. Include all fresh, frozen, canned and dried options in cooked or raw forms, including vegetable juices. Vegetables should be consumed in a nutrient-dense form, with limited additions such as salt, butter, or creamy sauces. The recommended amount of vegetables in the Healthy U.S.-Style Eating Pattern at the 2,000-calorie level is 2½ cup-equivalents per day.

- *Fruits*, especially whole fruits, which include fresh, canned, dried, or frozen fruits. The recommended amount of fruits in the Healthy U.S.-Style Eating Pattern at the 2,000-calorie level is 2 cup-equivalents per day.

- *Grains, at least half of which are whole grains.* The recommended amount of grains in the Healthy U.S.-Style Eating Pattern at the 2,000-calorie level is 6 ounce-equivalents per day. When refined grains are chosen, they should be enriched. See figures 9-5 and 9-6 for more information about grains.

- *Fat-free or low-fat dairy*, including milk, yogurt, cheese, and/or fortified soy beverages. Increasing the proportion of dairy intake that is fat-free or low-fat milk or yogurt and decreasing the proportion that is cheese

Figure 9-2 The Guidelines

1. **Follow a healthy eating pattern across the lifespan.** All food and beverage choices matter. Choose a healthy eating pattern at an appropriate calorie level to help achieve and maintain a healthy body weight, support nutrient adequacy, and reduce the risk of chronic disease.
2. **Focus on variety, nutrient density, and amount.** To meet nutrient needs within calorie limits, choose a variety of nutrient-dense foods across and within all food groups in recommended amounts.
3. **Limit calories from added sugars and saturated fats and reduce sodium intake.** Consume an eating pattern low in added sugars, saturated fats, and sodium. Cut back on foods and beverages higher in these components to amounts that fit within healthy eating patterns.
4. **Shift to healthier food and beverage choices.** Choose nutrient-dense foods and beverages across and within all food groups in place of less healthy choices. Consider cultural and personal preferences to make these shifts easier to accomplish and maintain.
5. **Support healthy eating patterns for all.** Everyone has a role in helping to create and support healthy eating patterns in multiple settings nationwide, from home to school to work to communities.

Figure 9-3 Key Recommendations

Consume a healthy eating pattern that accounts for all foods and beverages within an appropriate calorie level. A healthy eating pattern includes:

- A variety of vegetables from all of the subgroups—dark green, red and orange, legumes (beans and peas), starchy, and other
- Fruits, especially whole fruits
- Grains, at least half of which are whole grains
- Fat-free or low-fat dairy, including milk, yogurt, cheese, and/or fortified soy beverages
- A variety of protein foods, including seafood, lean meats and poultry, eggs, legumes (beans and peas), and nuts, seeds, and soy products
- Oils

A healthy eating pattern limits:

- Saturated fats and *trans* fats, added sugars, and sodium

  Key Recommendations that are quantitative are provided for several components of the diet that should be limited. These components are of particular public health concern in the United States, and the specified limits can help individuals achieve healthy eating patterns within calorie limits:

- Consume less than 10 percent of calories per day from added sugars
- Consume less than 10 percent of calories per day from saturated fats
- Consume less than 2,300 milligrams (mg) per day of sodium
- If alcohol is consumed, it should be consumed in moderation—up to one drink per day for women and up to two drinks per day for men—and only by adults of legal drinking age

In tandem with these recommendations, Americans of all ages—children, adolescents, adults, and older adults—should meet the Physical Activity Guidelines for Americans to help promote health and reduce the risk of chronic disease. Americans should aim to achieve and maintain a healthy body weight. The relationship between diet and physical activity contributes to calorie balance and managing body weight. As such, the Dietary Guidelines includes a Key Recommendation to:

- Meet the Physical Activity Guidelines for Americans

Figure 9-4 Principles of Healthy Eating Patterns

An eating pattern represents the totality of all foods and beverages consumed
▶ It is more than the sum of its parts; the totality of what individuals habitually eat and drink act synergistically in relation to health.

Nutritional needs should be met primarily from foods
▶ Individuals should aim to meet their nutrient needs through healthy eating patterns that include foods in nutrient-dense forms.

Healthy eating patterns are adaptable
▶ Any eating pattern can be tailored to the individual's socio-cultural and personal preferences.

(USDA & HHS, 2015)

would decrease saturated fats and sodium and increase potassium, vitamin A, and vitamin D provided from the dairy group. The recommended amount of dairy in the Healthy U.S.-Style Eating Pattern is based on age rather than calorie level. For adolescents ages 9 to 18 years and for adults, the recommendation is 3 cup-equivalents per day.

- *A variety of protein foods*, including seafood, lean meats and poultry, eggs, legumes (beans and peas), and nuts, seeds, and soy products. The recommendation for protein foods in the Healthy U.S.-Style Eating Pattern at the 2,000-calorie level is 5½ ounce-equivalents per day. See figure 9-7 for more information about seafood.

- *Oils* including: canola, corn, olive, peanut, safflower, soybean, and sunflower oils. Oils also are naturally present in nuts, seeds, seafood, olives, and avocados. Oils are fats that contain a high percentage of monounsaturated and polyunsaturated fats and are liquid a room temperature. Although they are not a food group, oils are emphasized as part of healthy eating patterns because they are a major source of essential fatty acids and vitamin E. The recommendation for oils in the Healthy U.S.-Style Eating Pattern at the 2,000-calorie level is 27 grams (about 5 teaspoons) per day.

Chapter 1 of the *2015-2020 Dietary Guidelines for Americans* policy document also includes discussion of the quantitative Key Recommendations for several components of the diet that should be limited. These components are of particular public health concern in the United States, and the specified limits can help individuals achieve healthy eating patterns within calorie limits:

- *Consume less than 10 percent of calories per day from added sugars*. The added sugars recommendation is a target based on food pattern modeling and national data on intakes of calories from added sugars. This target demonstrates the public health need to limit calories from added sugars to meet food group and nutrient needs within calorie limits. When added sugars exceed 10% of calories, a healthy eating pattern may be difficult to achieve.

- *Consume less than 10 percent of calories per day from saturated fats*. The recommendation to consume less than 10 percent of calories per day as saturated fats is a target based on evidence that replacing saturated fats with unsaturated fats is associated with reduced risk of cardiovascular disease. However, replacing saturated fats with carbohydrates is not associated with reduced risk of cardiovascular disease. Individuals should limit intake of *trans* fats to as low as possible by limiting foods that contain synthetic sources of *trans* fats, such as partially hydrogenated oils, and by limiting other solid fats. See figure 9-8 for more information about fat and cholesterol.

- *Consume less than 2,300 milligrams per day of sodium*. Americans are encouraged to follow the age- and sex-appropriate Tolerable Upper Intake Levels (ULs) for sodium set by the Institute of Medicine. The UL is 2,300 milligrams per day for individuals ages 14 years and older. The recommendations for children younger than 14 years of age are the IOM age- and sex-appropriate ULs, which vary from 1,500 to 2,200, depending on age. For adults with hypertension or prehypertension, further reduction to 1,500 mg per day can result in greater blood pressure reduction.

- *If alcohol is consumed, it should be consumed in moderation*—up to one drink per day for women and up to two drinks per day for men—and only by adults of legal drinking age. It is not recommended that individuals begin drinking or drink more for any reason, and there are many circumstances in which individuals should not drink, such as during pregnancy. See figure 9-9.

Shifting Toward Healthy Eating Patterns

Chapter 2 of the *2015-2020 Dietary Guidelines for Americans* policy document focuses on current food intakes among Americans and the shifts needed for Americans to align with healthy eating patterns. As such, chapter 2 focuses on the fourth Dietary Guideline: *Shift to healthier food and beverage choices*.

The typical eating patterns currently consumed by many in the United States do not align with the Dietary Guidelines. When compared to the Healthy U.S.-Style Eating Pattern:
- About three-fourths of the population has an eating pattern that is low in vegetables, fruits, dairy, and oils.
- More than half of the population is meeting or exceeding total grain and total protein foods recommendations, but are not meeting the recommendations for the subgroups within each of these food groups.
- Most Americans exceed the recommendations for added sugars, saturated fats, and sodium.

In addition, the eating patterns of many are too high in calories. Calorie intake over time, in comparison to calorie needs, is best evaluated by measuring body weight status. The high percentage of the population that is overweight or obese suggests that many in the United States overconsume calories. This overconsumption, when coupled with insufficient energy expenditure through regular physical activity, has resulted in more than two-thirds of all adults and nearly one-third of all children and youth in the United States being either overweight or obese.

Making changes to eating patterns can be overwhelming.

Figure 9-5 Understanding Grains

A food made from wheat, rice, oats, cornmeal, barley, or another cereal grain is called a grain product. Grains are categorized into two subgroups: whole grains and refined grains. Whole grains contain the entire grain kernel, which includes the bran, germ, and endosperm. **See figure 9-6**. Refined grains have been milled to remove the bran and germ giving them a smoother texture and a longer shelf life. The refining process also removes nutrients such as dietary fiber, iron, and many B vitamins. Most refined grains are 'enriched' when the B vitamins (thiamin, riboflavin, niacin, folic acid) and iron are added back in after the refining process. Multi-grain foods contain several types of grain; however, this does not indicate that it is a whole grain food. In fact, there may not be any whole grains in a multi-grain product.

Most Americans are likely to consume enough total grains; however, most of those consumed are refined grains rather than whole grains. Some research has indicated that increased whole grain consumption may reduce the risk of cardiovascular disease, is correlated with a lower body weight, and may reduce the incidence of type 2 diabetes. It is recommended that Americans strive to replace refined grain foods with whole grain foods so that at least half of the total daily grain intake is derived from nutrient-dense whole grain foods.

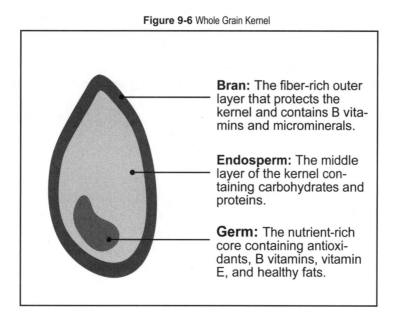

Figure 9-6 Whole Grain Kernel

Bran: The fiber-rich outer layer that protects the kernel and contains B vitamins and microminerals.

Endosperm: The middle layer of the kernel containing carbohydrates and proteins.

Germ: The nutrient-rich core containing antioxidants, B vitamins, vitamin E, and healthy fats.

Figure 9-7 About Seafood

Seafood, which includes fish and shellfish, are excellent sources of the heart-healthy omega-3 fatty acids including eicosapentaenoic acid (EPA) and docosahexaenoic acid (DHA). For the general population, consumption of about 8 ounces per week of a variety of seafood, which provide an average consumption of 250 mg per day of EPA and DHA, is associated with reduced cardiac deaths among individuals with or without preexisting cardiovascular disease (CVD). Strong research-based evidence has shown that eating patterns that include seafood are associated with reduced risk of CVD, and moderate evidence indicates these eating patterns are associated with reduced risk of obesity.

However, care must be used in the selection of seafood to avoid those high in methyl mercury. Women who are pregnant or breastfeeding should be particularly cautious and are encouraged to avoid tilefish, shark, swordfish, and king mackerel, which are all high in mercury. Seafood varieties commonly consumed in the United States that are higher in EPA and DHA, yet lower in methyl mercury include salmon, anchovies, herring, shad, sardines, Pacific oysters, trout, and Atlantic and Pacific mackerel.

Figure 9-8 Fat and Cholesterol

The National Academy of Medicine (formerly the Institute of Medicine) recommends that adults ages 19 years and older consume 20-35% of their daily calories from fat in order to reduce the risk of chronic diseases (IOM, 2005). The types of fatty acids consumed are perhaps more important than the total amount of fat in the diet with regard to risk of cardiovascular disease (USDA & HHS, 2010). A higher consumption of saturated fatty acids and *trans* fatty acids is associated with higher total blood cholesterol and low-density lipoprotein (LDL), the 'bad' cholesterol, both of which are associated with greater risk of cardiovascular disease. As noted in chapter 8, most fats containing a higher proportion of saturated or *trans* fatty acids are solid at room temperature and are therefore called solid fats. The most prominent sources of fatty acids in the American diet include full-fat cheese, pizza, grain-based desserts, dairy desserts, chicken and chicken mixed dishes, sausage, franks, bacon, and ribs (NCI, 2010).

Cholesterol is a waxy, fat-like substance found only in animal food products such as meats, poultry, organ meats, dairy products, and eggs. The human body also produces cholesterol in the liver at a level sufficient to fulfill its physiological and structural functions in the body. Therefore, it is not necessary to consume dietary sources of cholesterol. Nevertheless, cholesterol consumption exceeds recommended levels for many Americans, which increases blood cholesterol level, contributes to atherosclerosis of blood vessels, and the subsequent risk of cardiovascular disease. Individuals should eat as little dietary cholesterol as possible while consuming a healthy eating pattern. The Healthy U.S.-Style Eating Pattern contains approximately 100 to 300 mg of cholesterol across the 12 calorie levels (USDA & HHS, 2015).

Cholesterol is a major component of cell membranes and is needed for the formation of bile salts, vitamin D, and various hormones including estrogen and testosterone. Cholesterol is transported through the blood by molecules containing both fats and proteins, called lipoproteins. The lipoproteins are classified as low-density lipoproteins (LDLs) and high-density lipoproteins (HDLs) as well as very low-density lipoproteins (VLDLs). The combination of all lipoproteins in the blood represents the total serum cholesterol measured in milligrams per deciliter (mg/dL) of blood. The LDLs are the major carrier of cholesterol and lipids in the blood. LDLs have been labeled the 'bad' cholesterol since they contribute to the accumulation of plaque in the arteries causing atherosclerosis. Therefore, it is desirable to maintain a lower level of LDLs in the blood. The HDLs are considered to be the 'good' cholesterol and a higher level is desirable. HDLs are cholesterol scavengers working to transport cholesterol and lipids to the liver for metabolism and excretion. An individual's blood cholesterol profile is influenced by genetics as well as lifestyle behaviors such as diet and physical activity. Diets high in saturated fatty acids also tend to be high in cholesterol. Regular physical activity and exercise are associated with a reduction in total cholesterol, a reduction in LDLs, and an increase in HDLs, thus creating a healthier cholesterol profile. Table 9-1 provides the recommended blood cholesterol and triglyceride levels adopted from Cleeman et al., (2001).

Figure 9-9 Alcohol Consumption

Moderate alcohol consumption is defined as up to 1 drink per day for women and 2 drinks per day for men. One drink contains 0.6 fluid ounces of alcohol such as that contained in 12 fluid ounces of regular beer, 5 fluid ounces of wine, or 1.5 fluid ounces of 80 proof distilled spirits. When consumed in moderation, alcohol may provide some health benefits such as a lower risk of cardiovascular disease and a reduced risk of all-cause mortality among middle-aged and older adults (Nova et al., 2012). However, moderate alcohol consumption is also associated with adverse health effects and incidents such as increased risk of breast cancer, violence, drowning, and injuries sustained from falls or motor vehicle accidents. In addition, heavy alcohol consumption is associated with numerous health problems including cirrhosis of the liver, hypertension, stroke, various types of cancer, psychological disorders, and fetal alcohol syndrome (Rehm et al., 2010). Therefore, it is not recommended that non-drinkers begin to consume alcohol or that light-to-moderate drinkers increase their consumption.

Therefore, it is important to emphasize that every food choice is an opportunity to move toward a healthy eating pattern. Small shifts in food and beverage choices over the course of a week, a day, or even a meal can make a big difference. Here are a few examples (see also figure 9-10) of realistic shift strategies that can help people adopt healthy eating patterns:

- Increase vegetables in mixed dishes while decreasing the amounts of refined grains or meats high in saturated fat and/or sodium.
- Incorporate seafood in meals twice per week in place of meat, poultry, or eggs.
- Use vegetable oil in place of solid fats when cooking, and use oil-based dressings and spreads on foods instead of those made from solid fats.
- Choose beverages with no added sugars, such as water.
- Read the Nutrition Facts label to compare sodium content of foods and select the product with less sodium.

Figure 9-10 Healthy Shifts

High Calorie Snacks → Nutrient-Dense Snacks
Fruit Products with Added Sugars → Fruit
Refined Grains → Whole Grains
Snacks with Added Salt → Unsalted Snacks
Solid Fats → Oils
Beverages with Added Sugars → No-Sugar Added Beverages

Everyone Has a Role

Collective action is needed to create a new paradigm in which healthy lifestyle choices at home, school, work, and in the community are easy, accessible, affordable, and normative. Everyone has a role in helping individuals shift their everyday food, beverage, and physical activity choices to align with the Dietary Guidelines. Chapter 3 of the Dietary Guidelines policy document focuses on the fifth Guideline: *Support healthy eating patterns for all*.

As shown in the Social-Ecological Model (figure 9-11), a multitude of choices, messages, individual resources, and other factors affect the food and physical activity choices an individual makes, and these decisions are rarely made in isolation. The scientific literature has described a number of specific circumstances that can limit an individual's or family's capacity to choose a healthy diet. These contextual factors—food access, household food insecurity, and acculturation—are particularly important for millions of individuals living in the United States. As appropriate, fitness professionals can consider these critical factors when developing strategies and providing education to enhance the adoption of healthy eating patterns and regular physical activity.

Food Access - Having access to healthy, safe, and affordable food choices is crucial for an individual to achieve a healthy eating pattern. Food access is influenced by

Table 9-1 Cholesterol Guidelines

	Total Cholesterol	LDLs	HDLs	Triglycerides
Optimal	< 200	< 100	≥ 60	≤ 150
Borderline	200–239	100 – 159	40 – 59	150–199
High Risk	≥ 240	≥ 160	< 40	≥ 200

All values expressed in milliliters per deciliter (mg/dL) of blood. Adopted from the Third Report of the National Cholesterol Education Program Expert Panel on Detection, Evaluation, and Treatment of High Blood Cholesterol in Adults (2001).

diverse factors, including proximity to food retail outlets (e.g., distance to a store or the number of stores in an area), individual resources (e.g., income or personal transportation), and neighborhood-level resources (e.g., average income of the neighborhood and availability of public transportation). Race/ethnicity, socioeconomic status, geographic location, and the presence of a disability also may affect an individual's ability to access foods to support healthy eating patterns.

Household Food Insecurity - In the United States, about 48 million individuals live in households that experience food insecurity, which occurs when access to nutritionally adequate and safe food is limited or uncertain. Food insecurity can be temporary or persist over time. Living with food insecurity challenges a household's ability to obtain food and make healthy choices and can exacerbate stress and chronic disease risk. Government and nongovernment nutrition assistance programs play an essential role in providing food and educational resources to help individuals make healthy food choices within their budget.

Acculturation - Individuals who come to this country may adopt the attitudes, values, customs, beliefs, and behaviors of the new culture as well as its dietary habits. Healthy eating patterns are designed to be flexible in order to accommodate traditional and cultural foods. Individuals are encouraged to retain the healthy aspects of their eating and physical activity patterns and avoid adopting behaviors that are less healthy.

To shift from current eating patterns to those that align with the Dietary Guidelines, collective action across all segments of society is needed. As previously described, these actions must involve a broad range of sectors, occur across a variety of settings, and address the needs of individuals, families, and communities. These actions include identifying and addressing successful approaches for change; improving knowledge of what constitutes healthy eating and physical activity patterns; enhancing access to adequate amounts of healthy, safe, and affordable food choices; and promoting change in social and cultural norms and values to embrace, support, and maintain healthy eating and physical activity behaviors.

MyPlate

The Dietary Guidelines is developed and written for a professional audience. Therefore, its translation into actionable consumer messages and resources is crucial to help

Figure 9-5 Sample Label

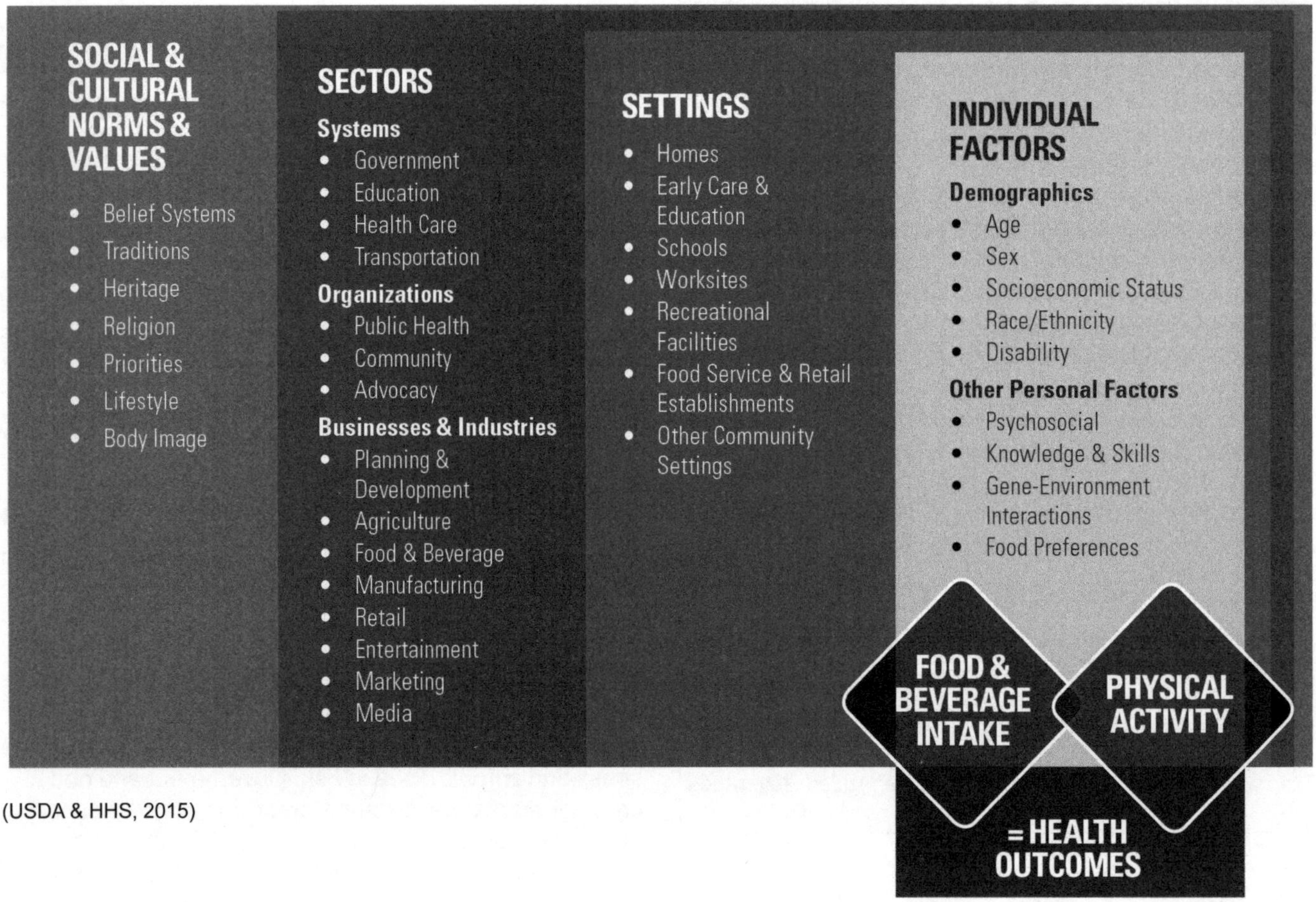

SOCIAL & CULTURAL NORMS & VALUES
- Belief Systems
- Traditions
- Heritage
- Religion
- Priorities
- Lifestyle
- Body Image

SECTORS
Systems
- Government
- Education
- Health Care
- Transportation

Organizations
- Public Health
- Community
- Advocacy

Businesses & Industries
- Planning & Development
- Agriculture
- Food & Beverage
- Manufacturing
- Retail
- Entertainment
- Marketing
- Media

SETTINGS
- Homes
- Early Care & Education
- Schools
- Worksites
- Recreational Facilities
- Food Service & Retail Establishments
- Other Community Settings

INDIVIDUAL FACTORS
Demographics
- Age
- Sex
- Socioeconomic Status
- Race/Ethnicity
- Disability

Other Personal Factors
- Psychosocial
- Knowledge & Skills
- Gene-Environment Interactions
- Food Preferences

FOOD & BEVERAGE INTAKE + PHYSICAL ACTIVITY = HEALTH OUTCOMES

(USDA & HHS, 2015)

individuals, families, and communities achieve healthy eating patterns. Over the years, the USDA has produced several consumer-oriented graphics to guide healthy dietary choices. See figure 9-12.

Beginning in 1992, the original Food Pyramid served as a teaching tool and resource to support the Dietary Guidelines (Post, 2011). In 2005, the original pyramid was replaced by the MyPyramid icon, which was intended to symbolize the nutrition principles of proportionality, variety, moderation, gradual improvement, physical activity, and personalization (Post, 2011). In response to criticism regarding the perceived complexity of this graphic, the MyPlate icon was introduced as a replacement in 2011. MyPlate was launched as a component of a larger communications initiative based on and in support of the *2010 Dietary Guidelines for Americans* to help consumers make better food choices. It is designed to remind Americans to eat healthfully, but alone is not intended to change consumer behavior. MyPlate illustrates the five food groups utilized in the USDA's Healthy U.S.-Style Eating Patterns using the familiar and simplistic mealtime place setting. To learn more about MyPlate and supporting resources, please visit http://www.choosemyplate.gov.

Nutrition Facts Label

The Nutrition Labeling and Education Act of 1990, which went into effect in May 1994, mandated that all pre-packaged foods display a nutrition label, with the exception of foods intended for immediate consumption (e.g., fresh produce) (Campos et al., 2011). Presently, the Food and Drug Administration (FDA) regulates the labeling on all packaged foods, as well as health claims and nutrient content claims. The current regulations require the Nutrition Facts label to include information on serving size, number of servings, total calories, calories from fat, total fat, saturated fat, cholesterol, sodium, carbohydrates, dietary fiber, sugar, protein, vitamin A, vitamin C, calcium, iron, and *trans* fat (Ollberding et al., 2010). Information regarding additional nutrients may be included on a voluntary basis. Please reference Figure 9-13 with regard to the following interpretation of a Nutrition Facts label.

Serving Size

This section is the basis for determining the number of calories, amount of each nutrient, and percent daily values (%DV) of a food. It is used to compare a serving size to the amount of food actually consumed. Serving sizes are given in familiar units, such as cups or pieces, followed by the metric unit (e.g., number of grams).

Amount of Calories

The amount of calories per serving is listed on the left side of the Nutrition Facts label. The right side of that panel indicates how many calories in one serving are derived from fat. In the sample label provided, there are 250 calories, 110 of which come from fat.

Percent (%) Daily Value

The column down the right side of the label indicates the percent of daily value (%DV) based on a 2,000-calorie diet. Each listed nutrient is based on 100% of the recommended amounts for that nutrient. For example, 20% for sodium indicates that one serving provides 20% of the total amount of sodium that you could consume in a day while staying within the recommended guidelines (i.e., upper limit of 2,300 mg/day). As a rule, 5%DV or less is considered 'low' and 20%DV or more is considered 'high' for one serving.

Limit these Nutrients

Consumption of too much total fat (including saturated fat and *trans* fat), cholesterol, or sodium may increase the risk of certain chronic diseases including heart disease, certain cancers, and high blood pressure. The goal is to stay below 100% DV for each of these nutrients each day.

Get Enough of these Nutrients

Many Americans don't consume enough dietary fiber, vitamin A, vitamin C, calcium, and iron in their diets. Eating enough of these nutrients may improve individual health and help reduce the risk of some diseases and conditions.

Footnote with Daily Values (DVs)

The footnote provides information about the DVs for important nutrients, including fats, sodium, and fiber. The DVs are listed for people who consume 2,000 or 2,500 calories per day. The amounts for total fat, saturated fat, cholesterol, and sodium are maximum amounts. Consumers should try to stay below the amounts listed for the corresponding caloric intake.

Calculating Macronutrients in Foods

The percent of calories represented by each macronutrient (i.e., fat, carbohydrates, and protein) can be calculated using the gram-to-calorie conversions presented in chapter 8. Remember, 1 gram of fat = 9 Calories; 1 gram of carbohydrate = 4 Calories; and 1 gram of protein = 4 Calories. The percentages derived from these calculations should not be confused with the percent Daily Values (%DV). The %DV represents the percent of fat or carbohydrates at the upper limit of the recommended macronutrient range based on a 2,000 calorie diet. The Acceptable Macronutrient Distribution Ranges (AMDR) for adults are 20-35% of total daily calories from fat, 45-65% from carbohydrates, and 10-35% from protein (see table 9-2). These recommendations should help to guide the selection of foods that support the maintenance of this overall macronutrient distribution in the daily diet. When perform-

Figure 9-13 Nutrition Facts Label

Nutrition Facts	
Serving Size 1 cup (228g)	
Servings Per Container 2	
Amount Per Serving	
Calories 250	Calories from Fat 110
	% Daily Value*
Total Fat 12g	18%
Saturated Fat 3g	15%
Trans Fat 1.5g	
Cholesterol 30mg	10%
Sodium 470mg	20%
Total Carbohydrate 31g	10%
Dietary Fiber 0g	0%
Sugars 5g	
Protein 5g	
Vitamin A	4%
Vitamin C	2%
Calcium	20%
Iron	4%

* Percent Daily Values are based on a 2,000 calorie diet. Your Daily Values may be higher or lower depending on your calorie needs:

	Calories:	2,000	2,500
Total Fat	Less than	65g	80g
Sat Fat	Less than	20g	25g
Cholesterol	Less than	300mg	300mg
Sodium	Less than	2,400mg	2,400mg
Total Carbohydrate		300g	375g
Dietary Fiber		25g	30g

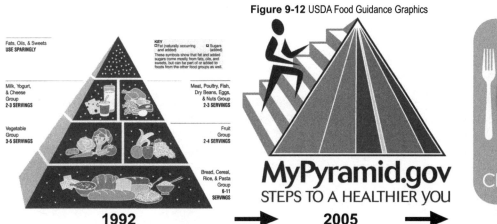

Figure 9-12 USDA Food Guidance Graphics

1992 → 2005 → 2011

ing the macronutrient calculations, we seek to answer the question, "What percent of the total calories in one serving of this food item are represented by fat, carbohydrates, or protein."

The sample Nutrition Facts label in figure 9-14 will be used to guide the sample macronutrient calculations provided in figure 9-15. Based on these calculations, one can conclude that this particular food item is significantly above the recommended range for fat, slightly below the lower limit of the recommended range for carbohydrates, and slightly below the lower limit recommendation for protein.

Table 9-2 AMDR

Acceptable Macronutrient Distribution Range (AMDR) for Adults (Percent of Total Daily Calories)		
Fat	Carbohydrates	Protein
20-35%	45-65%	10-35%

Updates to the Nutrition Facts Label

The Nutrition Facts label, introduced over 20 years ago, helps consumers make informed food choices and maintain healthy dietary practices. In May 2016, the U.S. Food and Drug Administration (FDA) announced the new Nutrition Facts label for packaged foods to reflect new scientific information, including the link between diet and chronic diseases such as obesity and heart disease (FDA, 2016). Food manufacturers will need to use the new label by July 26, 2018. However, manufacturers with less than $10 million in annual food sales will have an additional year to comply (FDA, 2016). The highlights of the new Nutrition Facts label (see figure 9-16) are provided below.

1. Features a Refreshed Design
- The "iconic" look of the label remains, but the FDA is making important updates to ensure consumers have access to the information they need to make informed decisions about the foods they eat. These changes include increasing the type size for "Calories," "servings per container," and the "Serving size" declaration, and bolding the number of calories and the "Serving size" declaration to highlight this information.
- Manufacturers must declare the actual amount, in addition to percent Daily Value of vitamin D, calcium, iron and potassium. They can voluntarily declare the gram amount for other vitamins and minerals.
- The footnote is changing to better explain what percent Daily Value means. It will read: "*The % Daily Value tells you how much a nutrient in a serving of food contributes to a daily diet. 2,000 calories a day is used for general nutrition advice."

Figure 9-14 Sample Label

Nutrition Facts

Serving Size 1 serving (251 g)
Servings Per Container 6

Amount Per Serving

Calories 198   **Calories from Fat** 90

% Daily Value*

Total Fat 10g	**15**%
Saturated Fat 2g	**10**%
Trans Fat 0g	
Cholesterol 0mg	**0**%
Sodium 220mg	**9**%
Total Carbohydrate 23g	**8**%
Dietary Fiber 6g	**24**%
Sugars 3g	
Proteins 4g	

Vitamin A 410%   •   Vitamin C 160%

Calcium 15%   •   Iron 25%

* Percent Daily Values are based on a 2,000 calorie diet. Your Daily Values may be higher or lower depending on your calorie needs:

	Calories:	2,000	2,500
Total Fat	Less than	65g	80g
Saturated Fat	Less than	20g	25g
Cholesterol	Less than	300mg	300mg
Sodium	Less than	2,400mg	2,400mg
Total Carbohydrate		300g	375g
Dietary Fiber		25g	30g

2. Reflects Updated Information about Nutrition Science
- "Added sugars," in grams and as percent Daily Value, will be included on the label. Scientific data shows that it is difficult to meet nutrient needs while staying within calorie limits if you consume more than 10 percent of your total daily calories from added sugar, and this is consistent with the *2015-2020 Dietary Guidelines for Americans*.
- The list of nutrients that are required or permitted to be declared is being updated. Vitamin D and potassium will be required on the label. Calcium and iron will continue to be required. Vitamins A and C will no longer be required, but can be included on a voluntary basis.

Figure 9-15 Sample Calculations

Sample Macronutrient Calculations:

Step One: **Grams of fat x 9 kcal/gram = Calories from fat**
10 grams x 9 kcal/gram = 90 Calories from fat

Step Two: **Grams of carbohydrates x 4 kcal/gram = Calories from carbohydrates**
23 grams x 4 kcal/gram = 92 Calories from carbohydrates

Step Three: **Grams of protein x 4 kcal/gram = Calories from protein**
4 grams x 4 kcal/gram = 16 Calories from protein

Step Four: **Macronutrient Calories ÷ total Calories = macronutrient percent of total Calories**
% from fat = 90 ÷ 198 = 45% of the total Calories are fat
% from carbohydrates = 92 ÷ 198 = 47% of the total Calories are carbohydrates
% from protein = 16 ÷ 198 = 8% of the total Calories are protein

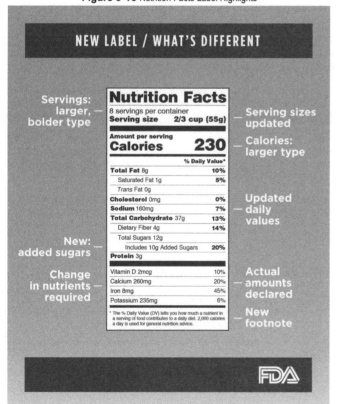

Figure 9-16 Nutrition Facts Label Highlights

Figure 9-17 Sample Dual Column Label

Nutrition Facts				
2 servings per container				
Serving size			1 cup (255g)	
	Per serving		Per container	
Calories	**220**		**440**	
		% DV*		% DV*
Total Fat	5g	6%	10g	13%
Saturated Fat	2g	10%	4g	20%
Trans Fat	0g		0g	
Cholesterol	15mg	5%	30mg	10%
Sodium	240mg	10%	480mg	21%
Total Carb.	35g	13%	70g	25%
Dietary Fiber	6g	21%	12g	43%
Total Sugars	7g		14g	
Incl. Added Sugars	4g	8%	8g	16%
Protein	9g		18g	
Vitamin D	5mcg	25%	10mcg	50%
Calcium	200mg	15%	400mg	30%
Iron	1mg	6%	2mg	10%
Potassium	470mg	10%	940mg	20%

* The % Daily Value (DV) tells you how much a nutrient in a serving of food contributes to a daily diet. 2,000 calories a day is used for general nutrition advice.

- While continuing to require "Total Fat," "Saturated Fat," and "*Trans* Fat" on the label, "Calories from Fat" is being removed because research shows the type of fat is more important than the amount.
- Daily values for nutrients like sodium, dietary fiber, and vitamin D are being updated based on newer scientific evidence from the Institute of Medicine and other reports such as the *2015 Dietary Guidelines Advisory Committee Report*, which was used in developing the *2015-2020 Dietary Guidelines for Americans*. Daily values are reference amounts of nutrients to consume or not to exceed and are used to calculate the percent Daily Value (% DV) that manufacturers include on the label. The % DV helps consumers understand the nutrition information in the context of a total daily diet.

3. Updates Serving Sizes and Labeling Requirements for Certain Package Sizes

- By law, serving sizes must be based on amounts of foods and beverages that people are actually eating, not what they should be eating. How much people eat and drink has changed since the previous serving size requirements were published in 1993. For example, the reference amount used to set a serving of ice cream was previously ½ cup, but is changing to ⅔ cup. The reference amount used to set a serving of soda is changing from 8 ounces to 12 ounces.
- Package size affects what people eat. So for packages that are between one and two servings, such as a 20-ounce soda or a 15-ounce can of soup, the calories and other nutrients will be required to be labeled as one serving because people typically consume it in one sitting.

For certain products that are larger than a single serving but that could be consumed in one sitting or multiple sittings, manufacturers will have to provide "dual column" labels to indicate the amount of calories and nutrients on both a "per serving" and "per package" or "per unit" basis. See figure 9-17. Examples would be a 24-ounce bottle of soda or a pint of ice cream. With dual-column labels available, people will be able to easily understand how many calories and nutrients they are getting if they eat or drink the entire package or unit at one time.

Chapter Summary

The Dietary Guidelines for Americans provide science-based recommendations to improve the overall health of the population. The Guidelines include balancing calories to manage weight, foods and food components to reduce, foods and nutrients to increase, and healthy eating patterns to adopt. Nutrition Facts labels can assist consumers to select healthier foods to stay within their caloric needs.

Chapter References

Campos, S., Doxey, J., & Hammond, D. (2011). Nutrition labels on pre-packaged foods: A systematic review. *Public Health Nutrition,* 14(8), 1496-1507.

Cleeman, J.I., Grundy, S.M., Becker, D., & Clark, L.T. (2001). Expert panel on Detection, Evaluation and Treatment of High Blood Cholesterol in Adults. Executive Summary of the Third Report of the National Cholesterol Education Program (NCEP) Adult Treatment Panel (ATP III). *Journal of the American Medical Association,* 285(19), 2486-2497.

Institute of Medicine (2005). Panel on Macronutrients, & Institute of Medicine (US). Standing Committee on the Scientific Evaluation of Dietary Reference Intakes. *Dietary reference intakes for energy, carbohydrate, fiber, fat, fatty acids, cholesterol, protein, and amino acids.* National Academy Press.

National Cancer Institute (2010). Top Food Sources of Saturated Fat among US Population, NHANES 2005-06. http://riskfactor.cancer.gov/diet/foodsources/sat_fat/sf.html#f_b. Updated May 24, 2010. Accessed March 8, 2013.

Nova, E., Baccan, G.C., Veses, A., Zapatera, B., & Marcos, A. (2012). Potential health benefits of moderate alcohol consumption: current perspectives in research. *The Proceedings of the Nutrition Society,* 71(2), 307-315.

Ollberding, N.J., Wolf, R.L., & Contento, I. (2010). Food label use and its relation to dietary intake among US adults. *Journal of the American Dietetic Association,* 110(8), 1233-1237.

Post, R.C. (2011). A new approach to dietary guidelines communications: Make MyPlate, your plate. *Childhood Obesity (Formerly Obesity and Weight Management),* 7(5), 349-351.

Rehm, J., Baliunas, D., Borges, G L., Graham, K., Irving, H., Kehoe, T., ... & Taylor, B. (2010). The relation between different dimensions of alcohol consumption and burden of disease: An overview. *Addiction,* 105(5), 817-843.

U.S. Department of Agriculture and U.S. Department of Health and Human Services (2015). *2015-2020 Dietary Guidelines for Americans,* 8th edition. Available at https://health.gov/dietaryguidelines/.

U.S. Department of Agriculture and U.S. Department of Health and Human Services (2010). *Dietary Guidelines for Americans, 2010.* 7th edition, Washington, DC: U.S. Government Printing Office.

U.S. Food and Drug Administration (2016). Changes to the Nutrition Facts Label. Available at: http://www.fda.gov/Food/GuidanceRegulation/GuidanceDocumentsRegulatoryInformation/LabelingNutrition/ucm385663.htm. Accessed on August 9, 2016.

Watts, M.L., Hager, M.H., Toner, C.D., & Weber, J.A. (2011). The art of translating nutritional science into dietary guidance: History and evolution of the Dietary Guidelines for Americans. *Nutrition Reviews,* 69(7), 404-412.

Recommended Reading

U.S. Department of Agriculture and U.S. Department of Health and Human Services (2015). *2015-2020 Dietary Guidelines for Americans,* 8th edition. Available at https://health.gov/dietaryguidelines/.

Chapter 9 Review Questions

1. A candy bar has 14 grams of fat, 25 grams of carbohydrates, and 6 grams of protein. What percent of the total calories are fat?
    - A. 50 %
    - B. 40 %
    - C. 22 %
    - D. 10 %

2. It is recommended to reduce daily sodium intake to _____ or less among those who are 51 years and older, and those of any age who are African American or have hypertension, diabetes, or chronic kidney disease.
    - A. 2,300 mg
    - B. 4,700 mg
    - C. 1,500 mg
    - D. 1,900 mg

3. It is recommended that Americans consume less than _____ of daily calories from saturated fats by replacing them with mono- and polyunsaturated fatty acids.
    - A. 35 %
    - B. 10 %
    - C. 40 %
    - D. 20 %

4. The Percent Daily Values (%DV) provided on a Nutrition Facts label are based on a _____ calorie diet.
    - A. 1,200
    - B. 3,000
    - C. 2,500
    - D. 2,000

5. The Adequate Intake (AI) of dietary fiber for an adult female is currently set at _____ per day.
    - A. 14 grams
    - B. 38 grams
    - C. 25 grams
    - D. 45 grams

6. A banana-walnut muffin contains 450 calories, 46 grams of carbohydrates, and 6 grams of protein. What percent of the total calories come from fat?
    - A. 54 %
    - B. 27 %
    - C. 14 %
    - D. 40 %

Answers to Review Questions on Page 384

Note: Review questions are intended to reinforce learning and comprehension of subject matter presented in the corresponding chapter. The review questions are not intended to be representative of actual certification exam questions in terms of style, content, or difficulty.

10
Weight Management

Introduction

The achievement and maintenance of a healthy body weight is perhaps the most common goal among those seeking the services of a fitness professional. Weight management can be defined as the desire to lose, gain, or maintain body weight. Weight management principles are similar regardless of an individual's goal and are based on the concept of energy balance (i.e., caloric balance). This chapter reviews principles and guidelines related to safe and effective weight management. With the growing epidemic of both adult and childhood obesity in the United States, fitness professionals play a key role in assisting clients toward the achievement of a healthy weight.

The Prevalence and Impact of Obesity

Obesity is a chronic disease of complex, multifactorial origin including the interaction of genetics, lifestyle behaviors, and environmental factors. Among adults, obesity is commonly defined as a *body mass index (BMI)* greater than or equal to 30 kg/m². Body mass index will be discussed further in chapter 13. *Prevalence* represents the number or rate of individuals within a population who have a condition (e.g., obesity) at a specific time or over a period of time. Over the last several decades, the prevalence of obesity among adults, youth, and adolescence in the United States has grown at an alarming rate. Beginning in the 1960s, the National Health and Nutrition Examination Survey (NHANES) has been conducted as a series of surveys and physical examinations focusing on a nationally-representative sample of adults and children in the U.S. The objective of the survey is to identify biometric information, health status, dietary habits, physical activity patterns, and lifestyle behaviors (HHS, 2012). Using the measured height and weight from NHANES participants, BMI is calculated and classified as normal, overweight, or obese. The NHANES data for 2013-14 indicates the age-adjusted prevalence of obesity among adults in the United States was 37.7% (Flegal et al., 2016). This is a significant increase from the data collected previously through both the NHANES in 1988-1994 and 1999-2000, which indicated an age-adjusted adult obesity rate of 22.9% and 30.5%, respectively (Flegal et al., 2002).

The Centers for Disease Control and Prevention provides adult obesity prevalence maps based on data collected through the Behavioral Risk Factor Surveillance System (BRFSS) between 1990 and 2010 (CDC, 2011). Unlike NHANES, which utilizes a measured height and weight, the BRFSS calculates BMI using self-reported height and weight. Adults are known to underreport weight and over report height, which leads to BMI values biased toward lower than actual values (Gorber et al., 2007). Subsequently, the actual obesity rates based on BRFSS data may be higher than reported. Nevertheless, the trends over time clearly demonstrate a rise in obesity among U.S. adults.

Beginning in 2011, several methodological changes were implemented with the BRFSS, which are likely to have altered obesity prevalence estimates in comparison to data

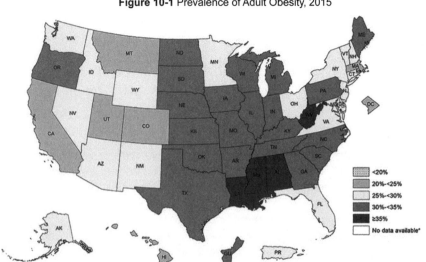

Figure 10-1 Prevalence of Adult Obesity, 2015

derived prior to these changes. For example, beginning with 2011 BRFSS data, records with the following were excluded: self-reported height <3 feet or ≥8 feet, self-reported height <50 pounds or ≥650 pounds, calculated BMI <12 kg/m² or ≥100 kg/m², or women who reported being pregnant (CDC, 2016b). Due to these and other changes, the obesity prevalence maps from 2011 and forward cannot be compared to those from 2010 and earlier.

Figure 10-1 indicates the U.S. obesity prevalence map for 2015. In 2015, no state had a prevalence of adult obesity less than 20%, 21 states had a prevalence of obesity between 30% and <35%, and 4 states (Alabama, Louisiana, Mississippi and West Virginia) had a prevalence of obesity of 35% or greater (CDC, 2016a; CDC, 20156).

The prevalence of obesity among children and adolescents is lower in comparison to adults; however, the youth obesity rates still pose a significant public health concern. Obesity among children and adolescents is defined as a BMI at or above the sex-specific 95th percentile on the U.S. Centers for Disease Control and Prevention (CDC) BMI-for-age growth charts (Ogden et al., 2016). The 2011-14 NHANES survey indicates that 17.0% of children and adolescents aged 2 through 19 years were obese (Ogden et al., 2016). Obesity during childhood is associated with elevated blood pressure, abnormal glucose and lipid levels, increased risk of adult obesity, and subsequent obesity-related chronic disease (Ogden et al., 2016).

Health Implications
The increased prevalence of obesity presents a significant health concern both in the United States and worldwide. Obesity increases the risk of many chronic diseases such as type 2 diabetes, hypertension (high blood pressure), dyslipidemia (high blood cholesterol), cardiovascular disease, gallbladder disease, and several forms of cancer (Shamseddeen et al., 2011; Wang et al., 2011; Withrow & Alter, 2010). Obesity may also increase the risk of stroke, osteoarthritis, asthma, enlarged prostate, sleep apnea, and infertility (Wang et al., 2011). In addition, obesity is associated with increased absenteeism, reduced occupational productivity, decreased quality of life, decreased number of disability-free years, and increased premature mortality (Wang et al., 2011).

Economic Impact
The direct and indirect costs associated with obesity and obesity-related comorbidities are quite substantial. It has been estimated that the health problems related to obesity cost our country an estimated $117 billion a year due to direct health care costs, as well as the indirect economic costs of lost productivity (Soto & White, 2010). Based on the review of eight studies, obese individuals were found to have medical expenditures approximately 30% to 42% higher than their normal-weight peers (Wang et al., 2011; Withrow & Alter, 2010). The additional medical costs associated with obesity in the U.S. were estimated to be $75 billion in 2003 (Wang et al., 2011) and $147 billion in 2008 (Shamseddeen et al., 2011). The annual indirect cost of obesity related to absenteeism has been estimated to be $4.3 billion (Shamseddeen et al., 2011).

Given the substantial health implications and the economic burden associated with obesity, one of the national health objectives for the Healthy People 2020 initiative is to reduce the prevalence of obesity among adults to 30.5% (HHS, Healthy People 2020, 2011).

Metabolism
The biochemical process of breaking down macronutrients (i.e., carbohydrates, fats, and protein) to provide the energy necessary to sustain life and activity is known as **metabolism**. The energy utilized by the body is often measured in terms of calories. A **calorie** is a unit of energy defined as the amount of heat necessary to raise the temperature of 1 gram of water 1 degree Celsius. The

Figure 10-2 Total Daily Energy Expenditure

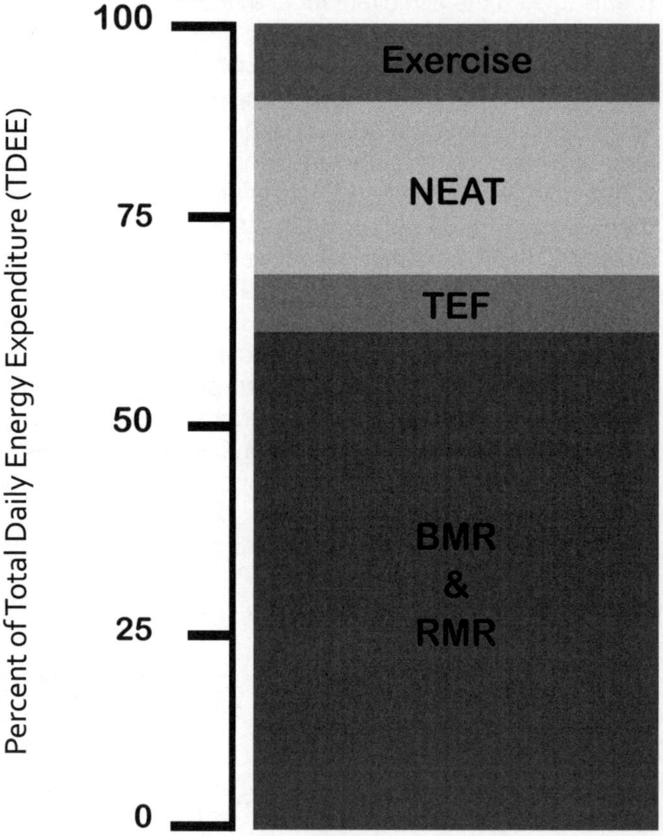

'calories' we refer to with regard to the energy content of food and the energy expended through exercise are technically **kilocalories (kcal)**. A kilocalorie is 1,000 calories or the amount of heat required to raise the temperature of 1 kilogram of water 1 degree Celsius. In both dietetics and fitness, it is common to interchange the terms 'calorie' and 'kilocalorie', although in both cases the actual unit of energy is a kilocalorie.

The total amount of energy (i.e., calories) burned throughout the course of a day is known as the **total daily energy expenditure (TDEE)**. The TDEE is composed of various sources of both involuntary and voluntary caloric expenditure. See figure 10-2. Approximately 60% of the TDEE is represented by the **basal metabolic rate (BMR)**. The basal metabolic rate is defined as the minimum amount of energy needed to sustain basic life functions (e.g., respiration, heart rhythm, blood circulation, brain activity, etc.) while lying at complete rest, in the morning, after sleep, and in a fasted state. The **resting metabolic rate (RMR)** is typically about 10% higher than the BMR and represents the energy expenditure in a resting and fasted state. The **thermal effect of food (TEF)** is the energy expenditure above RMR related to the digestion, absorption, and storage of the food we eat. The TEF contributes approximately 10% to 15% of the total daily energy expenditure. The BMR, RMR, and TEF can all be considered involuntary components of daily metabolism.

The voluntary component of total daily energy expenditure is represented by *activity thermogenesis*, which includes energy expenditure from exercise-related activity and **non-exercise activity thermogenesis (NEAT)**. Exercise-related activities include both structured, intentional exercise as well as leisure time physical activity (e.g., dancing, recreational sports, walking). Non-exercise activity thermogenesis is the energy we expend during everything we do that is not sleeping, eating, structured exercise, or leisure-time physical activity (Levine, 2004). NEAT includes energy expenditure associated with activities of daily living (ADLs), occupational activity, fidgeting, toe-tapping, spontaneous muscular contraction, communication, transportation, and maintenance of posture (Levine, 2004; Levine et al., 1999). NEAT represents the most variable component of daily energy expenditure, ranging from 15% of TDEE in very sedentary individuals to more than 50% of TDEE in highly active individuals (Levine, 2004).

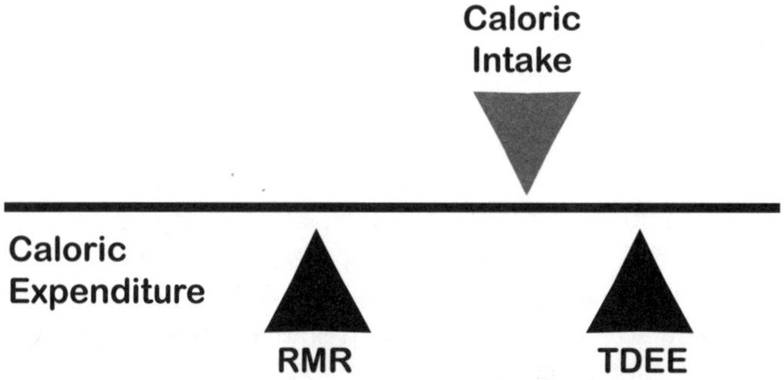

The fundamental principle of weight management is based on the first law of thermodynamics. This physical law relates to the conservation of energy and states that when energy (i.e., calories) are added to a system (i.e., the human body), the energy is either stored or used to perform physical work (Levine et al., 2006). When the consumption of calories via the food we eat exceeds the total daily energy expenditure, the excess energy will be stored as body fat. This is known as a *positive energy balance*, which results in weight gain. See figure 10-4. Conversely, when the total daily energy expenditure exceeds the caloric intake a *negative energy balance* occurs, resulting in weight loss. See figure 10-5. If the caloric intake is consistently equal to the caloric expenditure then the body remains in a state of energy balance and body weight is maintained. See figure 10-3.

Figure 10-3 Caloric Balance

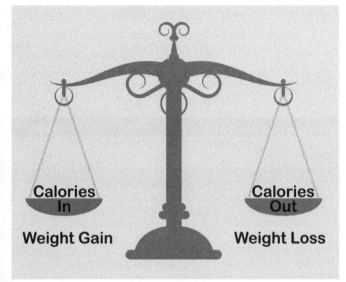

Figure 10-4 Positive Caloric Balance

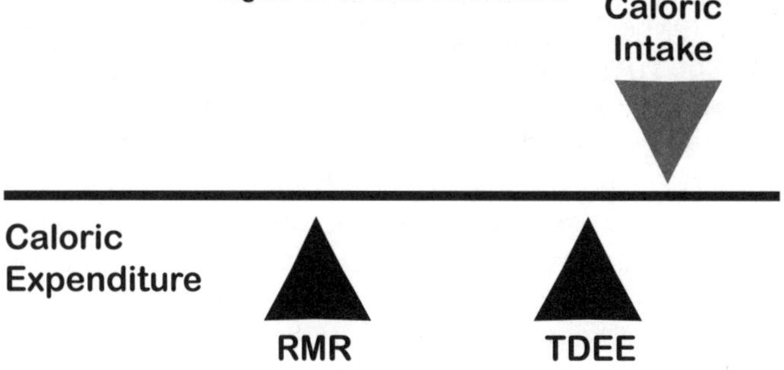

Figure 10-5 Negative Caloric Balance

Figure 10-6 Severe Caloric Restriction

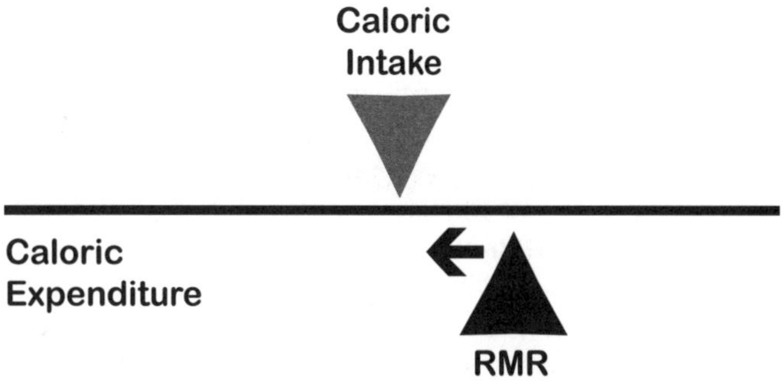

Safe and effective weight loss is achieved through a negative caloric balance of 500 to 1,000 calories per day (ACSM, 2018). An appropriate caloric deficit should result in a gradual weight loss of 1 to 2 pounds per week. Since 1 pound of fat contains 3,500 calories, a daily caloric deficit of 500 calories times 7 days equals 3,500 calories or 1 pound of weight loss per week. The daily caloric deficit should be achieved through a combination of modest reductions in caloric intake and increased voluntary energy expenditure through leisure-time physical activity and exercise. For many years, it was generally accepted that a safe weight loss program should not permit a caloric intake less than 1,200 kcal/day. Of greater importance is the need to maintain a caloric intake greater than the individual's resting metabolic rate. It has been suggested that a caloric intake restricted to levels below an individual's resting metabolic rate may cause metabolic distress, ultimately resulting in a significant reduction of RMR (Foster et al., 1990; Martin et al., 2012; Waddell et al., 1990). See figure 10-6. Although, severely restricting caloric intake may result in short-term weight loss, very low calorie diets are likely to impede long-term maintenance of weight loss and contribute to weight regain often observed upon return to a normal caloric intake pattern (Schwartz & Doucet, 2009). Therefore, for successful long-term weight loss and weight management, it is recommended that caloric intake remains above RMR, yet reasonably below TDEE.

Calculating Resting Metabolic Rate

Resting metabolic rate is best determined through indirect calorimetry using gas exchange analysis during which oxygen consumption and carbon dioxide production at rest are measured by a metabolic analyzer. In the absence of the appropriate equipment, time, and trained personnel, RMR is more often estimated using any number of prediction equations. Among these, two commonly used equations to predict RMR include the Mifflin-St Jeor equation (Mifflin et al., 1990) and the Harris-Benedict equation (Harris & Benedict, 1918).

For Example, using the Mifflin-St Jeor equation for men, the resting metabolic rate for a 38-year-old male who weighs 190 pounds (86.3 kg) and is 6 feet 0 inches (182.9 cm) tall is calculated as follows:

RMR = (9.99 x wt in kg) + (6.25 x ht in cm) - (4.92 x age in yrs) + 5

RMR = (9.99 x 86.3 kg) + (6.25 x 182.9 cm) - (4.92 x 38 yrs) + 5

RMR = (862.1) + (1,143.1) - (187.0) + 5

RMR = 1,823 kcals/day

The accuracy of the resting metabolic rate predictions from these equations varies based on many factors such as age, gender, body composition, and ethnicity, particularly if the individual is not similar to the subjects from which these equations were developed. Studies have been conflicting with regard to the best equation for accurate prediction of resting metabolic rate (Frankenfield et al., 2005; Hasson, 2011; Livingston & Kohlstadt, 2005).

An individual's total daily energy expenditure (TDEE) may be estimated by multiplying the resting metabolic rate by the appropriate physical activity level (PAL) correction factor as indicated in table 10-1 adopted from Shetty et al. (1996) and Trumbo et al. (2002).

Estimated TDEE = RMR x PAL

Using the example above, assume this gentleman has a sedentary office job and performs no leisure-time physical activity. If we determine his PAL to be 1.5, then his total daily energy expenditure is calculated as follows:

TDEE = 1,823 x 1.5 = 2,735 kcals/day

Guidelines for Safe Weight Loss

Several authoritative organizations have published position statements and recommendations regarding safe and effective weight management strategies (Donnelly et al., 2009; Raynor et al., 2016; Turocy et al., 2011). The consensus among these recommendations is that weight loss is facilitated by a negative caloric balance achieved through both reductions in caloric intake and increased voluntary energy expenditure through physical activity. The following recommendations for safe weight loss and weight management programs have been endorsed by the American College of Sports Medicine and the Academy of Nutrition and Dietetics (formerly known as the American Dietetic Association) (ACSM, 2018; Donnelly et al., 2009; Raynor et al., 2016):

Mifflin-St Jeor Equations:

Men: RMR = (9.99 x weight in kg) + (6.25 x height in cm) - (4.92 x age in yrs) + 5

Women: RMR = (9.99 x weight in kg) + (6.25 x height in cm) - (4.92 x age in yrs) - 161

Harris-Benedict Equations:

Men: RMR = 66.47 + (13.75 x weight in kg) + (5.0 x height in cm) – (6.75 x age in yrs)

Women: RMR = 665.09 + (9.56 x weight in kg) + (1.84 x height in cm) – (4.67 x age in yrs)

Table 10-1 PALs

Lifestyle and Level of Activity	PAL
At rest, exclusively sedentary, chair-bound or bed-bound.	1.2
Seated work with no option of moving around, lightly active with little or no strenuous leisure-time activity.	1.4 - 1.5*
Sedentary activity/seated work with some discretion to move around and occasional requirements to walk or stand, moderately active, but little or no strenuous leisure activity.	1.6 - 1.7*
Predominately standing or walking at work.	1.8 - 1.9*
Heavy occupational work or highly active leisure-time activity.	2.0 - 2.4

* Add 0.3 PAL units for those performing significant amounts of sport or strenuous leisure-time activity (30-60 minutes, 4-5 times per week).

- Target a minimal reduction in body weight of at least 3% to 10% of initial body weight over a 3- to 6-month period.
- Achieve an energy deficit (i.e., negative energy balance) of 500 to 1,000 kcal/day for 1 to 2 pounds of weight loss per week.
- Unless under the supervision of a qualified health care provider, energy intake should not be restricted to less than 1,200 to 1,500 kcal/day for women and 1,500 to 1,800 kcal/day for men.
- Reduced energy intake should be combined with a reduction in dietary fat to less than 30% of total daily caloric intake.
- The ACSM's cardiorespiratory exercise training guidelines for healthy individuals are applicable to overweight and obese populations with an emphasis on greater duration and frequency of exercise to maximize caloric expenditure. See chapter 17.
- To prevent weight gain and facilitate modest weight loss, perform 150 to 250 minutes of moderate-intensity physical activity per week (equivalent to an energy expenditure of approximately 1,200 to 2,000 kcal/wk).
- For more substantial weight loss and enhanced prevention of weight regain, it is recommended to perform 250 to 300 minutes of moderate-intensity physical activity per week (≥ 2,000 kcal/wk).
- Consider resistance training to supplement the combination of aerobic exercise and modest reductions in energy intake to lose weight. The ACSM's resistance training guidelines for healthy individuals are applicable to overweight and obese populations. See chapter 18.
- Adopt healthy dietary and exercise habits, as sustained changes in both behaviors result in significant long-term weight loss.
- Include portion control as part of a comprehensive weight management program.
- Distribute total caloric intake throughout the day, with consumption of four to five meals or snacks per day including breakfast. Consumption of greater energy intake earlier in the day is preferable to consumption in the evening.
- Incorporate one or more strategies for behavioral change such as self-monitoring, motivational interviewing, goal-setting, problem solving, and relapse prevention.
- Incorporate opportunities to enhance communication between health care professionals, dieticians, and exercise professionals.

Motivational Interviewing and Weight Loss

On the surface, weight loss may appear to be simply a matter of maintaining a consistent negative caloric balance through decreased energy intake and increased energy expenditure. In reality, weight loss is often derailed by environmental, societal, and personal factors. A healthy meal plan and a well-designed exercise program are ineffective when a client will not or cannot adhere to the regimen.

As discussed in chapter 4, motivational interviewing (MI) can be an effective coaching style to help clients overcome ambivalence to behavioral change, such as adopting a healthy diet or physically-active lifestyle. Several research studies have demonstrated that motivational interviewing is more effective than traditional approaches to facilitate lifestyle changes and subsequent weight loss among youth, adults, and those with chronic disease (Armstrong et al., 2011; Bean et al., 2015; Van Dorsten, 2007). To learn more about motivational interviewing for nutrition and fitness see Clifford & Curtis (2016).

National Weight Control Registry

The National Weight Control Registry (NWCR) is an ongoing study to investigate the strategies and behaviors of individuals successful at long-term maintenance of weight loss. The NWCR was established in 1994 by Rena Wing, Ph.D., the director of the Weight Control and Diabetes Research Center at Brown University, and James Hill, Ph.D., the director of the Center for Human Nutrition at the University of Colorado (Butryn et al., 2007; Thomas et al., 2011). The NWCR was developed in part to identify and study the characteristics and strategies of those who have experienced successful maintenance of weight loss. Since its inception, more than 10,000 individuals have been included in the NWCR, making it the largest longitudinal prospective study of successful weight loss practices. To be eligible for inclusion, participants must be at least 18 years old and have maintained a minimum weight loss of 30 pounds for at least one year (Butryn et al., 2007; Thomas et al., 2011).

The NWCR has identified many common behavioral characteristics among successful weight losers. Consistent with the recommendations of many organizations, the vast majority (89%) of NWCR members utilize a combination of dietary modification and physical activity to achieve their weight loss (Thomas et al., 2011). Among the most common dietary strategies is the restriction of certain types of foods such as those high in simple sugars and dietary fat. (Thomas et al., 2011). Participants indicate an overall average consumption of 1,380 kcal/day (± 573 kcal/day) with men consuming approximately 428 kcal/day more than women (Thomas et al., 2011). The approximate daily average of macronutrient calories among NWCR members studied from 1995-2003 was 26.6% fat, 53.4% carbohydrates, and 18.6% protein (Soleymani et al., 2016, Phelan et al., 2006). NWCR members tend to eat regularly, averaging nearly 5 meals/snacks per day, with 78% reporting they consume breakfast routinely with an overall average of 6.3 times/week (Phelan et al., 2006; Thomas et al., 2011; Soleymani et al., 2016). Most of their meals are prepared at home, fast food is rarely consumed, and most participants report very little variation in their food choices and patterns (Thomas et al., 2011).

National Weight Control Registry members report a significantly high level of weekly physical activity. Overall, 85.3% of men and 89.3% of women included on the registry indicate physical activity as a primary weight loss strategy (Catenacci et al., 2008). The caloric expenditure derived from physical activity averages over 2,600 kcal/wk among NWCR members (Catenacci et al., 2008; Phelan et al., 2006; Soleymani et al., 2016). This is equivalent to approximately 60-75 minutes of moderate-intensity physical activity per day or walking over 25 miles per week. Walking is the most commonly reported mode of activity and resistance training is the second most commonly reported, with 52.2% and 29.2% of NWCR members reporting these activities, respectively (Catenacci et al., 2008).

Finally, two other notable behaviors have been identified among registry participants. First, they regularly monitor their body weight, allowing them to make appropriate modifications to dietary and exercise habits in response to significant weight fluctuations. Surveys have revealed that 36% of successful weight losers indicated weighing themselves daily, and 79% weigh themselves at least weekly (Butryn et al., 2007). Second, NWCR members minimize the time spent in sedentary activities such as watching television. Sixty-three percent (63%) report watching less than 10 hours of television per week, in comparison to approximately 28 hours per week of TV 'screen time' for the typical American (Thomas et al., 2011).

> **Good to Know**
> **National Weight Control Registry Members Were Found To:**
> - Perform a high level of physical activity expending over 2,600 kcal/wk, the equivalent of >300 minutes of moderate-intensity physical activity per week.
> - Maintain a low-calorie intake (~1,300 kcal/day for women; ~1,725 kcal/day for men) with less than 30% of daily calories from fat.
> - Eat regularly (5 meals/snacks per day) including breakfast, which was consumed daily by 78% of NWCR participants.
> - Monitor body weight regularly (a least 1 time per week) to increase awareness of significant body weight fluctuations so that appropriate dietary and activity modifications can be made.
> - Minimize time spent in sedentary activities and limit television viewing time to less than 10 hours per week.

Calculation of Goal Body Weight

Since many clients may express goals related to weight loss, the fitness professional can provide predictions of goal body weight to facilitate goal setting, enhance motivation, and increase accountability. However, weight loss goals are outcome-oriented, resulting from the regular

---

Calculation of Goal Body Weight

Step One: Measure current body weight and body composition (i.e., % body fat)
Note: body composition analysis will be discussed in chapter 15.

Step Two: Calculate current fat weight
Fat Weight (lbs.) = Total Body Weight (lbs.) x % Body Fat

Step Three: Calculate current lean body weight
Lean Body Weight (lbs.) = Total Body Weight (lbs.) - Fat Weight (lbs.)

Step Four: Determine the goal percent lean body weight
Goal % Lean Body Weight = 100 – Goal % Body Fat

Step Five: Calculate the Goal Body Weight
Goal Body Weight (lbs.) = Current LBW (lbs.) ÷ Goal % LBW

For example, your client Bill currently weighs 205 pounds and has 20% body fat. His goal is to reduce his body fat to 15%. What is his goal body weight to achieve this target body composition?
  205 lbs. x 0.20 (% body fat) = 41 lbs. of body fat
  205 lbs. – 41 lbs. = 164 lbs. of lean body weight
  100% - 15% (goal % body fat) = 85% (or 0.85) goal lean body weight
  164 lbs. ÷ 0.85 = 193 lbs. (goal body weight)

achievement of action-oriented goals (e.g., decrease daily caloric intake, increase daily physical activity). Therefore, fitness professionals must be cautious and avoid placing too much emphasis on specific weight loss goals, but rather should encourage clients to focus attention on success measured through the adoption and maintenance of healthy behaviors.

The calculations outlined in the shaded box may be used when the fitness professional determines it to be necessary and appropriate to calculate goal body weight.

In the example provided in the box below, the client would need to lose 12 pounds to achieve the target weight, and theoretically, his goal percent body fat. Based on the recommended rate of safe weight loss (i.e., 1 to 2 pounds per week), it will take at least 6 to 12 weeks to achieve this goal. Although the use of these calculations provides an estimated goal body weight, there are some limitations to consider. First, the anchor point of these calculations is the current body weight and body composition of the client. Body weight can be easily and accurately obtained with a standardized scale. However, an accurate measurement of body composition and percent body fat may be more difficult to obtain. As will be discussed in chapter 15, it is generally accepted that hydrostatic (underwater) weighing provides the most accurate measurement of body composition. Since this technique is unlikely to be available in most fitness settings, body composition is more frequently estimated using skinfold testing or bioelectrical impedance analysis (BIA). Each of these techniques produces a larger margin of error in the estimation of percent body fat in comparison to the hydrostatic weighing. This error may be transferred into the calculation of goal body weight based on the measured body composition using these techniques.

A second source of error in the determination of goal body weight stems from the assumption inherent to these calculations that as an individual loses weight, this weight loss will be the result of changes (i.e., reductions) in fat mass with no changes in lean body mass. Ideally, we hope to see significant reductions in fat mass and maintenance, or perhaps even increases, in lean body mass. In cases of significant weight loss, it is likely that some lean body mass will also be lost. In a more favorable scenario, gains in lean body mass may be attained. Nevertheless, the calculations used above assume that lean body weight will remain unchanged. In the example provided, the client has 164 pounds of lean body weight at the initial assessment and reassessment visits. If the client's body fat is reassessed and found to be 15% as planned, but his body weight is 195 pounds versus the predicted 193 pounds, this may be best explained by a gain in lean body weight.

Chapter Summary

The rising prevalence of obesity in the United States has been declared an epidemic among adults, children, and adolescents. Obesity presents a significant public health concern with regard to its role in the development of many chronic diseases, the significant economic burden, and the negative impact on quality of life. This chapter presented information related to metabolism, recommendations for safe and effective weight management, and strategies utilized by the successful weight losers studied in conjunction with the National Weight Control Registry. The knowledge gained from this chapter can assist fitness professionals while guiding their clients and participants toward successful weight loss and weight maintenance.

Chapter References

American College of Sports Medicine (2018). *ACSM's Guidelines for Exercise Testing and Prescription*, 10th edition. Philadelphia, PA: Wolters Kluwer.

Armstrong, M.J., Mottershead, T.A., Ronksley, P.E., Sigal, R.J., Campbell, T.S., & Hemmelgarn, B.R. (2011). Motivational interviewing to improve weight loss in overweight and/or obese patients: A systematic review and meta-analysis of randomized controlled trials. *Obesity Reviews*, 12(9), 709-723.

Bean, M.K., Powell, P., Quinoy, A., Ingersoll, K., Wickham, E.P., & Mazzeo, S.E. (2015). Motivational interviewing targeting diet and physical activity improves adherence to pediatric obesity treatment: Results from the MI Values randomized controlled trial. *Pediatric Obesity*, 10(2), 118-125.

Butryn, M.L., Phelan, S., Hill, J.O., & Wing, R.R. (2007). Consistent self-monitoring of weight: A key component of successful weight loss maintenance. *Obesity*, 15(12), 3091-3096.

Catenacci, V.A., Ogden, L.G., Stuht, J., Phelan, S., Wing, R.R., Hill, J.O., & Wyatt, H.R. (2008). Physical activity patterns in the national weight control registry. *Obesity*, 16(1), 153-161.

Centers for Disease Control and Prevention (CDC) (2011). The history of the increase in state obesity prevalence as depicted in a PowerPoint slide presentation format. Available at: https://www.cdc.gov/obesity/data/prevalence-maps.html. Accessed on August 17, 2016.

Centers for Disease Control and Prevention (CDC) (2016a). Prevalence of self-reported obesity among U.S. adults by state and territory, BRFSS, 2015. Available at: https://www.cdc.gov/obesity/data/prevalence-maps.html. Accessed on October 15, 2016.

Centers for Disease Control and Prevention (CDC) (2016b). The adult obesity prevalence for states and territories in 2011-2015 as depicted in a PowerPoint slide presentation format. Available at: https://www.cdc.gov/obesity/data/prevalence-maps.html. Accessed on October 15, 2016.

Clifford, D., & Curtis, L. (2016). *Motivational Interviewing in Nutrition and Fitness*. New York, NY: The Guilford Company.

Donnelly, J.E., Blair, S.N., Jakicic, J.M., Manore, M.M., Rankin, J.W., & Smith, B.K. (2009). American College of Sports Medicine Position Stand. Appropriate physical activity intervention strategies for weight loss and prevention of weight regain for adults. *Medicine and Science in Sports and Exercise*, 41(2), 459-471.

Flegal, K.M., Kruszon-Moran, D., Carroll, M.D., Fryar, C.D., & Ogden, C.L. (2016). Trends in obesity among adults in the United States, 2005 to 2014. *Journal of the American Medical Association (JAMA)*, 315(21), 2284-2291.

Flegal, K.M., Carroll, M.D., Ogden, C.L., & Johnson, C.L. (2002). Prevalence and trends in obesity among US adults, 1999-2000. *Journal of the American Medical Association*, 288(14), 1723-1727.

Foster, G.D., Wadden, T.A., Feurer, I.D., Jennings, A.S., Stunkard, A.J., Crosby, L.O., ... & Mullen, J.L. (1990). Controlled trial of the metabolic effects of a very-low-calorie diet: Short-and long-term effects. *The American Journal of Clinical Nutrition*, 51(2), 167-172.

Frankenfield, D., Roth-Yousey, L., & Compher, C. (2005). Comparison of predictive equations for resting metabolic rate in healthy nonobese and obese adults: A systematic review. *Journal of the American Dietetic Association*, 105(5), 775-789.

Gorber, S.C., Tremblay, M., Moher, D., & Gorber, B. (2007). A comparison of direct vs. self-report measures for assessing height, weight and body mass index: A systematic review. *Obesity Reviews*, 8(4), 307-326.

Harris, J.A., & Benedict, F.G. (1918). A biometric study of human basal metabolism. *Proceedings of the National Academy of Sciences of the United States of America*, 4(12), 370-373.

Hasson, R.E., Howe, C.A., Jones, B.L., & Freedson, P.S. (2011). Accuracy of four resting metabolic rate prediction equations: Effects of sex, body mass index, age, and race/ethnicity. *Journal of Science and Medicine in Sport*, 14(4), 344-351.

Levine, J.A. (2004). Non-Exercise Activity Thermogenesis (NEAT). *Nutrition Reviews*, 62(s2), S82-S97.

Levine, J.A., Eberhardt, N.L., & Jensen, M.D. (1999). Role of non-exercise activity thermogenesis in resistance to fat gain in humans. *Science*, 283(5399), 212-214.

Levine, J.A., Vander Weg, M.W.; Hill, J.O., & Klesges, R.C. (2006). Non-exercise activity thermogenesis the crouching tiger hidden dragon of societal weight gain. A*rteriosclerosis, Thrombosis, and Vascular Biology*, 26(4), 729-736.

Livingston, E.H., & Kohlstadt, I. (2005). Simplified resting metabolic rate—predicting formulas for normal-sized and obese individuals. *Obesity Research*, 13(7), 1255-1262.

Martin, C.K., Heilbronn, L.K., Jonge, L., DeLany, J.P., Volaufova, J., Anton, S.D., ... & Ravussin, E. (2012). Effect of calorie restriction on resting metabolic rate and spontaneous physical activity. *Obesity*, 15(12), 2964-2973.

Mifflin, M.D., St Jeor, S.T., Hill, L.A., Scott, B.J., Daugherty, S.A., & Koh, Y.O. (1990). A new predictive equation for resting energy expenditure in healthy individuals. *The American Journal of Clinical Nutrition*, 51(2), 241-247.

Ogden, C.L., Carroll, M.D., Lawman, H.G., Fryar, C.D., Kruszon-Moran, D., Kit, B.K., & Flegal, K.M. (2016). Trends in obesity prevalence among children and adolescents in the United States, 1988-1994 through 2013-2014. *Journal of the American Medical Association (JAMA)*, 315(21), 2292-2299.

Phelan, S., Wyatt, H.R., Hill, J.O., & Wing, R.R. (2006). Are the eating and exercise habits of successful weight losers changing?. *Obesity*, 14(4), 710-716.

Raynor, H.A., & Champagne, C.M. (2016). Position of the Academy of Nutrition and Dietetics: Interventions for the Treatment of Overweight and Obesity in Adults. *Journal of the Academy of Nutrition and Dietetics*, 116(1), 129-147.

Schwartz, A., & Doucet, E. (2009). Relative changes in resting energy expenditure during weight loss: A systematic review. *Obesity Reviews*, 11(7), 531-547.

Shamseddeen, H., Getty, J.Z., Hamdallah, I.N., & Ali, M.R. (2011). Epidemiology and economic impact of obesity and type 2 diabetes. *The Surgical Clinics of North America*, 91(6), 1163-1172.

Shetty, P.S., Henry, C.J., Black, A.E., & Prentice, A.M. (1996). Energy requirements of adults: An update on basal metabolic rates (BMRs) and physical activity levels (PALs). *European Journal of Clinical Nutrition, 50*, S11-23.

Soleymani, T., Daniel, S., & Garvey, W.T. (2016). Weight maintenance: Challenges, tools and strategies for primary care physicians. *Obesity Reviews,* 17(1), 81-93.

Soto, C., & White, J.H. (2010). School health initiatives and childhood obesity: BMI screening and reporting. *Policy, Politics, & Nursing Practice*, 11(2), 108-114.

Thomas, J.G., Bond, D.S., Hill, J.O., & Wing, R.R. (2011). The National Weight Control Registry: A study of "successful losers". *ACSM's Health & Fitness Journal*, 15(2), 8-12.

Trumbo, P., Schlicker, S., Yates, A.A., & Poos, M. (2002). Dietary reference intakes for energy, carbohydrate, fiber, fat, fatty acids, cholesterol, protein and amino acids. *Journal of the American Dietetic Association*, 102(11), 1621-1630.

Turocy, P.S., DePalma, B.F., Horswill, C.A., Laquale, K.M., Martin, T.J., Perry, A.C., ... & Utter, A.C. (2011). National Athletic Trainers Association Position Statement: Safe weight loss and maintenance practices in sport and exercise. *Journal of Athletic Training*, 46(3), 322-336.

U.S. Department of Health and Human Services (HHS) (2012). National Health and Nutrition Examination Survey, 2011-2012: *Overview*. Retrieved from http://www.cdc.gov/nchs/nhanes/about_nhanes.htm. Updated September 9, 2012. Accessed March 15, 2013.

U.S. Department of Health and Human Services, Healthy People 2020. (2011, June 29). *Nutrition and Weight Status*. Retrieved from http://www.healthypeople.gov/2020/topicsobjectives2020/objectiveslist.aspx?topicId=29. Updated October 30, 2012. Accessed March 15, 2013.

Van Dorsten, B. (2007). The use of motivational interviewing in weight loss. *Current Diabetes Reports*, 7(5), 386-390.

Wadden, T.A., Foster, G.D., Letizia, K.A., & Mullen, J.L. (1990). Long-term effects of dieting on resting metabolic rate in obese outpatients. *Journal of the American Medical Association*, 264(6), 707-711.

Wang, Y.C., McPherson, K., Marsh, T., Gortmaker, S.L., & Brown, M. (2011). Health and economic burden of the projected obesity trends in the USA and the UK. *The Lancet*, 378(9793), 815-825.

Withrow, D., & Alter, D.A. (2010). The economic burden of obesity worldwide: A systematic review of the direct costs of obesity. *Obesity Reviews*, 12(2), 131-141.

Chapter 10 Review Questions

1. The number of calories expended throughout the course of a day is referred to as the
   A. resting metabolic rate.
   B. basal metabolic rate.
   C. total daily energy expenditure.
   D. non-exercise activity thermogenesis.

2. Which of the following represents a negative caloric balance?
   A. Daily calories expended = 1,523; daily calories consumed = 1,865
   B. Daily calories expended = 1,758; daily calories consumed = 1,758
   C. Daily calories expended = 1,934; daily calories consumed = 1,705
   D. Daily calories expended = 1,860; daily calories consumed = 2,135

3. According to the National Weight Control Registry (NWCR), which of the following has been identified as a common strategy utilized by successful weight losers?
   A. Consume a diet with ≥ 60 percent of total calories from protein
   B. Maintain a very low calorie diet of ≤ 1,200 calories per day
   C. Weigh themselves one time per month to avoid the frustration of daily and weekly weight fluctuations
   D. Perform regular moderate-intensity physical activity often > 300 minutes per week

4. Your new male client currently weighs 196 pounds and has 24% body fat based on skinfold measurements. He would like to reduce his body fat to 18% over the next twelve weeks. Using the information provided, what is his goal body weight?
   A. 149 lbs.
   B. 176 lbs.
   C. 182 lbs.
   D. 172 lbs.

5. Which of the following is recommended for safe and effective weight loss?
   A. Target a daily caloric intake not to exceed 1,200 calories for women and 1,500 for men.
   B. To prevent weight regain after weight loss, perform 150 minutes of moderate-intensity physical activity per day.
   C. To facilitate substantial weight loss, perform 250 to 300 minutes of moderate-intensity physical activity per week.
   D. Perform resistance training exercises 3-5 days per week as a primary weight loss strategy.

6. What is the maximum amount of weight loss that should be recommended to a client wishing to lose 'as much weight as possible' by her class reunion in 12 weeks?
   A. 12 pounds
   B. 24 pounds
   C. 36 pounds
   D. 18 pounds

Answers to Review Questions on Page 384

Note: Review questions are intended to reinforce learning and comprehension of subject matter presented in the corresponding chapter. The review questions are not intended to be representative of actual certification exam questions in terms of style, content, or difficulty.

11
Eating Disorders

Introduction

Disordered eating is characterized by a broad range of maladaptive dietary behaviors, weight loss practices, and psychological disorders. The behaviors and practices associated with disordered eating fall along a continuum of severity with four clinically diagnosable **eating disorders (ED)** representing the end of this continuum. See figure 11-1. These eating disorders include anorexia nervosa (AN), bulimia nervosa (BN), binge-eating disorder (BED), and feeding or eating disorders not elsewhere classified (FED-NEC). 'Disordered eating' refers to an entire spectrum of unhealthy dietary habits and abnormal behaviors, whereas 'eating disorder' is preferred when a definite clinical diagnosis has been made (Bonci et al., 2008). Medical professionals recognize that not every case fits into a specific diagnostic category as some patients may exhibit major signs and symptoms of an eating disorder, yet do not meet specific diagnostic criteria. Each disease has its own characteristics and underlying psychological challenges, which need to be addressed individually, along with other disordered eating behaviors. Fitness professionals should become knowledgeable about risk factors, characteristics, signs, and symptoms indicative of eating disorders in order to facilitate early detection and referral to the appropriate health care provider. The rapport and personal relationships established with their clients and participants place fitness professionals in a unique, yet often challenging, position to identify and initiate conversations regarding unhealthy dietary behaviors.

Prevalence of Eating Disorders

The exact frequency and distribution of eating disorders is unknown as the result of the high number of cases that go unreported or undetected due to the sensitive nature and secretive behaviors associated with these conditions (Ozier & Henry, 2011). The prevalence of eating disorders is known to be higher among females than males, and athletes compared to non-athletes (Bratland-Sanda & Sundgot-Borgen, 2013). Among athletes, the highest prevalence is seen among females participating in endurance (e.g., distance running) and aesthetic sports (e.g., gymnastics, diving, cheerleading, dance), whereas EDs are highest among male athletes participating in weight-class sports such as wrestling or boxing (Bratland-Sanda & Sundgot-Borgen, 2013). In the United States, it is estimated that anorexia and bulimia affect nearly 10 million females and 1 million males; however, the actual prevalence may be substantially higher since EDs are believed to be undiagnosed in up to 50% of cases (Bonci et al., 2008). This may be particularly true of males who are reluctant to discuss disordered eating behaviors due to feelings of shame and embarrassment over possibly having a disorder which has been stereotypically associated with females (Bonci et al., 2008). Eating disorders primarily affect adolescents and young adults with the highest incidence rates observed between the ages of 15 and 20 years (Smink et al., 2012).

General Risk Factors

The risk factors for development of eating disorders are multifactorial. Among the many factors that may predispose individuals to eating disorders are psychological characteristics including dissatisfaction with body image, low self-esteem, personality traits like perfectionism, and negative mood states such as depression, shame, inadequacy, guilt, or helplessness (Bratland-Sanda & Sundgot-Borgen, 2013; Bonci et al., 2008). Sociocultural factors may also influence the development of eating disorders. These factors include peer pressure, a history of being bullied, physical or sexual abuse, intentional or unintentional pressure created by a sports coach, and perceived expectations to attain unrealistic standards of thinness influ-

Figure 11-1 Eating Behavior Continuum

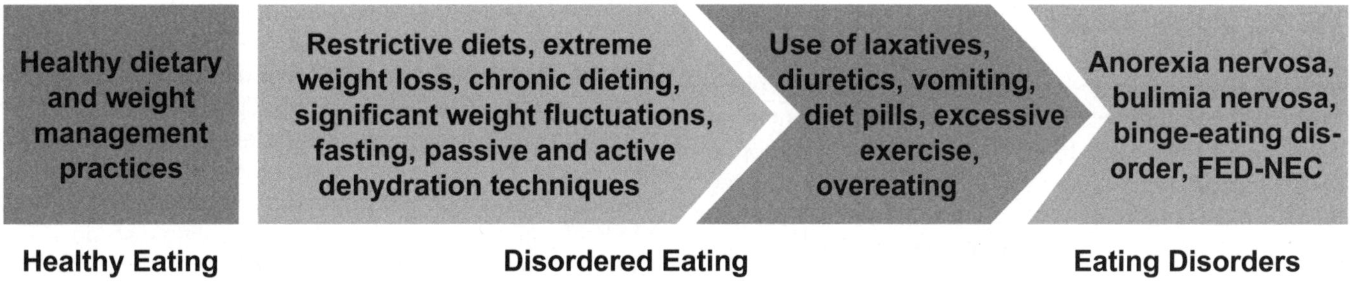

Healthy dietary and weight management practices	Restrictive diets, extreme weight loss, chronic dieting, significant weight fluctuations, fasting, passive and active dehydration techniques	Use of laxatives, diuretics, vomiting, diet pills, excessive exercise, overeating	Anorexia nervosa, bulimia nervosa, binge-eating disorder, FED-NEC
Healthy Eating	**Disordered Eating**		**Eating Disorders**

enced by the media (Bratland-Sanda & Sundgot-Borgen, 2013; Bonci et al., 2008). The onset of an eating disorder may be triggered by a traumatic event or injury as well as a negative comment regarding body weight, shape, or appearance. Athletes who participate in sports that emphasize appearance, a low body mass index, or require weight classifications are especially vulnerable to eating disorders (Bonci et al., 2008). Finally, biological factors including genetics, (e.g., family history of eating disorder), age (e.g., adolescence and young adults), and gender increase the risk of developing an eating disorder. Although women are more likely to develop eating disorders, men are also at risk, especially when they are self-driven for muscularity. The preoccupation with muscular development and leanness, known as *muscle dysmorphia*, may result in unsafe dieting, extreme exercise behaviors, and an increased risk of anabolic steroid use (Bratland-Sanda & Sundgot-Borgen, 2013).

Anorexia Nervosa

Anorexia nervosa (AN) is a serious mental illness characterized by self-starvation, failure to maintain a minimally normal weight, an irrational fear of gaining weight or becoming fat, and a preoccupation with body shape (Attia, 2010). Anorexia is present in only about 0.5% to 1% of females and about one tenth as many males (Attia, 2010). It is most prevalent in cultures where food is abundant and thinness is the cultural ideal. Individuals who are at the highest risk of developing anorexia nervosa are females (especially Caucasian and Asian), who are from an upper-level socioeconomic status, who demonstrate a marked preoccupation with thinness, who constantly discuss food and body image, and who may be seriously involved in activities requiring a low body weight (e.g., gymnastics, ballet, diving, modeling, and running).

In the United States most anorexics are female, in their mid-teens, middle-class, and of a well-educated family. Individuals suffering from anorexia nervosa tend to be highly-competitive and strive for perfection. The 'perfect body' is the ultimate goal, and in their minds is seemingly unattainable. Weight loss becomes an obsession, losing control becomes a great fear, and self-imposed starvation takes over. Exercise is often used in conjunction with caloric restriction to enhance weight loss. The use of laxatives is also common.

Anorexia is very difficult to treat and should be dealt with by qualified professionals. A study from the Renfrew Center in Philadelphia, a foundation that works on advancing the education, prevention, research, and treatment of eating disorders, reported that females with eating disorders often begin dieting much earlier than their peers (average age of 15 years). The prognosis for treatment is fairly good with early intervention; however, if left untreated, it is associated with early death.

Characteristics of Anorexia Nervosa

The following criteria are summarized from the *Diagnostic and Statistical Manual of Mental Disorders* (DSM-5) of the American Psychiatric Association:

- Restriction of energy intake relative to requirements leading to a significantly low body weight in the context of age, sex, developmental trajectory, and physical health. Significantly low weight is defined as a weight that is less than minimally normal, or for children and adolescents, less than that minimally expected.
- Intense fear of gaining weight or becoming fat, or persistent behavior that interferes with weight gain, even though at a significantly low weight.
- Disturbance in the way in which one's body weight or shape is experienced, undue influence of body weight or shape on self-evaluation, or persistent lack of recognition of the seriousness of the current low body weight.

There are many signs and symptoms associated with anorexia nervosa including physical, physiological, and psychological indicators. These signs and symptoms may include:

- Dramatic weight loss, including degenerative loss of skeletal muscle tissue (i.e., sarcopenia)
- Dry skin, which is sometimes tinged yellow from an accumulation of stored vitamin A
- Growth of fine body hair (i.e., lanugo)
- Intolerance to cold
- Low blood pressure (i.e., hypotension) and slow basal metabolic rate
- Low red blood cell count (i.e., anemia) caused by iron and vitamin B12 deficiencies
- Various hormonal changes
- Retarded bone growth and loss of bone mineral density
- Cessation of menstrual cycle (i.e., amenorrhea)

Bulimia Nervosa

Bulimia nervosa (BN) is characterized by frequent cycles of binge-eating and inappropriate compensatory purge behaviors intended to prevent weight gain. Purge behaviors include self-induced vomiting, abuse of diuretics, laxatives or enemas, fasting, and excessive exercise. According to the American Psychiatric Association, exercise may be considered excessive when it interferes with important activities, is done at inappropriate times or in inappropriate places, or when the individual exercises despite injury or medical complications. As with other eating disorders, bulimia may be exacerbated by our cultural obsession with thinness. In addition, unhealthy purging behaviors may be perpetuated by approval or unintentional indications of support by coaches or significant others, or initial 'success' found through these behaviors (Bratland-Sanda & Sundgot-Borgen, 2013). The obsession with body image and weight gain have an unhealthy correlation with the bulimic's self-worth and self-esteem. Those suffering from bulimia have a morbid fear of fatness. The body mass index (BMI) of bulimics is generally in the normal to normal-high range (Hudson et al., 2007). Ninety percent of the people suffering from bulimia are white females, ranging from 15 to 30 years of age. There are very few reports of males with bulimia. It is not uncommon for someone suffering from bulimia to eat as much as 6,000 calories in one sitting. Many fear that they won't be able to stop binge-eating voluntarily. During binges, they may have low self-esteem, feel out of control, guilty, or shameful. They report feeling depressed after a binge episode, even though the binge-eating may have resulted from depression.

To control fluctuations in body weight, purging behaviors often follow binge-eating. This cycle may produce a variety of health complications with potentially life-threatening consequences. Binge-eating can cause dilation and possible rupture of the gastrointestinal tract due to excessive food intake within a short period of time. Involuntary or self-induced vomiting after an episode of binging may damage tooth enamel, and upset the body's electrolyte balance. Repeated use of syrup of ipecac to induce vomiting can cause myocardial abnormalities. Abuse of laxatives by bulimics may promote a sense of purging, but seldom prevents the absorption of calories.

Characteristics of Bulimia Nervosa
The following criteria are summarized from the *Diagnostic and Statistical Manual of Mental Disorders* (DSM-5) of the American Psychiatric Association:

- Recurrent episodes of binge-eating. An episode of binge-eating is characterized by both of the following:
    1. Eating, in a discrete period of time (e.g., within any 2-hour period), an amount of food that is definitely larger than most people would eat during a similar period of time and under similar circumstances.
    2. A sense of lack of control over eating during the episode (e.g., a feeling that one cannot stop eating or control what or how much one is eating).
- Recurrent inappropriate compensatory behavior in order to prevent weight gain, such as self-induced vomiting; misuse of laxatives, diuretics, or other medications, fasting; or excessive exercise.
- The binge-eating and inappropriate compensatory behaviors both occur, on average, at least once a week for 3 months.

- Self-evaluation is unduly influenced by body shape and weight.
- The disturbance does not occur exclusively during episodes of anorexia nervosa.

Binge-Eating Disorder
In 1994, **binge-eating disorder (BED)** was introduced as a provisional diagnosis and the fourth edition of the *Diagnostic and Statistical Manual of Mental Disorders* (DSM-IV) still placed BED under the category of "eating disorders not otherwise specified," which may contribute to the increased and common use of this diagnosis (Striegel-Moore & Franko, 2008; White et al., 2011). In the updated fifth edition (DSM-5), binge-eating disorder was elevated to its own diagnostic label. Binge-eating disorder is defined as recurring episodes of eating significantly more food in a short period of time than most people would eat under similar circumstances, with episodes marked by feelings of lack of control (APA, 2013). Binge-eating disorder, also commonly known as 'compulsive overeating,' is the most common eating disorder. It represents about 25–30% of the individuals seeking treatment in a clinic-based weight management program. BED is similar to bulimia nervosa except that individuals with BED do not use the compensatory purge behaviors. Individuals with BED are almost always overweight. Binges may be triggered by stressful situations, negative moods, or eating tiny amounts of 'forbidden' foods. The binges bring on feelings of shame and self-loathing, which only seem to keep the negative cycle in motion.

Characteristics of Binge-Eating Disorder
The following criteria are summarized from *Diagnostic and Statistical Manual of Mental Disorders* (DSM-5) of the American Psychiatric Association:

- Recurrent episodes of binge-eating. An episode of binge-eating is characterized by both of the following:
    1. Eating, in a discrete period of time (e.g., within any 2-hour period), an amount of food that is definitely larger than most people would eat in a similar period of time under similar circumstances
    2. A sense of lack of control over eating during the episode (e.g., a feeling that one cannot stop eating or control what or how much one is eating)
- The binge-eating episodes are associated with three (or more) of the following:
    1. Eating much more rapidly than normal
    2. Eating until feeling uncomfortably full
    3. Eating large amounts of food when not feeling physically hungry
    4. Eating alone because of feeling embarrassed by how much one is eating
    5. Feeling disgusted with oneself, depressed, or very guilty afterwards

- Marked distress regarding binge-eating is present.
- The binge-eating occurs, on average, at least once a week for three months. The binge-eating is not associated with the recurrent use of inappropriate compensatory behavior (e.g., purging) and does not occur exclusively during the course of bulimia nervosa or anorexia nervosa.

Feeding or Eating Disorders Not Elsewhere Classified

The fourth edition of the *Diagnostic and Statistical Manual of Mental Disorders* (DSM-IV) identified another diagnosable eating disorder referred to as *eating disorder not otherwise specified (EDNOS)*. "Eating disorder not otherwise specified" had become the most common diagnosis of EDs used by physicians and psychiatrists for eating disorders of clinical severity meeting many, but not all of the criteria for anorexia nervosa or bulimia nervosa (Smink et al., 2012). EDNOS was also a popular diagnosis since at that time it included binge-eating disorder.

In DSM-5, this diagnostic category has been replaced by a label termed "feeding or eating disorders not elsewhere classified." **Feeding or Eating Disorders Not Elsewhere Classified (FED-NEC)** is characterized as disturbances in eating behavior that do not necessarily fall into the specific diagnoses of anorexia, bulimia, or binge-eating disorder. Warning signs and related health and psychological conditions of FED-NEC are similar to, and just as serious as, those for the other eating disorders. Some of the conditions that may fall under the category of FED-NEC include:

- Atypical Anorexia Nervosa: All of the criteria for Anorexia Nervosa are met, except that, despite significant weight loss, the individual's weight is within or above the normal range.
- Subthreshold Bulimia Nervosa (low frequency or limited duration): All of the criteria for Bulimia Nervosa are met, except that the binge-eating and inappropriate compensatory behaviors occur, on average, less than once a week and/or for less than for 3 months.
- Subthreshold Binge Eating Disorder (low frequency or limited duration): All of the criteria for binge-eating disorder are met, except that the binge-eating occurs, on average, less than once a week and/or for less than for 3 months.
- Purging Disorder: Recurrent purging behavior to influence weight or shape, such as self-induced vomiting, misuse of laxatives, diuretics, or other medications, in the absence of binge-eating. Self-evaluation is unduly influenced by body shape or weight or there is an intense fear of gaining weight or becoming fat.
- Night Eating Syndrome: Recurrent episodes of night eating, as manifested by eating after awakening from sleep or excessive food consumption after the evening meal. There is awareness and recall of the eating. The night eating is not better accounted for by external influences such as changes in the individual's sleep/wake cycle or by local social norms. The night eating is associated with significant distress and/or impairment in functioning. The disordered pattern of eating is not better accounted for by binge-eating disorder, another psychiatric disorder, substance.

Female Athlete Triad

The **female athlete triad** refers to the interrelated combination of low energy availability, amenorrhea, and reduced bone mineral density which may be seen among female athletes (Nattiv et al., 2007). See figure 11-2. Low energy availability may result from an inadequate intake of calories below the level necessary to support exercise, daily activities, and even basal metabolic needs. An unhealthy negative caloric balance may also arise from a combination of insufficient caloric intake and excessive energy expenditure through exercise. Chronic low energy availability may occur with or without an underlying eating disorder. When energy availability is regularly below the level needed for basic body functions, physiological mechanisms attempt to compensate by reducing the amount of energy used for cellular function, regulation of body temperature, growth and repair of tissue, and reproduction (Nattiv et al., 2007). Low energy availability may lead to amenorrhea, defined as the absence of menstrual cycles lasting more than three months. Amenorrhea indirectly impairs bone mineral density by reducing the activity of hormones that promote bone formation (Nattiv et al., 2007). The effect of amenorrhea on the bone density of young female athletes is of great concern. Bone density of the lumbar spine is lower among amenorrheic athletes, and tibial and metatarsal stress fractures are also more common. Since adolescence and young adulthood represent a critical window for women to accumulate optimal bone mineral density, the negative impact of amenorrhea on bone health increases the risk of developing osteoporosis later in life. (Bonci et al., 2008; Nattiv et al., 2007).

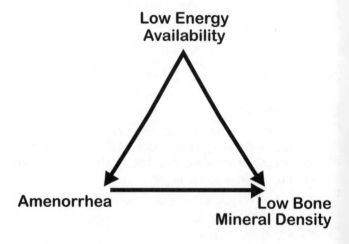

Figure 11-2 Female Athlete Triad

Table 11-1 Eating Disorder Professional Resources

National Eating Disorders Association 603 Stewart Ave., Suite 803 Seattle, WA 98101 Phone: (800) 931-2237 or (206) 382-3587 www.nationaleatingdisorders.org	**Academy for Eating Disorders** 6728 Old McLean Village Drive McLean, VA 22101 Phone: (703) 556-9222 www.acadeatdis.org
International Association of Eating Disorder Professionals P.O. Box 1295 Pekin, IL 61555 Phone: (800) 800-8126 www.iaedp.com	**National Association of Anorexia Nervosa and Associated Disorders** 750 E. Diehl Road #127 Naperville, IL 60563 Phone: (630) 577-1333 www.anad.org

Professional Ethics

It is of utmost importance that fitness professionals refer an individual that is suspected of having an eating disorder to a qualified health care provider. Fitness professionals must be careful not to overstep professional boundaries or fail to act in an ethical manner. Although it is important to have knowledge of the signs and symptoms of eating disorders, fitness professionals do not diagnose these illnesses or any other medical conditions. However, fitness professionals are in a position to recognize possible eating disorders, communicate genuine concern, and provide individuals with a list of community resources or referral to a health care provider. Peer support and encouragement is very important when guiding those with eating disorders to seek treatment. The initial conversation with an individual suspected of having an eating disorder should be facilitated by a trusted authority figure who has established the best rapport with the member or participant. When initiating this conversation be prepared to approach the individual with sensitivity and respect; indicate specific observations of concern; expect responses of denial, anger, or resistance; ensure confidentiality; and have resource and referral information readily available to share with the individual (Bonci et al., 2008). Table 11-1 provides a list of organizations that may serve as a source of information with regard to eating disorders. For more information about eating disorders and strategies for how to intervene, see the National Eating Disorders Association (NEDA) *Coaches & Trainers Toolkit*.

Chapter Summary

This chapter provided an overview of disordered eating and eating disorders including anorexia nervosa, bulimia nervosa, binge-eating disorder, and feeding or eating disorders not elsewhere classified. Information regarding the prevalence and risk factors was presented as well as signs and symptoms related to each of the diagnosable eating disorders. A related condition referred to as the female athlete triad was also reviewed. When working with individuals suspected of having an eating disorder, it is important to be sensitive and empathetic to their situation, maintain professionalism, and to encourage evaluation and treatment from a qualified health care provider.

Chapter References

Attia, E. (2010). Anorexia nervosa: Current status and future directions. *Annual Review of Medicine*, 61, 425-435.

American Psychiatric Association (2013). *Diagnostic and Statistical Manual of Mental Disorders*, 5th edition (DSM-5). Washington, DC: American Psychiatric Publishing.

Bonci, C.M., Bonci, L.J., Granger, L.R., Johnson, C.L., Malina, R.M., Milne, L.W., ... & Vanderbunt, E.M. (2008). National Athletic Trainers Association position statement: Preventing, detecting, and managing disordered eating in athletes. *Journal of Athletic Training*, 43(1), 80-108.

Bratland-Sanda, S., & Sundgot-Borgen, J. (2013). Eating disorders in athletes: Overview of prevalence, risk factors and recommendations for prevention and treatment. *European Journal of Sport Science*, 13(5), 449-508.

Hudson, J.I., Hiripi, E., Pope Jr, H.G., & Kessler, R.C. (2007). The prevalence and correlates of eating disorders in the National Comorbidity Survey Replication. *Biological Psychiatry*, 61(3), 348-358.

National Eating Disorders Association (NEDA): *Coaches & Trainers Toolkit*. Available at: https://www.nationaleatingdisorders.org/sites/default/files/Toolkits/CoachandTrainerToolkit.pdf.

Nattiv, A., Loucks, A.B., Manore, M.M., Sanborn, C.F., Sundgot-Borgen, J., & Warren, M.P. (2007). American College of Sports Medicine position stand. The female athlete triad. *Medicine and Science in Sports and Exercise*, 39(10), 1867-1882.

Ozier, A.D., & Henry, B.W. (2011). Position of the American Dietetic Association: Nutrition intervention in the treatment of eating disorders. *Journal of the American Dietetic Association*, 111(8), 1236-1241.

Smink, F.R., van Hoeken, D., & Hoek, H.W. (2012). Epidemiology of eating disorders: Incidence, prevalence and mortality rates. *Current Psychiatry Reports*, 14(4), 406-414.

Striegel-Moore, R.H., & Franko, D.L. (2008). Should binge eating disorder be included in the DSM-V? A critical review of the state of the evidence. *Annual Review of Clinical Psychology*, 4, 305-324.

White, S., Reynolds-Malear, J.B., & Cordero, E. (2011). Disordered eating and the use of unhealthy weight control methods in college students: 1995, 2002, and 2008. *Eating Disorders*, 19(4), 323-334.

Chapter 11 Review Questions

1. Which of the following is a common characteristic of individuals with eating disorders?
    A. High self-efficacy
    B. Low self-esteem
    C. Narcissism
    D. High sense of responsibility

2. According to the DSM-5 diagnostic criteria, which of the following is associated with anorexia nervosa?
    A. Recurrent episodes of binge-eating
    B. Normal to high-normal body mass index
    C. Intense fear of gaining weight or becoming fat, even though at a significantly low weight
    D. Repeatedly chewing and spitting out, but not swallowing, large amounts of food

3. Which of the following statements would be best to initiate a conversation with a class participant, who you suspect has an eating disorder?
    A. "You are going to have to be hospitalized if you keep starving yourself."
    B. "I can't allow you to attend my class any longer unless you start eating more."
    C. "I am very concerned that you may be harming yourself."
    D. "You really should eat more because you look too skinny."

4. Which of the following is included in the female athlete triad?
    A. Binge-eating
    B. Muscle dysmorphia
    C. Amenorrhea
    D. Electrolyte imbalance

5. Which of the following sports may place athletes at an increased risk for the development of an eating disorder?
    A. Softball
    B. Basketball
    C. Soccer
    D. Wrestling

6. The prevalence of eating disorders is highest among which of the following groups?
    A. Male athletes
    B. Female non-athletes
    C. Female athletes
    D. Male non-athletes

Answers to Review Questions on Page 384

Note: Review questions are intended to reinforce learning and comprehension of subject matter presented in the corresponding chapter. The review questions are not intended to be representative of actual certification exam questions in terms of style, content, or difficulty.

Section IV

Health and Fitness Assessments

The evaluation of a client's initial health and fitness is a crucial step in the process of delivering personal training services. The appropriate selection, administration, and interpretation of health and fitness assessments are important professional responsibilities for personal trainers and other fitness professionals. A thorough preparticipation screening process and a comprehensive series of health and fitness assessments are necessary components of the personal trainer's overall risk management plan. The information obtained from these assessments and screening protocols may assist to minimize liability exposures (see chapter 26) by allowing the fitness professional to identify those participants in need of further medical evaluation. In addition, the data obtained provides guidance for the safe and effective development of individualized exercise programs.

Chapter 12 reviews the components of preparticipation screening, which should be completed prior to fitness assessments and exercise participation. The preparticipation screening process is intended to determine the client's physical readiness for exercise, to categorize their level of risk for the development of chronic disease (e.g., coronary artery disease), and to identify those who should be advised to consult with a health care provider prior to beginning an exercise program.

Chapter 13 reviews health screening protocols that should be conducted by fitness professionals with all clients as a component of risk stratification. These screening protocols include measurements of resting heart rate, resting blood pressure, body mass index, and waist-to-hip ratio.

Chapter 14 introduces both static and dynamic postural analysis. The observation of postural and joint alignment obtained through functional movement screens may allow the fitness professional to identify possible muscle imbalances and postural distortion patterns to be considered and addressed when designing an exercise program.

Chapter 15 provides an overview of health-related physical fitness assessments addressing body composition, cardiorespiratory endurance, muscular fitness (i.e., strength and endurance), and flexibility. Various fitness assessment protocols are provided including normative data, which may be used in the evaluation and classification of a client's level of fitness.

12
Initial Intake & Preparticipation Screening

Introduction

For most adults, the benefits of physical activity and exercise far outweigh the potential risks and dangers. The long-term risks associated with a sedentary lifestyle are significantly greater in terms of chronic disease development, reduced quality of life, and increased economic burden, than the immediate risks associated with exercise. Nevertheless, fitness professionals have a duty to ensure safe exercise participation by screening all individuals prior to conducting physical fitness assessments or beginning an exercise program. In addition to completing an informed consent, the preparticipation process should also utilize tools such as the Physical Activity Readiness Questionnaire (PAR-Q), a Health Risk Appraisal (HRA), and a Health and Lifestyle Questionnaire (HLQ). These tools are used to gather relevant information regarding past and present medical conditions, lifestyle behaviors, risk factors for chronic disease, and signs or symptoms suggestive of disease. Guided by this information, the fitness professional is able to determine the need for medical clearance or if it is safe for a participant to proceed with an appropriate exercise program. The overarching purpose of preparticipation screening is to identify individuals who may be at elevated risk for exercise-related sudden cardiac death and/or acute myocardial infarction (i.e., heart attack) (ACSM, 2018; Magal & Riebe, 2016; Riebe et al., 2015). In addition, the information gathered during the preparticipation screening process will guide the fitness professional's decision-making when developing a safe and effective individualized exercise program.

Informed Consent

Prior to fitness testing and participation in an exercise program, it is important both legally and ethically to obtain a participant's **informed consent**. The exact language contained within the informed consent document may vary based on the exercise setting and the type of assessments being administered. However, the fitness professional must ensure that all participants clearly understand the inherent risks, dangers, and potential discomforts associated with the planned fitness assessments and subsequent exercise program. Although the benefits of exercise far exceed the potential risks for most individuals, it is still necessary to communicate the known risks and dangers to all participants. When developing an informed consent document, the following information must be included:

- **Explanation of the purpose and procedures**. The participant must have a clear understanding of the objective for each assessment, how the results will be used, and how the information or data will be obtained. In addition, the participant must understand the components of the exercise program and a general overview of activities to be incorporated into a fitness routine.

- **Explanation of the inherent risks, dangers, and potential discomforts**. The risks may include unlikely events such as abnormal blood pressure responses, irregular heart rate (i.e., arrhythmia), lightheadedness or fainting, musculoskeletal injury (e.g., sprains, strains, fractures), and in rare cases, heart attack, stroke, or even death. The discomforts may include shortness of breath, fatigue, and muscle soreness.

- **Expected benefits and outcomes**. The benefits of exercise are well-documented and for most individuals, far outweigh the risks. The informed consent should highlight some of the known benefits related to regular physical activity. In addition, the document should review the outcomes expected for each fitness assessment and the benefit of obtaining this objective information with regard to program design. Also discuss specific benefits as they relate to the individual goals and needs of the participant.

- **Responsibilities of the participant**. To facilitate appropriate decision-making, the participant must provide important and relevant information to the fitness professional. This includes personal information obtained during the preparticipation screening process (e.g., PAR-Q, HRA, HLQ) as well as reports of any unusual responses, sensations, or symptoms experienced during, or in response to the fitness assessments or the exercise program.

- **Confidentiality and use of information**. The participant should be assured that the information provided to the fitness professional and the data collected through fitness assessments will be treated as confidential and privileged information, not to be shared with any unauthorized person without the participant's consent.

- **Questions and inquiries.** The participant must be given the opportunity to ask any questions regarding the assessment process and/or exercise program.
- **Assumption of risk/freedom of consent.** Having now been informed and fully understanding the purpose of the assessments and/or program, the associated risks and benefits, and the participant responsibilities, the individual is agreeing to voluntarily participate in the designated activities and may discontinue at any time, for any reason.

After the participant has reviewed the informed consent and all questions have been answered, it should be signed, dated, and kept on file. Since laws differ from state to state, it is highly recommended that the informed consent document is reviewed by a qualified attorney prior to implementation. Sample informed consent documents may be referenced in *ACSM's Health/Fitness Facility Standards and Guidelines*, 4th edition (2012), or *ACSM's Guidelines to Exercise Testing and Prescription*, 10th edition (2018).

Physical Activity Readiness Questionnaire

The *Physical Activity Readiness Questionnaire (PAR-Q)* is a popular self-screening tool developed by the Canadian Society for Exercise Physiology. This questionnaire is also used by many fitness professionals as the minimum screening tool for identification of those participants with elevated health risk who should consult with a physician or other qualified health care provider prior to exercise participation. The PAR-Q is not designed to provide great detail with regard to the participant's health history or detect serious medical considerations. The simplicity and ease of use has contributed to its wide-spread popularity. The PAR-Q is most appropriate for adults who plan to begin a low- to moderate-intensity exercise program. The PAR-Q has been validated as a reliable tool to identify at-risk individuals (Chisholm et al., 1978).

The PAR-Q includes seven closed-ended questions to be answered with either a 'yes' or 'no' response. The specific questions include:

1. Has your doctor ever said that you have a heart condition and that you should only do physical activity recommended by a doctor?
2. Do you feel pain in your chest when you do physical activity?
3. In the past month, have you had chest pain when you were not doing physical activity?
4. Do you lose your balance because of dizziness or do you ever lose consciousness?
5. Do you have a bone or joint problem (for example, back, knee, or hip) that could be made worse by a change in your physical activity?
6. Is your doctor currently prescribing drugs (for example, water pills) for your blood pressure or heart condition?
7. Do you know of any other reason why you should not do physical activity?

Questions #1, 2 and 3 are designed to identify known or suspected heart disease. Question #4 is designed to establish if there are any symptoms that may indicate a neurological disorder. Question #5 is designed to identify any musculoskeletal disorders. Question #6 is designed to identify hypertension. Question #7 is a very general question that is designed to identify any other issues that may limit exercise participation.

If the participant responds 'yes' to any of the questions on the PAR-Q, then they should be directed to consult with a health care provider and obtain medical clearance prior to beginning an exercise program. Please see page 357 for a sample of the PAR-Q. You are encouraged to copy this form, provided it is not altered in any way.

Physical Activity Readiness Questionnaire for Everyone

Although the original version of the PAR-Q has been validated and is widely utilized by fitness professionals, it has also received some criticism. To minimize risks, the original PAR-Q was intentionally conservative; however, this does result in many 'false positives' and incorrectly identifies some people as at-risk for whom increased levels of physical activity would be safe (Jamnik et al., 2011). These false-positives indicate the need for certain individuals to seek medical consultation and clearance, which is frequently an unnecessary obstacle that may deter many from becoming more physically active. For example, such situations often arise in response to question #5 - "Do you have a bone or joint problem (for example, back, knee, or hip) that could be made worse by a change in your physical activity?" A participant may respond 'yes' with thoughts of an old injury that is presently asymptomatic and unproblematic. However, this situation should not preclude exercise participation.

In addition, the current PAR-Q has been validated only for persons between the ages of 15 and 69. However, there are few exercise contraindications for youth under the age of 15 or persons over the age of 69, many of whom are already physically active and are generally of much better health status than was the case 25 years ago when the original PAR-Q was launched (Jamnik et al., 2011).

Subsequently, the PAR-Q has recently been revised into the *Physical Activity Readiness Questionnaire for Everyone (PAR-Q+)* (Warburton et al., 2011). The 4-page PAR-Q+ has improved detail and enhanced specificity, which includes formalized questions to further investigate 'yes' responses and determine the true need for medical evaluation and clearance. The PAR-Q+, including the follow-up questions, can be found on pages 358–361. You are again encouraged to photocopy the PAR-Q+; however, you must use the entire questionnaire and no changes are permitted.

Personal Health & Lifestyle Questionnaire

Although the PAR-Q and PAR-Q+ are convenient minimum screening tools, they may still lack the detail necessary to complete a thorough evaluation of health status. Therefore, a more comprehensive health & lifestyle questionnaire should also be administered with new participants. It is important for the fitness professional to collect a thorough health and lifestyle history from clients before conducting fitness assessments or beginning an exercise program. The use of appropriate questionnaires helps the fitness professional to identify those who may require additional medical evaluation and clearance prior to engaging in physical activity. In addition, this information provides invaluable insight to guide the fitness professional through their needs analysis and decision-making.

Fitness professionals and fitness facilities may develop a unique questionnaire to address the specific needs of their environment and clientele or you may utilize a pre-existing document, provided permission to reproduce has been granted. A complete personal health & lifestyle questionnaire should address the following areas:

- Medical diagnoses and history of medical procedures
- Previous physical examination findings (e.g., heart murmurs, ankle edema, hypertension, abnormal pulmonary sounds)
- Recent laboratory findings (e.g., blood glucose, serum lipids and lipoproteins)
- History of signs or symptoms suggestive of disease
- Recent illness, hospitalization, new diagnoses, or surgical procedures
- Orthopedic problems
- Medication use (including dietary/nutritional supplements) and drug allergies
- Other habits including caffeine, alcohol, tobacco, or drug use
- Exercise and physical activity history
- Work/occupational history
- Family history of chronic diseases

The personal health & lifestyle questionnaire should be completed prior to beginning fitness assessments or an exercise program and should be updated periodically (e.g., every 6-12 months) to document any changes in the participant's health status. A sample questionnaire can be found on pages 366–369.

ACSM Preparticipation Screening Recommendations

In 2015, the ACSM published updated exercise preparticipation health screening recommendations (Riebe et al., 2015). The updated recommendations determine the need for medical clearance based on an individual's current level of exercise; the presence of major signs or symptoms of and/or known cardiovascular, metabolic, or renal disease; and the desired exercise intensity (ACSM, 2018; Magal & Riebe, 2016; Riebe et al., 2015).

Regular Exercise

Sedentary individuals are at greater total risk for acute cardiac events compared to their physically active counterparts (Riebe et al., 2015). Studies have demonstrated that the risk of nonfatal heart attack and sudden cardiac death is significantly higher during vigorous-intensity physical activity compared to rest. However, research also reveals that the likelihood of exercise-related cardiovascular incidents and death during or immediately following vigorous exercise is lower among those who engage in regular physical activity (Riebe et al., 2015). Therefore, the first step in the updated preparticipation screening process is to determine if an individual participates in regular exercise - defined as performing planned, structured physical activity at least 30 minutes at a moderate-intensity on at least 3 days per week for at least the last 3 consecutive months (ACSM, 2018; Magal & Riebe, 2016; Riebe et al., 2015).

Signs or Symptoms Suggestive of Disease

The next step is to identify the presence of known cardiovascular, metabolic, or renal disease, or major signs or symptoms suggestive of disease. The recognition of diagnosed cardiovascular, metabolic, and renal disease, and the identification of major signs or symptoms suggestive of these diseases is an important component of the preparticipation screening process and determination of the need for medical clearance (ACSM, 2018; Magal & Riebe, 2016; Riebe et al., 2015). At rest or during activity, major signs or symptoms include (ACSM, 2018; Magal & Riebe, 2016; Riebe et al., 2015):

- Pain or discomfort in the chest, neck, jaw, arms, or other areas that may result from ischemia (inadequate blood supply to the heart);
- Shortness of breath (i.e., dyspnea) at rest or with mild exertion;
- Dizziness or syncope (fainting or loss of consciousness);
- Orthopnea (shortness of breath while at rest in a reclined position that is promptly relieved by sitting upright or standing) or paroxysmal nocturnal dyspnea (shortness of breath beginning usually 2-5 hours after the onset of sleep, which is relieved by sitting upright on the side of the bed or getting out of bed);
- Ankle edema (swelling);
- Palpitations (an unpleasant awareness of the forceful or rapid beating of the heart) or tachycardia (abnormally rapid resting heart rate, usually greater than 100 b/min);

- Intermittent claudication (the pain that occurs in a muscle with inadequate blood supply, often the lower leg muscles when walking, which is relieved 1-2 minutes after exercise is stopped);
- A known heart murmur; or
- Unusual fatigue or shortness of breath with usual activities.

Desired Exercise Intensity

In comparison to rest, light-, and moderate-intensity physical activity, vigorous-intensity exercise does present a small but measurable acute risk of adverse cardiovascular complications (Riebe et al., 2015). Therefore, the desired exercise intensity is an important consideration when determining the need for referral to and medical clearance from a health care provider prior to beginning or progressing an exercise program.

Exercise intensity may be defined using a number of different terms including a percentage of heart rate reserve (HRR) or oxygen consumption reserve (VO_2R), metabolic equivalents (METs), or rating of perceived exertion (RPE). Light-intensity exercise or physical activity is defined as 30 to <40% of HRR or VO_2R, 2 to <3 METs, or an RPE of 9 to 11 on the category scale or 2 to 4 on the category-ratio scale. Moderate-intensity exercise or physical activity is defined as 40 to <60% of HRR or VO_2R, 3 to <6 METs, or an RPE of 12 to 13 on the category scale or 5 to 6 on the category-ratio scale. Vigorous-intensity exercise or physical activity is defined as $\geq$60% of HRR or VO_2R, $\geq$6 METs, or an RPE of $\geq$14 on the category scale or $\geq$7 on the category-ratio scale. Classification and monitoring of physical activity and exercise intensity are discussed in greater detail in chapters 16 and 17.

Medical Clearance

Medical clearance refers to written approval from a qualified health care provider to engage in exercise. The need to refer a participant to a health care provider and to obtain medical clearance is based on the participant's current level of exercise, the presence of signs or symptoms or known cardiovascular, metabolic, or renal disease, and the desired exercise intensity. The logic model illustrated in figure 12-1 may be used to guide decision-making with regard to the need for medical clearance (ACSM, 2018 Magal & Riebe, 2016; Riebe et al., 2015).

For individuals who currently participate in regular exercise:
1. If the individual is asymptomatic without known cardiovascular, metabolic, or renal disease, then medical clearance is not necessary. Continue with a moderate- to vigorous-intensity exercise program, progressing gradually according to ACSM's published exercise program guidelines.
2. If the individual is asymptomatic with known cardiovascular, metabolic, or renal disease, then medical clearance is recommended (within the last 12 months) before engaging in vigorous-intensity exercise; however, medical clearance is not necessary to continue with moderate-intensity exercise.
3. If the individual is symptomatic with or without known cardiovascular, metabolic, or renal disease, then the individual should discontinue exercise and obtain medical clearance from an appropriate health care provider.

For individuals who currently inactive (i.e., sedentary):
1. If the individual is asymptomatic without known cardiovascular, metabolic, or renal disease, then medical clearance is not necessary prior to beginning a light- to moderate-intensity exercise program. The individual may progress gradually to vigorous-intensity exercise according to ACSM's published exercise program guidelines.
2. If the individual is asymptomatic with known cardiovascular, metabolic, or renal disease, then medical clearance is recommended before beginning a light- to moderate-intensity exercise program. The individual may gradually progress as tolerated, following ACSM's published exercise program guidelines.
3. If the individual is symptomatic with or without known cardiovascular, metabolic, or renal disease, then medical clearance is recommended before beginning a light- to moderate-intensity exercise program. The individual may gradually progress as tolerated, following ACSM's published exercise program guidelines.

Risk Factors

The identification of risk factors for cardiovascular or other chronic diseases is an important component of the preparticipation screening process. Unlike the previous guidelines (ACSM, 2014; ACSM & AHA, 1998), the updated ACSM preparticipation screening recommendations do not include the identification of CVD risk factors or risk stratification (ACSM, 2018 Magal & Riebe, 2016; Riebe et al., 2015). Nevertheless, as noted by Magal & Riebe (2016), exercise professionals should continue to complete a CVD risk factor appraisal with their clients, even though it is no longer part of the decision-making logic model used to identify those clients who may require medical clearance prior to exercise.

Epidemiologic studies have revealed several risk factors having a strong association with the development of cardiovascular disease. Some risk factors, such as age and family history, are uncontrollable. Other factors are directly or indirectly related to lifestyle behaviors, such as cigarette smoking, physical inactivity, and obesity. These are considered controllable risk factors. The major risk factors for CVD, as defined by the ACSM (2018) are listed in table 12-1.

Table 12-1 Risk Factors for Cardiovascular Disease

Positive Risk Factors	Definition
Age	Men ≥45 years Women ≥55 years
Family History	Myocardial infarction, coronary revascularization, or sudden death before the age of 55 years in father or other male first-degree relative, or before 65 years of age in mother or other female first-degree relative
Cigarette Smoking	Current cigarette smoker or those who quit within the previous six months or exposure to environmental tobacco smoke
High Blood Pressure (Hypertension)	Systolic blood pressure ≥140 mmHg and/or diastolic pressure ≥90 mmHg, confirmed by measurements on at least two separate occasions, or on antihypertensive medication
High Cholesterol (Dyslipidemia)	LDL-C ≥130 mg/dL or HDL-C ≤40 mg/dL, or on lipid-lowering medication. If total serum cholesterol is all that is available, use ≥200 mg/dL
Diabetes	Fasting plasma glucose ≥126 mg/dL or 2-hour plasma glucose values in oral glucose tolerance test (OGTT) ≥200 mg/dL or HbA1C ≥6.5%
Obesity	BMI ≥30 kg/m² or waist circumference >102 cm (40 inches) for men and >88 cm (35 inches) for women
Sedentary Lifestyle	Not participating in at least 30 minutes of moderate-intensity physical activity on at least three days per week for at least three months
Negative Risk Factor	**Definition**
HDL Cholesterol	HDL-C ≥60 mg/dL

Source: American College of Sports Medicine (2018).

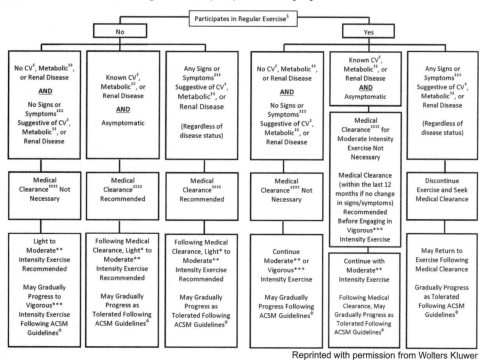

Figure 12-1 Preparticipation Screening Logic Model

Reprinted with permission from Wolters Kluwer

Footnotes for Preparticipation Screening Logic Model

§Exercise participation, performing planned, structured physical activity at least 30 min at moderate intensity on at least 3 d/wk for at least the last 3 months.

*Light-intensity exercise, 30% to <40% HRR or VO₂R, 2 to <3 METs, 9–11 RPE, an intensity that causes slight increases in HR and breathing.

**Moderate-intensity exercise, 40% to <60% HRR or VO₂R, 3 to <6 METs, 12–13 RPE, an intensity that causes noticeable increases in HR and breathing.

***Vigorous-intensity exercise ≥60% HRR or VO₂R, ≥6 METs, ≥14 RPE, an intensity that causes substantial increases in HR and breathing.

‡CVD, cardiac, peripheral vascular, or cerebrovascular disease.

‡‡Metabolic disease, type 1 and 2 diabetes mellitus.

‡‡‡Signs and symptoms, at rest or during activity; includes pain, discomfort in the chest, neck, jaw, arms, or other areas that may result from ischemia; shortness of breath at rest or with mild exertion; dizziness or syncope; orthopnea or paroxysmal nocturnal dyspnea; ankle edema; palpitations or tachycardia; intermittent claudication; known heart murmur; or unusual fatigue or shortness of breath with usual activities.

‡‡‡‡Medical clearance, approval from a health care professional to engage in exercise.

ΦACSM Guidelines, see *ACSM's Guidelines for Exercise Testing and Prescription*, 10th edition, 2018.

Positive risk factors are those that increase the risk of cardiovascular disease. Certain risk factors are likely to place an individual at greater risk than others. The presence of multiple risk factors may increase the overall risk for CVD exponentially. In some cases, a participant may not know their current biomarker levels (e.g., resting blood pressure, serum cholesterol levels, blood glucose). If the presence or absence of a CVD risk factor is not disclosed, is unknown, or is not available, then that risk factor should be counted as being present (ACSM, 2018).

Although physical inactivity is among the traditional risk factors for CVD, a low level of cardiorespiratory fitness (CRF) is not currently included among the risk factors identified by the ACSM and the American Heart Association (AHA). It is well-documented that low cardiorespiratory fitness increases the risk of CVD and all-cause premature mortality. Research supports the inclusion of measured or self-reported cardiorespiratory fitness (e.g., VO_2max, MET capacity) as an important risk factor for CVD, independent of traditional risk factors (Gupta et al., 2011; Holtermann et al., 2015; Lavie et al., 2012; Myers et al., 2015; Swift et al., 2013). Therefore, exercise professionals may also consider recognition of low CRF when assessing the overall risk of CVD.

Negative risk factors are those that decrease the risk of cardiovascular disease. A high-density lipoprotein cholesterol (HDL-C) level ≥60 mg/dL is a negative risk factor. In other words, a high HDL level is associated with reduced risk of cardiovascular disease. Presently, a high HDL cholesterol is the only negative risk factor for which a definition is recognized. However, a growing body of research supports the recognition of both regular physical activity and a high level of cardiorespiratory fitness as independent negative risk factors for CVD (Gupta et al., 2011; Holtermann et al., 2015; Lavie et al., 2012; Myers et al., 2015; Swift et al., 2013). A meta-analysis conducted by Kodama et al. (2009) indicates that subjects with a maximal aerobic capacity (i.e., cardiorespiratory fitness) ≥7.9 METs had substantially lower rates of CVD compared to those with an aerobic capacity <7.9 METs. In addition, for each one MET increase in CRF, CVD-related mortality is reduced by 15% (Kodama et al., 2009).

Chapter Summary
This chapter introduced common health questionnaires used in exercise settings and reviewed the updated preparticipation screening recommendations. The Physical Activity Readiness Questionnaire (PAR-Q) and the more recent PAR-Q+ are recommended as minimum screening tools. In addition, fitness professionals should administer a health & lifestyle questionnaire and health risk appraisal to ascertain more detail regarding a participants past and present medical status. The updated ACSM preparticipation screening recommendations guide exercise professionals to identify those individuals who should be referred to a health care provider for medical clearance prior to engage in an exercise program. As noted by Magal & Riebe (2016), these updated screening recommendations should not replace sound judgement, and decisions regarding referral and the need for medical clearance, which should continue to be made on an individual basis.

Chapter References
American College of Sports Medicine (2014). *ACSM's Guidelines for Exercise Testing and Prescription*, 9th edition. Baltimore, MD: Lippincott, Williams, and Wilkins.

American College of Sports Medicine (2018). *ACSM's Guidelines to Exercise Testing and Prescription*, 10th edition. Philadelphia, PA: Wolters Kluwer.

American College of Sports Medicine and American Heart Association (1998). Position Stand: Recommendations for cardiovascular screening, staffing, and emergency policies at heath/fitness facilities. *Medicine & Science in Sports & Exercise*, 30(6),1009-18.

Chisholm, D.M., Collis, M.L., Kulak, L.L., Davenport, W., Gruber, N., Stewart, G.W., et al., (1978). PAR-Q validation report: The evaluation of a self-administered pre-exercise screening questionnaire for adults. Victoria, BC: BC Ministry of Health and Health and Welfare Canada.

Gupta, S., Rohatgi, A., Ayers, C.R., Willis, B.L., Haskell, W.L., Khera, A., ... & Berry, J.D. (2011). Cardiorespiratory fitness and classification of risk of cardiovascular disease mortality. *Circulation*, 123(13), 1377-1383.

Holtermann, A., Marott, J.L., Gyntelberg, F., Søgaard, K., Mortensen, O.S., Prescott, E., & Schnohr, P. (2015). Self-reported cardiorespiratory fitness: Prediction and classification of risk of cardiovascular disease mortality and longevity—a prospective investigation in the Copenhagen City Heart Study. *Journal of the American Heart Association*, 4(1), e001495.

Jamnik, V.K., Warburton, D.E.R., Makarski, J., McKenzie, D.C., Shephard, R.J., Stone, J.A., Charlesworth, S., & Gledhill, N. (2011). Enhancing the effectiveness of clearance for physical activity participation: Background and overall process. *Applied Physiology, Nutrition, and Metabolism*, 36(S1), S3-S13.

Kodama, S., Saito, K., Tanaka, S., Maki, M., Yachi, Y., Asumi, M., ... & Yamada, N. (2009). Cardiorespiratory fitness as a quantitative predictor of all-cause mortality and cardiovascular events in healthy men and women: A meta-analysis. *Journal of the American Medical Association*, 301(19), 2024-2035.

Lavie, C.J., Swift, D.L., Johannsen, N.M., Arena, R., & Church, T.S. (2012). Physical fitness-an often forgotten cardiovascular risk factor. *Journal of Glycomics & Lipidomics*, 2(2), 1000e104.

Magal, M., & Riebe, D. (2016). New preparticipation health screening recommendations: What exercise professionals need to know. *ACSM's Health & Fitness Journal*, 20(3), 22-27.

Myers, J., McAuley, P., Lavie, C.J., Despres, J.P., Arena, R., & Kokkinos, P. (2015). Physical activity and cardiorespiratory fitness as major markers of cardiovascular risk: Their independent and interwoven importance to health status. *Progress in Cardiovascular Diseases*, 57(4), 306-314.

Riebe, D., Franklin, B.A., Thompson, P.D., Garber, C.E., Whitfield, G.P., Magal, M., & Pescatello, L.S. (2015). Updating ACSM's recommendations for exercise preparticipation health screening. *Medicine & Science in Sports & Exercise*, 47(11), 2473-2479.

Swift, D.L., Lavie, C.J., Johannsen, N.M., Arena, R., Earnest, C.P., O'Keefe, J.H., ... & Church, T.S. (2013). Physical activity, cardiorespiratory fitness, and exercise training in primary and secondary coronary prevention. *Circulation Journal*, 77(2), 281-292.

Warburton, D.E.R., Jamnik, V.K., Bredin, S.S.D., and Gledhill, N. on behalf of the PAR-Q+ Collaboration (2011). The Physical Activity Readiness Questionnaire (PAR-Q+) and Electronic Physical Activity Readiness Medical Examination (ePARmed-X+). *Health & Fitness Journal of Canada*, 4(2), 3-23.

Recommended Reading

American College of Sports Medicine (2018). Chapter 2: Exercise Preparticipation Health Screening. In, *ACSM's Guidelines to Exercise Testing and Prescription*, 10th edition. Philadelphia, PA: Wolters Kluwer.

Chapter 12 Review Questions

1. A 44-year-old sedentary individual is planning to begin a moderate-intensity exercise program under the supervision of a personal trainer. The individual is asymptomatic and does not have any known chronic diseases. According to the updated ACSM (2015) preparticipation screening recommendations, which of the following is the most appropriate for this individual?
   A. Medical clearance is recommend prior to beginning an exercise program.
   B. A graded exercise test (GXT) is recommended prior to beginning an exercise program.
   C. Medical clearance is not necessary prior to beginning an exercise program.
   D. Referral to a qualified health care provider for a complete medical examination is required prior to beginning an exercise program.

2. Your new client is a 42-year-old male with a BMI of 26.3. He does not currently perform any leisure-time physical activity and has a sedentary occupation. He is a non-smoker. His resting blood pressure is 136/98 mmHg, his fasting blood glucose is 94 mg/dL, his LDL cholesterol is 170 mg/dL and his HDL is 45 mg/dL. He does not have any known diseases, no family history of chronic disease, and does not report any major signs or symptoms suggestive of disease. Based on the information provided, how many major risk factors for CVD does this client have?
   A. 1
   B. 2
   C. 3
   D. 4

3. According to the updated ACSM (2015) preparticipation screening recommendations, for which of the following scenarios is medical clearance recommended?
   A. An asymptomatic individual without known cardiovascular, metabolic, or renal disease does not participate in regular exercise, but would like to begin a moderate-intensity exercise program
   B. An asymptomatic individual with known metabolic disease does not participate in regular exercise, but would like to begin a moderate-intensity exercise program
   C. An asymptomatic individual without known cardiovascular, metabolic, or renal disease participates in regular moderate-intensity physical activity, but would like to progress to vigorous-intensity exercise
   D. An asymptomatic individual with known cardiovascular disease would like to continue participation in a regular moderate-intensity exercise program

4. The phrase 'assumption of risk' refers to
   A. allowing a client to perform an activity or exercise that is contraindicated.
   B. an agreement to compensate for injuries resulting from a fitness assessment.
   C. the participant is voluntarily accepting the known dangers of exercise participation.
   D. the responsibility one accepts for another person who is involved in a high-risk activity.

5. Which of the following is considered to be a controllable risk factor for cardiovascular disease?
   A. Body mass index of 18.9 to 28.5 kg/m^2
   B. Resting systolic blood pressure of >130 mmHg
   C. Men ≥45 years old or women ≥55 years old
   D. No participation in moderate-intensity physical activity of at least 30 minutes on at least 3 days per week for at least 3 months

6. Which of the following forms is utilized to communicate the known risks and dangers associated with exercise participation?
   A. Health & Lifestyle Questionnaire
   B. Physical Activity Readiness Questionnaire
   C. Informed Consent
   D. Medical Clearance Form

Answers to Review Questions on Page 384

Note: Review questions are intended to reinforce learning and comprehension of subject matter presented in the corresponding chapter. The review questions are not intended to be representative of actual certification exam questions in terms of style, content, or difficulty.

13
Health Screening Assessments

Introduction
Several health screening assessments are recommended and commonly performed by fitness professionals in conjunction with preparticipation screening and initial health and fitness assessment procedures. These screening assessments are not intended to be diagnostic. Screening assessments are used by the fitness professional to assist with risk classification, determination of health status, and to identify those who may need to visit their physician for further evaluation and possible diagnosis. The screening assessments often performed by fitness professionals include resting heart rate, resting blood pressure, body mass index, and waist-to-hip ratio. This chapter reviews the proper administration and interpretation of these screening assessments.

Resting Heart Rate
Resting heart rate (RHR) can be manually counted by palpating either the radial or carotid pulse. See figure 13-1 and 13-2. Although the carotid pulse may be easier to locate, pressing too hard may cause a reflexive slowing of the heart rate. Measuring the resting heart rate involves feeling the pulse by using the first and second fingers to count the number of beats per minute. Resting heart rate is most accurately measured by counting the number of beats for a full minute, first thing in the morning before getting out of bed, and averaging that measurement over three consecutive days. Normal resting heart rate for an adult ranges from 60 to 90 beats per minute. Generally speaking, those with a higher level of cardiorespiratory fitness have a lower resting heart rate. A resting heart rate greater than 100 beats per minute is called *tachycardia* and may be an indication of serious cardiac dysfunction. A longitudinal study following over 4,700 subjects for 12 years indicated that an elevated resting heart rate, independent of other cardiovascular risk factors, was associated with increased all-cause mortality and cardiovascular mortality (Mensink & Hoffmeister, 1997). In addition, more recent research has demonstrated that a resting heart rate elevated above 90 beats per minute increases the risk of cardiovascular disease by two times in men and three times in women (Cooney et al., 2010). Since any number of conditions may cause an abnormally elevated resting heart rate, it is important to advise participants to consult with their physician for proper evaluation and diagnosis when consistent elevations in resting heart rate are identified.

Resting Blood Pressure
The assessment of **resting blood pressure (RBP)** is an essential component of a complete health and fitness evaluation. Blood pressure is the measure of the pressure, or resistance to blood flow, within the arterial vascular system. Blood pressure is expressed in terms of the systolic pressure (top number of a blood pressure measurement) and diastolic pressure (bottom number). **Systolic blood pressure (SBP)** represents the pressure exerted against the arterial vessel walls during the left ventricular contraction. **Diastolic blood pressure (DBP)** represents the pressure in the arterial vascular system during the relaxation phase of the cardiac cycle. A normal, healthy resting blood pressure for an adult is a systolic pressure of less than 120 mmHg and a diastolic pressure of less than 80 mmHg.

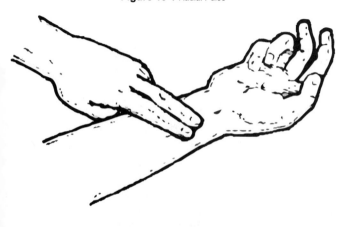

Figure 13-1 Radial Pulse

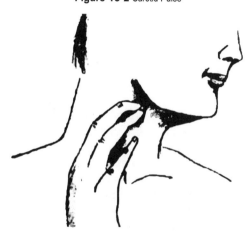

Figure 13-2 Carotid Pulse

High blood pressure, known as **hypertension**, is defined as a systolic pressure ≥140 mmHg and/or a diastolic blood pressure ≥90 mmHg, which has been confirmed on at least two separate occasions. Anyone taking a prescribed antihypertensive medication is also considered to be hypertensive, although their resting blood pressure may be within a normal range under the influence of this medication.

According to the Centers for Disease Control and Prevention, hypertension affects 1 out of 3 adults or approximately 68 million Americans (CDC, 2011). Hypertension is a controllable risk factor for cardiovascular disease; however, it is estimated that only 46% of those known to have high blood pressure have it under control (CDC, 2011). Hypertension contributes to one out of every seven deaths in the United States and can lead to coronary heart disease, congestive heart failure, stroke, kidney failure, and many other serious health problems (Carriker & Kravitz, 2013; CDC, 2011).

The adoption of healthy lifestyle behaviors is effective for the prevention and management of hypertension. These healthy behaviors include limit sodium and alcohol intake, perform regular physical activity, abstain from cigarettes and other tobacco products, maintain a healthy body weight, and manage stress effectively (Carriker & Kravitz, 2013). In addition, antihypertensive medications (e.g., beta-blockers, calcium channel blockers, diuretics) are often prescribed to help treat hypertension.

As with any health or fitness assessment, accuracy is essential for maintaining the reliability and effectiveness of blood pressure screening. Potential errors may arise from an improperly calibrated sphygmomanometer, an improperly sized blood pressure cuff (e.g., too large or too small), and error resulting from inexperienced screeners. To maximize accuracy, the following procedures should be followed when measuring resting blood pressure (ACSM, 2018; Bushman, 2016):

1. The participant should be seated quietly for at least 5 minutes in a chair with back support with their feet on the floor and the arm supported at heart level. The participant should refrain from ingesting caffeine for at least 30 minutes preceding the measurement.
2. Wrap the blood pressure cuff firmly around upper arm at heart level; align cuff with brachial artery. The appropriate cuff size must be used to ensure accurate measurement. The bladder within the cuff should encircle at least 80% of the upper arm. Many adults require a large adult cuff.
3. Insert the stethoscope earpieces into your ears. Place the diaphragm side of the stethoscope chest piece against the participant's arm below the antecubital space over the brachial artery.
4. Quickly inflate cuff pressure to 180-200 mmHg or at least 20 mmHg above the anticipated systolic pressure.
5. Turning the bulb valve to the left, slowly deflate the cuff to release pressure at a rate of approximately 2-3 mmHg per second.
6. Listening with the stethoscope, the systolic blood pressure (SBP) is the point at which the first of two or more Korotkoff sounds is heard, and the diastolic blood pressure (DBP) is the point before the disappearance of Korotkoff sounds. Note the SBP and DBP to the nearest mmHg.
7. At least two measurements should be obtained (minimum of one minute apart), and the average should be recorded.

Table 13-1 provides the classifications of blood pressure for adults adopted from the Joint National Committee on Prevention, Detection, Evaluation, and Treatment of High Blood Pressure (Chobanian et al., 2003).

Table 13-1 Classification of Blood Pressure

Classification	Systolic (mmHg)		Diastolic (mmHg)
Normal	<120	and	<80
Prehypertension	120-139	or	80-89
Stage 1 hypertension	140-159	or	90-99
Stage 2 hypertension	≥160	or	≥100

National Committee on the Prevention, Detection, Evaluation, and Treatment of High Blood Pressure (2003).

Body Mass Index

Body mass index (BMI) is a calculation used to assess body weight relative to height. BMI may be used as one of several risk indicators for the development of chronic diseases such as cardiovascular disease and type 2 diabetes. Body mass index is determined by taking the individual's weight in kilograms divided by their height in meters squared.

$$BMI = Weight\ (kg) / Height^2\ (m^2)$$

Note: 1 lb. = 0.45 kg. and 1 in. = 0.0254 m.

For example, the BMI for a client weighing 185 lbs. (83.25 kg) with a height of 75 in. (1.905 m) is calculated as follows:

$$BMI = 83.25\ kg / (1.905\ m)^2 = 22.9\ kg/m^2$$

In general, as body mass index increases, the level of risk for health problems also increases. A BMI from 25.0 to 29.9 is classified as 'overweight' and a BMI >30.0 is classified as 'obesity.' Table 13-2 provides the summary of body mass index classifications adopted from the National Heart, Lung, and Blood Institute (NHLBI, 1998).

Table 13-2 Classification of Overweight and Obesity

Classification	BMI (kg/m²)	Risk of Disease
Underweight	<18.5	—
Normal	18.5 - 24.9	Low
Overweight	25.0 - 29.9	Increased
Class 1 Obesity	30.0 - 34.9	High
Class 2 Obesity	35.0 - 39.9	Very High
Class 3 Obesity	≥40.0	Extremely High

National Heart, Lung, and Blood Institute (1998).

Despite the wide-spread use of body mass index for the classification of overweight and obesity, BMI has been scrutinized as a valid indicator of health risk due to the inability of this measurement to differentiate fat weight from lean body weight (Okorodudu et al., 2010; Romero-Corral et al., 2008). In certain cases, an individual may have a healthy body composition (i.e., low percent of body fat), yet may also have a high BMI due to a larger proportion of lean body mass. See figure 13-3. This may be especially true among athletic populations. Therefore, BMI should be used as one health indicator among other methods of body composition analysis.

Figure 13-3 BMI Comparison

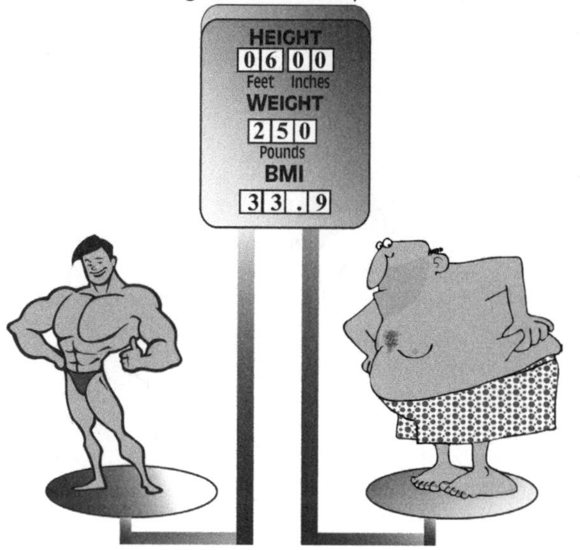

Waist-to-Hip Ratio

The **waist-to-hip ratio (WHR)** is a measurement used to assess an individual's regional fat distribution. Weight distribution patterns have been identified as an important indicator of health risks. Those who store more body fat through the central region of the body (i.e., abdominal fat), known as *android obesity*, are at an increased risk of hypertension, type 2 diabetes, dyslipidemia, cardiovascular disease, and premature death as compared to *gynoid obesity*, which is fat distributed in the hips and thighs. Therefore, the 'apple' body type presents more risk compared to the 'pear' body type. In fact, compared to body mass index, an elevated waist-to-hip ratio appears to be more strongly associated with cardiovascular disease, metabolic risk factors, and premature death (de Koning et al., 2007).

The waist-to-hip ratio is calculated by dividing the waist circumference by the hip circumference. See table 13-4 for the description of measurement sites. For example, if a client has a waist measurement of 35 inches and a hip measurement of 38 inches, the WHR is calculated as follows:

$$WHR = 35 \text{ inches} / 38 \text{ inches} = 0.92$$

In general, the risk of chronic health problems increase as the waist-to-hip ratio increases. For men this level of risk increases significantly at a WHR greater than 0.95 and for women at a WHR greater than 0.86. It has been shown that a 0.01 increase in waist-to-hip ratio is associated with a 5% increase in risk for cardiovascular disease (de Koning et al., 2007). Table 13-3 provides a detailed summary of health risk stratification based on waist-to-hip ratio. Considering the relative simplicity of determining WHR and the strong association as a predictor of risk, it is recommended that WHR is included among the screening assessments performed by fitness professionals.

Table 13-3 Waist-to-Hip Risk Classification

Disease Risk	Men	Women
Very Low	<0.85	<0.80
Low	0.85 to 0.89	0.80 to 0.84
Moderate	0.90 to 0.99	0.85 to 0.95
High	1.00 to 1.10	0.96 to 1.05
Very High	>1.10	>1.05

Hoeger & Hoeger (1994)

Circumference Measurements

Circumference or girth measurements can be used to determine a baseline from which to track changes in body size at various anatomical sites. Initial changes in body composition may not be readily evident through scale weight; however, a client may indicate that their clothes fit differently. Circumference measurements may help to quantify these changes and provide a valuable source of motivation. Circumference measurements are advantageous since they are quick and relatively simple to administer and do not require expensive equipment. These measurements also provide meaningful feedback relevant to many clients' goals. Table 13-4 provides the list and definition of standardized circumference sites. The following standardized procedures should be followed when performing circumference measurements:

1. All measurements should be obtained with a flexible yet inelastic tape measure. Use a tension-regulated tape measure (e.g., Gulick Tape Measure or MyoTape®) if available.

Table 13-4 Description of Circumference Locations

Location	Description
Abdominal	With the subject standing upright and relaxed, a horizontal measurement taken at the level of the umbilicus.
Calf	With the subject standing tall, a horizontal measurement taken at the maximal circumference between the knee and ankle, perpendicular to the long axis.
Forearm	With the subject standing and arms hanging downward and resting slightly away from the body, palms facing forward, a measurement taken perpendicular to the long axis of the forearm at the level of maximal circumference distal to the elbow.
Hips	With the subject standing, legs slightly apart (~10 cm), a horizontal measurement taken at the maximum circumference of the hips/buttocks.
Upper Arm	With the subject standing tall and arms hanging freely at the sides with the hands facing the hips, a horizontal measurement taken midway between the acromion and the olecranon processes.
Waist	With the subject standing, arms at the sides, feet together, and abdomen relaxed, a horizontal measurement taken at the narrowest circumference of the torso between the umbilicus and xiphoid process.
Mid Thigh	With the subject standing and one foot on a bench so the knee is flexed at 90 degrees, a measurement taken midway between the inguinal crease and the proximal border of the patella, perpendicular to the long axis.

Adopted from ACSM (2018)

2. The tape measure should be applied directly on the skin surface. When using a standard tape measure, pull to a proper and consistent level of tension without pinching the underlying skin or excessively compressing the subcutaneous adipose (i.e., fat) tissue.

3. Take 2 to 3 measurements at each site and retest if measurements are not within ¼ inch (5 mm) of each other.

4. Rotate through anatomical locations or allow time for skin and subcutaneous tissue to regain normal texture.

Waist circumference is a particularly important measurement as an indicator of health risk. As noted in chapter 12, a waist circumference >102 cm (40 inches) for men and >88 cm (35 inches) for women may be used as a classification of obesity with regard to coronary artery disease risk factors. It has been shown that each 1 cm (0.40 inch) increase in waist circumference is associated with a 2% increased risk of cardiovascular disease (de Koning et al., 2007).

Chapter Summary

As one component of the initial intake and assessment procedures for a new client, health screening assessments such as resting heart rate, resting blood pressure, body mass index, and waist-to-hip ratio should be administered by the fitness professional. Although these screening assessments are not intended to be diagnostic, they are necessary for the classification of health and risk status. Observations from these health screening assessments may also assist the fitness professional to identify those individuals who should visit their physician for further medical evaluation prior to exercise participation.

Chapter References

American College of Sports Medicine. (2018). *ACSM's Guidelines for Exercise Testing and Prescription*, 10th edition. Philadelphia, PA: Wolters Kluwer

Bushman, B.A. (2016). Blood pressure basics and beyond. *ACSM's Health & Fitness Journal*, 20(3), 5-9.

Carriker, C., & Kravitz, L. (2013). Exploring the amazing heart: Heart rate and blood pressure offer powerful clues to clients' fitness progress. *IDEA Fitness Journal*, 10(2), 36-43.

Centers for Disease Control and Prevention (2011). Vital signs: Prevalence, treatment, and control of hypertension – United States, 1999-2002 and 2005-2008, *Morbidity and Mortality Weekly Report*, 60(4), 103-108.

Chobanian, A.V., Bakris, G.L., Black, H.R., Cushman, W.C., Green, L.A., Izzo, J.L., ... & Roccella, E.J. (2003). Seventh report of the joint national committee on prevention, detection, evaluation, and treatment of high blood pressure. *Hypertension*, 42(6), 1206-1252.

Cooney, M.T., Vartiainen, E., Laakitainen, T., Juolevi, A., Dudina, A., & Graham, I.M. (2010). Elevated resting heart rate is an independent risk factor for cardiovascular disease in healthy men and women. *American Heart Journal*, 159(4), 612-619.

de Koning, L., Merchant, A.T., Pogue, J., & Anand, S.S. (2007). Waist circumference and waist-to-hip ratio as predictors of cardiovascular events: Meta-regression analysis of prospective studies. *European Heart Journal*, 28(7), 850-856.

Hoeger, W.K., & Hoeger, S.A. (1994). *Principles and Labs for Physical Fitness and Wellness*, 3rd edition. Englewood, CO: Morton Publishing Company.

Mensink, G.B.M., & Hoffmeister, H. (1997). The relationship between resting heart rate and all-cause, cardiovascular and cancer mortality. *European Heart Journal*, 18(9), 1404-1410.

National Heart, Lung, and Blood Institute (1998). *Clinical Guidelines on the Identification, Evaluation, and Treatment of Overweight and Obesity in Adults*. Bethesda, MD: Department of Health and Human Services, National Institutes of Health. NIH Publication No. 98-4083.

Okorodudu, D.O., Jumean, M.F., Montori, V.M., Romero-Corral, A., Somers, V.K., Erwin, P.J., & Lopez-Jimenez, F. (2010). Diagnostic performance of body mass index to identify obesity as defined by body adiposity: A systematic review and meta-analysis. *International Journal of Obesity*, 34(5), 791-799.

Romero-Corral, A., Somers, V.K., Sierra-Johnson, J., Thomas, R.J., Collazo-Clavell, M.L., Korinek, J., ... & Lopez-Jimenez, F. (2008). Accuracy of body mass index in diagnosing obesity in the adult general population. *International Journal of Obesity*, 32(6), 959-966.

Chapter 13 Review Questions

1. Your client is 5 feet 7 inches tall and currently weighs 166 pounds. Based on the information provided, what is the client's current body mass index (BMI) classification?
    A. Underweight
    B. Normal
    C. Overweight
    D. Obese

2. Calculate the waist-to-hip ratio for an individual having a waist circumference of 34 inches and a hip circumference of 37 inches.
    A. 0.83
    B. 1.10
    C. 0.92
    D. 0.88

3. When measuring blood pressure the first of two or more successive Korotkoff sounds represents the
    A. systolic blood pressure.
    B. rate pressure product.
    C. diastolic blood pressure.
    D. cardiac output.

4. During the initial health screening with a new client, you determine their resting heart rate to be 102 beats per minute. To confirm this measurement, you decided to reassess the client's resting heart rate the following morning. The client is instructed to refrain from caffeinated beverages and physical activity for at least 30 minutes prior to appointment. After sitting quietly for 10 minutes, the client's resting heart rate is reassessed to be 100 beats per minute. Based on the results of these measurements, which of the following is the most appropriate course of action?
    A. Refer the client to a more qualified and experienced personal trainer
    B. Encourage the client to begin a moderate-intensity exercise program to help lower the resting heart rate
    C. Encourage the client to sign up for a Bikram yoga class to help facilitate stress management and relaxation
    D. Advise the client to visit their physician for additional medical evaluations

5. Which of the following is considered to be a limitation of body mass index (BMI)?
    A. BMI is expensive and invasive for the participant
    B. Subjects often over-report their body weight
    C. BMI does not consider the relative proportions of fat and lean tissue
    D. BMI is poorly correlated to risk of chronic illnesses such as diabetes and heart disease

6. The amount of pressure exerted against the arterial walls during a left ventricular contraction is known as the
    A. diastolic blood pressure.
    B. rate-pressure product.
    C. hydrostatic transmural pressure.
    D. systolic blood pressure.

Answers to Review Questions on Page 384

Note: Review questions are intended to reinforce learning and comprehension of subject matter presented in the corresponding chapter. The review questions are not intended to be representative of actual certification exam questions in terms of style, content, or difficulty.

14
Postural Analysis

Introduction
This chapter covers concepts related to postural alignment, static and dynamic postural analysis, and common postural deviations. Maintenance of proper posture and alignment is critical to avoid unnecessary musculoskeletal and joint stress. Over time, poor posture may contribute to the onset of muscular imbalances, inefficient movement, and cumulative injuries resulting in shoulder, knee, neck, or lower back pain. During exercise, it is imperative to maintain appropriate posture and joint alignment in order to both maximize neuromuscular efficiency and to reduce the risk of orthopedic injuries. The fitness professional must have knowledge and skill in the analysis and interpretation of postural alignment.

Posture and the Kinetic Chain
Posture may be defined as the position of all body parts at any given time. Ideal posture aligns the body segments to minimize the muscular effort necessary to maintain the biomechanical efficiency of the neuromuscular and musculoskeletal systems. Although some individual variation exists, proper posture in the static standing position is typically defined with regard to the *plumb line*. See figure 14-1. Observed from a lateral view, the plumb line (sometimes referred to as the line of gravity) is the imaginary vertical line that drops from the ear through the center of the shoulder joint, along the lateral midline of the trunk, through the bodies of the lumbar vertebrae, slightly anterior to the sacroiliac joint, through the greater trochanter of the femur, anterior to the midline of the knee (posterior to the patella), and slightly anterior to the lateral malleolus of the ankle. This interconnected series of body segments and joints spanning from the feet, superiorly to the head, is often referred to as the **kinetic chain**. Although typically identified through skeletal landmarks and joints, the kinetic chain is actually an interrelated network that includes the skeletal system, the muscular system, and the nervous system. When screening posture, observations should also be conducted from both an anterior and lateral view to note alignment and symmetries (or asymmetries) of the shoulders, hips, and knees.

Proper postural alignment is crucial for the maintenance of structural integrity, which is necessary to overcome the various forces and loads applied to the body. When in proper alignment, the muscles are able to maintain their ideal length-tension relationship allowing for optimal force production (Clark et al., 2008). The *length-tension rela-* *tionship* refers to the length at which a muscle is capable of producing the greatest force. This suggests that when a muscle is moved through a range of motion, toward an overly-lengthened or an overly-shortened position, its ability to generate force will gradually diminish. When positioned in optimal alignment, the joints are also able to effectively absorb and distribute external forces, thus reducing stress on the joints (Clark et al., 2008). When an individual is chronically placing their body in a position of misalignment (i.e., poor posture), they are likely to develop muscle imbalances, inefficient or restricted movement patterns, and cumulative musculoskeletal injury.

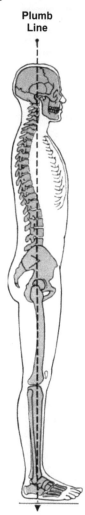

Figure 14-1 Plumb Line

Therefore, it is both important to screen and educate clients with regard to proper postural alignment. Fitness professionals should screen both static (i.e., stationary) and dynamic (i.e., moving) postural alignment to identify possible muscle weakness and tightness that may need to be addressed as a component of the overall fitness program. Although attempts have been made to place objective criteria in the postural screening protocol, there remains a high level of subjectivity in the fitness professional's ability to observe, interpret, and qualify postural alignment. When observing static posture, the postural screening checklist found in table 14-1 may be used to guide your screening procedures. Static posture may also be subjectively rated using table 14-2.

Pelvic Alignment

The lumbo-pelvic-hip (LPH) region is affected by numerous muscles that attach to, cross over, and influence the position of the pelvis. A **neutral** lumbo-pelvic-hip position (i.e., 'neutral pelvis') is characterized by vertical alignment of the anterior-superior iliac spine (ASIS) and the pubic bone of the pelvis. In the neutral position, the lumbar spine maintains a natural lordotic curve. During an **anterior pelvic tilt**, the ASIS moves anteriorly (i.e., forward) relative to the pubic bone. This anteriorly tilted pelvic position causes an increase lordodic curvature of the lumbar spine. An anterior pelvic tilt is accompanied by shortening of the iliopsoas and erector spinae muscle groups. When performing a **posterior pelvic tilt**, the ASIS moves posteriorly (i.e., backward) relative to the pubic bone. A posterior pelvic tilt is accompanied by shortening of the hamstrings and rectus abdominis. Figure 14-2 illustrates neutral pelvis, anterior pelvic tilt, and posterior pelvic tilt.

> **Good to Know**
>
> **Keys to Postural Alignment**
> - Ear is vertically aligned over the center of the shoulder.
> - Scapula are slightly retracted and depressed to position the center of the shoulder directly over the hip.
> - Neutral position is maintained through the lumbar spine with the core muscles engaged.
> - Knees are soft (not locked) with the patella facing forward and in-line vertically with the center of the foot.
> - Feet are positioned hip-width apart with toes pointing forward. Normal arches are maintained through medial aspect of feet.

medical conditions such as spinal osteoporosis, vertebral fractures, degenerative disc disease, and Scheuermann's disease (Bruno et al., 2012; Kado et al., 2013; Tsirikos & Jain, 2011). **Lordosis** is characterized by excessive anterior curvature (arching) of the lumbar spine. See figure 14-3. Lumbar lordosis is accompanied by an anterior pelvic tilt, which is associated with weakness of the core abdominal muscles and tightness of the erector spinae and hip flexor muscle groups. **Flat-back** spinal posture is characterized by flexion of the upper thoracic spine, straightening of the lower thoracic spine, flexion (flattening) of the lumbar spine and a posterior pelvic tilt. See figure 14-4. Tight and overactive hamstring muscles are commonly seen with flat-back posture. **Sway-back** posture is characterized by a forward head position, rounding of the thoracic spine, displacement of the anterior ribs behind the hips, a posterior pelvic tilt, forward swaying of the pelvis over the feet, and hyperextended knees. See figure 14-6. **Scoliosis** is a lateral curvature of the spine frequently accompa-

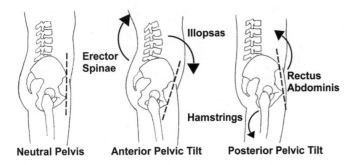

Figure 14-2 Pelvic Alignment

Neutral Pelvis   Anterior Pelvic Tilt   Posterior Pelvic Tilt

Spinal Misalignments

As the result of either structural anomalies or muscle imbalances, several misalignments of the spinal column may be observed. **Kyphosis** is characterized by excessive posterior curvature (rounding) of the thoracic spine. See figure 14-3. Kyphosis is associated with rounded shoulders, sunken chest, and forward head position accompanied by hyperextension of the cervical spine. In more advanced cases of kyphosis, a characteristic 'humpback' may be present. Kyphosis may be attributed to poor posture and the resulting muscle imbalances, as well as more serious

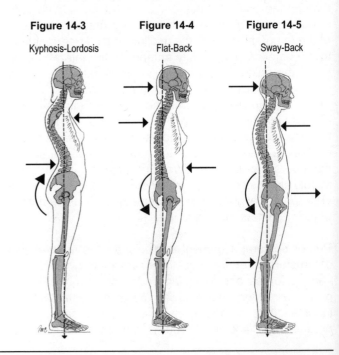

Figure 14-3 Kyphosis-Lordosis   **Figure 14-4** Flat-Back   **Figure 14-5** Sway-Back

Table 14-1 Static Postural Screen Checklist

Anatomic Checkpoint (view)	Observation	No	Yes	Left	Right
Head (anterior)	Is the head tilted or rotated to one side?				
Head (lateral)	Is the head/chin flexed/protracted forward?				
Shoulders (anterior)	Is one shoulder higher than the other?				
Shoulders (lateral)	Is the center of shoulder aligned with plumb line?				
Shoulders (lateral)	Are the shoulders rounded forward?				
Upper Back (posterior)	Is one scapula higher than the other?				
Upper Back (posterior)	Are the scapula elevated and/or protracted?				
Upper Back (lateral)	Is there excessive rounding of the thoracic spine?				
Lower Back (lateral)	Is there excessive arching of the lumbar spine?				
Lower Back (lateral)	Is there excessive flattening of the lumbar spine?				
Core (lateral)	Is the abdomen protruding or core muscles disengaged?				
Hips (anterior)	Is one hip lower than the other?				
Hips (anterior)	Are the hips internally rotated?				
Hips/Knees (anterior)	Are the hips/knees adducted (inward toward midline)?				
Knees (anterior)	Are the patella pointing medially or laterally?				
Knees (lateral)	Are the knees locked or hyperextended?				
Ankles/Feet (anterior)	Are the feet pointing inward or outward?				
Ankles/Feet (anterior)	Are the arches flattened or excessively arched?				

Table 14-2 Static Posture Rating

Anatomic Site (view)	Good	Fair	Poor
Head (anterior)	Head is erect, gravity line passes directly though the center.	Head is slighted tilted or turned to one side.	Head is significantly tilted or turned to one side.
Neck (lateral)	Neck is erect, chin slightly retracted and head directly above shoulders.	Neck and chin slightly protracted.	Neck and chin significantly protracted.
Shoulders (anterior)	Both shoulders are level (horizontally).	One shoulder is slightly higher than the other.	One shoulder is significantly higher than the other.
Upper Back (lateral view)	Normal rounding consistent with upper thoracic curvature.	Slightly more rounding than typical thoracic curvature.	Significant rounding and kyphosis.
Spine (posterior)	Spine is in a straight line.	Spine is slightly curved laterally (scoliosis).	Spine is significantly curved laterally (scoliosis).
Spine/Trunk (lateral)	Trunk is erect and aligned directly over the pelvic girdle.	Trunk is leaning slightly forward.	Trunk is leaning significantly forward.
Abdomen (lateral)	Abdomen is flat or slightly rounded.	Abdomen is protruding.	Abdomen is protruding and sagging.
Lower Back (lateral)	Lower back has a normal 'S' curvature consistent with the lumbar vertebrae.	Lower back appears slightly hollow. Slight exaggeration of the lumbar curvature.	Lower back is significantly curved causing a 'sway back' or lordosis.
Hips (anterior)	Both hips are level (horizontally).	One hip is slightly higher than the other.	One hip is significantly higher than the other
Ankles and Feet (anterior)	Feet point straight forward with ankles directly above the heel.	Feet turned outward, slightly pronated, or slightly supinated.	Feet significantly turned outward, pronated, or supinated.

nied by rotation of vertebrae. See figure 14-6. Scoliosis may be evident by asymmetry in the level of the hips and shoulders in which one side appears lower than the other.

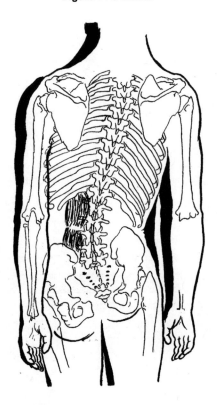

Figure 14-6 Scoliosis

Dynamic Posture

In addition to static posture, it is also important for fitness professionals to observe the client's dynamic postural control and the ability to maintain alignment throughout the kinetic chain during movement and exercise. Research has provided some evidence that several biomechanical compensations and misalignments may increase the risk of various exercise-related injuries (Neely, 1998).

Tightness in either the gastrocnemius and/or soleus muscles may limit ankle dorsiflexion. Clients may compensate for this limited range of motion by rotating their feet outward in an attempt to find a pathway of motion offering less restriction. This often leads to excessive pronation (i.e., flattened arches) of the feet as well as compensation at other joints along the kinetic chain. Subsequently, individuals, particularly runners, are at greater risk of repetitive injuries such as shin splints or iliotibial band friction syndrome (Messier & Pittala, 1988).

Further up the kinetic chain another biomechanical abnormality that is frequently observed is internal rotation of the hips (i.e., femur), which has been implicated in the development of patellofemoral (anterior knee) pain (Neely, 1998).

Affected by these biomechanical alterations at the joints both above and below the knee, a commonly seen movement compensation at the knee is adduction (inward movement toward the midline of the body), which is observed during a squat, leg press, or related exercises, and when landing from a jump. This poor structural alignment, known as *valgus torque*, creates excessive and potentially damaging shearing and compressive forces on the knee joint (Neely, 1998). Coupled with poor neuromuscular control of the lower extremities, valgus loading of the knee has been suggested to be a main contributing factor leading to non-contact ACL injuries, especially among female athletes (Hewett et al., 2005).

The risk of injury related to biomechanical and structural misalignments is not limited to just athletic populations. Poor posture and movement compensations can negatively affect both those involved in fitness activities as well as sedentary populations. The negative effect is not only demonstrated by acute and chronic injuries, but also by the more subtle impact on inefficient training and sub-optimal results achieved from exercise programs. To ensure both safe and effective training, it's important for fitness professionals to evaluate dynamic postural control. Some commonly-used dynamic postural assessments (also known as *functional movement screens*) include the body weight squat, the upper body push, and the upper body pull. The purpose of these assessments is to evaluate dynamic range of motion (i.e., flexibility) as well as neuromuscular control to maintain proper body segment and joint alignment. The observations made during these assessments will assist the fitness professional to identify potentially tight and overactive muscles, as well as weak and functionally inhibited muscles. The procedures and observational checklists for the body weight squat, upper body push, and upper body pull are listed in tables 14-3, 14-4, and 14-5, respectively. Table 14-6 can be used to assist in the possible interpretations of observations made during these movement screens.

Postural Distortion Patterns

The combination of several postural and/or structural misalignments and the ensuing neuromuscular dysfunction is referred to as a *postural distortion pattern* (Clark et al., 2008). These postural distortion patterns can lead to fairly predictable muscle imbalances (i.e., weakness coupled with tightness). Clients who have developed postural distortion patterns may have trouble correctly performing certain exercises, which can reduce the effectiveness of their program and may lead to cumulative injury (Blievernicht, 2000). Understanding these postural distortion patterns and the related muscle imbalances will allow the fitness professional to identify safe and effective exercises to be incorporated into the client's program. Two commonly seen postural distortion patterns are upper cross syndrome and lower cross syndrome.

Table 14-3 Body Weight Squat Screen

Procedures:
1. The participant begins by standing tall with feet positioned hip-width apart and toes pointing directly forward.
2. Arms are raised overhead (if able) in a parallel position with the elbows fully extended. Arms should be bisecting the ears.
3. Instruct the participant to squat down as though sitting into a chair, pause, and return to the starting position with arms still reaching overhead. Repeat 5-10 repetitions.
4. Observe the participant from the anterior and lateral views noting position and changes in alignment of feet, ankles, knees, torso, arms, and head.
5. Note observations on the checklist below.

Anatomic Checkpoint (view)	Observation	No	Yes	Left	Right
Ankles and Feet (anterior)	Do the feet turn outward?				
Ankles and Feet (anterior)	Do the feet flatten?				
Heels (lateral)	Do the heels elevate off the floor?				
Knees (anterior)	Do the knees move inward (adduction)?				
Knees (anterior)	Do the knees rotate inward?				
Trunk (lateral)	Does the torso lean excessively forward?				
Lower Back (lateral)	Does the low back arch or round?				
Arms (lateral)	Do the arms fall forward?				
Head (lateral)	Does the head fall forward out of alignment with torso?				

Table 14-4 Upper Body Push Screen

Procedures:
1. Select an appropriate chest press exercise such as a selectorized machine or cable-based equipment (e.g., cable column, FreeMotion®).
2. Instruct participant to sit or stand, depending on mode of pushing exercise, with feet hip-width apart, toes pointing forward, lower back in neutral position with abdominals activated, shoulder vertically aligned with hip (lateral view), scapula retracted and depressed (neutral starting position), and ear vertically aligned with center of shoulder (lateral view).
3. Using a light resistance, instruct the participant to slowly press the handles forward and return to starting position (elbows at 90 degrees, upper arms abducted in the frontal plane), performing 10-15 repetitions in a slow and controlled manner.
4. Observe the participant from the anterior and lateral views noting position and changes in alignment of lower back, shoulders, scapula, and head.
5. Note observations on the checklist below.

Anatomic Checkpoint (view)	Observation	No	Yes	Left	Right
Lower Back (lateral)	Does the low back arch or round?				
Shoulders (anterior)	Do the shoulders elevate?				
Scapula (lateral)	Do the scapula protract when pushing?				
Head (lateral)	Does the head protrude forward?				

Table 14-5 Upper Body Pull Screen

Procedures:
1. Select an appropriate rowing exercise such as a selectorized machine or cable-based equipment (e.g., cable column, FreeMotion®).
2. Instruct participant to sit or stand, depending on mode of pulling exercise, with feet hip-width apart, toes pointing forward, lower back in neutral position with abdominals activated, shoulder vertically aligned with hip (lateral view), scapula retracted and depressed (neutral starting position), and ear vertically aligned with center of shoulder (lateral view).
3. Using a light resistance, instruct the participant to slowly pull the handles through a full range of motion and return to starting position, performing 10-15 repetitions in a slow and controlled manner.
4. Observe the participant from the anterior and lateral views noting position and changes in alignment of lower back, shoulders, scapula, and head.
5. Note observations on the checklist below.

Anatomic Checkpoint (view)	Observation	No	Yes	Left	Right
Lower Back (lateral)	Does the low back arch or round?				
Torso (lateral)	Does the torso drift forward or backward?				
Shoulders (anterior)	Do the shoulders elevate?				
Upper Back (lateral)	Does the upper back round forward?				
Head (lateral)	Does the head protrude forward?				

Table 14-6 Movement Screen Observational Interpretation

Observation	Possible Tight, Dominant, or Overactive Muscles	Possible Weak, Passive, or Underactive Muscles
Feet turn outward	Soleus, Lateral Gastrocnemius, Biceps Femoris	Medial Gastrocnemius, Medial Hamstrings, Gracilis, Sartorius
Feet flatten	Gastrocnemius, Peroneals	Tibialis Anterior, Tibialis Posterior, Gluteus Medius
Heels elevate during squat	Gastrocnemius, Soleus	Tibialis Anterior, Tibialis Posterior
Knees adduct inward (valgus)	Adductor Group, Tensor Fascia Latae	Gluteus Medius, Gluteus Maximus
Torso leans forward excessively	Iliopsoas, Abdominals	Gluteus Maximus, Erector Spinae
Low back arches	Iliopsoas, Erector Spinae, Latissimus Dorsi	Gluteus Maximus, Hamstrings, Core Stabilizers
Low back flattens or rounds	Rectus Abdominis, External Obliques, Hamstrings	Gluteus Maximus, Gluteus Medius, Erector Spinae
Arms fall forward during squat	Latissimus Dorsi, Pectoralis Major, Teres Major	Middle/Lower Trapezius, Rhomboids, Rotator Cuff
Shoulders elevate	Upper Trapezius, Levator Scapulae	Lower Trapezius
Scapula protract during push	Pectoralis Minor/Major, Latissimus Dorsi	Rhomboids, Middle/Lower Trapezius
Upper back rounds	Pectoralis Minor/Major, Latissimus Dorsi	Rhomboids, Middle/Lower Trapezius, Posterior Deltoid, Teres Minor, Infraspinatus
Heads protrudes forward	Upper Trapezius, Sternocleidomastoid, Scalenes	Deep Cervical Flexors

Upper cross syndrome, also known as *rounded shoulder syndrome*, is characterized by a forward (i.e., protracted) head position, protracted and elevated scapula, increased *kyphosis*, and forward-rounded shoulders. This postural deviation is typical of sedentary individuals and those who spend a great deal of time sitting at a desk, but can also result from overemphasis of one muscle group in training (e.g., chest), compensation due to injury, or even emotional distress (Blievernicht, 2000). Upper cross syndrome typically involves functionally tight or overactive muscles as well as weak or inhibited muscles. This is physiologically explained through a neuromuscular concept called reciprocal inhibition. **Reciprocal inhibition** is the process whereby a tight, overactive agonist muscle will decrease or inhibit the neurological activation of its antagonist muscle, which results in functional weakness of this antagonist. Put simply, muscles that are shortened are over-stimulated by the nervous system and become dominant, whereas muscles that are lengthened are under-stimulated by the nervous system and become weak or passive (Blievernicht, 2000). For example, prolonged sitting with poor posture (e.g., at a computer) places the pectoralis major muscle in a chronically shortened position resulting in tightness and dominance. As a result, there is decreased activation of the antagonist muscles (i.e., rhomboids, middle trapezius, posterior deltoids) causing inhibition of muscle recruitment and subsequent weakness. Table 14-7 lists the muscles that are likely to be dominant and passive in those who exhibit upper cross syndrome and figure 14-7 provides an illustration.

Lower cross syndrome is often characterized by an anterior pelvic tilt and a corresponding increase in lumbar *lordosis*, internally rotated hips, adducted (i.e., valgus) knees, and outwardly rotated feet (Sahrmann, 2002). Lower cross syndrome also involves functionally tight and weak muscles as discussed previously with regard to upper cross syndrome. Many indications of these muscle imbalances may be observed when performing the body weight squat screen. In particular, lower cross syndrome typically involves tightness in the hip flexors (i.e., iliopsoas), hamstrings, hip adductors, lower back, and calves (i.e., gastrocnemius, soleus). The corresponding weak muscles groups may include the gluteus maximus and medius, rectus abdominis, quadriceps, and tibialis anterior. Table 14-8 lists the muscles that are likely to be tight and weak in those who display lower cross syndrome and figure 14-8 provides an illustration.

When designing an exercise program with those exhibiting postural misalignment or movement compensations, the fitness professional should incorporate specific exercises to address these possible muscle imbalances. Exercises should be selected to activate and strengthen those muscles believed to be weak or inhibited and to lengthen those muscles believed to be tight or overactive.

Table 14-7 Upper Cross Syndrome

Tight/Dominant Muscles	Weak/Passive Muscles
Upper Trapezius	Deep Cervical Flexors
Levator Scapulae	Serratus Anterior
Sternocleidomastoid	Rhomboids
Pectoralis Major & Minor	Posterior Deltoid
Latissimus Dorsi	Middle & Lower Trapezius
Subscapularis	Infraspinatus & Teres Minor

Note: The tight muscles are not intended to be paired with the corresponding weak muscle in this table since a clear correlation does not always exist.

Table 14-8 Lower Cross Syndrome

Tight/Dominant Muscles	Weak/Passive Muscles
Iliopsoas	Gluteus Maximus
Hamstrings	Quadriceps (Rectus Femoris)
Hip Adductors	Gluteus Medius & Minimus
Gastrocnemius	Tibialis Anterior
Soleus	Rectus Abdominis
Erector Spinae	Transverse Abdominis
Iliotibial Band	Internal & External Obliques

Note: The tight muscles are not intended to be paired with the corresponding weak muscle in this table since a clear correlation does not always exist.

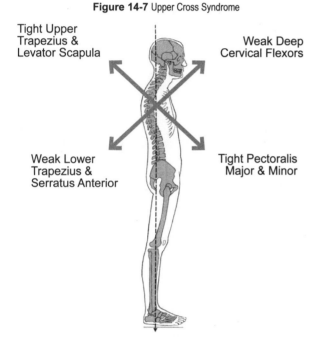

Figure 14-7 Upper Cross Syndrome

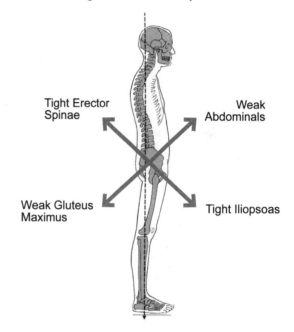

Figure 14-8 Lower Cross Syndrome

Chapter Summary

The information presented in this chapter provides the basic knowledge for fitness professionals to instruct and coach their clients with regard to proper postural alignment. In addition, this chapter introduces strategies to assess static and dynamic posture as well as postural deviations and common movement compensations. To maximize the safety and effectiveness of exercise programming, it is necessary for fitness professionals to understand appropriate body alignment, recognize postural deviations, and select the appropriate exercises corresponding to the client's needs.

Chapter References

Blievernicht, J.A. (2000). Round shoulder syndrome. *IDEA Health & Fitness Source*, 2001(6). September.

Bruno, A.G., Anderson, D.E., D'Agostino, J., & Bouxsein, M.L. (2012). The effect of thoracic kyphosis and sagittal plane alignment on vertebral compressive loading. *Journal of Bone and Mineral Research*, 27(10), 2144-2151.

Clark, M.A., Lucett, S., & Corn, R.J. (2008). *NASM Essentials of Personal Fitness Training*, 3rd edition. Philadelphia, PA: Lippincott Williams & Wilkins.

Hewett, T.E., Myer, G.D., Ford, K.R., Heidt, R.S. Jr., Colosimo, A.J., McLean, S.G., van den Bogert, A.J., Paterno, M.V., and Succop, P. (2005). Biomechanical measures of neuromuscular control and valgus loading of the knee predict anterior cruciate ligament injury risk in female athletes. *The American Journal of Sports Medicine*. 33(4), 492-501.

Kado, D.M., Huang, M.H., Karlamangla, A.S., Cawthon, P., Katzman, W., Hillier, T.A., ... & Cummings, S.R. (2013). Factors associated with kyphosis progression in older women: 15 years' experience in the study of osteoporotic fractures. *Journal of Bone and Mineral Research*, 28(1), 179-187.

Messier, S.P., & Pittala, K.A. (1988). Aetiological factors associated with selected running injuries. *Medicine and Science in Sports & Exercise*, 20(5), 501-505.

Neely, F.G. (1998). Biomechanical risk factors for exercise-related lower limb injuries. *Sports Medicine*, 26(6), 395-413.

Sahrmann, S.A. (2002). *Diagnosis and Treatment of Movement Impairment Syndromes*. St. Louis, MO: Mosby.

Tsirikos, A.I., & Jain, A.K. (2011). Scheuermann's kyphosis: Current controversies. *Journal of Bone & Joint Surgery*, British Volume, 93(7), 857-864.

Recommended Reading
Cook, E.G. (2010). *Movement: Functional Movement Systems: Screening, Assessment, Corrective Strategies*. Aptos, CA: On Target publications.

Chapter 14 Review Questions

1. Which of the following muscles is typically tight and overactive in those with upper cross syndrome?
    A. Rhomboids
    B. Hamstrings
    C. Pectoralis major
    D. Gluteus medius

2. Which of the following exercises are most appropriate for a client with lower cross syndrome?
    A. Hamstring stretches and core strengthening
    B. Quadriceps stretches and hamstring strengthening
    C. IT band stretches and erector spinae strengthening
    D. Iliopsoas stretches and hamstring strengthening

3. During the body weight squat screen, you observe that you client's heels elevate slightly off the floor during the eccentric phase of the exercise. Which of the following is most likely to contribute to this movement compensation?
    A. Tightness through the anterior tibialis muscle
    B. Weakness through the iliopsoas muscles
    C. Tightness through the gastrocnemius and soleus muscles
    D. Weakness through the adductor muscle group

4. Which spinal misalignment is characterized by flexion of the upper thoracic spine, straightening of the lower thoracic spine, flexion (flattening) of the lumbar spine and a posterior pelvic tilt?
    A. Lordosis
    B. Flat-back
    C. Sway-back
    D. Kyphosis

5. Bilateral tightness of the hamstring muscle group is likely to contribute to a _____.
    A. posterior pelvic tilt
    B. neutral pelvic position
    C. anterior pelvic tilt
    D. asymmetric hip shift

6. Based on the concept of reciprocal inhibition, an overactive and tight iliopsoas muscle group will cause inhibition and weakness of the _____.
    A. quadriceps
    B. rectus abdominis
    C. gluteus maximus
    D. gastrocnemius

Answers to Review Questions on Page 384

Note: Review questions are intended to reinforce learning and comprehension of subject matter presented in the corresponding chapter. The review questions are not intended to be representative of actual certification exam questions in terms of style, content, or difficulty.

15
Health-Related Physical Fitness Assessments

Introduction and Overview

The health-related components of physical fitness include body composition, cardiorespiratory endurance, muscular strength, muscular endurance, and flexibility. This chapter will review fitness assessment protocols commonly used by fitness professionals to obtain measurements for each of these components of fitness.

There are many objectives related to the administration of fitness assessments. The data obtained from fitness assessments provide the baseline measurements from which realistic and attainable goals may be established, and progress toward these goals will be monitored. In addition, assessments provide insight and education to the client regarding the strengths and weaknesses within their personal fitness profile. In some cases, fitness assessments may serve as a motivational tool as well as a strategy to enhance adherence and accountability to an exercise program. Finally, perhaps the most obvious purpose of fitness assessments is to provide guidance for the fitness professional to design safe and effective individualized exercise programs.

Just as the exercise program must be individually designed for each client, the selection of health and fitness assessment protocols must also be tailored to the specific goals, needs, and limitations of the client. This individualized approach to both the initial fitness assessments and the subsequent exercise program is one of the many factors adding value to the services of a personal trainer.

Many of the health and fitness assessments must be performed prior to the initiation of an exercise program. However, in the early stages of behavioral change (e.g., adopting a more active lifestyle), many clients will have apprehension, anxiety, and even fear regarding participation with fitness assessments and the results obtained. In these cases, it is important to recognize and remain sensitive to the client's feelings and preferences. It may be most appropriate to postpone nonessential assessments (i.e., those not included in preparticipation decision making) until a later date. In doing so, the personal trainer will have greater success in establishing rapport and trust with the new client. In addition, this thoughtfulness is more likely to create a positive experience for the participant, which may increase adherence to the exercise program and facilitate greater long-term outcomes.

Best Practices

To ensure valid and reliable assessment data as well as a meaningful and professional experience, the following best-practice strategies should be observed.

Practice and prepare: The time to learn how to perform an assessment is not with your client in front of you. Practice conducting fitness assessments with coworkers, friends, or family members to perfect your skills and abilities before assessing your clients. Having greater skill and confidence will increase your credibility and professionalism. In addition, you can be certain that the measurements you obtain are both valid and reliable.

Set the stage: Take a few moments to organize the area (e.g., fitness testing office, space in the fitness center, group exercise studio) you plan to utilize for the fitness assessments and the necessary equipment before your client arrives. Make sure the assessment space is large enough to accommodate the planned assessments and the environment is comfortable for your client. Provide your client with an appropriate level of privacy when conducting assessments. Check the equipment to ensure it is in good working order and properly calibrated when necessary. Finally, before conducting the fitness assessments, clearly articulate the purpose and objectives to your client.

Pick proper protocols: As stated above, some assessment and screening tools will be routinely performed with all clients. Others will be individually selected based on the goals, needs, and limitations of the client. It will be necessary to discuss the client's overall goals and objectives to guide you in the selection of relevant fitness assessment options. Consider important factors such as time, space, equipment, and abilities of the participant as you explore the many fitness assessment options.

Create consistency: Reliable comparisons between initial and re-assessment measurements are only possible if the data is obtained in a consistent manner. Therefore, it is very important to adhere to the established protocols and standardized procedures for each assessment. In addition, do everything possible to replicate the same testing experience by using the same equipment, communicating standardized pretest instructions, ensuring similar environmental conditions, and conducting the same assessment protocols in the same sequence. When performing a series of fitness assessments during the same appointment the following order is recommended:

1. Resting measurements (e.g., blood pressure, heart rate)
2. Biometric and anthropometric measurements (e.g., height, weight, body mass index, waist-to-hip ratio)
3. Body composition analysis
4. Cardiorespiratory endurance assessment
5. Dynamic postural assessments
6. Muscular fitness assessments (e.g., strength, endurance)
7. Flexibility assessments

It may not be possible to replicate the exact conditions during each subsequent re-assessment appointment, but the more consistency, the better!

Emphasize the individual: Throughout this chapter, we will present normative data and fitness classifications related to many assessment protocols and components of physical fitness. Although some clients may find this information interesting, useful, and even motivating, others may find their fitness ratings discouraging and disappointing. Highly fit and competitive individuals may thrive on comparisons to others as they seek to enhance performance and 'win'. On the other hand, sedentary or less-fit individuals are likely to experience negative emotions in response to 'below average' or 'poor' fitness ratings. This information may be counter-productive by reducing self-efficacy and desire to pursue fitness goals. Therefore, it is important to empathize with the client and understand their personal sources of motivation (or demotivation). When establishing goals, place emphasis on the improvement of individual health and fitness, rather than competition with and comparisons to others.

Explore the options: The collection of fitness assessments provided in this chapter is not an all-inclusive list. Although this manual provides a significant number of assessments, many others also exist. Take the time to familiarize yourself with the vast menu of options including those that go beyond basic assessments of physical fitness and into parameters of performance (e.g., speed, power, agility). Refer to the references and recommended reading sections of this chapter for additional fitness assessment resources.

Assessment of Body Composition

Using the two-compartment model, **body composition** is defined as the relative amount of fat mass and lean body mass throughout the body and is expressed as a percent of body fat (%BF). Body composition may be measured or estimated using a number of different techniques. Among these, underwater weighing (also called hydrostatic weighting or hydrodensitometry) is considered to be the 'gold standard' for the assessment of body composition. This method of measuring body composition is based on Archimedes principle that states when an object (i.e., body) is submerged in water it is buoyed by a counterforce equal to the weight of the water displaced by the object (ACSM, 2018). The difference between body weight on land and immersed in water is used to calculate the body volume. Since lean body tissue (e.g., bone, muscle) is more dense than water, an individual with a higher proportion of lean body mass will demonstrate a smaller difference in underwater weight compared to land weight (i.e., the lean individual tends to sink in water). On the other hand, since fat tissue is less dense than water, an individual with a higher proportion of fat mass will reflect a greater difference between underwater and land weight (i.e., the individual with more body fat will be more buoyant in water). Based on the information collected during this assessment, the individual's body density and subsequently their percentage of body fat may be calculated.

In addition to underwater weighing, other reliable and accurate methods to assess body composition include: air displacement plethysmography (BOD POD®), dual energy X-ray absorptiometry (DEXA), total body electrical conductivity (TOBEC), and near-infrared interactance (NIR). However, like underwater weighing, the equipment necessary for all of these methods of testing is expensive and rarely accessible in the health club setting. *Bioelectrical impedance analysis (BIA)* does offer a cost-effective, non-invasive, and user-friendly method to assess body composition. BIA sends a small electrical current through the body. Based on the resistance (i.e., impedance) to this current as measured by the BIA analyzer, the individual's body composition may be estimated. Although BIA testing offers a simple method for the assessment of body composition, accuracy of results can only be ensured if pretest instructions and assessment protocols are strictly followed.

Skinfold Measurement

Considering the limitations and barriers presented by the preceding methods for body composition analysis, skinfold measurement techniques offer the most practical alternative for fitness professionals. The skinfold technique is based upon the assumption that the amount of subcutaneous fat (i.e., under the skin) is proportional (~1:3) to the total body fat with some variations based on age, gender, and ethnicity. By measuring the subcutaneous fat (i.e., skinfold thickness) using skinfold calipers, the individual's percent of body fat may be estimated using appropriate regression equations. This method can be quite accurate in comparison to hydrostatic weighing; however, it is highly dependent upon the skill and experience of the test administrator as well as the selection of population-specific protocols.

To ensure a valid and reliable estimation of body composition, the following standardized procedures should be used when performing skinfold testing (ACSM, 2018):

- All measurements should be taken on the right side of the body with the subject standing upright.
- Caliper should be placed directly on the skin surface, 1 cm from the thumb and finger, perpendicular to the skinfold, and halfway between the crest and base of the fold.
- The pinch should be maintained while reading the caliper.
- Wait 1-2 seconds, but not longer, before reading the caliper.
- Take duplicate measurements at each site, and retest if the measurements are not within 1-2 mm.
- Rotate through skinfold sites or allow time for the skin and subcutaneous tissue to regain normal texture and thickness.

The description of standardized skinfold sites are listed in table 15-1. Figures 15-1, 15-2, and 15-3 illustrate a proper pinch and caliper placement on a skinfold.

Two commonly used protocols involving three skinfold sites have been validated for both men (Jackson & Pollock, 1978) and women (Jackson et al., 1980). For men, this protocol utilizes skinfold measurements taken at the chest, abdominal, and thigh. For women the three skinfold sites include the triceps, suprailiac, and thigh. In accordance with the standardized skinfold testing procedures, several (e.g., 2–3) measurements are obtained at each anatomical location until a consistent (i.e., within 1–2 mm) number is obtained. The average measurement obtained at each of the three skinfold sites is then totaled together. The sum of the three skinfold sites is then located in the gender-specific table (15-2 for women; 15-4 for men) corresponding to the subject's age range. This indicates the estimated percent of body fat for this subject.

For example, the following skinfold measurements were obtained from a 46-year-old female subject who currently weighs 157 pounds. Using table 15-2, the estimated percentage of body fat is determined by cross-referencing the sum of the three skinfold sites with the age category corresponding to the subject's age.

Table 15-1 Skinfold Locations

	Description of Standardized Skinfold Sites
Abdominal	Vertical fold; 2 cm to the right of the umbilicus
Triceps	Vertical fold; on the posterior midline of the upper arm, halfway between the acromion and olecranon processes, with the arm held freely to the side of the body
Chest	Diagonal fold; one-half of the distance between the anterior axillary line and the nipple for men or one-third of the distance for women
Medial Calf	Vertical fold; at the maximum circumference of the calf on the midline of its medial border
Midaxillary	Vertical fold; on the midaxillary line at the level of the xiphoid process of the sternum
Suprailiac	Diagonal fold; in line with the natural angle of the iliac crest taken in the anterior axillary line immediately superior to the iliac crest
Thigh	Vertical fold; on the anterior midline of the thigh, midway between the proximal border of the patella and inguinal crease (hip)
Subscapular	Diagonal fold (45° angle) taken 1-2 cm below the inferior angle of the scapula

Figure 15-1

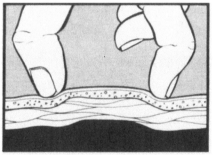

Figure 15-2

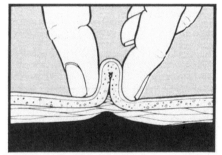

Figure 15-3

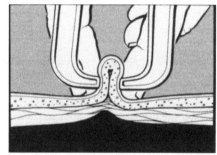

Figures 15-1, 15-2, and 15-3 are excerpted and reprinted with permission from, Donoghue, W.C., (2009). *How To Measure Your % Bodyfat: An Instruction Manual For Measuring % Bodyfat Using Skinfold Calipers*, 7th edition. Ann Arbor, MI: Creative Health Products.

Table 15-2 Estimated Body Fat for Women (Sum of Triceps, Suprailiac, & Thigh)

Sum of Skinfolds (mm)	Age < 22	Age 23-27	Age 28-32	Age 33-37	Age 38-42	Age 43-47	Age 48-52	Age 53-55	Age >57
23-25	9.7	9.9	10.2	10.4	10.7	10.9	11.2	11.4	11.7
26-28	11.0	11.2	11.5	11.7	12.0	12.3	12.5	12.7	13.0
29-31	12.3	12.5	12.8	13.0	13.3	13.5	13.8	14.0	14.3
32-34	13.6	13.8	14.0	14.3	14.5	14.8	15.0	15.3	15.5
35-37	14.8	15.0	15.3	15.5	15.8	16.0	16.3	16.5	16.8
38-40	16.0	16.3	16.5	16.7	17.0	17.2	17.5	17.7	18.0
41-43	17.2	17.4	17.7	17.9	18.2	18.4	18.7	18.9	19.2
44-46	18.3	18.6	18.8	19.1	19.3	19.6	19.8	20.1	20.3
47-49	19.5	19.7	20.0	20.2	20.5	20.7	21.0	21.2	21.5
50-52	20.6	20.8	21.1	21.3	21.6	21.8	22.1	22.3	22.6
53-55	21.7	21.9	22.1	22.4	22.6	22.9	23.1	23.4	23.6
56-58	22.7	23.0	23.2	23.4	23.7	23.9	24.2	24.4	24.7
59-61	23.7	24.0	24.2	24.5	24.7	25.0	25.2	25.5	25.7
62-64	24.7	25.0	25.2	25.5	25.7	26.0	26.2	26.4	26.7
65-67	25.7	25.9	26.2	26.4	26.7	26.9	27.2	27.4	27.7
68-70	26.6	26.9	27.1	27.4	27.6	27.9	28.1	28.4	28.6
71-73	27.5	27.8	28.0	28.3	28.5	28.8	29.0	29.3	29.5
74-76	28.4	28.7	28.9	29.2	29.4	29.7	29.9	30.2	30.4
77-79	29.3	29.5	29.8	30.0	30.3	30.5	30.8	31.0	31.3
80-82	30.1	30.4	30.6	30.9	31.1	31.4	31.6	31.9	32.1
83-85	30.9	31.2	31.4	31.7	31.9	32.2	32.4	32.7	32.9
86-88	31.7	32.0	32.2	32.5	32.7	32.9	33.2	33.4	33.7
89-81	32.5	32.7	33.0	33.2	33.5	33.7	33.9	34.2	34.4
92-94	33.2	33.4	33.7	33.9	34.2	34.4	34.7	34.9	35.2
95-97	33.9	34.1	34.4	34.6	34.9	35.1	35.4	35.6	35.9
98-100	34.6	34.8	35.1	35.3	35.5	35.8	36.0	36.3	36.5
101-103	35.3	35.4	35.7	35.9	36.2	36.4	36.7	36.9	37.2
104-106	35.8	36.1	36.3	36.6	36.8	37.1	37.3	37.5	37.8
107-109	36.4	36.7	36.9	37.1	37.4	37.6	37.9	38.1	38.4
110-112	37.0	37.2	37.5	37.7	38.0	38.2	38.5	38.7	38.9
113-115	37.5	37.8	38.0	38.2	38.5	38.7	39.0	39.2	39.5
116-118	38.0	38.3	38.5	38.8	39.0	39.3	39.5	39.7	40.0
119-121	38.5	38.7	39.0	39.2	39.5	39.7	40.0	40.2	40.5
122-124	39.0	39.2	39.4	39.7	39.9	40.2	40.4	40.7	40.9
125-127	39.4	39.6	39.9	40.1	40.4	40.6	40.9	41.1	41.4
128-130	39.8	40.0	40.3	40.5	40.8	41.0	41.3	41.5	41.8

Table 15-3 Body Composition Norms for Women

Age	20-29	30-39	40-49	50-59	60+
Excellent	<15	<16	<17	<18	<19
Good	16-19	17-20	18-21	19-22	20-23
Fair	20-28	21-29	22-30	23-31	24-32
Poor	29-31	30-32	31-33	32-34	33-35
Very Poor	>32	>33	>34	>35	>36

Table 15-4 Estimated Body Fat for Men (Sum of Chest, Abdominal, & Thigh)

Sum of Skinfolds (mm)	Age < 22	Age 23-27	Age 28-32	Age 33-37	Age 38-42	Age 43-47	Age 48-52	Age 53-55	Age >57
8-10	1.3	1.8	2.3	2.9	3.4	3.9	4.5	5.0	5.5
11-13	2.2	2.8	3.3	3.9	4.4	4.9	5.5	6.0	6.5
14-16	3.2	3.8	4.3	4.8	5.4	5.9	6.4	7.0	7.5
17-19	4.2	4.7	5.3	5.8	6.3	6.9	7.4	8.0	8.5
20-22	5.1	5.7	6.2	6.8	7.3	7.9	8.4	8.9	9.5
23-25	6.1	6.6	7.2	7.7	8.3	8.8	9.4	9.9	10.5
26-28	7.0	7.6	8.1	8.7	9.2	9.8	10.3	10.9	11.4
29-31	8.0	8.5	9.1	9.6	10.2	10.7	11.3	11.8	12.4
32-34	8.9	9.4	10.0	10.5	11.1	11.6	12.2	12.8	13.3
35-37	9.8	10.4	10.9	11.5	12.0	12.6	13.1	13.7	14.4
38-40	10.7	11.3	11.8	12.4	12.9	13.5	14.1	14.6	15.2
41-43	11.6	12.2	12.7	13.3	13.8	14.4	15.0	15.5	16.1
44-46	12.5	13.1	13.6	14.2	14.7	15.3	15.9	16.4	17.0
47-49	13.4	13.9	14.5	15.1	15.6	16.2	16.8	17.3	17.9
50-52	14.3	14.8	15.4	15.9	16.5	17.1	17.6	18.2	18.8
53-55	15.1	15.7	16.2	16.8	17.4	17.9	18.5	19.1	19.7
56-58	16.0	16.5	17.1	17.7	18.2	18.8	19.4	20.0	20.5
59-61	16.9	17.4	17.9	18.5	19.1	19.7	20.2	20.8	21.4
62-64	17.6	18.2	18.8	19.4	19.9	20.5	21.1	21.7	22.2
65-67	18.5	19.0	19.6	20.2	20.8	21.3	21.9	22.5	23.1
68-70	19.3	19.9	20.4	21.0	21.6	22.2	22.7	23.3	23.9
71-73	20.1	20.7	21.2	21.8	22.4	23.0	23.6	24.1	24.7
74-76	20.9	21.5	22.0	22.6	23.2	23.8	24.4	25.0	25.5
77-79	21.7	22.2	22.8	23.4	24.0	24.6	25.2	25.8	26.3
80-82	22.4	23.0	23.6	24.2	24.8	25.4	25.9	26.5	27.1
83-85	23.2	23.8	24.4	25.0	25.5	26.1	26.7	27.3	27.9
86-88	24.0	24.5	25.1	25.7	26.3	26.9	27.5	28.1	28.7
89-81	24.7	25.3	25.9	26.5	27.1	27.6	28.2	28.8	29.4
92-94	25.5	26.0	26.6	27.2	27.8	28.4	29.0	29.6	30.2
95-97	26.1	26.7	27.3	27.9	28.5	29.1	29.7	30.3	30.9
98-100	26.9	27.4	28.0	28.6	29.2	29.8	30.4	31.0	31.6
101-103	27.5	28.1	28.7	29.3	29.9	30.5	31.1	31.7	32.3
104-106	28.2	28.8	29.4	30.0	30.6	31.2	31.8	32.4	33.0
107-109	28.9	29.5	30.1	30.7	31.3	31.9	32.5	33.1	33.7
110-112	29.6	30.2	30.8	31.4	32.0	32.6	33.2	33.8	34.4
113-115	30.2	30.8	31.4	32.0	32.6	33.2	33.8	34.5	35.1
116-118	30.9	31.5	32.1	32.7	33.3	33.9	34.5	35.1	35.7
119-121	31.5	32.1	32.7	33.3	33.9	34.5	35.1	35.7	36.4
122-124	32.1	32.7	33.3	33.9	34.5	35.1	35.8	36.4	37.0
125-127	32.7	33.3	33.9	34.5	35.1	35.8	36.4	37.0	37.6

Table 15-5 Body Composition Norms for Men

Age	20-29	30-39	40-49	50-59	60+
Excellent	<10	<11	<13	<14	<15
Good	11-13	12-14	14-16	15-17	16-18
Fair	14-20	15-21	17-23	18-24	19-25
Poor	21-23	22-24	24-26	25-27	26-28
Very Poor	>24	>25	>27	>28	>29

Triceps: 18, 20, 19 = 19 mm
Suprailiac: 12, 13, 12 = 12 mm
Thigh: 33, 32, 32 = 32 mm

Sum of Three Sites = 63 mm
Estimated Body Fat = 26.0%

When appropriate, the subject's estimated body fat percentage may be classified based on the normative data provided in table 15-3. Body composition for male subjects may be similarly estimated from skinfold measurements using table 15-4 and classified according to male normative data provided in table 15-5.

Assessment of Cardiorespiratory Endurance

Cardiorespiratory endurance is the capacity of the circulatory and respiratory systems to deliver oxygen and nutrients to the working muscles in support of continuous aerobic activity. Cardiorespiratory endurance is not only a component of health-related physical fitness, but is also highly correlated to a decreased risk of obesity, multiple chronic diseases, and premature death.

Cardiorespiratory endurance is typically measured or estimated by oxygen consumption. *Oxygen consumption* is the amount of oxygen that is utilized (i.e., consumed) by the skeletal muscles during a specific level of activity. Oxygen consumption may be expressed in relative terms as milliliters of oxygen per kilogram of body weight per minute of activity (mL/kg/min) or in absolute terms as liters of oxygen per minute (L/min). The best indication of cardiorespiratory fitness is maximal oxygen consumption (VO_2max), defined as the highest amount of oxygen that can be utilized by the skeletal muscles during maximal, exhaustive exercise.

Maximal oxygen consumption may be measured directly through gas exchange analysis or estimated from the heart rate response during a *graded exercise test (GXT)*. Graded exercise test protocols are typically performed on a treadmill or stationary cycle during which the exercise intensity (i.e., workload) is gradually increased at set time intervals (typically 2–3 minutes) as the physiological responses of the body are monitored. Maximal GXTs are performed up to the physiological maximum oxygen consumption, as defined by a plateau in VO_2max despite further increases to the exercise workload, or to the point of volitional fatigue. Submaximal GXTs are performed up to a predetermined end-point, typically 85% of age-predicted maximum heart rate. The heart rate response to this submaximal assessment is then used to predict the VO_2max that would have been attained had the subject continued to their theoretical age-predicted maximum heart rate. During both maximal and submaximal graded exercise testing, the test is also terminated if adverse cardiovascular responses are observed or if the subject requests to stop.

The level of medical supervision during graded exercise testing is dependent upon the end-point of the exercise test (e.g., submaximal or maximal) as well as other considerations regarding the subject, the fitness professional, and the facility. According to ACSM (2018), appropriately trained nonphysician staff can safely administer maximal exercise tests when a qualified physician is in the immediate vicinity and available for emergencies. Likewise, the American Heart Association (AHA) requires that a physician is physically present during graded exercise testing of high-risk individuals (Myers et al., 2014). During exercise testing of moderate-risk participants, it is also recommended that a physician is readily available, but is not necessary based on the health and risk status of the participant, the training and experience of the fitness staff, and local policies (ACSM, 2014). Graded exercise testing of low-risk participants may be conducted by qualified fitness professionals without the immediate availability of a physician (ACSM, 2014). The AHA indicates that graded exercise tests for low- or moderate-risk individuals can be safely supervised by nonphysician health professionals if the individual meets competency requirements for exercise testing, is trained in emergency cardiac care, and is supported by a physician skilled in exercise testing (Myers et al., 2014). A comprehensive understanding of exercise physiology is perhaps the most important competency area for health and exercise professionals conducting graded exercises tests (Myers et al., 2014). In addition, the safety of exercise testing depends on understanding and identifying test indications and contraindications, selecting an appropriate test protocol, knowing when to terminate the test, and emergency preparedness (Myers et al., 2014). The decision to administer graded exercise testing should consider the legal implications for the fitness facility if a complication or adverse event were to occur during exercise testing that is not physician or professionally supervised.

Graded exercise testing, particularly involving the use of direct gas exchange analysis, requires expensive testing equipment as well as significant technical training and skill for the test administrator. Although a GXT offers greater precision, validity, and reliability, it is often not a feasible option in most health club settings. However, cardiorespiratory fitness and VO_2max may also be estimated through a variety of field tests, which tend to be more cost-effective, convenient, and easy to administer. Subsequently, many fitness professionals implement field tests to evaluate cardiorespiratory endurance. These field tests utilize various modes of exercise, such as walking, running, and stepping, performed at a submaximal intensity. Field tests may be performed in a non-laboratory setting and require only minimal equipment. The specific protocol selected should be appropriate based on the participant's goals, current level of fitness, health status, skill, and limitations. Several common field tests to assess cardiorespiratory endurance are presented in this chapter.

Rockport One-Mile Walk Test

The Rockport One-Mile Walk Test is recommended for nearly all populations including those with a low level of fitness. Since walking is a mode of physical activity familiar to most, this test tends to be well-tolerated and a more reliable indicator of cardiorespiratory fitness as compared to step tests, particularly when the subject is able to walk briskly enough to elevate their heart rate over 120 beats per minute. The fitness professional may utilize the information obtained from this test to estimate the subject's VO_2max. In addition, the participant can also easily understand the primary measurement outcome, time to complete a one-mile walk, which provides motivation and allows progress to be readily self-monitored as fitness levels improve.

Equipment: stopwatch, a flat one-mile course (preferable) or treadmill.

Procedure:
1. Allow participant a short warm-up period (5 minutes).
2. Instruct participant to walk the one-mile course as quickly as possible. The subject may not run. Walking is defined as having one foot in contact with the ground at all times.
3. Upon completion of the one-mile walk, record the elapsed time and,
4. Immediately take heart rate (at the radial pulse site, see page 149) for 15 seconds. Multiply the number of beats counted for 15 seconds by 4 to determine the recovery heart rate in beats per minute.
5. The subjects VO_2max may be estimated from the recovery heart rate using the formula provided in the box below developed by Kline et al. (1987).
6. The subject's fitness category may be classified according to the time to complete the one-mile walk using table 15-6.

Table 15-6 One-Mile Walk Time to Completion

Rating	Men <40	Men >40	Women <40	Women >40
Excellent	13:00 or less	14:00 or less	13:30 or less	14:30 or less
Good	13:01 – 15:30	14:01 – 16:30	13:31 – 16:00	14:31 – 17:00
Average	15:31 – 18:00	16:31 – 19:00	16:01 – 18:30	17:01 – 19:30
Below Average	18:01 – 19:30	19:01 – 21:30	18:31 – 20:00	19:31 – 22:00
Low	19:31 or more	21:31 or more	20:01 or more	22:01 or more

12-Minute Walk/Run Test

The 12-Minute Walk/Run Test was developed by Cooper (1968) as a method of predicting cardiorespiratory fitness based on the maximal distance covered in 12 minutes. Similar to the one-mile walk test, this field test is a convenient and cost-effective option requiring minimal equipment or skill. However, this test may be more appropriate for conditioned individuals who are accustomed to moderate- to vigorous-intensity physical activity.

Equipment: stopwatch, 400-meter Olympic track (preferable), flat course with a measured distance, or treadmill.

Procedure:
1. Allow participant a short warm-up period (5-10 minutes).
2. Instruct the participant to run/walk as far as possible in 12 minutes. The objective is to cover as much distance as possible within the allotted time. Walking is permitted, but the subject should be encouraged to challenge themselves as much as possible.
3. Upon the completion of 12 minutes, record the total distance covered in meters.

Estimation of VO_2max from Rockport One-Mile Walk Test

VO_2max = 132.853 – (0.1692 x weight) – (0.3877 x age) + (6.315 for men only) – (3.2649 x time) – (0.1565 x HR)

Notes:
Weight = kilograms (1 pound = 0.4536 kilograms)
Age = years
Time = minutes to nearest hundredth of a minute (e.g., 15 min 45 sec = 15.75 minutes)
Heart rate (HR) = recovery heart rate in beats per minute

For example: if a 32-year-old male participant weighing 175 lbs. (79.4 kg) completed the one-mile walk test in 13 minutes and 45 seconds with a recovery heart rate of 140 b/min (35 beats for 15 seconds), then his VO_2max is estimated as follows:

VO_2max = 132.853 – (0.1692 x 79.4) – (0.3877 x 32) + (6.315) – (3.2649 x 13.75) – (0.1565 x 140)

VO_2max = 132.853 – 13.43 – 12.41 + 6.315 – 44.89 – 21.91

VO_2max = 46.5 mL/kg/min

Estimation of VO₂max from 12-Minute Walk/Run Test

$$VO_2max = (0.0268 \times meters) - 11.3$$

For example: if a 45-year-old female is able to complete 3.50 laps (1,400 meters) around a standard track in 12 minutes, then her estimated VO₂max would be calculated as follows:

$$VO_2max = (0.0268 \times 1,400) - 11.3$$

$$VO_2max = 26.2 \text{ mL/kg/min}$$

Table 15-7 Men: Fitness Classification Based on Walk/Run Distance (meters) in 12 Minutes

Fitness Classification	17-19 yrs.	20-29 yrs.	30-39 yrs.	40-49 yrs.	50+ yrs.
Excellent	> 3,000	> 2,800	> 2,700	> 2,500	> 2,400
Above Average	2,700-3,000	2,400-2,800	2,300-2,700	2,100-2,500	2,000-2,400
Average	2,500-2,699	2,200-2,399	1,900-2,299	1,700-2,099	1,600-1,999
Below Average	2,300-2,499	1,600-2,199	1,500-1,899	1,400-1,699	1,300-1,599
Poor	< 2,300	< 1,600	< 1,500	< 1,400	< 1,300

Table 15-8 Women: Fitness Classification Based on Walk/Run Distance (meters) in 12 Minutes

Fitness Classification	17-19 yrs.	20-29 yrs.	30-39 yrs.	40-49 yrs.	50+ yrs.
Excellent	> 2,300	> 2,700	> 2,500	> 2,300	> 2,200
Above Average	2,100-2,300	2,200-2,700	2,000-2,500	1,900-2,300	1,700-2,200
Average	1,800-2,099	1,800-2,199	1,700-1,999	1,500-1,899	1,400-1,699
Below Average	1,700-1,799	1,500-1,799	1,400-1,699	1,200-1,499	1,100-1,399
Poor	< 1,700	< 1,500	< 1,400	< 1,200	<1,100

4. The subjects VO₂max may be estimated from the total distance covered in meters using the equation provided in the shaded box.

5. The subject's fitness category may be classified based on distance covered in meters using table 15-7 for men and table 15-8 for women.

Cooper 1.5-Mile Run

The Cooper 1.5-Mile Run test is an appropriate field test for individuals who are known to have a higher level of cardiorespiratory fitness. Participants should be able to jog or run for a minimum of 15 continuous minutes to obtain a reasonable estimation of VO₂max from this test. This test in not appropriate for deconditioned individuals, novice exercisers, or those classified as moderate- or high-risk with regard to cardiovascular disease (ACSM, 2005).

Equipment: stopwatch and a flat 1.5-mile course.

Procedure:
1. Allow the participant a short warm-up (5 minutes).
2. Instruct the participant to run the 1.5-mile course as quickly as possible.
3. Record the time upon completion of the 1.5-mile run.
4. Allow the client a cool-down period.
5. The subject's VO₂max may be estimated from the time to completion of the 1.5 mile run using the equation provided in the box below.
6. The subject's fitness category may be classified based on time to completion using table 15-9 for men and table 15-10 for women.

Estimation of VO₂max from Cooper 1.5-Mile Run

$$VO_2max = 88.01 - (0.1656 \times weight) - (2.76 \times time) + (3.716 \times gender)$$

Notes:
Weight = kilograms (1 pound = 0.4536 kilograms)
Time = minutes to nearest hundredth of a minute (e.g., 9 min 30 sec = 9.50 minutes)
Gender = 0 for female and 1 for male

For example: If a male client who weighs 185 lbs. (83.9 kg) completed the 1.5-mile run in 12 minutes and 45 seconds, his estimated VO₂max is calculated as follows:

$$VO_2max = 88.01 - (0.1656 \times 83.9) - (2.76 \times 12.75) + (3.716 \times 1)$$

$$VO_2max = 88.01 - 13.89 - 35.19 + 3.716$$

$$VO_2max = 42.6 \text{ mL/kg/min}$$

Table 15-9 Cooper 1.5-Mile Run Fitness Ranking for Men

Rating & %tile		Age 20-29	Age 30-39	Age 40-49	Age 50-59	Age 60+
Elite	99	7:29	7:11	7:42	8:44	9:30
	95	8:13	8:44	9:30	10:40	11:20
Excellent	90	9:09	9:30	10:16	11:18	12:20
	85	9:45	10:16	11:18	12:20	13:22
	80	10:16	10:47	11:44	12:51	13:53
Good	75	10:42	11:18	11:49	13:22	14:24
	70	10:47	11:34	12:34	13:45	14:53
	65	11:18	11:49	12:51	13:03	15:19
	60	11:41	12:20	13:14	14:24	15:29
Average	55	11:49	12:38	13:22	14:40	15:55
	50	12:18	12:51	13:53	14:55	16:07
	45	12:20	13:22	14:08	15:08	16:27
	40	12:51	13:36	14:29	15:26	16:43
Below Average	35	13:06	13:53	14:47	15:53	16:58
	30	13:22	14:08	14:56	15:57	17:14
	25	13:53	14:24	15:26	16:23	17:32
	20	14:13	14:52	15:41	16:43	18:00
Low	15	14:24	15:20	15:57	16:58	18:31
	10	15:10	15:52	16:28	17:29	19:15
	5	16:12	16:27	17:23	18:31	20:04
	1	17:48	18:00	18:51	19:36	20:57

The Cooper Institute for Aerobics Research

Table 15-10 Cooper 1.5-Mile Run Fitness Ranking for Women

Rating & %tile		Age 20-29	Age 30-39	Age 40-49	Age 50-59	Age 60+
Elite	99	8:33	10:05	10:47	12:28	12:36
	95	10:47	11:49	12:51	14:20	14:06
Excellent	90	11:43	12:51	13:22	14:55	14:55
	85	12:20	13:06	14:06	15:29	15:57
	80	12:51	13:43	14:31	15:57	16:20
Good	75	13:22	14:08	14:57	16:05	16:27
	70	13:53	14:24	15:16	16:27	16:58
	65	14:08	14:50	15:41	16:51	17:29
	60	14:24	15:08	15:57	16:58	17:46
Average	55	14:35	15:20	16:12	17:14	18:00
	50	14:55	15:26	16:27	17:24	18:16
	45	15:10	15:47	16:34	17:29	18:31
	40	15:26	15:57	16:58	17:55	18:44
Below Average	35	15:48	16:23	16:59	18:09	18:54
	30	15:57	16:35	17:24	18:23	18:59
	25	16:26	16:58	17:29	18:31	19:02
	20	16:33	17:14	18:00	18:49	19:21
Low	15	16:58	17:29	18:21	19:02	19:33
	10	17:21	18:00	18:31	19:30	20:04
	5	18:14	18:31	19:05	19:57	20:23
	1	19:25	19:27	20:04	20:47	21:06

The Cooper Institute for Aerobics Research

YMCA 3-Minute Step Test

The YMCA 3-Minute Step Test may be used to categorize an individual's level of cardiorespiratory fitness based on recovery heart rate following this standardized step test. The YMCA step test uses a 12-inch high step with a stepping rate of 24 step cycles per minute (96 foot contacts per minute), which is equivalent to an oxygen consumption of 25.8 mL/kg/min. This test is appropriate for nearly all populations, although caution is warranted for those with knee and balance issues.

Equipment: stopwatch, metronome, 12-inch step

Procedure:
Set metronome to 96 beats per minute (24 step cycles per minute).
1. Allow the participant to practice for a short time to establish proper stepping cadence ("up, up, down, down").
2. Instruct the participant to step for 3 minutes keeping pace with the metronome.
3. Upon conclusion of 3 minutes of stepping, the participant immediately sits down and recovery heart rate is counted for one (1) full minute. Counting of recovery heart rate must begin within 5 seconds of the end of stepping.
4. Use the normative data provided in table 15-11 for men and 15-12 for women to categorize the participant's level of cardiorespiratory fitness.

Assessment of Muscular Strength

Muscular strength is defined as the ability of a muscle or group of muscles to exert maximal force against an external resistance. Muscular strength may be expressed in terms of the absolute amount of weight lifted or relative to the individual's body weight. Muscular strength has traditionally been assessed using a one-repetition maximum (1-RM) testing protocol, usually performed on the bench press for upper body strength and the squat for lower body strength. As an alternative, 1-RM testing may also be performed on a Universal machine bench press or a Universal leg press, respectively. Prediction equations have been developed for 1-RM conversions between the free weight and Universal exercises (Simpson et al., 1997). Muscular strength is highly specific to the individual muscle groups, type of muscle action (e.g., isometric vs. isotonic), speed of movement, and joint position; therefore, a single measurement representative of total body muscular strength does not exist (ACSM, 2005).

Regardless of the type of equipment utilized and the muscle group tested, one-repetition maximum tests consist of having the participant lift, through trial and error to progressively heavier workloads, as much weight as possible for one repetition using good form and technique. However, caution is advised when conducting 1-RM testing protocols since the risk of musculoskeletal injury increases with greater workloads. Participants must be instructed on appropriate execution of the planned exercises and proper technique must be observed at all times. In addition, a spotter must be present during all lifts. Skill and neuromuscular coordination are necessary to properly perform the exercises, particularly when utilizing free weights; therefore, valid data is more likely to be obtained from those experienced in the exercises to be tested.

Table 15-11 YMCA Step Test Fitness Classification for Men

Fitness Category	Age 18 - 25	Age 26 - 35	Age 36 - 45	Age 46 - 55	Age 56 - 65	Age 65+
Excellent	<79	<81	<83	<87	<86	<88
Good	79-89	81-89	83-96	87-97	86-97	88-96
Above Average	90-99	90-99	97-103	98-105	98-103	97-103
Average	100-105	100-107	104-112	106-116	104-112	104-113
Below Average	106-116	108-117	113-119	117-122	113-120	114-120
Poor	117-128	118-128	120-130	123-132	121-129	121-130
Very Poor	>128	>128	>130	>132	>129	>130

Table 15-12 YMCA Step Test Fitness Classification for Women

Fitness Category	Age 18 - 25	Age 26 - 35	Age 36 - 45	Age 46 - 55	Age 56 - 65	Age 65+
Excellent	<85	<88	<90	<94	<95	<90
Good	85-98	88-99	90-102	94-104	95-104	90-102
Above Average	99-108	100-111	103-110	105-115	105-112	103-115
Average	109-117	112-119	111-118	116-120	113-118	116-122
Below Average	118-126	120-126	119-128	121-126	119-128	123-128
Poor	127-140	127-138	129-140	127-135	129-139	129-134
Very Poor	>140	>138	>140	>135	>139	>134

Predicting One-Repetition Maximum Strength

As noted earlier, there is significant risk of musculoskeletal injury when performing a one-repetition maximum test, especially for an unskilled or deconditioned participant. Subsequently, a number of methods have been established to predict one-repetition maximum strength based on a submaximal resistance lifted for several repetitions to fatigue (Dohoney et al., 2002; Reynolds et al., 2006). These prediction equations are based on the assumption that an inverse linear relationship exists between the amount of weight lifted and the number of repetitions that can be performed to fatigue as indicated by the strength-endurance continuum illustrated in figure 15-4. As the weight increases, the number of repetitions that can be performed decreases.

Figure 15-4 Strength–Endurance Continuum

High Intensity	Moderate Intensity		Low Intensity	
1RM 5RM	8RM	10RM	12RM 15RM	20+RM
100% 85%	75%		65%	55%

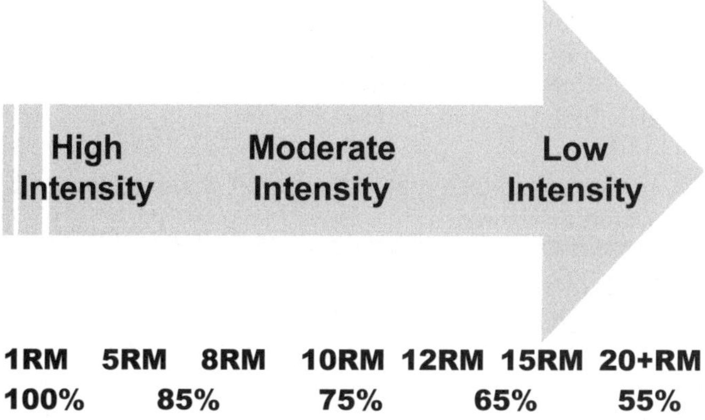

One of the commonly used formulas to estimate 1-RM is known as the Brzycki Equation (Brzycki, 1993). This formula is as follows:

$$\text{Predicted 1-RM} = \frac{\text{Weight Lifted}}{1.0278 - (0.0278 \times \text{reps to fatigue})}$$

For example, if a participant was able to lift 220 pounds on the bench press for 6 repetitions to muscle fatigue (i.e., unable to complete a 7th repetition), then one-repetition maximum is predicted as follows:

$$\text{Predicted 1-RM} = \frac{220 \text{ lbs}}{1.0278 - (0.0278 \times 6 \text{ reps})} = 255 \text{ lbs}$$

This particular formula was developed to predict 1-RM for males so it has the highest validity when testing similar subjects; however, it may be applied to females as well, provided the assessment procedures are consistent when testing and retesting. The validity of this prediction is also increased if the number of repetitions performed to fatigue is 10 or less. When more than 10 repetitions are performed, the assessment tends to be more reflective of muscular endurance versus strength. Table 15-13 was developed from the Brzycki Equation and may be used as a quick reference prediction of 1-RM without completing the previous calculations.

Assessment of Muscular Endurance

Muscular endurance is defined as the ability of a muscle or a group of muscles to perform multiple repetitions against a submaximal resistance. Subsequently, assessments of muscular endurance involve performing the maximum number of repetitions possible during a particular resistance training exercise. The mode of exercise may be similar to those used for one-repetition maximum testing; however, the objective is maximal repetitions versus maximal resistance. Assessments of muscular endurance may utilize an absolute workload (i.e., the same submaximal resistance for all subjects), a relative workload (i.e., a percent of the individual subject's 1-RM), or the subject's own body weight. Similar to muscular strength testing, the risk-to-benefit ratio must be considered for each participant to determine the appropriateness of various assessment protocols. Some examples of common assessments utilized to quantify muscular endurance include the YMCA Bench Press Endurance Test, the Push-Up Test, and the Partial Curl-Up Test.

YMCA Bench Press Endurance Test

The YMCA Bench Press Endurance Test provides an assessment of muscular endurance using the same absolute workload for men (80 lbs) and women (35 lbs), respectively (YMCA, 2000). Generally speaking, the bench press endurance test is appropriate for all individuals who are able to tolerate the designated workload as a submaximal effort. Those who are unfamiliar with the bench press exercise must receive proper instruction and be provid-

Table 15-13 Predicted One-Repetition Maximum

Weight Lifted	50	60	70	80	90	100	110	120	130	140	150	160	170	180	190	200	210	220	230	240	250
Repetitions																					
1	50	60	70	80	90	100	110	120	130	140	150	160	170	180	190	200	210	220	230	240	250
2	51	62	72	82	93	103	113	123	134	144	154	165	175	185	195	206	216	226	237	247	257
3	53	64	74	85	95	106	116	127	138	148	159	169	180	191	201	212	222	233	244	254	265
4	55	65	76	87	98	109	120	131	142	153	164	175	185	196	207	218	229	240	251	262	273
5	56	67	79	90	101	112	124	135	146	157	169	180	191	202	214	225	236	247	259	270	281
6	58	70	81	93	105	116	128	139	151	163	174	186	197	209	221	232	244	255	267	279	290
7	60	72	84	96	108	120	132	144	156	168	180	192	204	216	228	240	252	264	276	288	300
8	62	74	87	99	112	124	137	149	161	174	186	199	211	223	236	248	261	273	286	298	310
9	64	77	90	103	116	129	141	154	167	180	193	206	219	231	244	257	270	283	296	309	321
10	67	80	93	107	120	133	147	160	173	187	200	213	227	240	253	267	280	293	307	320	333

Brzycki (1993)

ed with time to establish the neuromuscular coordination needed to safely execute the exercise. This test may be contraindicated for individuals with pre-existing shoulder injuries (e.g., shoulder impingement syndrome, history of shoulder subluxations, rotator cuff tendonitis) or other orthopedic concerns that may be worsened by this exercise.

Equipment: flat bench, barbell (80 lbs. for men, 35 lbs. for women), metronome

Procedure:
1. Allow participant to complete proper warm-up and familiarization of equipment and testing procedures.
2. Set metronome to a cadence of 60 beats/min (30 repetitions/minute).
3. Instruct the participant to perform as many repetitions as possible keeping pace with the metronome. ('beep" = up, "beep" = down, etc.). The bar should be lowered to lightly touch the chest with the elbows flexed, and then raised to the starting position with the elbows fully extended.
4. The tester counts the number of repetitions performed until the participant can no longer maintain the pace with good form and technique due to muscular fatigue.
5. Tables 15-14 and 15-15 may be used to determine the fitness classification for men and women, respectively.

Push-Up Test

The push-up test is a commonly used field test to assess upper body muscular endurance. The push-up test is suitable for most populations with some considerations. Safe execution of the push-up test does require adequate shoulder complex and core stabilization. However, this test may serve a secondary objective to provide insight into the subject's ability to stabilize the shoulder complex and core. The push-up test may be contraindicated for those with pre-existing shoulder injuries, wrist injuries, or other orthopedic limitations.

Equipment: floor mat (optional)

Procedure:
1. Allow the participant a proper warm-up period.
2. For men, the participant should be in the full-body push-up position with the body in a straight line from shoulders to ankles and arms fully extended. For women, the protocol is the same except the participant performs the push-ups in the modified position with knees on the mat.
3. Hands can be placed where most comfortable (approximately shoulder-width apart).
4. Subject lowers their body while maintaining a straight line from shoulders to ankles until elbows reach a 90° angle of flexion.
5. The participant then returns to the starting position with the elbows fully extended.
6. The tester counts the maximum number of repetitions performed to exhaustion with good body alignment and technique.
7. Table 15-16 for men and 15-17 for women may be used to determine the participant's fitness classification and percentile rank based on total number of push-ups completed.

Partial Curl-Up Test

The partial curl-up test may be used to assess abdominal muscular endurance. Generally, this assessment is well-tolerated by most individuals; however, care should be used with those having lower back and neck injuries. In addition to the protocol presented below, several other variations of this assessment have also been developed (Diener et al., 1995; Faulkner et al., 1989; Payne et al., 2000)

Equipment: exercise mat, metronome, masking tape, ruler or tape measure

Procedure:
1. Mark off two sets of masking tape lines approximately six inches long and 8 cm apart (one for left hand and one for right).
2. Set a metronome to 40 beats/min (curl-ups to be done at a rate of 1 per 3 seconds, 20/min).
3. Testing subject starts in the supine position with knees bent at 90 degrees.
4. The tester cradles the subject's neck while kneeling behind the subject's head (optional).
5. Subject begins with finger tips on the closest piece of masking tape and curls up until the finger tips reach the second piece of tape on the mat (8 cm apart).
6. Return to starting position until the back of the subject's head reaches the tester's cradled hands and the finger tips return to the first piece of tape.
7. Continue without pausing until subject can no longer perform the curl-ups at the prescribed rate established by the metronome and/or loses form, up to a maximum of 75 curl-ups.

Compare the total number of curl-ups completed to the normative data provided in table 15-18.

Table 15-14 YMCA Bench Press Endurance Test Norms for Men

Fitness Classification	18–25 yrs.	26–35 yrs	36–45 yrs.	46–55 yrs.	56–65 yrs.	65+ yrs.
Excellent	44-64	41-61	36-55	28-47	24-41	20-36
Good	34-41	30-37	26-32	21-25	17-21	12-16
Above Average	29-33	26-29	22-25	16-20	12-14	9-10
Average	24-28	21-24	18-21	12-14	9-11	7-8
Below Average	20-22	17-20	14-17	9-11	5-8	4-6
Poor	13-17	12-16	9-12	5-8	2-4	2-3
Very Poor	0-10	0-9	0-6	0-2	0-1	0-1

YMCA (2000)

Table 15-15 YMCA Bench Press Endurance Test Norms for Women

Fitness Classification	18–25 yrs.	26–35 yrs	36–45 yrs.	46–55 yrs.	56–65 yrs.	65+ yrs.
Excellent	42-66	40-62	33-57	29-50	24-42	18-30
Good	30-38	29-34	26-30	20-24	17-21	12-16
Above Average	25-28	24-28	21-24	14-18	12-14	8-10
Average	20-22	18-22	16-20	10-13	8-10	5-7
Below Average	16-18	14-17	12-14	7-9	5-6	3-4
Poor	9-13	9-13	6-10	2-6	2-4	0-2
Very Poor	0-6	0-6	0-4	0-1	0-1	0

YMCA (2000)

Table 15-16 Full Body Push-Up Endurance Test Norms for Men

Fitness Classification	%tile Rank	20–29 yrs	30–39 yrs.	40–49 yrs.	50–59 yrs.	60–69 yrs.
Well Above Average	90	41	32	25	24	24
	80	34	27	21	17	16
Above Average	70	30	24	19	14	11
	60	27	21	16	11	10
Average	50	24	19	13	10	9
	40	21	16	12	9	7
Below Average	30	18	14	10	7	6
	20	16	11	8	5	4
Well Below Average	10	11	8	5	4	2

ACSM (2005)

Table 15-17 Modified Push-Up Endurance Test Norms for Women

Fitness Classification	%tile Rank	20–29 yrs	30–39 yrs.	40–49 yrs.	50–59 yrs.	60–69 yrs.
Well Above Average	90	32	31	28	23	25
	80	26	24	22	17	15
Above Average	70	22	21	18	13	12
	60	20	17	14	10	10
Average	50	16	14	12	9	6
	40	14	12	10	5	4
Below Average	30	11	10	7	3	2
	20	9	7	4	1	0
Well Below Average	10	5	4	2	0	0

ACSM (2005)

Table 15-18 Partial Curl Up Test Norms

Rating	Number of Repetitions Completed					
	Men			Women		
Age	<35	35–44	>45	<35	35–44	>45
Excellent	60	50	40	50	40	30
Good	45	40	25	40	25	15
Marginal	30	25	15	25	15	10
Poor	15	10	5	10	6	4

Faulkner et al. (1989)

Assessment of Flexibility

Flexibility is defined as the ability of a joint to move through a full, pain-free range of motion (ROM). Range of motion is measured in degrees of movement with the anatomical position serving as the beginning point of reference. Table 15-19 provides the normative range of motion values for adults at various joints of the body.

Table 15-19 Range of Motion Values

Shoulder	ROM	Hip	ROM
Flexion	90-120°	Flexion	90-135°
Extension	20-60°	Extension	10-30°
Abduction	80-100°	Abduction	30-50°
Adduction	40-50°	Adduction	10-30°
Horizontal Abduction	30-45°	Horizontal Abduction	NA
Horizontal Adduction	90-135°	Horizontal Adduction	NA
Internal Rotation	70-90°	Internal Rotation	30-45°
External Rotation	70-90°	External Rotation	45-60°
Knee	**ROM**	**Elbow**	**ROM**
Flexion	130-140°	Flexion	135-160°
Extension	5-10°	Extension	NA
Trunk	**ROM**	**Ankle**	**ROM**
Flexion	120-150°	Dorsiflexion	15-20°
Extension	20-45°	Plantar Flexion	30-50°
Lateral Flexion	10-35°	Inversion	10-30°
Rotation	20-40°	Eversion	10-20°

ACSM (2018)

The range of motion can be accurately measured using a relatively inexpensive device called a goniometer or a more technical piece of equipment called an inclinometer. However, these methods of assessment can be time-consuming and require significant experience and skill to reach an acceptable level of accuracy and reliability. In fitness settings, flexibility is more commonly assessed through linear measurements of movement. This involves moving a body segment in a specified direction, during which the range of motion may be objectively measured or subjectively assessed. Flexibility is highly specific to the body segment, joint, and even individual movements around a joint; therefore, no single assessment can accurately represent total body flexibility. A variety of flexibility tests are recommended based on the goals and needs of the participant. Common field tests that may be utilized by fitness professionals include the Sit-and-Reach Test, the Shoulder Flexibility Test, and the Trunk Extension Test.

Sit-and-Reach Flexibility Test

The Sit-and-Reach Test is perhaps one of the most commonly used flexibility assessments among fitness professionals. This assessment is intended to reflect collective flexibility of the hamstrings, posterior hip, and lower back. Several modifications of the Sit-and-Reach Test have also been developed (Baltaci et al., 2003; CIAR, 1994; CSEP, 2003; YMCA, 2000).

Equipment: Sit-and-Reach box

Procedure:
1. Allow the participant a 5-10 minute light cardiorespiratory warm-up prior to testing.
2. Instruct the participant to remove their shoes and sit on the floor with legs fully extended and feet up against the edge of the box (15 inch line).
3. The participant slowly reaches forward with both hands, one on top of the other, sliding the marker along the ruler. Knees should remain fully extended throughout each trial.
4. When the maximum distance is reached the participant must hold momentarily, then relax and return to the starting position.
5. Record the best score of three consecutive trials.
6. The subject's fitness classification may be determined using table 15-20 for men and 15-21 for women.

Shoulder Flexibility Test

The Shoulder Flexibility Test may be used to assess mobility through the shoulder complex. Movements at the glenohumeral joint include shoulder flexion, extension, abduction, adduction, external rotation and internal rotation. Movements at the scapulothoracic joint include scapular protraction, retraction, upward rotation, and downward rotation (Karageanes, 2005). The combination of movements utilized during this test does make it difficult to isolate the specific cause of any observed limitation to range of motion. Muscular tightness is likely to contribute limited range of motion; however, tightness within the joint capsule and/or ligaments may also play a role in reduced mobility. Similarly, the Apley Back Scratch Test may also be used as a general assessment of shoulder range of motion (House & Mooradian, 2010).

Equipment: tape measure

Procedure:
1. Allow the participant a 5-10 minute light cardiorespiratory warm-up prior to testing.
2. Instruct the participant to reach one arm overhead, attempting to place the hand down between the shoulder blades.
3. The participant then reaches with the opposite arm behind the back, attempting to move the hand upward between the shoulder blades toward the other hand.
4. Encourage the participant to touch/clasp the fingertips of both hands together between the shoulder blades.
5. Perform the assessment on both the right and left sides.
6. Table 15-22 may be used to rate the observations from the Shoulder Flexibility Test.

Table 15-20 Sit-and-Reach Norms (Distance in Inches) for Men

Fitness Classification	18-25 yrs.	26-35 yrs.	36-45 yrs.	46-55 yrs.	56-65 yrs.	65+ yrs.
Excellent	>20	>20	>19	>19	>17	>17
Good	18-20	18-19	17-19	16-17	14-17	13-16
Above Average	17-18	16-17	15-17	14-15	12-14	11-13
Average	15-16	15-16	13-15	12-13	10-12	9-11
Below Average	13-14	12-14	11-13	10-11	8-10	8-9
Poor	10-12	10-12	9-11	7-9	5-8	5-7
Very Poor	<10	<10	<8	<7	<5	<5

Table 15-21 Sit-and-Reach Norms (Distance in Inches) for Women

Fitness Classification	18-25 yrs.	26-35 yrs.	36-45 yrs.	46-55 yrs.	56-65 yrs.	65+ yrs.
Excellent	>24	>23	>22	>21	>20	>20
Good	21-23	20-22	19-21	18-20	18-19	18-19
Above Average	20-21	19-20	17-19	17-18	16-17	16-17
Average	18-19	18	16-17	15-16	15	14-15
Below Average	17-18	16-17	14-15	14-15	13-14	12-13
Poor	14-16	14-15	11-13	11-13	10-12	9-11
Very Poor	<13	<13	<10	<10	<9	<8

Table 15-22 Shoulder Flexibility Test Rating

Rating	Observation
Good	Fingertips are able to touch
Fair	Fingertips cannot touch, but are less than 2 inches apart
Poor	Fingertips are more than 2 inches apart

Prone Trunk Extension Test

The Prone Trunk Extension Test is used to qualify spinal extensibility. When lying in a prone position and extending the torso, the anterior-superior iliac spines (ASISs) should remain in contact with the support surface (e.g., stretching table, floor, mat). Elevation of the hips indicates range of motion is also gained from hip extension and suggests reduced spinal extensibility (Kendall et al., 2005). This assessment may be contraindicated for those with pre-existing low back injuries or acute lower back pain as well as those unable to lay in the prone position.

Equipment: tape measure, floor mat

Procedure:
1. Allow the participant a 5-10 minute light cardiorespiratory warm-up prior to testing.
2. Instruct the subject to lay prone on a mat with both hands placed directly under shoulders.
3. Instruct the participant to press chest and torso away from the mat by straightening both arms.
4. Encourage the participant to keep hips in contact with the mat while straightening the arms.
5. Measure the distance from the anterior-superior iliac spine (ASIS) to the mat surface while arms are fully extended.
6. Table 15-23 may be used to rate the observation and measurement from the Trunk Extension Flexibility Test.

Table 15-23 Trunk Extension Test Rating

Rating	Observation
Good	Hips (i.e., ASISs) remain in contact with the mat
Fair	Hips elevate from the mat 2 inches or less
Poor	Hips elevate greater than 2 inches from the mat

Chapter Summary

The administration of health-related physical fitness assessments is a crucial component of the exercise program development process. This chapter presented a small sampling of the many fitness assessment protocols that may be utilized with clients. Fitness professionals must have knowledge and skill in the selection, administration, and interpretation of fitness assessments. Just as each exercise program must be tailored to the unique goals, needs, and limitations of the participant, the choice of fitness assessments must also be individualized. Fitness professionals are encouraged to explore other fitness assessment options beyond those reviewed in this manual. Refer to the list of recommended reading provided for this chapter.

Chapter References

American College of Sports Medicine (2014). *ACSM's Guidelines for Exercise Testing and Prescription*, 9th edition. Baltimore, MD: Lippincott, Williams, and Wilkins.

American College of Sports Medicine (2018). *ACSM's Guidelines to Exercise Testing and Prescription*, 10th edition. Philadelphia, PA: Wolters Kluwer.

American College of Sports Medicine (2005). *ACSM's Health-Related Physical Fitness Assessment Manual*. Baltimore, MD: Lippincott, Williams, and Wilkins.

Baltaci, G., Un, N., Tunay, V., Besler, A., & Gerçeker, S. (2003). Comparison of three different sit and reach tests for measurement of hamstring flexibility in female university students. *British Journal of Sports Medicine*, 37(1), 59-61.

Brzycki, M. (1993). Strength testing-predicting a one-rep max from reps-to-fatigue. *Journal of Physical Education Recreation and Dance*, 64(1), 88.

Canadian Society for Exercise Physiology (2003). *The Canadian Physical Activity, Fitness & Lifestyle Approach*: CSEP-Health & Fitness Programs' Health-Related Appraisal and Counseling Strategy, 3rd edition. Ottawa, Ontario: Canadian Society for Exercise Physiology.

Cooper Institute for Aerobics Research (1994). *The Prudential FITNESSGRAM test administration manual*. Dallas, TX: Cooper Institute for Aerobics Research.

Cooper, K.H. (1968). A means of assessing maximal oxygen uptake. *Journal of the American Medical Association*, 203(3), 201-204.

Diener, M.H., Golding, L.A., & Diener, D. (1995). Validity and reliability of a one-minute half sit-up test of abdominal strength and endurance. *Research in Sports Medicine: An International Journal*, 6(2), 105-119.

Dohoney, P., Chromiak, J.A., Lemire, D., Abadie, B.R., & Kovacs, C. (2002). Prediction of one repetition maximum (1-RM) strength from a 4-6 RM and a 7-10 RM submaximal strength test in healthy young adult males. *Journal of Exercise Physiology*, 5(3), 54-59.

Faulkner, R.A., Sprigings, E.J., McQuarrie, A., & Bell, R.D. (1989). A partial curl-up protocol for adults based on an analysis of two procedures. *Canadian Journal of Sport Science*, 14(3), 135.

House, J., & Mooradian, A. (2010). Evaluation and management of shoulder pain in primary care clinics. *Southern Medical Journal*, 103(11), 1129-1137.

Jackson, A.S., & Pollock, M.L. (1978). Generalized equations for predicting body density of men. *British Journal of Nutrition*, 40(3), 497–502.

Jackson, A.S., Pollock, M.L., & Ward, A. (1980). Generalized equations for predicting body density of women. *Medicine and Science in Sports and Exercise*, 12(3), 175–82.

Karageanes, S.J. (2005). *Principles of Manual Sports Medicine*, Philadelphia, PA: Lippincott Williams & Wilkins.

Kendall, F.P., McCreary, E.K., Provance, P.G., Rodgers, M.M., & Romani, W.A. (2005). *Muscles Testing and Function with Poster and Pain* (5th edition). Baltimore, MD: Lippincott Williams & Wilkins.

Kline, G.M., Porcari, J.P., Hintermeister, R., Freedson, P.S., Ward, A., McCarron, R.F., Ross, J., & Rippe, J.M. (1987). Estimation of VO_2 max from a one-mile track walk, gender, age, and body weight. *Medicine and Science in Sports and Exercise*, 19(3), 253-259.

Myers, J., Forman, D.E., Balady, G.J., Franklin, B.A., Nelson-Worel, J., Martin, B.J., Herbert, W.G., Guazzi, M., & Arena, R. (2014). Supervision of exercise testing by nonphysicians: A scientific statement from the American Heart Association. *Circulation*, 130(12), 1014-1027.

Payne, N., Gledhill, N., Katzmarzyk, P.T., Jamnik, V.K., & Keir, P.J. (2000). Canadian musculoskeletal fitness norms. *Canadian Journal of Applied Physiology*, 25(6), 430-442.

Reynolds, J.M., Gordon, T.J., & Robergs, R.A. (2006). Prediction of one repetition maximum strength from multiple repetition maximum testing and anthropometry. *The Journal of Strength & Conditioning Research*, 20(3), 584-592.

Simpson, S.R., Rozenek, R., Garhammer, J., Lacourse, M., & Storer, T. (1997). Comparison of one repetition maximums between free weight and Universal machine exercises. *The Journal of Strength & Conditioning Research*, 11(2), 103-106.

YMCA of the USA, Golding, L.A. (Ed.), (2000). *YMCA Fitness Testing and Assessment Manual*, 4th edition. Champaign, IL: Human Kinetics.

Recommended Reading

American College of Sports Medicine (2014). *ACSM's Health-Related Physical Fitness Assessment Manual*, 4th edition. Philadelphia, PA: Wolters Kluwer.

Golding, L.A. (Ed.). (2000). *YMCA Fitness Testing and Assessment Manual*, 4th edition. Champaign, IL: Human Kinetics.

Heyward, V.H., & Gibson, A.L. (2014). *Advanced Fitness Assessment and Exercise Prescription*, 7th edition. Champaign, IL: Human Kinetics.

Hoffman, J. (2006). *Norms for Fitness, Performance, and Health*. Champaign, IL: Human Kinetics.

American College of Sports Medicine (2018). Chapter 4: Health-Related Physical Fitness Testing and Interpretation. In, *ACSM's Guidelines to Exercise Testing and Prescription*, 10th edition. Philadelphia, PA: Wolters Kluwer.

Chapter 15 Review Questions

1. When conducting a series of fitness assessments, it is recommended that the assessments are performed in the following order:
   A. Sit-and-Reach Test, Resting Blood Pressure, Partial Curl-Up Test, One Mile Walk Test, Body Composition via Skinfold Test
   B. 3-Minute Step Test, Apley Back Scratch Test, Resting Blood Pressure, Body Composition via Skinfold Test, Push-Up Test
   C. Resting Blood Pressure, Body Composition via Skinfold Test, 3-Minute Step Test, Push-up Test, Sit-and-Reach Test
   D. Body Composition via Skinfold Test, Sit-and-Reach Test, Cooper 1.5 Mile Run, Push-Up Test, Resting Blood Pressure

2. According to standardized procedures, skinfold caliper measurements are taken on the _____ side of the body.
   A. lateral
   B. posterior
   C. left
   D. right

3. A 48-year-old male client has an average abdominal skinfold measurement of 28 mm, a thigh measurement of 15 mm, and a chest measurement of 9 mm. What is this client's estimated percent body fat?
   A. 22.1%
   B. 15.0%
   C. 17.6%
   D. 18.3%

4. A 34-year-old female client achieves a maximum distance of 19 inches on the Sit-and-Reach Test. This places her in the _____ fitness category.
   A. excellent
   B. average
   C. above average
   D. good

5. Your 26-year-old male client is able to complete 6.25 laps around a standard Olympic track during the 12-minute Walk/Run Assessment. Based on the results of this assessment, what is the client's estimated maximal oxygen consumption (VO_2max)?
   A. 26.2 mL/kg/min
   B. 55.7 mL/kg/min
   C. 38.9 mL/kg/min
   D. 42.6 mL/kg/min

6. Referring to the client in question #5, based on the results of the 12-minute Walk/Run Assessment, what is this client's fitness classification for cardiorespiratory endurance?
   A. Excellent
   B. Poor
   C. Good
   D. Above Average

Answers to Review Questions on Page 384

Note: Review questions are intended to reinforce learning and comprehension of subject matter presented in the corresponding chapter. The review questions are not intended to be representative of actual certification exam questions in terms of style, content, or difficulty.

Section V
Fitness Programming

Individuals engage in physical activity and structured exercise for a variety of reasons including the countless physical and psychological health benefits, increased fitness, and enhanced athletic performance. In order to guide clients toward the achievement of these desired outcomes, fitness professionals must have an understanding of the guidelines for physical activity and exercise, and the application of training principles fundamental to the development of safe and effective fitness programs.

Chapter 16 summarizes the many health benefits of regular physical activity. The historical and present day physical activity recommendations for improved health will be reviewed including absolute and relative measurements of physical activity intensity. This chapter will also provide an introduction to the health-related and performance-related components of fitness as well as the fundamental principles of exercise training.

Chapter 17 reviews considerations for cardiorespiratory exercise programming. Topics include the ACSM guidelines for cardiorespiratory exercise, methods to monitor exercise intensity, and basic programming strategies.

Chapter 18 addresses guidelines and programming considerations to improve muscular strength and/or endurance. Included in this chapter are topics such as the ACSM guidelines for resistance training, strategies for program design, and an assortment of resistance training exercises including instructions and illustrations.

Chapter 19 covers topics related to flexibility training including underlying physiologic mechanisms that lead to increased range of motion as well as guidelines for safe and effective stretching. In addition, research is presented with regard to the effects of stretching on injury prevention and athletic performance. Finally, recommended stretching exercises and foam roller techniques are introduced to enhance flexibility.

16
Physical Activity & Health

Introduction
According to the World Health Organization, **health** does not merely represent the absence of disease, but also reflects a state of optimal physical, social, and psychological well-being. Health is impacted by many interrelated factors such as the environment, genetics, socioeconomic status, and modifiable lifestyle behaviors. Lifestyle behaviors include use of tobacco products, alcohol consumption, safety practices, dietary habits, and physical activity. **Physical activity** has been defined as any bodily movement produced by the use of skeletal muscles that increases energy expenditure above the resting level (Caspersen et al., 1985; HHS, 2008; Pate et al., 1995). Physical activity is comprised of 4 major domains including: domestic physical activity (e.g., yard work, house work, chores, child care); transportation physical activity (e.g., walking, biking); occupational physical activity (e.g., work-related); and leisure-time physical activity (e.g., recreation, sports, exercise, hobbies) (Jamnik et al., 2011). Among the subsets of leisure-time physical activity, **exercise** is defined as planned, structured, and repetitive bodily movement performed to improve or maintain one or more components of physical fitness (Caspersen et al., 1985; Pate et al., 1995). **Physical fitness** is a set of attributes possessed or attained by an individual that contribute to the ability to perform physical activity with vigor and without undue fatigue (Caspersen et al., 1985; HHS, 2008; Pate et al., 1995). This chapter will focus primarily on physical activity recommendations intended for the improvement of overall health. In addition, the components of physical fitness and the basic principles of exercise training will be introduced.

Health Benefits of Physical Activity
Countless scientific and epidemiologic research studies provide an overwhelming body of evidence regarding the many health benefits associated with regular physical activity. Although physical activity and exercise do present some risks, for the vast majority of individuals, the health benefits of a physically-active lifestyle far outweigh the potential risks. For adults, there is strong scientific evidence to support the health benefits of physical activity including:

- Reduces the risk of all-cause premature death
- Reduces the risk of coronary heart disease and stroke
- Reduces the risk of developing type 2 diabetes
- Reduces the risk of high blood pressure (i.e., hypertension)
- Lowers blood pressure in people who already have hypertension
- Reduces the risk of developing colon cancer and breast cancer
- Reduces feelings of depression and anxiety
- Helps to achieve and maintain a healthy body weight
- Helps build and maintain healthy bones, muscles, and joints
- Improves cardiorespiratory endurance
- Promotes psychological well-being and improved cognitive function

The benefits of regular physical activity are indisputable. As stated by Booth et al. (2000), "Indeed, with the possible exception of diet modifications, we know of no single intervention with greater promise than physical exercise to reduce the risk of virtually all chronic diseases, simultaneously."

Physical Activity Recommendations for Improved Health
The health benefits of physical activity have been promoted for several decades. Among the first population-based physical activity recommendations were those jointly published by the Centers for Disease Control and Prevention and the American College of Sports Medicine in 1995 (Pate et al., 1995). This consensus statement recommended that, "Every US adult should accumulate 30 minutes or more of moderate-intensity physical activity on most, preferably all, days of the week" (Pate et al., 1995). Shortly thereafter, a very similar recommendation was stated in *Physical Activity and Health: A Report of the Surgeon General* (HHS, 1996). This recommendation indicated that, "Significant health benefits can be obtained by including a moderate amount of physical activity on most, if not all, days of the week. Through a modest increase in daily activity, most Americans can improve their health and quality of life" (HHS, 1996). In comparison to previous guidelines focused on the exercise-fitness model,

these recommendations were unique given their broader application to the physical activity-health model (Pate et al., 1995). In contrast to exercise guidelines, which tended to focus on vigorous-intensity continuous exercise, the physical activity recommendations emphasized the health benefits of moderate-intensity activity performed in shorter intermittent bouts (Pate et al., 1995). In addition, the physical activity recommendations also highlight the dose-response effect, demonstrating that health benefits are obtained in proportion to total weekly energy expenditure such that greater levels of physical activity confer greater health benefits (Pate et al., 1995).

In 2007, the American College of Sports Medicine (ACSM) and the American Heart Association (AHA) updated the physical activity recommendations for adults (Haskell et al., 2007). The primary recommendation of this report states, "To promote and maintain health, all healthy adults aged 18 to 65 years need moderate-intensity aerobic (endurance) physical activity for a minimum of 30 minutes on five days each week or vigorous-intensity aerobic physical activity for a minimum of 20 minutes on three days each week. Combinations of moderate- and vigorous-intensity activity can be performed to meet this recommendation. The recommended amount of aerobic activity is in addition to routine activities of daily living of light intensity (e.g., self-care, cooking, casual walking or shopping) or lasting less than 10 minutes in duration (e.g., walking around home or office, walking from the parking lot)" (Haskell et al., 2007). Although the fundamental message of this updated recommendation is largely similar to the original recommendation, it does provide several enhancements and clarifications. These include, the recommended frequency of moderate-intensity activity is now specified as five days per week; vigorous-intensity activity is explicitly included in the new recommendation; the type of physical activity is specified to be aerobic-type (endurance) activity in addition to activities of daily living (ADLs); and the minimum length of short bouts of activity is clarified as at least 10 minutes (Haskell et al., 2007). In addition, the updated recommendations also include a statement regarding muscle-strengthening activities, "It is recommended that 8-10 exercises be performed on two or more nonconsecutive days each week using the major muscle groups. To maximize strength development, a resistance (weight) should be used that allows 8-12 repetitions of each exercise resulting in volitional fatigue" (Haskell et al., 2007).

Physical Activity Guidelines for Americans

In recognition of the strong scientific evidence demonstrating a positive association between physical activity and health, the U.S. Department of Health and Human Services issued the *2008 Physical Activity Guidelines for Americans (PAGA)*. See figure 16-1. The content of the *Physical Activity Guidelines* is intended to complement the *Dietary Guidelines for Americans* (see chapter 9). Together these two publications provide direction to policy makers and health professionals regarding the promotion of physical activity and healthy dietary practices (HHS, 2008). The PAGA include guidelines for adults as well as other groups within the population including children and adolescents, older adults, women during pregnancy and the postpartum period, adults with disabilities, and people with chronic medical conditions. Fitness professionals are encouraged to review the full PAGA document which, may be accessed at http://www.health.gov/paguidelines/. The key physical activity guidelines for adults are summarized below (HHS, 2008).

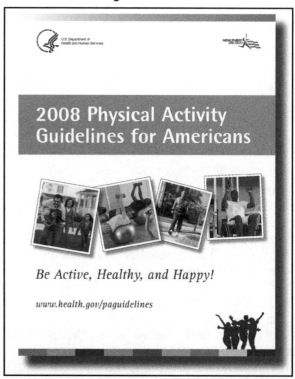

Figure 16-1 PAGA

- All adults should avoid inactivity. Some physical activity is better than none, and adults who participate in any amount of physical activity gain some health benefits.

- For substantial health benefits, adults should do at least 150 minutes (2 hours and 30 minutes) a week of moderate-intensity, or 75 minutes (1 hour and 15 minutes) a week of vigorous-intensity aerobic physical activity, or an equivalent combination of moderate- and vigorous-intensity aerobic activity. Aerobic activity should be performed in episodes of at least 10 minutes, and preferably, it should be spread throughout the week.

- For additional and more extensive health benefits, adults should increase their aerobic physical activity to 300 minutes (5 hours) a week of moderate-intensity, or 150 minutes a week of vigorous-intensity aerobic physical activity, or an equivalent combination of moderate- and vigorous-intensity activity. Additional health benefits are gained by engaging in physical activity beyond this amount.

- Adults should also do muscle-strengthening activities that are moderate- or high-intensity and involve all major muscle groups on 2 or more days a week, as these activities provide additional health benefits.

The second edition of the PAGA is scheduled to be released in late 2018. The 2018 Physical Activity Guidelines Advisory Committee is responsible for reviewing the body of scientific and medical evidence in physical activity and health. Using this evidence, the Advisory Committee will prepare a scientific report that documents the background and rationale for its recommendations for the second edition of the Physical Activity Guidelines for Americans. For more information regarding the development of the forthcoming 2018 PAGA, please visit https://health.gov/paguidelines/second-edition/.

Physical Activity Intensity & METs

The recommendations and guidelines for physical activity utilize terms such as moderate- and vigorous-intensity. The two approaches to define and monitor the intensity of physical activity include *relative intensity* and *absolute intensity*. Relative intensity is based on the level of individual effort required to perform a certain activity. This approach is synonymous to rating of perceived exertion (RPE), which will be discussed further in chapter 17. Generally speaking, less fit individuals require a subjectively higher level of effort than well-conditioned individuals to perform the same activity. The relative intensity or effort can be estimated using a scale of 0 to 10, where sitting quietly resting is 0 and the maximal possible effort is 10. Using this scale, moderate-intensity is equivalent to a rating of 5 or 6; vigorous-intensity is equivalent to a rating of 7 or 8.

However, the physical activity guidelines have been established based on absolute measures of intensity since scientific research largely demonstrates that the health benefits of physical activity are dependent upon the total weekly amount of energy expended. A **metabolic equivalent**, or **MET,** is the unit of measurement used to define the absolute energy expenditure of a specific activity. A MET is the rate of energy expenditure during an activity (i.e., activity metabolic rate) divided by the rate of energy expenditure at rest (i.e., resting metabolic rate) (Ainsworth et al., 2011; DHHS, 2008). One MET is equal to an oxygen consumption of approximately 3.5 milliliters of oxygen per kilogram of body weight per minute (3.5 mL/kg/min). For example, walking on a flat surface at 4.0 mph requires an energy expenditure (i.e., oxygen consumption) of 17.5 mL/kg/min. The MET level for this activity is calculated as follows:

$$17.5 \text{ mL/kg/min} \div 3.5 \text{ mL/kg/min} = 5.0 \text{ METs}$$

In other words, walking on a flat surface at 4 mph requires 5.0 METs or approximately 5 times the energy expenditure at rest. Table 16-1 provides the definition of absolute intensity of physical activity based on METs.

Table 16-1 Absolute Intensity of PA

Intensity	MET Level
Sedentary	1.0–1.5
Light	1.6–2.9
Moderate	3.0–5.9
Vigorous	≥6.0

Ainsworth et al. (2011)

The Compendium of Physical Activities has been established as a resource to estimate and classify the energy costs of various physical activities (Ainsworth et al., 2011). The Compendium includes a comprehensive list of physical activities and their respective MET values for 21 major categories of activities. See table 16-2. Table 16-3 provides a sample of physical activities found in the Compendium. The Compendium may be accessed at https://sites.google.com/site/compendiumofphysicalactivities/.

To further quantify the total amount of energy expended through physical activity, the concept of **MET-minutes** has been adopted. MET-minutes represent the average MET level for a specific physical activity multiplied by the number of minutes the activity was performed. For example, running on a flat surface at 6.0 mph (10 minute per mile pace) is equivalent to 9.8 METs. If this pace is maintained for 20 continuous minutes, then the total energy expenditure is 196 MET-minutes.

$$9.8 \text{ METs} \times 20 \text{ minutes} = 196 \text{ MET-minutes}$$

Table 16-2 Compendium Categories

Major Categories in the Compendium of Physical Activities		
1—Bicycling	8—Lawn and garden	15—Sports
2—Conditioning exercises	9—Miscellaneous	16—Transportation
3—Dancing	10—Music playing	17—Walking
4—Fishing and hunting	11—Occupation	18—Water activities
5—Home activity	12—Running	19— Winter activities
6—Home repair	13—Self-care	20—Religious activities
7—Inactivity	14—Sexual activity	21—Volunteer activities

Ainsworth et al. (2011)

Table 16-3 Sample of 2011 Compendium of Physical Activities

Code	METs	Major Heading	Specific Activities
01003	14.0	bicycling	bicycling, mountain, uphill, vigorous
01018	3.5	bicycling	bicycling, leisure, 5.5 mph
01019	5.8	bicycling	bicycling, leisure, 9.4 mph
02011	3.5	conditioning exercise	bicycling, stationary, 30-50 watts, very light to light effort
02012	6.8	conditioning exercise	bicycling, stationary, 90-100 watts, moderate to vigorous effort
02013	8.8	conditioning exercise	bicycling, stationary, 101-160 watts, vigorous effort
02022	3.8	conditioning exercise	calisthenics (e.g., push-ups, sit-ups, pull-ups, lunges), moderate effort
02048	5.0	conditioning exercise	elliptical trainer, moderate effort
02052	5.0	conditioning exercise	resistance (weight) training, squats, slow or explosive effort
02054	3.5	conditioning exercise	resistance (weight) training, multiple exercises, 8-15 reps at varied resistance
02071	4.8	conditioning exercise	rowing, stationary, general, moderate effort
02101	2.3	conditioning exercise	stretching, mild
02105	3.0	conditioning exercise	Pilates, general
02110	6.8	conditioning exercise	teaching exercise class (e.g., aerobic, water)
02120	5.3	conditioning exercise	water aerobics, water calisthenics, water exercise
03015	7.3	dancing	aerobic, general
03018	5.5	dancing	aerobic, step, with 4-inch step
03020	5.0	dancing	aerobic, low impact
03021	7.3	dancing	aerobic, high impact
17170	3.0	walking	walking, 2.5 mph, level, firm surface
17190	3.5	walking	walking, 2.8 to 3.2 mph, level, moderate pace, firm surface
17200	4.3	walking	walking, 3.5 mph, level, brisk, firm surface, walking for exercise
17210	5.3	walking	walking, 2.9 to 3.5 mph, uphill, 1 to 5% grade
17211	8.0	walking	walking, 2.9 to 3.5 mph, uphill, 6% to 15% grade
17220	5.0	walking	walking, 4.0 mph, level, firm surface, very brisk pace
17231	8.3	walking	walking, 5.0 mph, level, firm surface
17235	9.8	walking	walking, 5.0 mph, uphill, 3% grade
12050	9.8	running	running, 6 mph (10 min/mile)
12060	10.5	running	running, 6.7 mph (9 min/mile)
12080	11.5	running	running, 7.5 mph (8 min/mile)
12090	11.8	running	running, 8 mph (7.5 min/mile)
12110	12.8	running	running, 9 mph (6.5 min/mile)

Accessed from https://sites.google.com/site/compendiumofphysicalactivities/compendia on March 16, 2017.

According to the ACSM/AHA 2007 consensus statement, adults can fulfill their physical activity recommendations through a combination of moderate- and vigorous-intensity physical activity totaling a minimum of 450 to 750 MET-minutes per week (Pate et al., 2007). However, recommendations published in the *2008 Physical Activity Guidelines for Americans* and a statement published in 2011 by the ACSM recommends a total weekly volume of accumulated physical activity within the range of 500 to 1,000 MET-minutes (Garber et al., 2011; DHHS, 2008).

Physical Activity Epidemiology

In the United States, several ongoing national surveys are in place to monitor and track health behaviors such as physical activity. Among these, the three largest surveillance systems collecting information about the physical activity habits of adults include the National Health Interview Survey (NHIS), the National Health and Nutrition Examination Survey (NHANES), and the Behavioral Risk Factor Surveillance System (BRFSS) (Carlson et al., 2009; Dishman et al., 2012).

The NHIS is a large face-to-face survey conducted throughout the year with a random sample of U.S. households. Since 1957, the NHIS has been administered continuously by the National Center for Health Statistics (NCHS), a division of the Centers for Disease Control and Prevention (CDC). The NHIS is used to track progress toward the Healthy People 2010 and 2020 objectives outlined by the U.S. Department of Health and Human Services (Dishman et al., 2012).

NHANES, also managed by the NCHS, utilizes both a face-to-face survey and a physical examination conducted in a mobile examination center to collect statistics regarding health, nutrition, and physical activity behaviors. The physical examination includes an assessment of cardiorespiratory endurance and a musculoskeletal fitness test, which previously provided the only national data available on the physical fitness of adults (Dishman et al., 2012). In 2014, the Fitness Registry and the Importance of Exercise: A National Data Base (FRIEND) was established as a multi-institutional initiative to track and establish normative cardiorespiratory fitness values among adults in the U.S. (Kaminsky et al., 2013; Kaminsky et al., 2015).

The BRFSS is a population-based telephone survey that provides estimates of national and state trends regarding physical activity, obesity, and other health indicators. The BRFSS is conducted by state and territorial health departments with support from the National Center for Chronic Disease Prevention and Health Promotion of the CDC (Carlson et al., 2009).

Using data from these surveys, many epidemiological studies have reported the prevalence of physical activity behaviors among adults in the United States. The findings of these studies indicate that as a group, Americans generally fall short of the recommended physical activity levels. Data from the 2009 BRFSS indicate an estimated 51.0% of adults in the U.S. attained the recommended level of physical activity, defined as at least 30 minutes of moderate-intensity activity five or more days per week, or vigorous-intensity activity for at least 20 minutes three or more times per week (CDC, 2016a). According to more recent data from the NHIS, in 2015 49.0% of U.S. adults aged 18 and over met the 2008 federal physical activity guidelines for aerobic activity (Ward et al., 2016). The annual percentage of adults who met the 2008 physical activity guidelines for aerobic activity increased from 41.4% in 2006 to 49.5% in 2012 and has remained stable through 2015 (CDC, 2016b; Ward et al., 2016). In 2015, 20.9% of U.S. adults met the guidelines for both aerobic and muscle-strengthening activities (Ward et al., 2016). The annual percentage of adults who met both the aerobic and muscle-strengthening activity guidelines increased from 16.0% in 2006 to 20.4% in 2010, and has since remained stable through 2015 (Ward et al., 2016).

Other studies have investigated physical activity levels using more objective measurements obtained from accelerometers. Troiano et al. (2008) utilized a representative sample of the U.S. population from the 2003-04 NHANES to collect accelerometer data. The data obtained from nearly 5,000 participants having four or more days of valid monitor use revealed that less than 5% of adults attained the minimum level of physical activity. Another study looked at self-reported physical activity levels ascertained from over 3,000 participants in the 2005-06 NHANES in comparison to the accelerometer data obtained from the same participants (Tucker et al., 2011). The self-reported information indicated that 66.1% of men and 58.2% of women achieved the 2008 PAGA threshold (Tucker et al., 2011). In contrast, the objective accelerometer data indicated that only 10.6% of men and 8.7% of women achieved the recommended minimum level of physical activity (Tucker et al., 2011).

Regardless of the methods used to monitor and quantify physical activity behaviors, it is evident that the vast majority of American adults will greatly benefit from the adoption and maintenance of a more physically-active lifestyle. Fitness professionals are well-positioned to facilitate physical activity and exercise programs for adults seeking improved health, fitness, or athletic performance. The subsequent chapters will introduce guidelines and parameters that should be observed when designing individualized fitness programs. Looking forward to these guidelines for exercise programming, we will first define the various components of physical fitness and the underlying principles of exercise training.

Components of Physical Fitness

As illustrated in figure 16.2, physical fitness is built upon the foundation of health. Athletic performance is then development upon the combined foundation created by the maintenance of health and fitness. The components of physical fitness may be categorized as health-related and performance-related. The five components of **health-related physical fitness** include cardiorespiratory endurance, body composition, muscular strength, muscular endurance, and flexibility. The components of **performance-related physical fitness** include agility, coordination, balance, power, reaction time, and speed. The components of performance-related physical fitness may also be referred to as *skill-related*. Some, or perhaps all, of the components of health-related physical fitness are necessary for optimal performance. Likewise, certain components of performance-related physical fitness (e.g., balance, reaction time) may also be necessary for fitness and even health. Table 16-4 provides the definitions for each of the components of physical fitness.

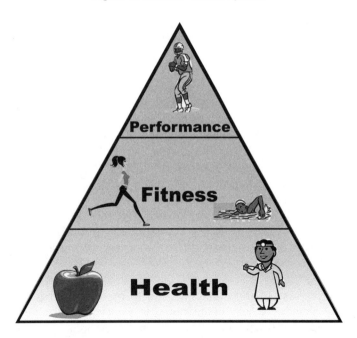

Figure 16-2 Health—Fitness Pyramid

Individuals participating in exercise programs or seeking the services of fitness professionals are striving toward the achievement of various personal goals. For many, these goals are focused on health, which may include prevention or management of chronic disease, recovery from an injury, enhanced quality of life, or improved psychological well-being. For others, their personal goals may focus on higher levels of fitness such as enhanced flexibility, a reduction in body fat, or increased strength. A smaller segment of the population may aspire to achieve athletic endeavors such as running a 10-kilometer race, making the varsity basketball team, or improving their golf game. In many cases, the outcome of an exercise program may positively impact each level of the health-fitness pyramid. For example, the loss of significant body weight improves health through a reduced risk of hypertension, heart disease, and type 2 diabetes. Fitness is increased as seen by a reduced percentage of body fat (i.e., improved body composition). Likewise, in many cases athletic performance is enhanced through a reduction in body weight, such as improved running economy resulting in faster race times. The positive effects of physical activity and exercise are rarely limited to just one outcome.

Principles of Training

Inherent to any exercise program is the objective to improve health as well as develop one or more components of physical fitness. The stimulus provided by an exercise program causes a *training effect,* which refers to the physiological and physical adaptations resulting from exercise. There are three underlying principles of training which are characteristic of any exercise program and are influential upon the training effect. These principles include overload, progression, and specificity.

The **principle of overload** refers to the application of a physiologic or physical stress greater than that to which the body or targeted body system is normally subjected. This greater-than-normal stress may be applied through any number of variables including an increase in exercise intensity, duration, or volume, as well as choice of exercise or manipulation of rest periods. For example, within a resistance training program, overload may be applied by lifting a heavier weight, performing more repetitions, completing additional sets, or reducing the rest periods between sets. The cardiorespiratory system may be subjected to an overload stimulus by exercising at a higher heart rate, extending the duration of the exercise, or increasing the frequency of exercise (i.e., number of days per week).

The **principle of progression** indicates that as the body adapts and becomes accustomed to a specific level of exercise, the training stimulus must be increased in order to apply sufficient overload. To minimize the risk of injury, the magnitude of the progression must be gradual and appropriate to the health status, level of fitness, and capabilities of the participant. Since overload and progression are closely related to one another, they are often referred to collectively as the *principle of progressive overload*.

The **principle of specificity** indicates that the training effect is specific to the training stimulus or stress applied to the body. The principle of specificity is also referred to as the *S.A.I.D. principle - Specific Adaptations to Imposed Demands*. The physiologic and physical adaptations are specific to the demands (i.e., stress or stimulus) imposed upon the targeted system or body part. In resistance training, the principle of specificity is seen by the manipulation of the workload and the corresponding repetitions. For example, lifting heavy weights (i.e., 85-100% of 1-RM) for a low number of repetitions (i.e., 1-8 RM) results in muscular strength improvements. On the other hand, lifting relatively light weights (i.e., 50-70% of 1-RM) for a high number of repetitions (i.e., 15-25 RM) elicits improvements in muscular endurance. Another example can be seen when training the various energy systems of the body. The training stimulus created by short bursts of high-intensity activity cause adaptations and improvements specific to the phosphagen and anaerobic glycolysis systems; whereas, relatively low-intensity, long-duration continuous activity stimulates improvements within the aerobic metabolic pathways (i.e., aerobic glycolysis, fatty acid oxidation). The mode of exercise also creates specific adaptations. Physical adaptations and biomechanical efficiency achieved through regular running may have limited crossover to cycle performance, and vice versa.

In addition to the three fundamental principles of training, some additional principles should also be considered as part of a well-designed exercise program. Just as the body will adapt in the presence of a training stimulus, the adaptations and improvements will also be lost if the training

Table 16-4 Components of Physical Fitness

Health-Related Components	
Cardiorespiratory Endurance:	The ability of the circulatory and respiratory systems to supply oxygen to the muscles during sustained physical activity or exercise. Cardiorespiratory endurance is typically expressed in terms of maximal oxygen consumption (VO_2max).
Body Composition:	The relative amount of lean body tissues (e.g., muscle, bone) and adipose tissue (i.e., fat) throughout the body. Body composition is typically expressed in terms of percentage of body fat (BF%).
Muscular Strength:	The ability of a muscle or group of muscles to exert maximal force against an external resistance. Muscular strength is typically expressed in terms of one-repetition maximum (1-RM).
Muscular Endurance:	The ability of a muscle or group of muscles to exert repeated or continuous submaximal force without fatigue. Muscular endurance is typically expressed in terms of the number of repetitions performed against a designated workload.
Flexibility:	The ability to move a joint through a full, pain-free range of motion. Flexibility is typically expressed in terms of degrees or inches of movement around a joint in a specific direction.
Performance-Related Components	
Agility:	The ability to start, stop, and change the position of the body in space with speed and accuracy.
Coordination:	The ability to integrate several movements of the body simultaneously and sequentially to achieve a complex task.
Balance:	The ability to control the position of the body in a state of equilibrium against external forces while stationary or moving.
Power:	The ability to produce the greatest amount of force in the shortest possible time.
Reaction Time:	The time elapsed between stimulation and the onset of movement in response to this stimulation.
Speed:	The ability to perform a movement in a specified direction as fast as possible.

Adopted from ACSM (2018) and HHS (2008)

stimulus is removed for an extended period of time. This detraining effect, or the gradual loss of conditioning in the absence of a training stimulus, is commonly referred to as the **principle of reversibility**. The rate and magnitude of the adaptations observed with a training program are specific to the individual. Likewise, the detraining effects of inactivity are also influenced by individual characteristics, the presence of injury or illness, personal level of fitness, and other lifestyle activity. In some cases, a planned regression in the training stimulus may produce desirable outcomes (e.g., the taper before a marathon); however, generally speaking, during prolonged abstinence from exercise, "if you don't use it, you will lose it."

Another important consideration is the **principle of variation**, which as the name implies, involves strategic and meaningful variety within an exercise program. Variety may be created by the choice of exercise modality or through alterations in training intensity and volume. In addition, variety is also important to maintain participant interest, motivation, and adherence to an exercise program. Regardless of the intention, appropriate variety within an exercise program can enhance the training outcomes while reducing the likelihood of plateaus or overtraining. In a very structured exercise regimen, variety may be incorporated through the use of periodization. **Periodization** is the systematic manipulation of acute program variables (e.g., workload, intensity, volume, rest periods, exercise modality) intended to optimize gains while avoiding overuse, overtraining, and plateaus. The concept of periodization will be discussed in greater detail in chapter 18.

Chapter Summary

To attain optimal health, adults should adopt and maintain a physically-active lifestyle including the weekly accumulation of 150 minutes of moderate-intensity, or 75 minutes of vigorous-intensity physical activity, or an equivalent combination of moderate- and vigorous-intensity leisure-time physical activity totaling 500 to 1,000 MET-minutes per week. Despite the numerous well-document benefits of physical activity, many American adults fail to attain sufficient levels of physical activity. In addition to the health benefits of regular physical activity, a more structured exercise program provides additional improvements among health-related and performance-related components of physical fitness. Understanding the fundamental principles of training allows the fitness professional to construct safe and effective exercise programs to achieve a variety of health, fitness, and performance goals.

Chapter References

Ainsworth, B.E., Haskell, W.L., Herrmann, S.D., Meckes, N., Bassett, D.R., Tudor-Locke, C., ... & Leon, A.S. (2011). 2011 compendium of physical activities: A second update of codes and MET values. *Medicine and Science in Sports and Exercise*, 43(8), 1575-1581.

American College of Sports Medicine (2018). *ACSM's Guidelines for Exercise Testing and Prescription*, 10th edition. Philadelphia, PA: Wolters Kluwer.

Booth, F.W., Gordon, S.E., Carlson, C.J., & Hamilton, M.T. (2000). Waging war on modern chronic diseases: primary prevention through exercise biology. *Journal of Applied Physiology*, 88(2), 774-787.

Carlson, S.A., Densmore, D., Fulton, J.E., Yore, M.M., & Kohl, H.W. (2009). Differences in physical activity prevalence and trends from 3 US surveillance systems: NHIS, NHANES, and BRFSS. *Journal of Physical Activity & Health*, 6(Suppl 1), S18-S27.

Caspersen, C.J., Powell, K.E., & Christenson, G.M. (1985). Physical activity, exercise, and physical fitness: Definitions and distinctions for health-related research. *Public Health Reports*, 100(2), 126-131.

Centers for Disease Control and Prevention (2016a). National Center for Chronic Disease Prevention and Health Promotion, Division of Population Health. BRFSS Prevalence & Trends Data [online]. Accessed August 25, 2016 from http://www.cdc.gov/brfss/brfssprevalence/.

Centers for Disease Control and Prevention (2016b). QuickStats: Percentage of U.S. adults who met the 2008 Federal physical activity guidelines for aerobic and strengthening activity, by sex — National Health Interview Survey, 2000–2014. Morbidity and Mortality Weekly Report (MMWR), 65:485.

Dishman, R.K., Heath, G.W., & I-Min Lee (2013). *Physical Activity Epidemiology*, 2nd edition. Champaign, IL: Human Kinetics.

Garber, C.E., Blissmer, B., Deschenes, M.R., Franklin, B.A., Lamonte, M.J., Lee, I.M., ... & Swain, D.P. (2011). American College of Sports Medicine position stand. Quantity and quality of exercise for developing and maintaining cardiorespiratory, musculoskeletal, and neuromotor fitness in apparently healthy adults: Guidance for prescribing exercise. *Medicine and Science in Sports and Exercise*, 43(7), 1334-1359.

Haskell, W.L., Lee, I., Pate, R.R., Powell, K.E., Blair, S.N., Franklin, B.A., ... & Bauman, A. (2007). Physical activity and public health: Updated recommendation for adults from the American College of Sports Medicine and the American Heart Association. *Medicine and Science in Sports and Exercise*, 39(8), 1423-1434.

Jamnik, V.K., Warburton, D.E., Makarski, J., McKenzie, D.C., Shephard, R.J., Stone, J.A., ... & Gledhill, N. (2011). Enhancing the effectiveness of clearance for physical activity participation: Background and overall process. *Applied Physiology, Nutrition, and Metabolism*, 36(S1), S3-S13.

Kaminsky, L.A., Arena, R., Beckie, T.M., Brubaker, P.H., Church, T.S., Forman, D.E., ... & Patel, M.J. (2013). The importance of cardiorespiratory fitness in the United States: The need for a national registry a policy statement from the American Heart Association. *Circulation*, 127(5), 652-662.

Kaminsky, L.A., Arena, R., & Myers, J. (2015). Reference standards for cardiorespiratory fitness measured with cardiopulmonary exercise testing: Data from the Fitness Registry and the Importance of Exercise National Database. *Mayo Clinic Proceedings*, 90(11), 1515-1523.

Nelson, M.E., Rejeski, W.J., Blair, S.N., Duncan, P.W., Judge, J.O., King, A.C., ... & Castaneda-Sceppa, C. (2007). Physical activity and public health in older adults: Recommendation from the American College of Sports Medicine and the American Heart Association. *Medicine and Science in Sports and Exercise*, 39(8), 1435-1445.

Pate, R.R., Pratt, M., Blair, S.N., Haskell, W.L., Macera, C.A., Bouchard, C., ... & Wilmore, J.H. (1995). Physical activity and public health. *The Journal of the American Medical Association*, 273(5), 402-407.

Tucker, J.M., Welk, G.J., & Beyler, N.K. (2011). Physical activity in US adults: Compliance with the physical activity guidelines for Americans. *American Journal of Preventive Medicine*, 40(4), 454-461.

Troiano, R.P., Berrigan, D., Dodd, K.W., Mâsse, L.C., Tilert, T., & McDowell, M. (2008). Physical activity in the United States measured by accelerometer. *Medicine and Science in Sports and Exercise*, 40(1), 181-188.

U.S. Department of Health and Human Services (1996). *Physical Activity and Health: A Report of the Surgeon General*. Atlanta, GA: U.S. Department of Health and Human Services, Public Health Service, Centers for Disease Control and Prevention, President's Council on Physical Fitness & Sports, National Center for Chronic Disease Prevention and Health Promotion.

U.S. Department of Health and Human Services (2008). *2008 Physical Activity Guidelines for Americans*. ODPHP Publication No. U0036.

Ward, B.W., Clarke, T.C., Nugent, C.N., & Schiller, J.S. (2016). Early release of selected estimates based on data from the 2015 National Health Interview Survey. National Center for Health Statistics. Available from: http://www.cdc.gov/nchs/nhis.htm.

Chapter 16 Review Questions

1. A new club member participates in a low-impact aerobics class including 40 minutes of continuous activity. Using information from the Compendium of Physical Activities, what is the estimated number of MET-minutes completed during this class?
    A. 150 MET-minutes
    B. 200 MET-minutes
    C. 5 MET-minutes
    D. 40 MET-minutes

2. Using the information from question #1, in order to achieve the minimum recommendation of the *2008 Physical Activity Guidelines for Americans*, how many additional MET-minutes of physical activity will this individual need to complete within the week?
    A. 300 MET-minutes
    B. 500 MET-minutes
    C. 110 MET-minutes
    D. 250 MET-minutes

3. Based on absolute intensity, which of the following activities is classified as a vigorous-intensity physical activity?
    A. Riding a bicycle at an average speed of 8.0 mph
    B. Aerobic step class using a 4-inch step
    C. Resistance training including multiple exercises at 10-15 repetitions
    D. Walking at an average speed of 3.5 mph at 7% grade

4. Performing 6 x 400 meter sprints on an Olympic track with 45 seconds of active recovery between sprints provides the training stimulus to increase the participant's anaerobic threshold. Which principle of training is represented by this scenario?
    A. Principle of progression
    B. Principle of specificity
    C. Principle of variation
    D. Principle of recovery

5. Which of the following training approaches is most likely to improve muscular strength?
    A. Resistance training with a workload at 90% of 1-RM for 5 repetitions per set
    B. Repeated plyometric drop-jumps from a 24 inch box
    C. Resistance training with a workload of 75% 1-RM for 15 repetitions per set
    D. Push-ups performed to volitional fatigue including 3 sets of 20-25 repetitions

6. In comparison to the physical activity levels self-reported on questionnaires and obtained through surveys, the objective measurements of physical activity from accelerometer data are _____.
    A. slightly higher
    B. about the same
    C. significantly lower
    D. inaccurate

Answers to Review Questions on Page 384

Note: Review questions are intended to reinforce learning and comprehension of subject matter presented in the corresponding chapter.
The review questions are not intended to be representative of actual certification exam questions in terms of style, content, or difficulty.

17
Cardiorespiratory Fitness Programming

Introduction
Cardiorespiratory endurance is defined as the ability of the circulatory and respiratory systems to supply oxygen to the muscles during sustained physical activity or exercise. Cardiorespiratory endurance is typically expressed in terms of maximal oxygen consumption (VO_2max). The training stimulus necessary to increase cardiorespiratory endurance is provided by exercise that is primarily aerobic in nature and involves the use of large muscle groups in a rhythmic and continuous manner. During cardiorespiratory exercise (i.e., aerobic exercise), the demand for oxygen increases in response to the energy needs of the working muscles, thereby creating an overload stimulus on the circulatory, respiratory, and muscular systems. When applied regularly, this overload leads to specific physiologic and physical adaptations (see chapter 7), which over time increases cardiorespiratory endurance. This chapter will present guidelines and programming considerations with regard to cardiorespiratory exercise (CRE) training.

Elements of the Cardiorespiratory Exercise Session
An individual session of cardiorespiratory exercise includes three elements: a warm-up, the conditioning phase, and a cool-down. The warm-up includes at least 5 to 10 minutes of light- to moderate-intensity aerobic activity and dynamic flexibility exercises. The warm-up serves to prepare the body physically, physiologically, and psychologically for the higher relative intensity of exercise that will be performed during the conditioning phase of the session. The specific objectives and effects of the warm-up are summarized in table 17-1.

The **conditioning phase** of the session provides the primary training stimulus to increase cardiorespiratory endurance. The conditioning phase typically represents 20 to 60 minutes of the session during which aerobic-type exercise is performed. This may include exercises such as walking, jogging, running, cycling, elliptical training, stair climbing, rowing, and any other mode of exercise that is primarily aerobic in nature and involves the use of large muscle groups in a rhythmic and continuous manner. The specific parameters related to the conditioning phase and cardiorespiratory programming in general are typically outlined using the acronym F.I.T.T. – Frequency, Intensity, Time, and Type. The guidelines related to F.I.T.T. will be presented later in this chapter.

The **cool-down** follows the conditioning phase of the exercise session. Similar to the warm-up, the cool-down consists of 5 to 10 minutes of light- to moderate-intensity aerobic activity. In addition, the cool-down is often concluded with some stretching exercises. The purpose of the cool-down is to allow for the gradual return of cardiovascular variables (e.g., heart rate, blood pressure) back toward pre-exercise levels and to facilitate the removal of metabolic byproducts (e.g., lactate, carbon dioxide) from the skeletal muscles. The specific objectives and effects of the cool-down are summarized in table 17-2.

Table 17-1 Warm-Up

Objectives and Effects of the Warm-Up
• Allows for a gradual metabolic response, such as increased oxygen uptake, which enhances cardiorespiratory performance.
• Prevents premature onset of blood lactic acid accumulation and fatigue during higher levels of exercise.
• Minimizes the oxygen deficit at the onset of exercise.
• Causes a gradual increase in muscle temperature, which reduces the likelihood of muscle injury.
• Facilitates better neural transmission and motor unit recruitment.
• Improves coronary blood flow and lessens the potential for myocardial ischemia.
• Allows gradual redirection of blood flow to the exercising skeletal muscles.
• Increases the elasticity of the connective tissues and other muscle components.
• Provides mental preparation for higher levels of exercise, increases arousal, motivation, and focus.

Table 17-2 Cool-Down

Objectives and Effects of the Cool-Down
• Keeps the muscles actively pumping to facilitate venous return of blood to the heart to prevent post-exercise blood pooling in the extremities.
• Reduces potential for a sudden drop in blood pressure (i.e., hypotension), thereby reducing the likelihood of post-exercise lightheadedness and fainting.
• Ensures continued adequate circulation to the skeletal muscles, heart, and brain.
• Reduces tendency for immediate post-exercise muscle spasm and cramping.
• Reduces the concentration of exercise hormones, such as norepinephrine, thereby lowering the probability of post-exercise disturbances in cardiac rhythm.
• May reduce the severity and duration of delayed-onset muscle soreness (DOMS).
• Provides an opportunity for the practice of mental relaxation techniques.

Guidelines for Cardiorespiratory Exercise

Programs designed to increase cardiorespiratory endurance include the variables of frequency, intensity, time, and type of exercise. This collection of variables is often referred to as the **FITT principle**.

The **frequency** of exercise refers to the number of days per week that aerobic exercise is to be performed. This answers the question, "How often should I exercise?" It is recommended that cardiorespiratory exercise is performed 3 to 5 days per week in order to obtain and maintain health and fitness benefits (ACSM, 2018; Garber et al., 2011). The frequency of exercise is often influenced by the intensity such that vigorous-intensity exercise may be performed less frequently than moderate-intensity exercise.

The **intensity** of CRE answers the question, "How hard should I exercise?" The overload stimulus created during exercise and the subsequent training effects are highly correlated to the intensity of exercise. Several methods exist to establish and monitor exercise intensity including percentage of maximal oxygen consumption (VO_2max), percentage of maximal heart rate (HR_{max}), percentage of heart rate reserve (HRR), oxygen consumption reserve (VO_2R), rating of perceived exertion (RPE), and metabolic equivalents (METs). Presently, it is recommended that most adults perform moderate- and/or vigorous-intensity exercise; however, very deconditioned individuals may place initial focus on light- to moderate-intensity exercise (ACSM, 2018; Garber et al., 2011). The specific parameters related to these descriptors of exercise intensity are provided in table 17-3. A more detailed review of methods to establish exercise intensity will be presented later in this chapter.

The **time** (i.e., duration) of exercise answers the question, "How long should I exercise?" This represents the duration of time CRE is to be performed. Cardiorespiratory exercise may be performed continuously during one session or accumulated throughout the day in intermittent bouts each lasting a minimum of 10 minutes (ACSM, 2018). It is recommended to accumulate 30 to 60 minutes of moderate-intensity exercise, 20 to 60 minutes of vigorous-intensity exercise, or an equivalent combination of moderate- and vigorous-intensity exercise each day (ACSM, 2018; Garber et al., 2011). The duration of exercise will be influenced by personal goals, health and fitness status, scheduling constraints, and other individual factors.

The **type** or mode of exercise answers the question, "What kind of exercise should I perform?" Obviously, a wide variety of options are available with regard to the selection of cardiorespiratory exercise. Personal preferences, physical limitations, and equipment availability are among the factors likely to influence the choice of exercise. Cardiorespiratory exercise includes any mode of exercise that is primarily aerobic in nature and involves the use of large muscle groups in a rhythmic and continuous manner. As noted earlier, this may include activities such as walking, running, biking, dancing, group exercise classes, stair climbing, elliptical training, and many more. The 'best' exercise is likely to be the type that is safe and effective as well as enjoyable to the participant to ensure motivation and long-term adherence to the exercise program.

Table 17-3 Classification of CRE Intensity

Descriptor	%HRR/VO_2R	%HR_{max}	%VO_2max	RPE (6-20 scale)	RPE (0-10 scale)	METs
Light	30–39	57–63	37–45	9–11	2–4	2.0–2.9
Moderate	40–59	64–76	46–63	12–13	5–6	3.0–5.9
Vigorous	60–89	77–95	64–90	14–17	7–8	6.0–8.7
Near-maximal to maximal	≥90	≥96	≥91	18–20	9–10	≥8.8

ACSM (2018)

The widely-recognized guidelines for cardiorespiratory endurance training, which have been established by the American College of Sports Medicine, are summarized in table 17-4. Fitness professionals should be well-versed with these guidelines.

Methods to Monitor Exercise Intensity

Among the variables included within a cardiorespiratory exercise program, perhaps the most important in terms of safely and effectively creating a training stimulus is the intensity of exercise. The use of METs to categorize exercise intensity was introduced in chapter 16. In addition, this chapter will review several methods to establish and monitor exercise intensity using heart rate, as well as methods utilizing subjective ratings of perceived exertion.

Monitoring Intensity via Heart Rate

Heart rate may be determined by palpating the radial or carotid artery (see chapter 13, figures 13-1 and 13-2) and counting the number of beats. A ten-second count is multiplied by six or a fifteen-second count is multiplied by four to obtain the one-minute heart rate. The manual counting of pulse does present some challenges, especially during vigorous exercise. A number of companies sell personal heart rate monitors (sometimes called training computers), which provide convenient, accurate, and instantaneous feedback regarding exercise heart rate. Heart rate monitors typically include a chest strap, which transmits the electrical signal from the heart, and a wrist watch, which receives the signal and displays the user's exercise heart rate. Heart rate monitors also provide and track additional information such as exercise duration, estimates of caloric expenditure, time in target training zone, and the average and peak heart rate. Training computers with global positioning system (GPS) functions can also track routes, measure distance, and calculate pace. For many, these devices provide a source of motivation, accountability, and entertainment.

One of the most common approaches to monitor exercise intensity in the fitness setting is the **maximal heart rate (HR_{max}) method**. This method utilizes maximal heart rate as the anchor point from which the target heart rate (THR) is calculated as a straight percentage of the HR_{max}. Numerous formulas have been developed to estimate age-predicted maximum heart rate among various populations (ACSM, 2018; Robergs & Landwehr, 2002). Perhaps the most frequently used equation is that proposed by Fox et al. (1971). This equation is:

$$\text{Estimated } HR_{max} = 220 - \text{age}$$

The simplicity of this prediction equation has likely contributed to its widespread use among fitness professionals despite the many research studies that have noted a significant margin of error among HR_{max} values derived from this formula (Cleary et al., 2011; Gellish et al., 2007; Robergs & Landwehr, 2002; Tanaka et al., 2001). It has been reported that the "220 – age" formula tends to overestimate HR_{max} in adults younger than 40 years old and underestimates HR_{max} with increasing age over 40 (Tanaka et al., 2001). Table 17-5 provides some examples of equations that may serve to estimate maximal heart rate within a smaller margin of error. Each of these formulas was developed from studies utilizing a unique group of subjects intended to represent the broader population. As such, the accuracy of each equation will be greatest when applied to individuals having characteristics (e.g., age, health status, medications) similar to the group from which the equation was developed. Given the prevalent use of the traditional "220 – age" formula, we will utilize this prediction equation when presenting the following sample target heart rate calculations.

For example, calculate the target heart rate for a 42-year-old male who will be exercising at a moderate-intensity that corresponds to 70% of his age-predicted maximum heart rate.

$$220 - 42 = 178 \text{ b/min } (HR_{max})$$

$$178 \times 0.70 = 125 \text{ b/min (THR)}$$

Table 17-4 Cardiorespiratory FITT Guidelines

	Guidelines for Cardiorespiratory Exercise
Frequency	3 to 5 days per week of combined moderate- and vigorous-intensity exercise is recommended for most adults to achieve and maintain health/fitness benefits.
Intensity	Moderate- to vigorous-intensity exercise is recommended for most adults and light- to moderate-intensity exercise can be beneficial for those who are deconditioned.
Time	Most adults should accumulate 30 to 60 minutes per day of moderate-intensity exercise, 20 to 60 minutes per day of vigorous-intensity exercise, or an equivalent combination of moderate- and vigorous-intensity exercise.
Type	Exercise that is primarily aerobic in nature and involves the use of large muscle groups in a rhythmic and continuous manner.

ACSM (2018); Garber et al. (2011)

Another approach to determine the target heart rate is known as the **heart rate reserve (HRR) method**. This method was first introduced by the physiologist, Dr. M.J. Karvonen and has therefore come to be known as the **Karvonen Formula** (Karvonen et al., 1957). The calculation of target heart rate begins with the standard "220 – age" to estimate maximum heart rate. The next step is to calculate the heart rate reserve, which is the difference between the maximum heart rate and the resting heart rate (HRR = HR_{max} – RHR). The heart rate reserve is multiplied by the desired training percentage, and then the resting heart rate is added back in to obtain the target heart rate.

For example, using the Karvonen Formula, calculate the target heart rate for a 56-year-old female having a resting heart rate of 76 and wishing to exercise at a moderate-intensity of 60% of her heart rate reserve.

$$220 - 56 = 164 \text{ b/min } (HR_{max})$$

$$164 - 76 = 88 \text{ (HRR)}$$

$$88 \times 0.60 = 52.8 + 76 = 129 \text{ b/min (THR)}$$

Table 17-5 HR_{max} Equations

HR_{max} Prediction Equations	
Equation	**Source**
$HR_{max} = 205.8 - (0.685 \times age)$	Inbar et al. (1994)
$HR_{max} = 208.0 - (0.70 \times age)$	Tanaka et al. (2001)
$HR_{max} = 206.9 - (0.67 \times age)$	Gellish et al. (2007)
$HR_{max} = 211.0 - (0.64 \times age)$	Nes et al. (2013)

Monitoring Intensity via Perceived Exertion

The use of **rating of perceived exertion (RPE)** was first introduced by Gunnar Borg and has since become widely used in a variety of fitness and clinical exercise settings (Borg, 1982). The rating of perceived exertion provides a subjective indication regarding the difficulty of the exercise being performed by the participant. The original RPE scale, known as the *category scale*, includes a 15-point range of values from 6 to 20, which was intended to loosely correspond to heart rates ranging from 60 to 200 beats per minute (Borg, 1982). To ensure valid and reliable RPE values, it is recommended that the following instructions are communicated to the participant prior to exercise (ACSM, 2006). These instructions may be adapted to both fitness assessment and exercise training scenarios.

> "During the exercise (test) we want you to pay close attention to how hard you feel the exercise work rate is. This feeling should reflect your total amount of exertion and fatigue, combining all sensations and feelings of physical stress, effort, and fatigue. Don't concern yourself with any one factor such as leg pain, shortness of breath or exercise intensity, but try to concentrate on your total, inner feeling of exertion. Try not to underestimate or overestimate your feelings of exertion; be as accurate as you can."

The original rating of perceived exertion scale is provided in table 17-6. Using the original RPE scale, a rating of 12 to 13 is considered to be moderate-intensity and a rating of 14 to 17 is considered vigorous-intensity.

More recently, a revised rating of perceived exertion scale, known as the *category-ratio scale*, was introduced (Borg, 1982). This revised scale provides a range of values from 0 to 10. See table 17-7. Using the revised scale, a rating of 5 to 6 represents moderate-intensity exercise and a rating of 7 to 8 represents vigorous-intensity. The category-ratio scale has gained popularity due to its relative simplicity, which allows for ease of use and understanding by lay persons and fitness professionals. Similar 10-point scales have subsequently been developed for a variety of subjective measures.

Table 17-6 Original

Original RPE Scale	
6	
7	Very, very light
8	
9	Very light
10	
11	Fairly light
12	
13	Somewhat hard
14	
15	Hard
16	
17	Very hard
18	
19	Very, very hard
20	

Borg (1982)

Table 17-7 Revised

Revised RPE Scale	
0	Nothing at all
0.5	Very, very weak
1	Very weak
2	Weak
3	Moderate
4	Somewhat strong
5	Strong
6	
7	Very Strong
8	
9	
10	Very, very strong

Borg (1982)

An example of such a scale is the **OMNI Scale of Perceived Exertion**, which was originally developed for use with children and later was adapted for use with adults performing weight-bearing cardiorespiratory exercise such as walking and running (Robertson, 2004; Utter et al., 2004). Figure 17-1 illustrates the OMNI Walk/Run Scale. In addition, similar adult-oriented OMNI scales have been validated using depictions of cycling (Robertson et al., 2004), elliptical training (Mays et al., 2010), and resistance training (Robertson et al., 2003).

Another relatively simple and practical method often used as a general guide of exercise intensity is the talk test. The **talk test** is an indication of the participant's ability to comfortably converse during exercise (Persinger et al., 2004). As the participant is exercising, the talk test is performed by having the individual recite, from memory, a short familiar paragraph (e.g., Pledge of Allegiance). Immediately upon completion, the participant is asked, "Can you still speak comfortably?" If the answer is an unequivocal, "Yes", then one may be reliably certain that the exercise intensity is within the acceptable parameters for low- to moderate-intensity physical activity (Persinger et al., 2004). The talk test has also been found to correspond closely to the *ventilatory threshold*, which is an indicator of the client's anaerobic threshold (Foster et al., 2004; Quinn & Coons, 2011).

Strategies for Cardiorespiratory Programming

The foundation of cardiorespiratory endurance is a well-developed *aerobic base*. The aerobic base is often defined as the level at which the body utilizes fat most efficiently as a substrate for energy production during aerobic (i.e., oxygen-dependent) exercise. The aerobic base is developed through **steady state exercise** sessions. For most individuals seeking the health and general fitness benefits of cardiorespiratory exercise, this is the primary training strategy. During steady state exercise, a low-to-moderate-intensity is sustained at a fairly constant level over a continuous period of time. For example, following an appropriate 10-minute warm-up, the exercise intensity may be increased to the level eliciting a heart rate equivalent to 70% of HR_{max}, which is sustained for 30 minutes followed by a 5-minute cool-down period. See figure 17-2.

A well-developed aerobic base is critical for optimal performance during endurance sports. Within the category of steady state training, the vocabulary of endurance athletes (e.g., runners) often includes workouts such as 'long slow distance', 'tempo', and 'threshold' training. A *long slow distance (LSD)* workout involves a light-to-moderate (i.e., 55% to 75% HR_{max}) steady state pace maintained over an extended duration of time (i.e., 75 to 120+ minutes) or distance (i.e., 8 to 20 miles). LSD workouts are ideal for developing aerobic adaptations within the skeletal muscles as well as building tolerance to the musculoskeletal and psychologic stress of very long bouts of continuous exercise.

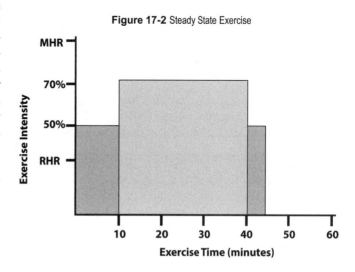

Figure 17-2 Steady State Exercise

Figure 17-1 OMNI Walk/Run Scale

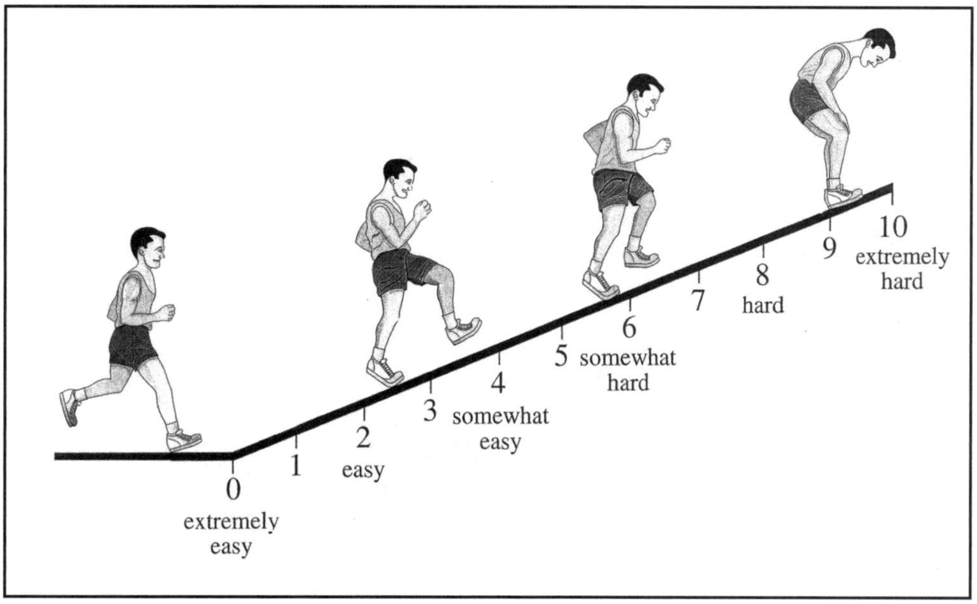

Threshold training is performed at the upper end of the aerobic range, just slightly below the anaerobic threshold, at approximately 85% to 90% of HR_{max}. During a threshold workout, a vigorous steady-state pace is maintained for about 20 to 40 minutes or 3 to 6 miles, at a speed about 25 to 30 seconds slower than 5-kilometer (3.1 mile) race pace (Karp, 2010).

On the steady-state continuum, *tempo training* falls somewhere between long slow distance and threshold training. Tempo workouts typically maintain a 'comfortably hard' intensity between 75% and 85% of HR_{max}, which is sustained for 40 to 75 minutes or 5 to 8 miles. Both threshold and tempo workouts are effective to increase cardiorespiratory endurance. In addition, endurance sport performance is enhanced by increasing the speed at which the anaerobic threshold occurs, subsequently allowing athletes to maintain a faster pace without the onset of limiting fatigue.

Having established a solid aerobic base through regular steady state exercise, interval training may also be used as an effective strategy to further increase cardiorespiratory endurance (i.e., VO_2max) and anaerobic threshold. An **interval training** session involves a series of relatively short vigorous-intensity bouts of exercise, called *work intervals*, which are alternated with low-intensity *active recovery intervals*. During the work interval, the exercise intensity is quickly elevated above the anaerobic threshold, typically 85% to 95% of HR_{max}, for approximately 10 seconds to 3 minutes. This bout of vigorous-intensity exercise is immediately followed by an active recovery interval performed at 50% to 60% of HR_{max}. Each pair of work and recovery intervals is called a *cycle*. Each interval cycle is expressed as a ratio of work-to-recovery (work:recovery). For example, a work interval lasting for 45 seconds followed by a 90-second recovery is expressed as a 1:2 work-to-recovery ratio. The duration of the work interval and the ratio of work-to-recovery are based on many factors such as the participant's level of fitness, motivation, and fitness goal, as well as the desired training effect. A very short interval (e.g., 10 to 20 seconds) will stimulate a training effect specific to the phosphagen system; whereas, relatively longer intervals (e.g., 30 seconds to 3 minutes) will lead to adaptations within the anaerobic glycolysis energy system. The intensity of the work interval and work-to-recovery ratios should allow for 5 to 8 cycles to be completed within a workout. The example provided in figure 17-3 illustrates a 40-minute interval workout beginning with a 10-minute warm-up, followed by seven cycles of 1-minute work and 2 minutes 30 seconds recovery, concluding with a 7-minute cool-down.

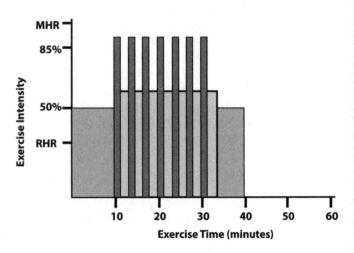

Figure 17-3 Interval Training

Chapter Summary

As one of the five components of health-related physical fitness, cardiorespiratory endurance is arguably the most important aspect of a well-rounded exercise program to promote overall health and prevention of chronic disease. Each cardiorespiratory exercise session consists of a warm-up, a conditioning phase, and a cool-down. The FITT principle outlines the guidelines for cardiorespiratory exercise including frequency, intensity, time, and type of activity. The training strategies often utilized to increase cardiorespiratory endurance include steady state exercise and interval training. Fitness professionals should incorporate cardiorespiratory exercise into the fitness program for each client based on their individual health and fitness goals.

Chapter References

American College of Sports Medicine (2006). *ACSM's Guidelines for Exercise Testing and Prescription*, 7th edition. Baltimore, MD: Lippincott, Williams, and Wilkins.

American College of Sports Medicine (2018). *ACSM's Guidelines for Exercise Testing and Prescription*, 10th edition. Philadelphia, PA: Wolters Kluwer.

Borg, G.A.V. (1982). Psychophysical bases of perceived exertion. *Medicine and Science in Sports and Exercise*, 14(5), 377-381.

Cleary, M.A., Hetzler, R.K., Wages, J.J., Lentz, M.A., Stickley, C.D., & Kimura, I.F. (2011). Comparisons of age-predicted maximum heart rate equations in college-aged subjects. *The Journal of Strength & Conditioning Research*, 25(9), 2591-2597.

Foster, C., Porcari, J. P., Anderson, J., Paulson, M., Smaczny, D., Webber, H., ... & Udermann, B. (2008). The talk test as a marker of exercise training intensity. *Journal of Cardiopulmonary Rehabilitation and Prevention*, 28(1), 24-30.

Fox, S.M., Naughton, J.P., & Haskell, W.L. (1971). Physical activity and the prevention of coronary heart disease. *Annals of Clinical Research*, 3(6), 404-432.

Garber, C.E., Blissmer, B., Deschenes, M.R., Franklin, B.A., Lamonte, M.J., Lee, I.M., ... & Swain, D.P. (2011). American College of Sports Medicine position stand. Quantity and quality of exercise for developing and maintaining cardiorespiratory, musculoskeletal, and neuromotor fitness in apparently healthy adults: Guidance for prescribing exercise. *Medicine and Science in Sports and Exercise, 43*(7), 1334-1359.

Gellish, R.L., Goslin, B.R., Olson, R.E., McDonald, A., Russi, G.D., & Moudgil, V.K. (2007). Longitudinal modeling of the relationship between age and maximal heart rate. *Medicine and Science in Sports and Exercise, 39*(5), 822-829.

Inbar, O., Oren, A., Scheinowitz, M., Rotstein, A., Dlin, R., & Casaburi, R. (1994). Normal cardiopulmonary responses during incremental exercise in 20-to 70-yr-old men. *Medicine and Science in Sports and Exercise, 26*(5), 538-246.

Karp, J.R. (2010). *101 Developmental Concepts & Workouts for Cross Country Runners*. Monterey, CA: Coaches Choice.

Karvonen, M., Kentala, E., & Mustala, O. (1957). The effects of training on heart rate: A longitudinal study. *Annales Medicinae Experimentalis et Biologiae Fenniae, 35*(3), 307-315.

Mays, R.J., Goss, F.L., Schafer, M.A., Kim, K.H., Nagle-Stilley, E.F., & Robertson, R.J. (2010). Validation of adult OMNI perceived exertion scales for elliptical erogometry 1, 2, 3. *Perceptual and Motor Skills, 111*(3), 848-862.

Nes, B.M., Janszky, I., Wisloff, U., Stoylen, A., & Karlsen, T. (2013). Age-predicted maximal heart rate in healthy subjects: The HUNT Fitness Study. *Scandinavian Journal of Medicine & Science in Sports*, 23(6), 697-704.

Persinger, R., Foster, C., Gibson, M., Fater, D.C., & Porcari, J.P. (2004). Consistency of the talk test for exercise prescription. *Medicine and Science in Sports and Exercise, 36*(9), 1632-1636.

Quinn, T.J., & Coons, B.A. (2011). The Talk test and its relationship with the ventilatory and lactate thresholds. *Journal of Sports Sciences, 29*(11), 1175-1182.

Robergs, R.A., & Landwehr, R. (2002). The surprising history of the "HRmax= 220-age" equation. *Journal of Exercise Physiology, 5*(2), 1-10.

Robertson, R.J. (2004). *Perceived Exertion for Practitioners: Rating Effort with the OMNI Picture System*. Champaign, IL: Human Kinetics.

Robertson, R.J., Goss, F.L., Dube, J., Rutkowski, J., Dupain, M., Brennan, C., & Andreacci, J. (2004). Validation of the adult OMNI scale of perceived exertion for cycle ergometer exercise. *Medicine and Science in Sports and Exercise, 36*(1), 102-108.

Robertson, R.J., Goss, F.L., Rutkowski, J., Lenz, B., Dixon, C., Timmer, J., ... & Andreacci, J. (2003). Concurrent validation of the OMNI perceived exertion scale for resistance exercise. *Medicine and Science in Sports and Exercise, 35*(2), 333-341.

Tanaka, H., Monahan, K.D., & Seals, D.R. (2001). Age-predicted maximal heart rate revisited. *Journal of the American College of Cardiology, 37*(1), 153-156.

Utter, A.C., Robertson, R.J., Green, J.M., Suminski, R.R., McAnulty, S.R., & Nieman, D.S. (2004). Validation of the Adult OMNI Scale of perceived exertion for walking/running exercise. *Medicine and Science in Sports and Exercise, 36*, 1776-1780.

Recommended Reading

American College of Sports Medicine (2018). Chapter 6: General Principles of Exercise Prescription. In, *ACSM's Guidelines to Exercise Testing and Prescription*, 10th edition. Philadelphia, PA: Wolters Kluwer.

Chapter 17 Review Questions

1. According to the American College of Sports Medicine (ACSM), it is recommended that adults perform moderate- to vigorous-intensity cardiorespiratory exercise _____ days per week.
    A. 2 to 3
    B. 3 to 5
    C. 5 to 7
    D. 4 to 6

2. Using the Karvonen formula, calculate the target heart rate for a 50-year-old male client, having a resting heart rate of 68, and wishing to exercise at 65% of his heart rate reserve.
    A. 111 beats per minute
    B. 156 beats per minute
    C. 134 beats per minute
    D. 149 beats per minute

3. Your 44-year-old female client is exercising on the elliptical trainer at a steady state heart rate of 123 beats per minute. Based on a percentage of her age-predicted maximum heart rate, her current exercise intensity is classified as _____.
    A. light
    B. moderate
    C. vigorous
    D. very vigorous

4. Your new female client is 55 years old. Although her lifestyle has been sedentary for many years, she is otherwise is good health with no medical considerations. Her primary goal is to increase her cardiorespiratory endurance. Which of the following is the MOST appropriate for this client's initial exercise program?
    A. Steady state exercise 3-4 days per week, 20 minutes per session, at 65-70% HRmax
    B. Steady state exercise 4-5 days per week, 30 minutes per session, at 80-85% HRmax
    C. Interval training 2-3 days per week, 30 minutes per session, 8 cycles at 3:1 work:recovery ratio
    D. Long slow distance training, 3-5 days per week, 75 minutes per session, at 75% HRmax

5. While walking on a treadmill at 3.8 mph and 4% grade, your client indicates a RPE of 7 on the category-ratio scale. This rating should correspond to an exercise intensity equivalent to _____ of the client's heart rate reserve.
    A. 64% to 90%
    B. 40% to 59%
    C. 60% to 89%
    D. 64% to 76%

6. Calculate the target heart rate at 80% of heart rate reserve for a 28-year-old client with a resting heart rate of 62.
    A. 166 b/min
    B. 192 b/min
    C. 130 b/min
    D. 154 b/min

Answers to Review Questions on Page 384

Note: Review questions are intended to reinforce learning and comprehension of subject matter presented in the corresponding chapter. The review questions are not intended to be representative of actual certification exam questions in terms of style, content, or difficulty.

18
Muscular Fitness Programming

Introduction

Among the five components of health-related physical fitness, two are directly related to muscular fitness including muscular strength and muscular endurance. **Muscular strength** is the ability of a muscle or group of muscles to exert maximal force against an external resistance. Muscular strength is typically expressed in terms of one-repetition maximum (1-RM). **Muscular endurance** is the ability of a muscle or group of muscles to exert repeated or continuous submaximal force without undue fatigue. Muscular endurance is typically measured in terms of the number of repetitions performed against a designated workload. Both muscular strength and endurance are enhanced through various resistance training exercises. Based on the principles of overload and specificity, the outcome of resistance training is highly correlated to the training stimulus, which is provided by the intensity of resistance training (expressed as a percentage of one-repetition maximum) and the number of *repetitions* performed to fatigue. As illustrated in figure 18-1, low- or light-intensity resistance training, characterized by less than 50% of 1-RM, will elicit improvements in muscular endurance. At the other end of the continuum, high- or vigorous-intensity resistance training, performed with workloads greater than 85% of 1-RM, will primarily stimulate increased muscular strength.

Figure 18-1 Strength-Endurance Continuum

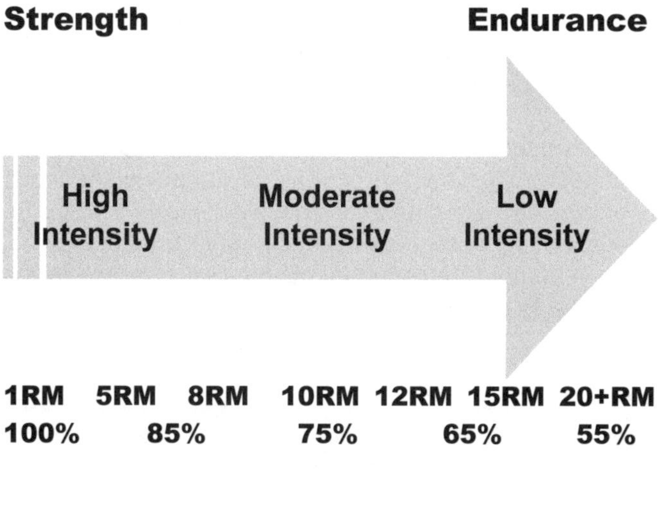

Strength → **Endurance**

High Intensity | Moderate Intensity | Low Intensity

1RM	5RM	8RM	10RM	12RM	15RM	20+RM
100%	85%		75%	65%		55%

The number of repetitions performed is inversely related to the amount of resistance. A low number of repetitions (e.g., 1 to 5) can be performed against a heavy resistance (e.g., 85% to 100% of 1-RM); whereas a relatively high number of repetitions (e.g., > 15) can be performed when a lighter resistance (e.g., 55% to 65% of 1-RM) is selected. In addition to the number of repetitions and the amount of resistance, several other factors must also be considered in the design of resistance training programs. These factors include the number of *sets*, *tempo* (i.e., speed of movement), length of rest periods, frequency of training, range of motion, and the choice of exercise. Collectively, these factors are referred to as the *acute training variables*, each of which can be manipulated to elicit a different training effect. The specific 'prescription' of these acute training variables within a resistance training program should reflect the unique goals, abilities, and potential limitations of each client.

Benefits of Resistance Training

A significant body of scientific evidence demonstrates the many benefits of regular resistance training (Garber et al., 2011; Williams et al., 2007; Winett & Carpinelli, 2001). Many of these health benefits are similar to those observed with regular cardiorespiratory exercise, yet some are unique benefits specific to resistance training. The mechanical loading applied to the bones during resistance training provides a stimulus to increase bone mineral density and subsequently lowers the risk of osteoporosis and fractures (Haskell et al., 2007). Among older adults, resistance training also reduces the risk of falling and injuries sustained from falls; reduces the risk of developing musculoskeletal disorders such as osteoarthritis; and preserves functional capacity, the ability to perform activities of daily living, independence, and quality of life (Graber et al., 2011; Nelson et al., 2007; Winett & Carpinelli, 2001). Table 18-1 lists a summary of the major health benefits associated with regular resistance training.

Types of Resistance Training

There are generally three types of resistance training exercise and/or resistance training equipment: isotonic, isometric, and isokinetic. **Isotonic** ('iso-' means 'equal' and '-tonic' means 'tension') resistance training involves both a concentric (i.e., shortening) and eccentric (i.e., lengthening) phase of muscle action (i.e., contraction) performed against a fixed workload. This is the most common type of resistance training utilized in fitness settings. Isotonic equipment includes free weights (e.g., dumbbells, barbells), plate-loaded equipment (e.g., Hammer Strength®), and selectorized resistance training machines (e.g., Nautilus®, Cybex®, Free Motion®).

Table 18-1 Resistance Training Benefits

Benefits of Resistance Training
• Increases lean body mass, increases resting metabolic rate, and improves body composition
• Increases bone mineral density, reduces risk of osteoporosis, and reduces the risk of hip fractures
• Reduces the incidence of falls and injuries sustained from falls among older adults
• Maintains functional capacity to perform activities of daily living
• Improves neuromuscular coordination and balance
• Reduces risk of non-exercise related musculoskeletal injuries
• Reduces the risk of developing musculoskeletal disorders such as osteoarthritis, reduces pain and disability for those with osteoarthritis
• Reduces the incidence and prevalence of low back pain
• Enhances athletic performance

Isometric ('-metric' means 'measurement') resistance training includes exercises during which muscular force is exerted against a resistance, but no movement or change in the muscle's length occurs. Isometric exercises may be performed by pushing against an immovable object (e.g., wall, door frame), attempting to lift an external resistance that exceeds the muscle's strength capacity, or simply resisting movement by pushing one limb against the other (e.g., pushing the palms of your hands together). Isometrics are often used when movement of a body part causes joint pain or if other types of equipment are not readily available. One limitation of isometric exercises is that the strength gains are highly specific to the joint angle at which the exercise is performed (Weir et al., 1995). However, isometric exercises performed at several joint angles appear to minimize this limitation and elicit strength improvements throughout the full range of motion (Folland et al., 2005). Another potential concern relates to the exaggerated rise in blood pressure elicited during isometric muscle actions when compared to isotonic or dynamic resistance training (Chrysant, 2010; Williams et al., 2007). In addition, due to the static nature, isometric exercises are likely to be accompanied by the Valsalva maneuver. The **Valsalva maneuver** is characterized by holding one's breath while attempting to forcibly exhale against a closed glottis, thus preventing the air to escape from the lungs. This causes a large increase to both intrathoracic pressure and arterial blood pressure, which is potentially dangerous for those with cardiovascular disease or underlying hypertension (ACSM, 2010). Therefore, dynamic (i.e., isotonic) resistance training exercises are preferable to static (i.e., isometric) exercises. Isometrics may be considered by many to be contraindicated (i.e., not recommended) for individuals with cardiovascular disease, hypertension, or retinopathy. In addition, the Valsalva maneuver should be avoided during both dynamic and static resistance training among all populations.

Isokinetic ('-kinetic' means 'movement') resistance training involves dynamic muscle contractions during which the speed of movement is controlled at a constant angular velocity, regardless of the amount of effort exerted by the user. This computerized equipment (e.g., Biodex, Cybex®, CSMi) is used to measure the force and torque generated by a muscle throughout a range of motion. Isokinetic equipment is uncommon in the typical fitness setting, but is more likely to be used for research in academic settings and rehabilitation in clinical settings.

Elastic resistance (also call rubber resistance) products include tubes and bands, which provide an external force through their property of elastic recoil. As the rubber material of this equipment is stretched it creates an increasing level of elastic resistance. Elastic resistance products are also available in various thicknesses (often color-coded), each of which generates a different level of resistance force. Elastic equipment was originally used in clinical settings for physical rehabilitation; however, over the last several decades its use has expanded into many fitness settings such as group exercise, personal training, and home exercise programs. Elastic resistance products are a convenient option for many due to their versatility, portability, and affordability, as well as the fact that the force created by these products is not dependent on gravity. Although exercises utilizing elastic resistance do involve both a concentric and an eccentric phase, the magnitude of external force generated by the rubber material will increase as it is stretched to greater lengths through an increasing range of motion.

Resistance training exercises may also be classified as open or closed kinetic chain exercises. **Closed kinetic chain** exercises are those during which the distal end (i.e., hand or foot) of the working body segment is in a fixed position and remains in constant contact with an immovable surface, typically the ground. For example, a barbell squat is considered a closed chain exercise since the feet are in contact with the ground. Likewise, a push-up is an example of a closed chain exercise for the upper body. Closed chain exercises often involve multiple body segments and joints such that the position of one joint will affect the other joints along the kinetic chain. During the barbell squat, it is impossible to flex the knee without also creating movement at the ankle and hip.

Open kinetic chain exercises are those during which the distal end (i.e., hand or foot) of the targeted body segment is 'open' to freely move through space. For example, the leg extension machine is an open chain exercise since the leg pad is able to move through space. A dumbbell biceps curl, dumbbell chest press, and dumbbell lateral raise are all examples of open chain exercises for the upper body. In each case, the hands are able to freely move the dumbbells through space. During open chain exercises, the joint(s) adjacent to the moving joint are not significantly affected by the movement. For instance, the movement at the knee during a leg extension occurs independently from the ankle and hip joints.

General Adaptation Syndrome

The **general adaptation syndrome (GAS)** was first proposed in the 1930s by Dr. Hans Selye to explain the physiologic response to an imposed stress such as the overload applied to muscles during resistance training (Selye, 1998). According to the GAS, the exerciser may experience three stages of adaptation in response to resistance training. The first stage, known as the *alarm stage*, involves the body's initial response to the physical stress imposed by the resistance training exercise. The immediate reaction is that of the 'fight or flight' response. During the 'fight or flight' response the sympathetic nervous system stimulates a release of stress hormones (i.e., catecholamines), causing an elevation in cardiovascular activity (e.g., heart rate, blood pressure) and a mobilization of energy substrates necessary to meet the demands being placed upon the body. The alarm stage is also characterized by symptoms such muscle fatigue, a temporary decrease in strength, muscle stiffness, and delayed onset muscle soreness. **Delayed onset muscle soreness (DOMS)** typically begins about 24 hours after a session of resistance training and peaks about 48 to 72 hours post-exercise. Many theories have been proposed to explain the cause of DOMS including lactic acid accumulation, muscle spasm, microtrama to muscle fibers, connective tissue damage, inflammation, and enzyme and electrolyte influx (Lewis et al., 2012). Perhaps the most widely accepted theory regarding the cause of DOMS is explained by structural damage inflicted upon the muscle and connective tissue, which results from the mechanical load applied primarily during the eccentric phase of a resistance exercise (Clarkson & Hubal, 2002). This initial microtrama is then exacerbated by subsequent inflammation, leading to more pronounced symptoms of DOMS (Clarkson & Hubal, 2002).

The second stage of the general adaptation syndrome is known as the *resistance stage*. During the resistance stage, the exerciser experiences several physiologic, physical, and perhaps even psychologic adaptations to the stress (Stone et al., 1982). These adaptations prepare the individual for future exposures to similar stresses (i.e., resistance training) and effectively lead to increased strength and performance. Both the alarm and resistance stages of the GAS may be seen in what is known as the 'super-compensation cycle'. See figure 18-2. In response to the first resistance training session, the participant's strength temporarily decreases below the initial baseline, representing the alarm stage. During the ensuing recovery period (i.e., the resistance stage), the muscles adapt and the strength increases back to the initial baseline, and then 'super compensates' to establish a new baseline of enhanced strength. It is at the peak of this super compensation (typically ≥48 hours post-exercise) that the next training session should be performed.

The third stage of the GAS is called the *exhaustion stage*. The exhaustion stage is characterized by extended periods of fatigue, decreased performance, lack of motivation, and possibly injury. The exhaustion stage is actually one to be avoided through proper program design and appropriate recovery strategies. Returning to the super compensation cycle in figure 18-2, if the subsequent training session is performed before strength returns to baseline or super compensation occurs, then performance will decrease. Chronically introducing overload beyond the body's ability to adapt or inadequately recovering on a regular basis may lead to *overtraining syndrome*. Overtraining includes a variety of signs and symptoms which are summarized in table 18-2. An important consideration in the design of resistance training programs in to incorporate adequate rest and recovery to ensure optimal performance and to decrease the risk of overtraining.

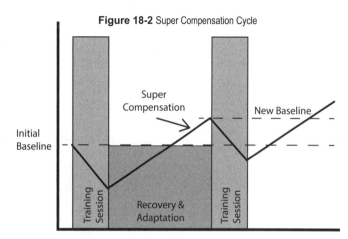

Figure 18-2 Super Compensation Cycle

Table 18-2 Overtraining

Signs & Symptoms of Overtraining	
Prolonged fatigue	Increased susceptibility to illness
Decrements in performance	Disturbed sleep
Elevated resting and submaximal heart rate	Loss of motivation
Change in appetite	Decreased mental concentration and focus
Unexplained weight loss	Mood disturbances

Meeusen et al. (2013)

Resistance Training Guidelines

According to the Physical Activity Guidelines for Americans, adults can obtain health benefits in addition to those derived from aerobic-type physical activity by performing muscle-strengthening (i.e., resistance training) activities that are moderate- or high-intensity and involve all major muscle groups on 2 or more days a week (HHS, 2008). The American College of Sports Medicine has published a more comprehensive set of resistance training guidelines intended to improve general muscle fitness (ACSM, 2018; Garber et al., 2011; Ratamess et al., 2009). The resistance training guidelines established by the ACSM are summarized in table 18-3.

Table 18-3 Resistance Training Guidelines

Guidelines for Resistance Training	
Frequency	• Each major muscle group should be trained 2 to 3 days per week.
Intensity	• 60% to 70% of 1-RM for novice to intermediate exercisers to improve strength • ≥80% of 1-RM for experienced exercisers to improve strength • 40% to 50% of 1-RM for older individuals beginning exercise to improve strength • 40% to 50% of 1-RM may be beneficial to improve strength in sedentary individuals beginning a resistance training program • <50% of 1-RM to improve muscular endurance
Time	• No specific duration of resistance training has been identified for effectiveness.
Type	• Resistance exercises involving each major muscle group are recommended. • Emphasize multi-joint exercises affecting more than one muscle group and target both agonist and antagonist muscle groups. • A variety of resistance training modalities, including free-weight, resistance machines, and body weight exercises, may be used.
Repetitions	• 8 to 12 repetitions are recommended to improve strength and power in most adults. • 10 to 15 repetitions are effective in improving strength in middle-aged and older individuals starting an exercise program. • 15 to 25 repetitions are recommended to improve muscular endurance.
Sets	• 2 to 4 sets are recommended for most adults to improve strength and power. • A single set of resistance exercise for each major muscle group can be effective, especially among older and novice exercisers. • ≤2 sets are effective in improving muscular endurance.
Recovery	• Rest intervals of 2 to 3 minutes between each set of repetitions are effective. • A rest of ≥48 hours between sessions for any single muscle group is recommended.
Exercise Order	• It is recommended that large muscle group exercises are performed before small muscle group exercises; multiple-joint exercises before single-joint exercises; higher-intensity exercises before lower-intensity exercises; or rotation of upper and lower body or agonist and antagonist muscle group exercises.
Tempo	• It is recommended that resistance exercises are performed in a slow-to-moderate speed in a controlled and deliberate manner. • Slow may be defined as a concentric phase of 2 seconds and an eccentric phase of 4 seconds (CON:ECC = 2:4) and moderate may be defined as a 1-2 second count for both the concentric and eccentric phases (1-2:1-2).
Technique	• All individuals should perform resistance training using correct form and technique. • Proper resistance exercise techniques utilize controlled and deliberate movements performed through a full range of motion, including both concentric and eccentric muscle actions.
Breathing	• Maintain a normal breathing pattern throughout the exercise. • Exhale during the concentric phase and inhale during the eccentric phase. • Avoid the Valsalva maneuver during static and dynamic resistance exercises.
Progression	• As muscles adapt to a resistance training program, the participant should continue to progressively overload the targeted muscles by gradually increasing resistance, repetitions, number of sets, or frequency of training.

ACSM (2018); Garber et al. (2011); Ratamess et al. (2009)

Resistance Training Program Design Models

Whereas the resistance training guidelines may be thought of as traffic laws, an individualized resistance training program represents a GPS route used to navigate the client toward their personal goal. Each client is likely to have a unique starting point as well as a different ending destination (i.e., goal). Subsequently, a seemingly infinite number of routes (i.e., exercise programs) may exist to arrive at the target destination. Regardless of the route taken, each will adhere to the same set of traffic laws (i.e., training guidelines) throughout the course of the journey. When creating a resistance training program, the decision-making process regarding the acute training variables is guided by the client's desired goal. Each session within the program is designed to provide a specific training stimulus. Over time, the training effects from the individual sessions provide cumulative adaptations, which support eventual achievement of the goal.

Training for Postural Stability

The initial stage of a resistance training program should place an emphasis on activating and conditioning muscles that function to stabilize postural alignment and joint position. The exercises selected during this stage of the program are generally unstable. The objectives of these exercises are to facilitate the activation of appropriate stabilizer muscles, increase neuromuscular coordination, enhance kinesthetic awareness, and improve postural stability during both static and dynamic activities. Resistance training exercises focused on stability typically use body weight or a relatively light external load as the source of resistance. Subsequently, stabilization exercises are performed at the endurance end of the strength-endurance continuum. See figure 18.1. Dynamic stability exercises (e.g., isotonic) are performed to a moderate-to-high number of repetitions and static exercises (i.e., isometric) are performed over a longer duration (i.e., time under tension). The 'overload' of a stability exercise is provided and progressed by the degree of instability, rather than significantly increasing the external resistance. Figure 18-3 illustrates progression strategies that may be used with stabilization-oriented resistance training exercises.

A common characteristic of stabilization-oriented exercises is that participants are challenged to maintain the position of non-moving body segments (e.g., spine, shoulder complex, supporting extremity) while force is produced to move, or resist movement, of an external load. For example, during a cable chest press performed while standing in a tandem stance, the user attempts to maintain the stable position of the lower extremities and the spinal column as the weight is concentrically lifted and eccentrically lowered. The movement of the upper extremities pressing against the external load creates a dynamic challenge to the participant's postural stability. The exercise may be progressed by reducing the participant's base of support to further challenge their ability to stabilize, rather than increasing the workload which requires greater force production. Considering the relatively low workloads and moderate-to-high repetition ranges used in conjunction with stabilization exercises, these exercises may also serve to enhance muscular endurance of agonist muscles.

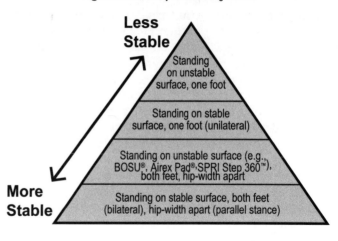

Figure 18-3 Stability Exercise Progressions

In order to decrease the risk of musculoskeletal injury and to maximize the effectiveness of the overall program, participants must demonstrate the ability to maintain postural stability and joint alignment before advancing to the next stage of a resistance training program.

Training for Muscular Strength

Traditionally, personal trainers and fitness enthusiasts have initiated resistance training programs to increase muscular strength without giving attention to the development of requisite postural stability. This approach may increase the risk of injury by over-emphasizing prime mover strength, while neglecting intrinsic stabilization. In essence, this is synonymous to attempting to build a sturdy house on a weak and fragile foundation.

Once the participant has demonstrated the ability to maintain postural alignment during both static and dynamic exercises, they may be progressed to exercises focused on the development of muscular strength. Resistance training exercises selected for the purpose of increasing muscular strength are inherently more stable, which allows the participant to utilize the heavier workloads necessary to elicit strength adaptations. Strength-oriented exercises include free weights, selectorized machines, and cable-based resistance training equipment. When performing strength exercises, the overload is progressed by increasing the external resistance applied to the targeted muscle group. The same exercises may also be used to elicit improvements in muscular endurance by selecting low-to-moderate workloads and performing a moderate-to-high number of repetitions.

Choice of Exercises

Among the many factors to consider when designing a resistance training program, the choice of exercise will have the most significant impact on the outward appearance of the program. The exercise selection is influenced by a number of factors such as the overall objective (e.g., stabilization, endurance, or strength), the availability of equipment, and the client's goals, preferences, abilities, and limitations. A well-designed program will represent all of the major muscle groups of the body including the legs, hips, back, chest, abdomen, shoulders, and arms (HHS, 2008). In addition, a resistance training program should include exercises representing each of four categories including: lower body, upper body push, upper body pull, and core/rotation.

> **Good to Know**
>
> **Resistance Training Progression Strategies**
>
> **Stability**: overload is progressed by increasing the degree of instability during the exercise.
>
> **Endurance**: overload is progressed by increasing the number of repetitions performed.
>
> **Strength**: overload is progressed by increasing the external resistance to be lifted.

Order of Exercises

The resistance training routine can also include a variety of strategies related to the sequence of exercises. As noted in the ACSM resistance training guidelines, it is recommended that large muscle group exercises are performed before small muscle group exercises, multiple-joint exercises before single-joint exercises, and higher-intensity exercises before lower-intensity exercises (Ratamess et al., 2009). It is also permissible to alternate exercises that target upper and lower body or agonist and antagonist muscle groups.

A time-efficient strategy that is used to elicit strength, endurance, and metabolic training effects is circuit training. A **circuit training** routine consists of a series of several exercises that are performed with minimal rest between exercises. Each set consists of 15 to 20 repetitions with a light-to-moderate (e.g., 55% to 65% of 1-RM) resistance. Alternatively, each exercise may be performed for a predetermined amount of time (e.g., 30 to 45 seconds) rather than to a specified number of repetitions. Figure 18-4 depicts a traditional approach to circuit training using only resistance exercises. The exercises are sequenced from large muscle groups to small, and alternates upper and lower body exercises. Figure 18-5 illustrates a circuit training program that alternates resistance training exercises with stations of cardiorespiratory activity. In this sample program both resistance and cardiorespiratory stations are performed for 45 seconds with a 15 second recovery and transition time between exercises.

Within resistance training programs, several approaches are also utilized with regard to the order of exercise. Some common examples include super-sets, compound-sets, tri-sets, and pyramids. A **super-set** consists of two exercises, each targeting antagonistic muscle groups, performed with minimal rest between sets. Some examples include a dumbbell biceps curl paired with a cable triceps pushdown; a chest press machine paired with a seated row; or a leg extension paired with a leg curl. Super-sets provide a time-efficient option and encourage balanced training for opposing muscle groups. As one muscle group works, the antagonistic muscle group is allowed to rest and vice versa. Another variation of super-setting involves a multiple-joint exercise paired with a single-joint exercise

Figure 18-4 Circuit Weight Training

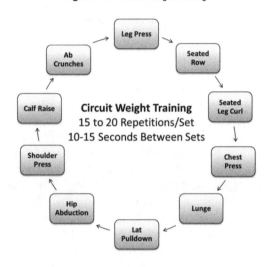

Figure 18-5 Cardio Circuit Weight Training

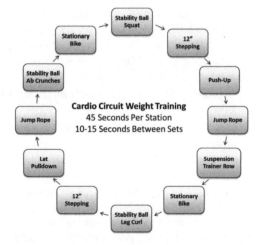

targeting an antagonistic muscle. For example, a chest press may be paired with a biceps curl (multi-joint push – single-joint pull), or a seated narrow row may be paired with a triceps pushdown (multi-joint pull – single-joint push).

Like a super-set, a **compound-set** also consists of two exercises performed with minimal rest between sets; however, in this case a different exercise targeting the same muscle group is selected for each set. For example, a dumbbell chest press is immediately followed by a standing cable fly, or a dumbbell shoulder press is followed by a dumbbell lateral raise. Although not necessary, it is common for the first exercise of a compound set to involve multiple joints; whereas, the second set is a single-joint exercise as represented in the examples above. The exercises may also be selected such that the first exercise of the compound-set is strength-oriented (i.e., stable); whereas, the second exercise is stabilization-oriented (i.e., unstable). For example, a seated leg press may be followed by a body weight squat performed on a BOSU® to create a compound set. Generally speaking, compound-sets provide a greater overload stimulus to the targeted muscle group. Therefore, this training strategy may be more appropriate for intermediate or advanced exercisers.

A **tri-set** functions much like a mini circuit of exercises. Tri-sets are characterized by three consecutive exercises targeting the same body part, each involving a different movement pattern. A lower body tri-set may include a stability ball squat, a stability ball leg curl, and hip abduction using resistance tubing. An upper body tri-set may include a cable chest press, a dumbbell lateral raise, and a wide-grip row. In both examples, the series of three exercises are performed in rapid succession followed by a rest period. Once adequately recovered, a second tri-set may be performed utilizing the same triad of exercises.

Pyramid training is a strategy often used by power lifters to develop strength and power specific to the bench press, dead lift, and squat. However, the pyramid concept can be applied to other exercises and used by other populations as well. A pyramid typically involves multiple sets (e.g., 4 to 7) of a specific exercise. The first set utilizes a moderate workload (e.g., 65% to 75% 1-RM) lifted for 10 to 12 repetitions. During subsequent sets, the resistance is increased and the corresponding number of repetitions performed to fatigue decreases, peaking with a set near-maximal workload, lifted for only 1 to 3 repetitions. This peak set may be followed by 1 or 2 additional sets at a reduced workload descending back down the opposite side of the pyramid. Figure 18-6 illustrates a classic pyramid model.

Periodization of Training

Periodization of training originated in Eastern Europe and has been used for many years by strength and conditioning coaches to optimize the performance of athletes. In recent years, periodized training programs have become more widely used by personal trainers guiding their clients to maximize gains in fitness (Fleck, 2011). Periodization of training refers to the planned and systematic changes in the acute program variables (Fleck, 2011; Gamble, 2006; Plisk & Stone, 2003). The primary goals of periodization are to maximize the training effect to promote optimal fitness and performance, and to manage fatigue to prevent training plateaus and overtraining (Plisk & Stone, 2003). The general adaptation syndrome provided the initial theoretical basis for periodization; however, the *fitness-fatigue model* has become more widely accepted as the prevailing theory of training adaptation and periodization (Gamble, 2006; Plisk & Stone, 2003; Turner, 2011). According to the fitness-fatigue model, performance is optimal when training strategies are focused on maximizing the training effect (i.e., fitness) while minimizing fatigue (Gamble, 2006; Plisk & Stone, 2003; Turner, 2011). In other words, it is the net effect of these two opposing outcomes, fitness versus fatigue, which determines the individual's performance with regard to a specific task (Gamble, 2006).

Periodized training programs are broken down into three primary components including the macrocycle, mesocycles, and microcycles. A **macrocycle** represents the entire training period, often ranging from 6 months to 1 year or longer. The macrocycle is comprised of several mesocycles each of which may last from several weeks to months and is focused on a specific training goal (e.g., endurance, strength, power). Each mesocycle is then made up of smaller **microcycles** that typically represent 1 week blocks of training or even individual workout sessions.

A key characteristic of periodized training programs is the systematic manipulation of the acute training variables. Among these, emphasis is placed on changes in training intensity and volume to elicit specific training adaptations. Training intensity is often inversely related to training volume such that as the intensity of training increases, the volume will decrease. In addition, rest periods are also adjusted to ensure adequate recovery in relation to the training stimulus. Higher intensity exercise will require longer rest periods to facilitate complete recovery and optimal adaptation. The choice of exercise may also be dictated by the phase of training and the desired training outcomes. Early mesocycles may be dedicated to outcomes specific to postural stability and endurance; whereas, later mesocycles may be intended to elicit strength or power adaptations.

Figure 18-6 Pyramid Training

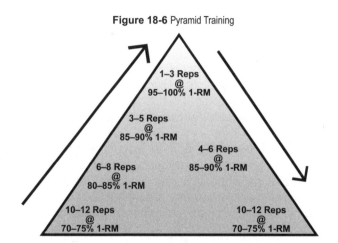

Generally speaking, two types of periodization are commonly utilized: linear periodization (also called *classic periodization*) and nonlinear periodization (also called *undulating periodization*). Linear periodization is often used by individual and team sport athletes for the purpose of achieving peak performance, corresponding to the competitive season or an important event. A program of linear periodization progressively increases training intensity as the corresponding training volume decreases. Early phases of training (i.e., mesocycles) emphasize general physical conditioning. Later phases seek to develop sport-specific adaptations.

Table 18-4 outlines the phases or cycles of a linear periodization model. The top row indicates the phases of a linear model using the typical European terminology; the second row indicates the phases using traditional American terminology, and the third row indicates the phases using the American strength/power model terminology. The bottom of the table provides the general parameters for the acute training variables as they correspond to the American strength/power linear periodization model. Keep in mind that many variations of these linear models have been developed for various sports and individual athletes. This table simply provides a schematic overview of common underlying models that guide most linear periodization training programs. Again, a key characteristic of linear periodization is an initial high volume and low intensity with gradual increases in intensity and decreases in volume within and across training periods (Harries et al., 2015). Linear periodization is often effectively applied to sport-specific training programs for athletes. A potential limitation to a well-designed linear program for health-seekers and fitness enthusiasts is inconsistency of training, which disrupts the linear progression and continuity of the program.

Nonlinear periodization is characterized by more frequent changes in training intensity and volume, often from one workout session to the next (Fleck, 2011). The convenience, flexibility, and variety offered by nonlinear periodization has contributed to its gain in popularity among participants seeking fitness-oriented goals. Using a nonlinear approach, the intensity of each session is altered by increasing or decreasing the target *repetition-maximum (RM)* range. For example, a range of 4 to 6 RM (able to perform up to a maximum of 6 repetitions with good technique) may be used to provide a strength stimulus; a range of 8 to 12 RM provides a strength-endurance stimulus; and a range of 15 to 20 RM provides an endurance stimulus. During each session, the volume of work performed is also adjusted by the number of sets performed for each exercise and for the session overall. Strength-oriented sessions will generally have a lower volume; whereas, endurance-oriented sessions will provide a higher volume.

Table 18-5 outlines some nonlinear periodization models. The intensity of each week or day (i.e., training session) is typically defined by the repetition-maximum (RM) target range applied to most exercise sets within the respective phase. For example, 12-15 RM sets may be conceptualized as a "low" intensity or "light" resistance; 8-10 RM may be considered a "moderate" intensity or resistance; and 4-6 RM a "high" intensity or "heavy" resistance. Similar to linear periodization, as the intensity increases, the volume decreases. So, the volume of training is high during a low-intensity week or day, on the other hand the volume of training is low on a high-intensity week or day. Rest periods between sets and exercises also correspond to intensity, such that low-intensity resistance training will require shorter rest periods (e.g., 20-60 seconds); whereas high-intensity resistance training will require longer rest periods (e.g., 2-3 minutes). The row labeled "weekly" indicates a nonlinear or undulating plan that cycles from low- to high- to moderate-intensity training each week. The row labeled "biweekly" indicates a nonlinear or undulating plan that follows the same low-high-moderate-intensity changes; however, each phase spans two weeks versus one. The "daily" nonlinear periodization reflects a change in intensity from day to day within the week. Daily periodization may also be implemented following the contemporary approach focused on stabilization-, strength-, and power-oriented training.

Harries et al. (2015) conducted a meta-analysis review of both linear and nonlinear periodized resistance training programs, which indicates no significant difference in strength gains attained from either models. These authors state, "It is reasonable to suggest that the novelty or variation in stimulus compared to the participants' previous training experience is of greater importance for eliciting strength improvements and overcoming accommodation than the specific type of periodization approach employed" (Harries et al., 2015). It is very likely that a novice exerciser will initially obtain significant gains from any resistance training program, regardless of methods and models, provided the program is performed consistently and does not injure the participant. Continued gains beyond the first 12-16 weeks of training will require more strategic and specific programming.

Regardless of the periodization strategy utilized, it is apparent that a program including planned and systematic changes among the acute training variables provides superior outcomes in comparison to resistance training programs that lack appropriate variety.

Common Resistance Training Exercises

The following section provides a library of resistance training exercises that are recommended for individuals wishing to increase muscular strength and/or endurance. The unique goals, needs, abilities, and physical limitations must be considered for each client when selecting safe and appropriate resistance training exercises. The 'joint actions' refers to the primary joint actions during the concentric phase of an exercise. The selection of exercises provided in this manual is not all-inclusive. Readers are encouraged to research other resources for additional resistance exercise options.

Table 18-4 Linear Periodization

	Linear Periodization Models				
European Terminology	Preparation Phase	First Transition		Competition Phase	Second Transition
Traditional American Terminology	Pre-Season			In-Season	Off-Season
American Strength/ Power Terminology	**Hypertrophy**	**Strength**	**Power**	**Peaking**	**Active Rest**
Sets/exercise	3-5	3-5	3-5	1-3	Light Physical Activity
Reps/set	8-12	2-6	2-3	1-3	
Intensity	Low	Moderate	High	Very High	
Volume	Very High	High	Moderate	Low	

Adapted from Fleck & Kraemer (2014)

Table 18-5 Nonlinear Periodization Models

	Nonlinear Periodization Models					
	Week 1	Week 2	Week 3	Week 4	Week 5	Week 6
Weekly	12-15 RM "Low"	4-6 RM "High"	8-10 RM "Moderate"	12-15 RM "Low"	4-6 RM "High"	8-10 RM "Moderate"
Biweekly	12-15 RM "Low"	12-15 RM "Low"	4-6 RM "High"	4-6 RM "High"	8-10 RM "Moderate"	8-10 RM "Moderate"
	Week 1			Week 2		
	Day 1	Day 2	Day 3	Day 1	Day 2	Day 3
Daily	12-15 RM "Low"	8-10 RM "Moderate"	4-6 RM "High"	12-15 RM "Low"	8-10 RM "Moderate"	4-6 RM "High"
Daily	Stabilization	Strength	Power	Stabilization	Strength	Power

Smith Squat

Primary Muscles:
- Quadriceps
- Gluteus Maximus
- Hamstrings

Joint Actions:
- Knee Extension
- Hip Extension

Alternative Exercises:
- Barbell Squat
- Dumbbell
- Stability Ball Squat
- Leg Press
- Hip Sled

Exercise Execution:
- Position the bar across the back of the shoulders resting comfortably on the trapezius muscle.
- Position feet hip-width apart with the toes pointing forward, patella vertically aligned over the center of the foot, and feet in front of the body's center of gravity.
- Lift, rotate, and disengage the bar from the support pins.
- Lower the weight to a position no more than 90 degrees of flexion in the hips and knees.
- Lift the weight back to the starting position without locking or hyperextending the knees.
- Maintain proper posture and neutral spinal alignment with the core muscles activated throughout the exercise.

⚠ **Caution:** Performing squat exercises lower than 90 degrees of knee flexion may cause potentially damaging patellofemoral stress.

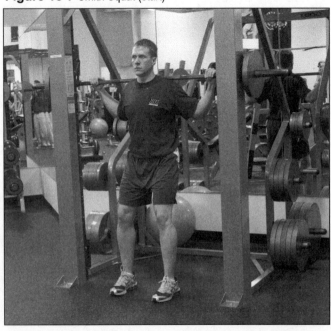

Figure 18-7 Smith Squat (start)

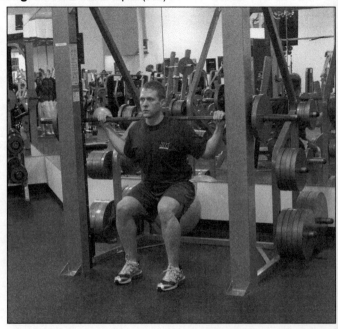

Figure 18-8 Smith Squat (end)

Vertical Leg Press

Primary Muscles:
- Quadriceps
- Gluteus Maximus
- Hamstrings

Joint Actions:
- Knee Extension
- Hip Extension

Alternative Exercises:
- Barbell Squat
- Dumbbell Squat
- Stability Ball Squat
- Smith Squat
- Hip Sled

Exercise Execution:
- Adjust the seat position so the knees and hips are at slightly less than 90 degrees.
- Position both feet on the foot plate hip-width apart with the patella vertically aligned over the center of the foot.
- Press the platform away from the body by extending the knees and hips through a full range of motion without locking or hyperextending the knees.
- Lower the platform back toward the torso to 90 degrees of knee flexion without allowing the weight plates to touch.
- Maintain proper posture and alignment throughout the exercise.

Figure 18-9 Vertical Leg Press (start)

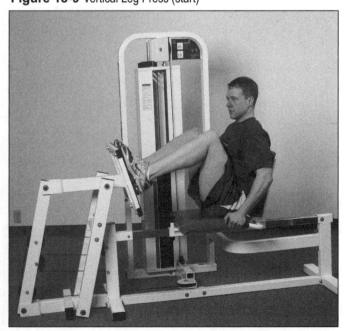

Figure 18-10 Vertical Leg Press (end)

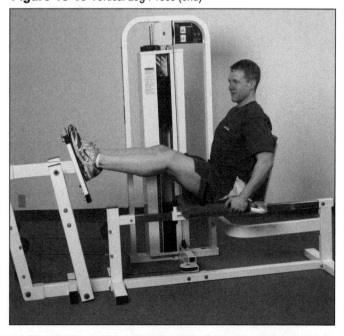

Stability Ball Squat

Primary Muscles:
- Quadriceps
- Gluteus Maximus
- Hamstrings

Joint Actions:
- Knee Extension
- Hip Extension

Alternative Exercises:
- Barbell Squat
- Dumbbell Squat
- Leg Press
- Smith Squat
- Hip Sled

Exercise Execution:
- Place the ball between the lower back and the wall.
- Position feet hip-width apart with the toes pointing forward, patella vertically aligned over the center of the foot, and feet in front of the body's center of gravity.
- Lower the body to a position no more than 90 degrees of flexion in the hips and knees.
- Rise back to the starting position without locking or hyperextending the knees.
- Maintain proper posture and neutral spinal alignment with the core muscles activated throughout the exercise.

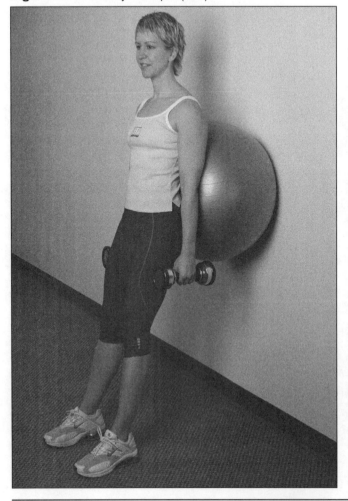

Figure 18-11 Stability Ball Squat (start)

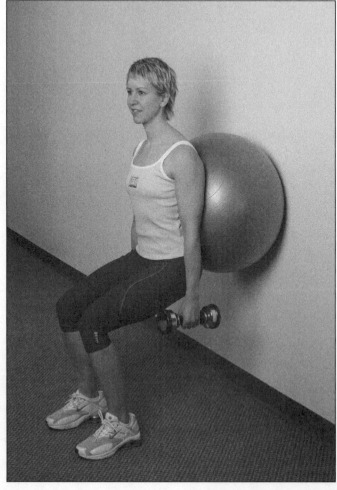

Figure 18-12 Stability Ball Squat (end)

Stationary Lunge

Primary Muscles:
- Quadriceps
- Gluteus Maximus
- Hamstrings

Joint Actions:
- Knee Extension
- Hip Extension

Alternative Exercises:
- Barbell Lunge
- Dumbbell Lunge
- Smith Lunge
- Striding Lunge
- Walking Lunge
- Stability Ball Lunge

Exercise Execution:
- Stand in a stride stance with feet positioned hip-width apart, toes pointing forward, patella vertically aligned over the center of the foot.
- Lower the body to a position no more than 90 degrees of flexion in the forward knee and hip.
- Return back to the starting position without locking or hyperextending the knee.
- Maintain proper posture and neutral spinal alignment with the core muscles activated throughout the exercise.
- Keep the forward knee vertically aligned over the center of the foot at all times.

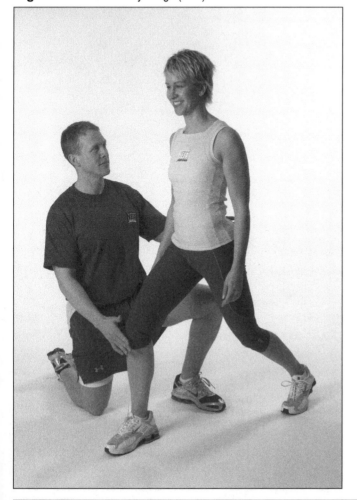

Figure 18-13 Stationary Lunge (start)

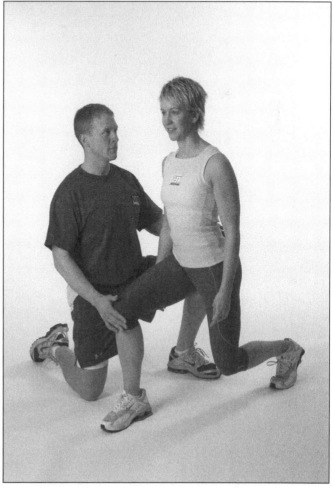

Figure 18-14 Stationary Lunge (end)

Leg Extension

Primary Muscles:
- Quadriceps

Joint Action:
- Knee Extension

Alternative Exercises:
- Supine Straight Leg Raise
- Squat variations
- Leg Press
- Lunge variations

Exercise Execution:
- Adjust the back rest to align the center of the knee joints with the axis of rotation of the machine.
- Adjust the leg pad to rest comfortably above the ankle joint.
- Extend the knees slowly to lift the lower legs to a point approximately 5-10 degrees short of full extension.
- Return to the starting position with the knees flexed at approximately 90 degrees.
- Maintain proper postural alignment throughout the exercise.
- ⚠ **Caution:** The leg extension exercise may place potentially harmful shearing force across the knee joint and upon the anterior cruciate ligament (ACL).

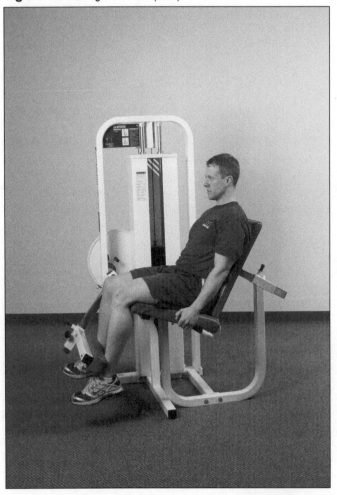

Figure 18-15 Leg Extension (start)

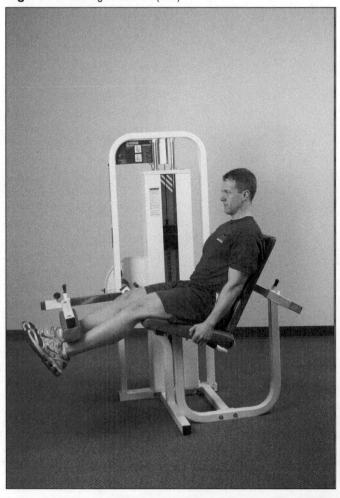

Figure 18-16 Leg Extension (end)

Prone Leg Curl

Primary Muscles:
- Hamstrings

Joint Action:
- Knee Flexion

Alternative Exercises:
- Seated Leg Curl
- Standing Cable Leg Curl
- Stability Ball Leg Curl
- Straight Leg Deadlift

Exercise Execution:
- Position the body to align the center of the knee joints with the axis of rotation of the machine.
- Adjust the leg pad to rest comfortably above the ankle joint, superior to the Achilles tendon.
- Bend the knees to raise the leg pad to a position slightly ≤90 degrees of knee flexion.
- Return to the starting position with the knees fully extended, but not locked or hyperextended.
- Maintain proper postural alignment throughout the exercise. Keep the anterior hip bones anchored on pad and core muscles activated to maintain neutral lower back.

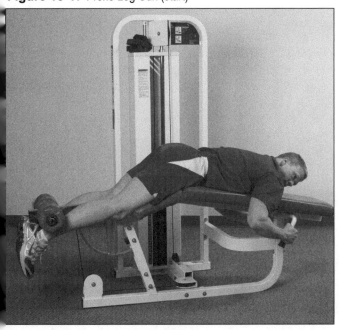

Figure 18-17 Prone Leg Curl (start)

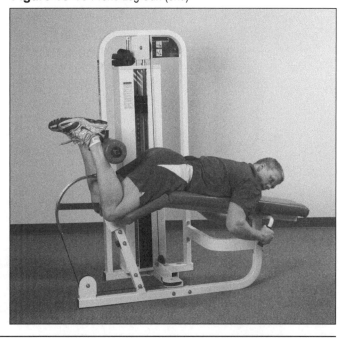

Figure 18-18 Prone Leg Curl (end)

Stability Ball Leg Curl

Primary Muscles:
- Hamstrings

Joint Action:
- Knee Flexion

Alternative Exercises:
- Seated Leg Curl
- Standing Cable Leg Curl
- Prone Leg Curl
- Straight Leg Deadlift

Exercise Execution:
- Lay in the supine position with both feet positioned on the top of the stability ball.
- Elevate the hips off the floor to bring ankle, knee, hips, and shoulders into alignment.
- Pull heels toward body until the knees are ≤90 degrees of knee flexion.
- Extend legs to return to starting position.
- Keep hips elevated and level throughout the exercise.

Figure 18-19 Stability Ball Leg Curl (start)

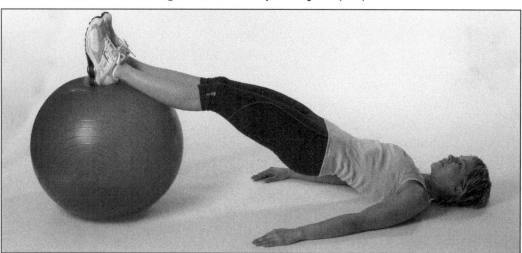

Figure 18-20 Stability Ball Leg Curl (end)

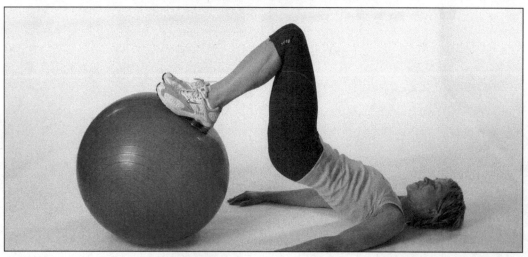

Straight Leg Deadlift

Primary Muscles:
- Gluteus Maximus
- Hamstrings

Joint Action:
- Hip Extension

Alternative Exercises:
- Seated Leg Curl
- Standing Cable Leg Curl
- Stability Ball Leg Curl
- Prone Leg Curl
- Glute Machine

Exercise Execution:
- Position feet hip-width apart with toes pointing forward.
- Hold the barbell in front of body with elbows straight, but not locked, and wrists in neutral position.
- Slowly lower the bar toward the floor to a point approximately midway along the lower leg.
- Return to the starting position.
- Maintain neutral spine, and a straight (not locked or hyperextended) position of the knees.

⚠ **Caution:** The deadlift exercise may place significant stress on the lumbar spine and the intervertebral discs. Maintain neutral spinal alignment at all times. Do not flex or arch the lumbar spine.

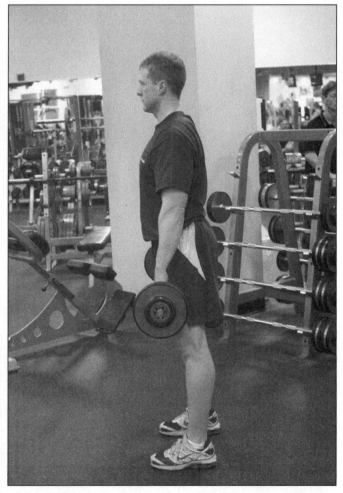

Figure 18-21 Straight Leg Deadlift (start)

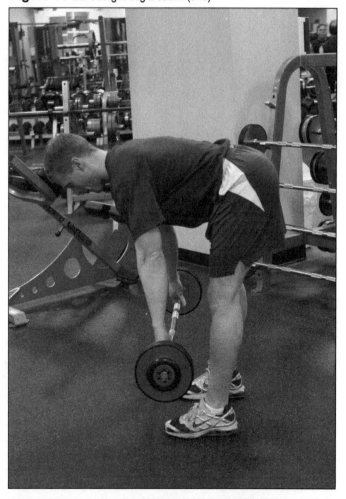

Figure 18-22 Straight Leg Deadlift (end)

Resistance Tubing Hip Abduction

Primary Muscles:
- Gluteus Medius
- Gluteus Minimus

Joint Action:
- Hip Abduction

Alternative Exercises:
- Lateral Stepping with Tubing
- Seated Hip Abduction Machine
- Standing Cable Hip Abduction
- Side-Lying Leg Lift (top leg)

Exercise Execution:
- Place tubing around mid-lower leg or ankles.
- Stand with feet positioned hip-width apart and toes pointing forward.
- Abduct one leg to ~30-40 degrees.
- Return to starting position without allowing targeted leg to contact the floor.
- Maintain postural alignment including level hip position throughout the exercise.

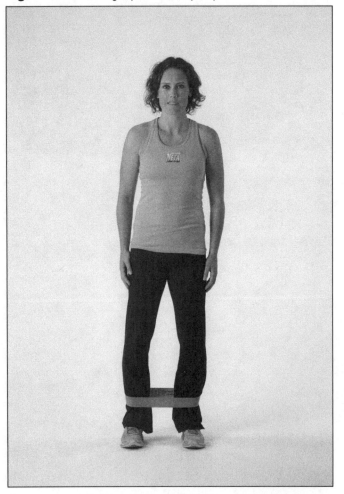

Figure 18-23 Tubing Hip Abduction (start)

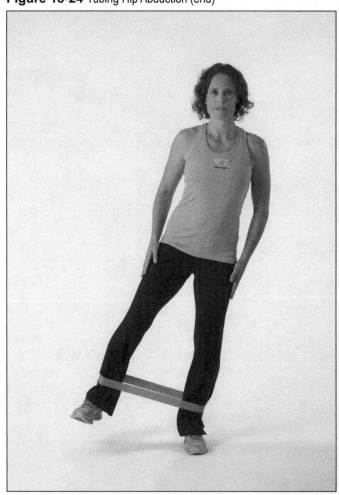

Figure 18-24 Tubing Hip Abduction (end)

Upward Torso Rotation

Primary Muscles:
- Core
  - Erector Spinae
  - External Obliques
  - Internal Obliques
  - Transverse Abdominis
- Shoulder Complex
- Lumbo-Pelvic-Hip Complex

Joint Actions:
- Multiple

Alternative Exercises:
- Medicine Ball Hay-Bailer
- Downward Torso Rotation
- Horizontal Torso Rotation

Exercise Execution:
- Secure cable pulley to lower position.
- Stand at angle in the direction of the pulley.
- Position feet in stride stance approximately hip-width apart and toes angled in the same direction.
- Grasp handle with both hands in interlocked position.
- Lift handle in a diagonal pattern across body above the opposite shoulder.
- Pivot feet, hips, and shoulders in unison as the torso is rotated to 'follow' the movement of the arms.
- Slowly return to the starting position without allowing the weights to touch the weight stack.
- Maintain neutral spinal alignment throughout the exercise.

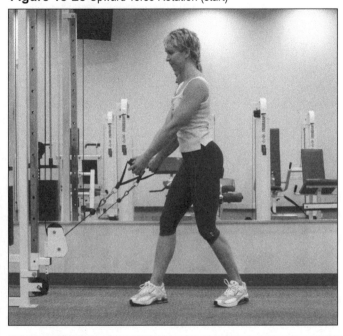

Figure 18-25 Upward Torso Rotation (start)

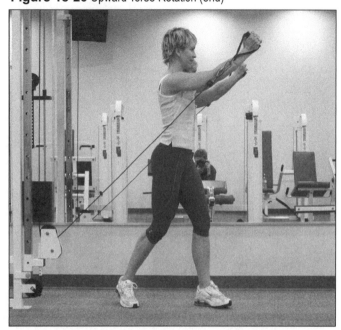

Figure 18-26 Upward Torso Rotation (end)

Seated Narrow Row

Primary Muscles:
- Latissimus Dorsi
- Teres Major
- Rhomboids
- Middle Trapezius
- Biceps Brachii

Joint Actions:
- Shoulder Extension
- Scapular Retraction
- Elbow Flexion

Alternative Exercises:
- Dumbbell One-Arm Row
- Cable One-Arm Row
- Seated Row Machine
- Wide Row
- Assisted Pull-Up
- Suspension Trainer Row

Exercise Execution:
- Sit with tall posture, feet positioned on floor with knees flexed to 90 degrees or on foot plate with knees slightly bent.
- Grasp handle with neutral hand position.
- Initiate movement by retracting the scapula, then pull the handle toward the torso by extending the shoulders and flexing the arms in the sagittal plane.
- Return to starting position.
- Maintain tall position with proper postural alignment at all times. Do not lean backwards or flex the lumbar spine.

⚠ **Caution:** Flexing or rounding the lumbar spine may place potentially harmful stress on the lower back. Maintain neutral spinal alignment at all times.

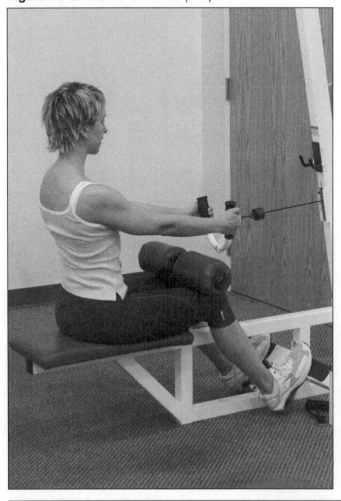

Figure 18-27 Seated Narrow Row (start)

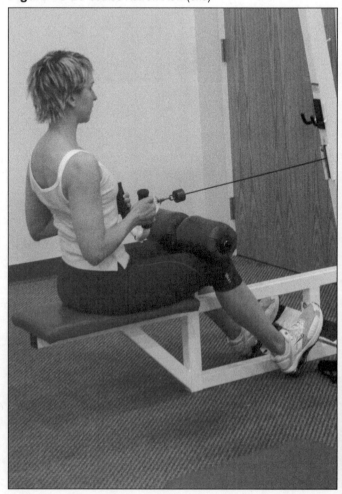

Figure 18-28 Seated Narrow Row (end)

Dumbbell One-Arm Row

Primary Muscles:
- Latissimus Dorsi
- Teres Major
- Rhomboids
- Middle Trapezius
- Biceps Brachii

Joint Actions:
- Shoulder Extension
- Scapular Retraction
- Elbow Flexion

Alternative Exercises:
- Seated Cable Narrow Row
- Cable One-Arm Row
- Seated Row Machine
- Wide Row
- Assisted Pull-Up
- Suspension Trainer Row

Exercise Execution:
- Position one knee on a flat bench directly under hip. Place the ipsilateral hand on bench directly below shoulder.
- Grasp the dumbbell with the opposite hand using a neutral grip.
- Initiate movement by retracting the scapula, then pull the dumbbell toward the hip by extending the shoulder and flexing the arm in the sagittal plane.
- Maintain proper postural alignment through hip, shoulder, and head. Keep the hips and shoulders level and maintain a neutral spine.

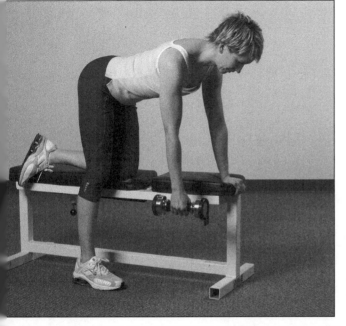

Figure 18-29 Dumbbell One-Arm Row (start)

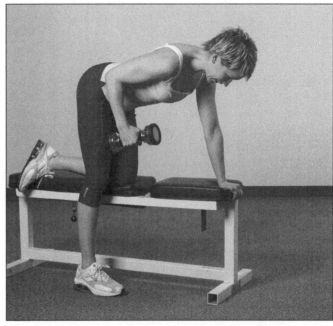

Figure 18-30 Dumbbell One-Arm Row (end)

Lat Pulldown

Primary Muscles:
- Latissimus Dorsi
- Teres Major
- Rhomboids
- Middle Trapezius
- Biceps Brachii

Joint Actions:
- Shoulder Adduction
- Scapular Retraction/Downward Rotation
- Elbow Flexion

Alternative Exercises:
- Assisted Pull-Up
- Lat Pulldown Machine
- Seated Cable Narrow Row
- Cable One-Arm Row
- Seated Row Machine
- Wide Row

Exercise Execution:
- Adjust the thigh pad to secure the lower body with feet flat on floor and knees at 90 degrees.
- Grasp handle in a position that creates a 90 degree angle in the elbows when the upper arm is parallel to the ground.
- Lean slightly backward (just enough so the bar does not hit the head).
- Pull the bar down in front of the head toward the upper region of the chest.
- Return to the starting position.
- Maintain parallel alignment between the cable and the forearms throughout the exercise.
- Maintain postural alignment at all times, do not lean excessively backward.

⚠ **Caution:** Do not perform the lat pulldown in the behind-the-head position. This places dangerous stress across the shoulder joint and may also result in injury to the cervical spine.

Figure 18-31 Lat Pulldown (start)

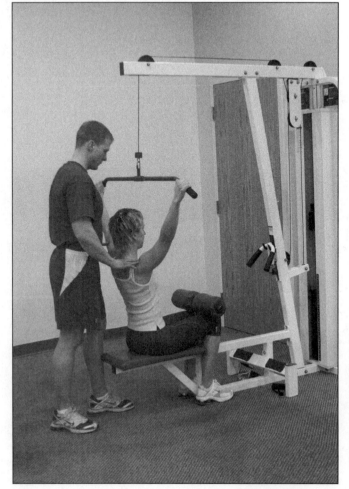

Figure 18-32 Lat Pulldown (end)

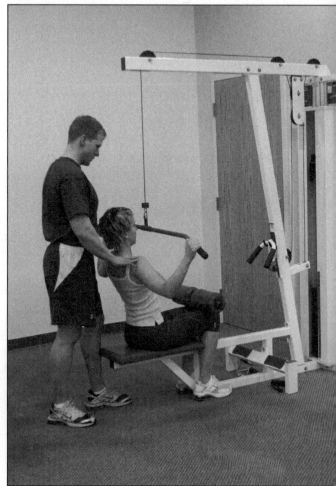

Assisted Pull-Up

Primary Muscles:
- Latissimus Dorsi
- Teres Major
- Rhomboids
- Middle Trapezius
- Biceps Brachii

Joint Actions:
- Shoulder Adduction
- Scapular Retraction/Downward Rotation
- Elbow Flexion

Alternative Exercises:
- Lat Pulldown
- Lat Pulldown Machine
- Seated Cable Narrow Row
- Cable One-Arm Row
- Seated Row Machine
- Wide Row

Exercise Execution:
- Grasp handle in a position that creates a 90 degree angle in the elbows when the upper arm is parallel to the ground.
- Step one foot at a time onto the assistance lever.
- Pull down, moving upward, until elbows are flexed to ≤90 degrees (eyes at level of handles).
- Return to the starting position.
- Maintain postural alignment throughout the exercise.
- Exit machine by stepping one foot at a time onto the top step, slowly lowering the weight back to the weight stack using the opposite foot.

⚠ **Caution:** Use caution when entering and exiting this exercise. Make sure the weight is resting on the weight stack before removing second foot from the assistance lever.

Figure 18-33 Assisted Pull-Up (start)

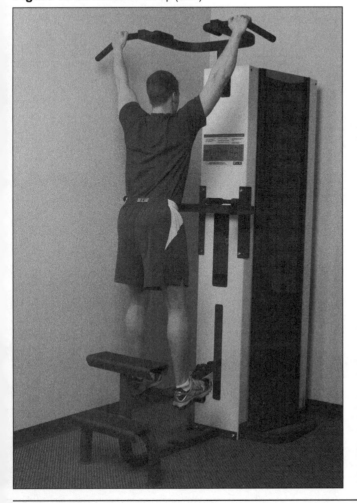

Figure 18-34 Assisted Pull-Up (end)

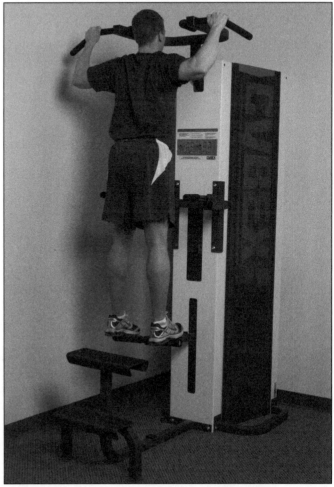

Bench Press

Primary Muscles:
- Pectoralis Major
- Anterior Deltoid
- Triceps

Joint Actions:
- Shoulder Horizontal Adduction
- Elbow Extension

Alternative Exercises:
- Incline Bench Press
- Dumbbell Chest Press
- Chest Press Machine
- Cable Chest Press
- Floor Push-Up
- Stability Ball Push-Up
- Cable Chest Fly
- Suspension Trainer Chest Press

Exercise Execution:
- Lie on bench with both feet positioned flat on floor, end of bench, or platform at end of bench.
- Grasp bar in a position that allows for 90 degrees of elbow flexion when the upper arms are parallel to the floor. Wrists are in neutral position.
- Lift bar off the support rack and position directly over the chest with the elbows extended, but not locked or hyperextended.
- Lower the bar toward the middle of the chest until the elbows are flexed to 90 degrees ('goal-post' position).
- Push the bar back up to the starting position.
- Keep head, scapula, and hips in contact with the bench at all times. Maintain neutral lumbar spine, do not arch the back.

⚠ **Caution:** Risk of shoulder injury increases as the bar is lowered below the 'goal-post' position. Do not bounce the bar off the chest. Do not arch or hyperextend the lumbar spine. Always use a spotter when performing the bench press.

Figure 18-35 Bench Press (start)

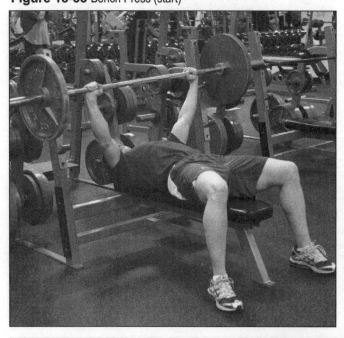

Figure 18-36 Bench Press (end)

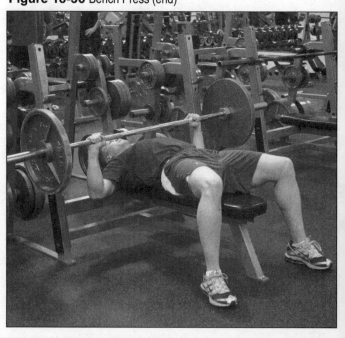

Chest Press Machine

Primary Muscles:
- Pectoralis Major
- Anterior Deltoid
- Triceps

Joint Actions:
- Shoulder Horizontal Adduction
- Elbow Extension

Alternative Exercises:
- Narrow Grip Chest Press Machine
- Bench Press
- Incline Bench Press
- Dumbbell Chest Press
- Cable Chest Press
- Floor Push-Up
- Stability Ball Push-Up
- Cable Chest Flys
- Suspension Trainer Chest Press

Exercise Execution:
- Adjust seat height to align horizontal handles through the middle of the chest.
- Use foot release (if available) to bring handles forward.
- Grasp horizontal hand grips in a position that allows for 90 degrees of elbow flexion when upper arms are directly to the sides of body. Remove feet from foot release.
- Push handles forward until arms are fully extended, but not locked or hyperextended.
- Return to the position of 90 degrees of elbow flexion.
- Use foot release (if available) to control weight as hands are removed from the handles.
- Maintain proper postural alignment throughout the exercise with head, scapula, and hips against the back rest.
- ⚠ **Caution:** Risk of shoulder injury increases as the handles are lowered past the 'goal-post' position. (i.e., elbows move posterior to the frontal plane).

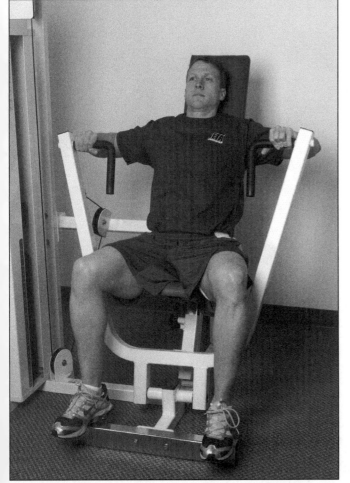

Figure 18-37 Chest Press Machine (start)

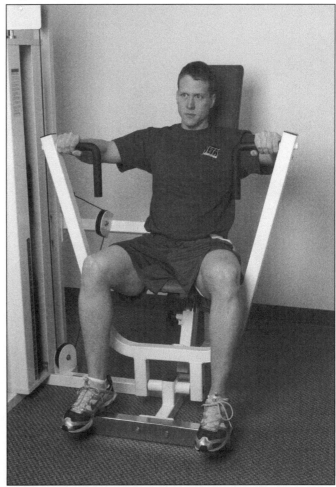

Figure 18-38 Chest Press Machine (end)

Dumbell Chest Press

Primary Muscles:
- Pectoralis Major
- Anterior Deltoid
- Triceps

Joint Actions:
- Shoulder Horizontal Adduction
- Elbow Extension

Alternative Exercises:
- Chest Press Machine
- Incline or Flat Bench Press
- Incline Dumbbell Chest Press
- Stability Ball Chest Press
- Cable Chest Press
- Floor Push-Up
- Stability Ball Push-Up
- Cable Chest Fly
- Suspension Trainer Chest Press

Exercise Execution:
- Sit on the end of the bench with the dumbbells resting on your thighs just above the knees.
- Roll back into a supine position on the bench, keeping the arms straight to position the dumbbells directly over the chest.
- Feet may be positioned on the end of the bench (as pictured) or flat on the floor.
- Holding the dumbbells in a barbell position, slowly lower the weights until the elbows are flexed to 90 degrees ('goal-post' position).
- Press the dumbbells back up to the starting position.
- Keep head, scapula, and hips in contact with the bench at all times. Maintain neutral lumbar spine, do not arch the back.
- To exit the exercise, bring both knees up to meet the dumbbells. With dumbbells touching thigh and arms straight, roll forward to the seated position.

⚠ **Caution:** Risk of shoulder injury increases as the dumbbells are lowered past the 'goal-post' position (i.e., elbows move posterior to the frontal plane).

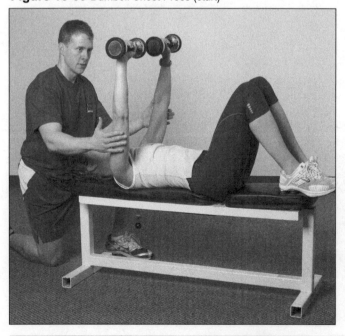

Figure 18-39 Dumbell Chest Press (start)

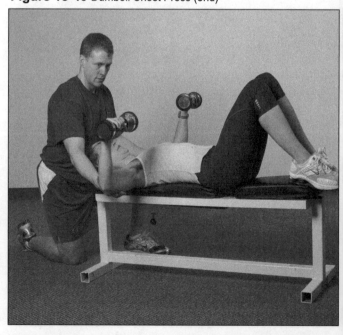

Figure 18-40 Dumbell Chest Press (end)

Stability Ball Dumbbell Chest Press

Primary Muscles:
- Pectoralis Major
- Anterior Deltoid
- Triceps

Joint Actions:
- Shoulder Horizontal Adduction
- Elbow Extension

Alternative Exercises:
- Chest Press Machine
- Incline or Flat Bench Press
- Incline or Flat Dumbbell Chest Press
- Cable Chest Press
- Floor Push-Up
- Cable Chest Fly
- Suspension Trainer Chest Press

Exercise Execution:
- Sit on the stability ball with dumbbells resting on thighs just above knees.
- Walk the feet forward rolling the ball up the back to a final position supporting the shoulders and head. Dumbbells are positioned over the chest with arms fully extended.
- Holding the dumbbells in a barbell position, slowly lower the weights until the elbows are flexed to 90 degrees ('goal-post' position).
- Press the dumbbells back up to the starting position.
- Walk the feet back toward the ball, rolling back into the seated position with the dumbbells resting on the thighs.
- ⚠ **Caution:** Risk of shoulder injury increases as the dumbbells are lowered past the 'goal-post' position (i.e., elbows move posterior to the frontal plane).

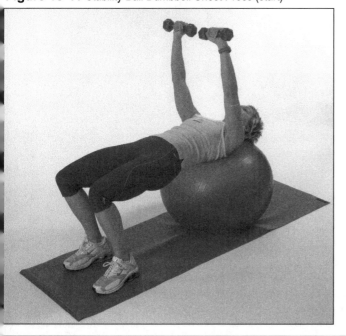

Figure 18-41 Stability Ball Dumbbell Chest Press (start)

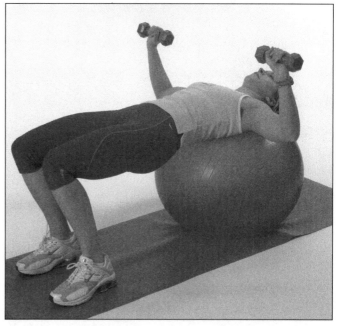

Figure 18-42 Stability Ball Dumbbell Chest Press (end)

Shoulder Press Machine

Primary Muscles:
- Anterior and Medial Deltoid
- Upper Trapezius
- Triceps

Joint Actions:
- Shoulder Abduction
- Scapular Upward Rotation
- Elbow Extension

Alternative Exercises:
- Barbell Shoulder Press
- Dumbbell Shoulder Press
- Cable Shoulder Press
- Dumbbell, Tubing, or Cable Lateral Raise
- Scaption

Exercise Execution:
- Adjust seat height so the horizontal hand grips are slightly below the top of the shoulders.
- Grasp the horizontal handles with a neutral wrist position.
- Press the handles overhead until the elbows are fully extended, but not locked.
- Lower the weight back down to near the staring position without allowing the weights to touch the weight stack.
- Maintain proper postural alignment throughout the exercise with head, scapula, and hips against the back rest. Do not arch the lower back.
- **Caution:** This exercise may not be appropriate for those with pre-existing shoulder considerations such as shoulder impingement or tendonitis.

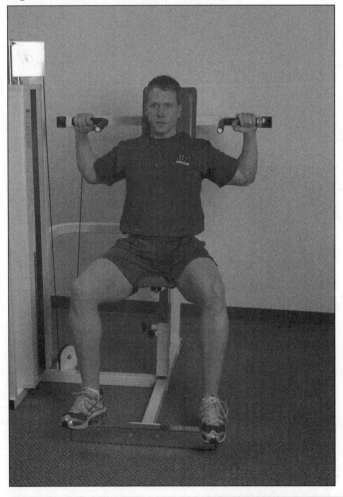

Figure 18-43 Shoulder Press Machine (start)

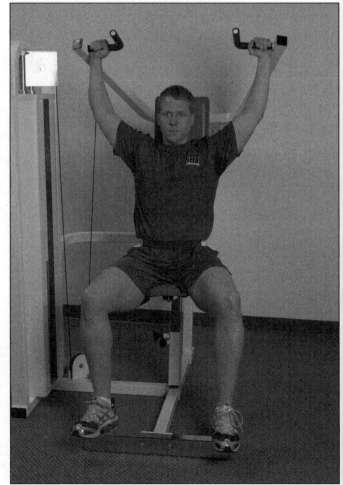

Figure 18-44 Shoulder Press Machine (end)

Dumbbell Shoulder Press

Primary Muscles:
- Anterior and Medial Deltoid
- Upper Trapezius
- Triceps

Joint Actions:
- Shoulder Abduction
- Scapular Upward Rotation
- Elbow Extension

Alternative Exercises:
- Barbell Shoulder Press
- Shoulder Press Machine
- Cable Shoulder Press
- Dumbbell, Tubing, or Cable Lateral Raise
- Scaption

Exercise Execution:
- Sit on a bench or stability ball (as pictured) with tall posture and feet flat on the floor.
- Raise the dumbbells into the starting position with elbows at 90 degrees and forearms perpendicular to floor (i.e., 'goal-post' position).
- Press the dumbbells overhead until the elbows are fully extended, but not locked.
- Lower the dumbbells back to the starting position.
- Maintain proper postural alignment throughout the exercise with head, shoulder, and hip in vertical alignment. Do not arch the lower back.
- ⚠ **Caution:** This exercise may not be appropriate for those with pre-existing shoulder considerations such as shoulder impingement or tendonitis.

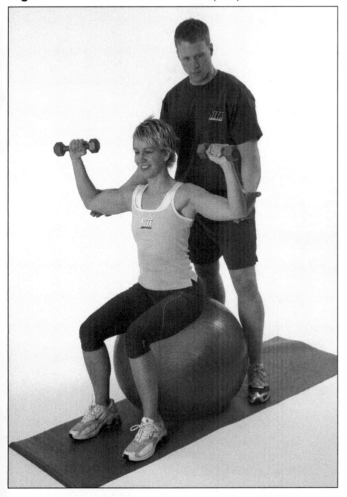

Figure 18-45 Dumbbell Shoulder Press (start)

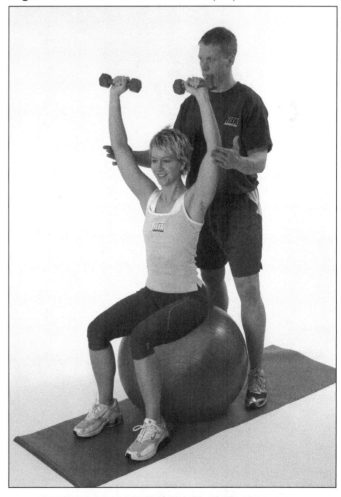

Figure 18-46 Dumbbell Shoulder Press (end)

Tubing Lateral Raise

Primary Muscles:
- Anterior and Medial Deltoid
- Upper Trapezius

Joint Actions:
- Shoulder Abduction
- Scapular Upward Rotation

Alternative Exercises:
- Barbell or Dumbbell Shoulder Press
- Shoulder Press Machine
- Cable Shoulder Press
- Dumbbell or Cable Lateral Raise
- Dumbbell, Tubing, or Cable Front Raise
- Scaption

Exercise Execution:
- Anchor the middle of resistance tubing under feet.
- Hold handles with arms at the sides of the body as pictured.
- Lift both arms laterally, away from the body in the frontal plane, until the arms are less than or equal to parallel to the floor.
- Maintain proper postural alignment throughout the exercise with head, shoulder, and hip in vertical alignment. Do not arch the lower back or elevate the shoulders.

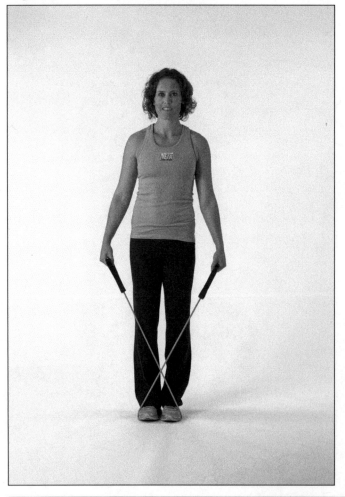

Figure 18-47 Tubing Lateral Raise (start)

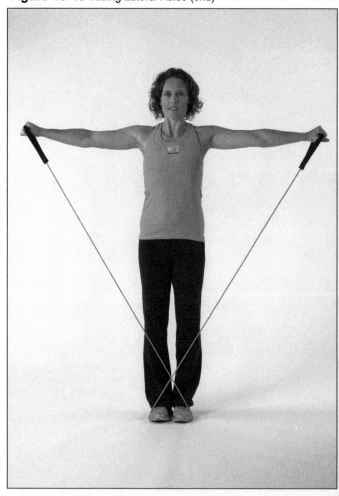

Figure 18-48 Tubing Lateral Raise (end)

Cable Shoulder Internal Rotation

Primary Muscles:
- Subscapularis

Joint Action:
- Shoulder Internal Rotation

Alternative Exercises:
- Tubing Shoulder Internal Rotation
- Side-Lying Dumbbell Internal Rotation

Exercise Execution:
- Adjust the pulley height to slighter higher than the elbow.
- Position the arm slightly off the side of the body (use rolled towel as needed) with the elbow flexed at 90 degrees.
- Pull the handle toward the torso rotating internally through the vertical axis of the humerus.
- Return to the starting position (approximately 45 degrees of external rotation)
- Keep the wrist neutral at all times. Do not allow the elbow to move away from the starting position.

Figure 18-49 Shoulder Internal Rotation (start)

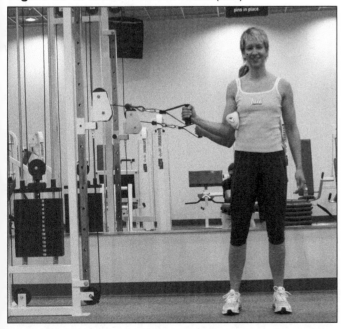

Figure 18-50 Shoulder Internal Rotation (end)

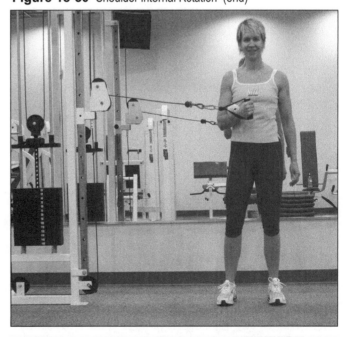

Cable Shoulder External Rotation

Primary Muscles:
- Infraspinatus
- Teres Minor

Joint Action:
- Shoulder External Rotation

Alternative Exercises:
- Cable Shoulder External Rotation
- Side-Lying Dumbbell External Rotation

Exercise Execution:
- Adjust the pulley height to slighter lower than the elbow.
- Position the arm slightly off the side of the body (use rolled towel as needed) with the elbow flexed at 90 degrees.
- Pull the handle away from the torso rotating externally through the vertical axis of the humerus to approximately 45 degrees of external rotation.
- Return to the starting position with the hand near the torso.
- Keep the wrist neutral at all times. Do not allow the elbow to move away from the starting position.

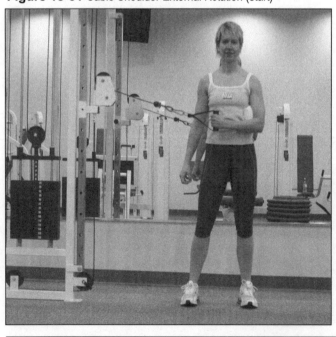

Figure 18-51 Cable Shoulder External Rotation (start)

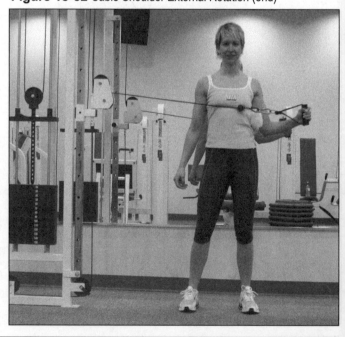

Figure 18-52 Cable Shoulder External Rotation (end)

Dumbbell Biceps Curl

Primary Muscles:
- Biceps Brachii

Joint Action:
- Elbow Flexion

Alternative Exercises:
- Barbell Biceps Curl
- Cable Biceps Curl
- Arm Curl Machine
- Preacher Curl
- Hammer Curl
- Tubing Biceps Curl

Exercise Execution:
- Sit on a bench or stability ball (as pictured) with tall posture and feet flat on the floor.
- Hold the dumbbells in the natural anatomical position.
- Lift the dumbbells toward the shoulders by flexing the elbows.
- Keep the upper arms stable at all times. Do not swing the arms.
- Maintain proper postural alignment throughout the exercise with head, shoulder, and hip in vertical alignment.

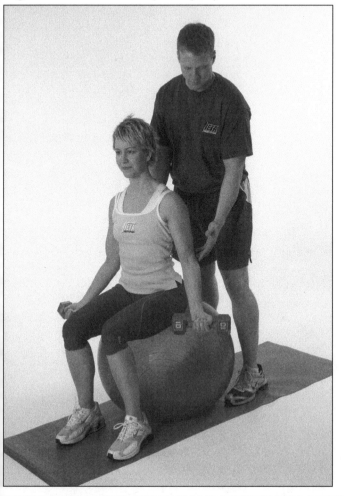

Figure 18-53 Dumbbell Biceps Curl (start)

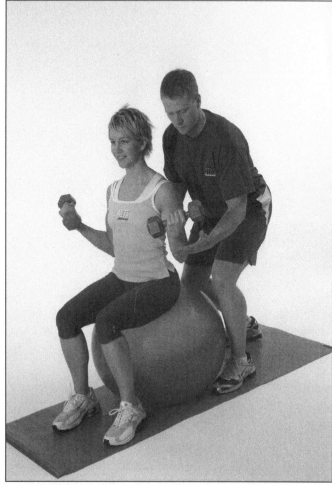

Figure 18-54 Dumbbell Biceps Curl (end)

Arm Curl Machine

Primary Muscles:
- Biceps Brachii

Joint Action:
- Elbow Flexion

Alternative Exercises:
- Barbell Biceps Curl
- Cable Biceps Curl
- Dumbbell Biceps Curl
- Preacher Curl
- Hammer Curl
- Tubing Biceps Curl

Exercise Execution:
- Adjust the seat height to position the arms flat on the arm pad with the center of the elbow aligned with the axis of rotation on the machine.
- Grasp the handles with a supinated grip keeping the wrists neutral throughout the exercise.
- Lift the handles toward the shoulders by flexing the elbows. Do not lean back or rock to move the weight.
- Maintain proper postural alignment throughout the exercise with head, shoulder, and hip in vertical alignment.

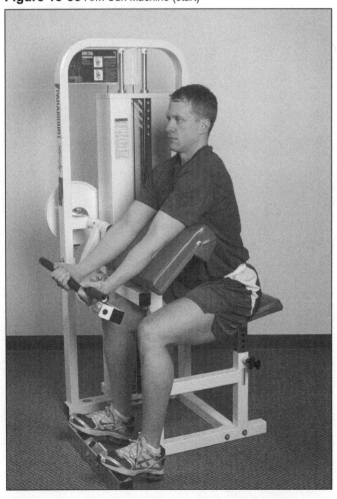

Figure 18-55 Arm Curl Machine (start)

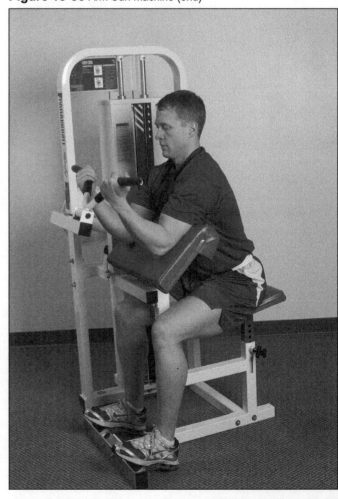

Figure 18-56 Arm Curl Machine (end)

Cable Triceps Push-Down

Primary Muscles:
- Triceps

Joint Action:
- Elbow Extension

Alternative Exercises:
- Supine Dumbbell Triceps Extension
- Supine Barbell Triceps Extension
- Overhead Cable Triceps Extension
- Arm Extension Machine
- Triceps Press-Down Machine
- Suspension Trainer Triceps Extension

Exercise Execution:
- Adjust the pulley to the top of the cable column.
- Stand facing the cable column with one foot forward in a stride stance.
- Grasp the rope with a neutral grip, leaning slightly forward. (other attachments such as straight bar, w-bar, or v-bar may also be used.)
- Push the rope handle down toward the top of the thigh until the elbows are fully extended.
- Return to the starting position with elbows flexed to <90 degrees.
- Keep upper arm stable at all times. Do not allow the elbow to drift forward or backward.
- Maintain proper postural alignment throughout the exercise with head, shoulder, and hip in vertical alignment.

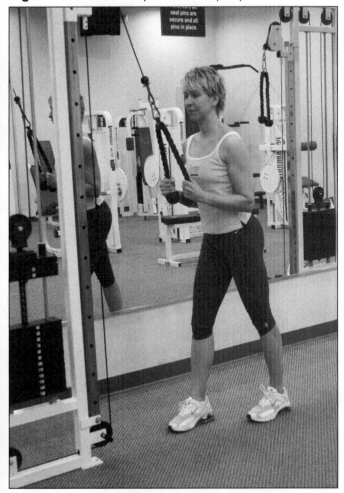

Figure 18-57 Cable Triceps Push-Down (start)

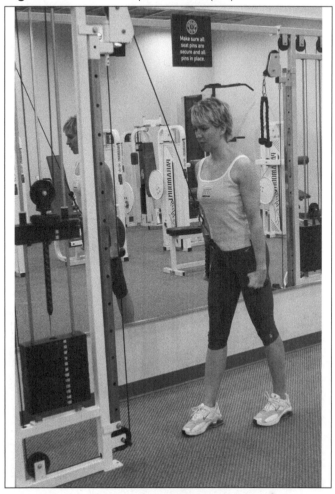

Figure 18-58 Cable Triceps Push-Down (end)

Triceps Press-Down Machine

Primary Muscles:
- Triceps

Joint Action:
- Elbow Extension

Alternative Exercises:
- Supine Dumbbell Triceps Extension
- Supine Barbell Triceps Extension
- Overhead Cable Triceps Extension
- Arm Extension Machine
- Cable Triceps Push-Down
- Suspension Trainer Triceps Extension

Exercise Execution:
- Adjust the seat height to allow for a comfortable range of motion without the weights hitting the weight stack.
- Grasp the handles with a neutral grip and wrist position.
- Press the handles down to full extension of the elbows.
- Return to the starting position with elbows flexed to ≤90 degrees.
- Maintain proper postural alignment throughout the exercise with head, scapula, and hips against the back rest.

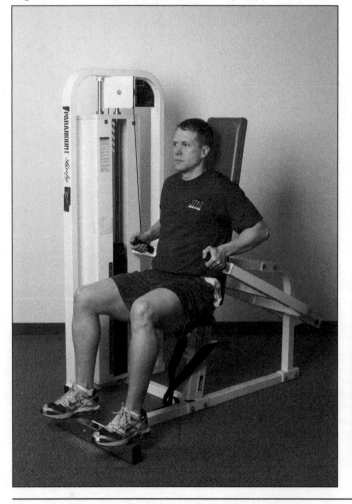

Figure 18-59 Triceps Press-Down Machine (start)

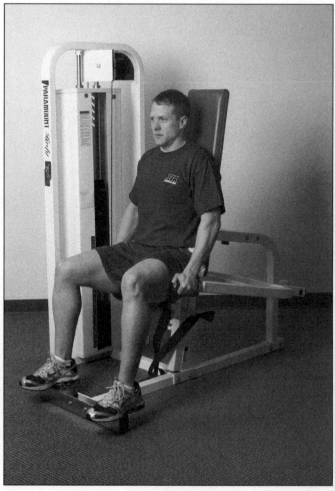

Figure 18-60 Triceps Press-Down Machine (end)

Prone Plank

Primary Muscles:
- Rectus Abdominis
- External/Internal Obliques
- Transverse Abdominis

Joint Action:
- Isometric Opposition to Spinal Extension

Alternative Exercises:
- Modified Prone Plank on Knees (pictured below)
- Plank with Leg Lift Progressions
- Stability Ball Plank
- Side-Lying Plank

Exercise Execution:
- Position body face down (prone) on mat with elbows resting on floor directly below the shoulders and on toes with feet together.
- Supporting weight on elbows and toes, raise the hips off the floor to align the ear, shoulder, hips, knee, and ankle in a straight line.
- Hold the position for a designated amount of time.
- Maintain proper kinetic chain alignment and normal breathing pattern throughout the exercise.

Figure 18-61 Modified Prone Plank

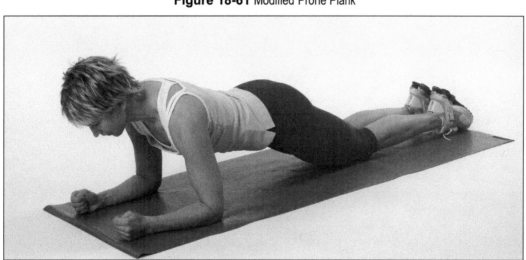

Figure 18-62 Full Body Prone Plank

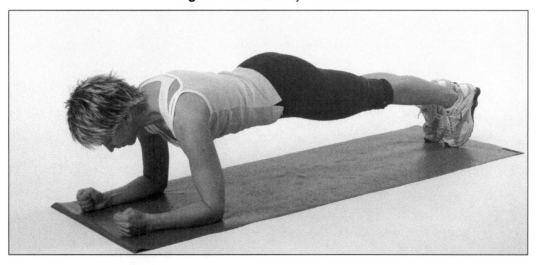

Side-Lying Plank

Primary Muscles:
- External/Internal Obliques
- Transverse Abdominis
- Quadratus Lumborum

Joint Action:
- Isometric Opposition to Spinal Lateral Flexion

Alternative Exercises:
- Side-Lying Plank with Hip Abduction
- Modified Side-Lying Plank on Knees (pictured below)
- Dumbbell or Cable Side Bends

Exercise Execution:
- Position body side-lying on the mat with the elbow directly under the shoulder and the feet in tandem position.
- Supporting weight on elbow and lateral/medial edges of feet, raise the hips off the floor to align the ear, shoulder, hips, knee, and ankle in a straight line.
- Hold the position for a designated amount of time.
- Maintain proper kinetic chain alignment and normal breathing pattern throughout the exercise.

Figure 18-63 Side-Lying Plank

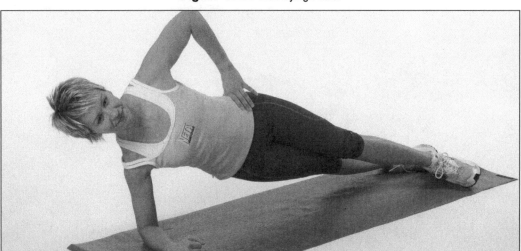

Figure 18-64 Modified Side-Lying Plank

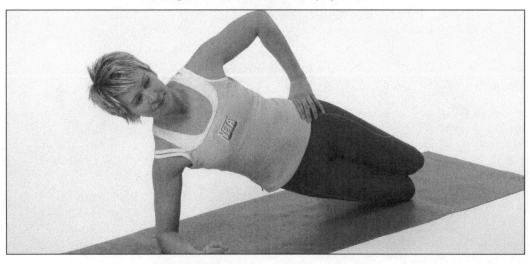

Abdominal Crunch

Primary Muscles:
- Rectus Abdominis
- External/Internal Obliques
- Transverse Abdominis

Joint Action:
- Spinal Flexion

Alternative Exercises:
- Stability Ball Abdominal Crunch
- Floor Oblique Crunch
- Stability Ball Oblique Crunch
- Abdominal Machine

Exercise Execution:
- Lie in supine position on mat with feet hip-width apart and knees flexed to 90 degrees.
- Perform a posterior pelvic tilt to gently press the lower back into the floor.
- While holding the pelvic tilt, flex the torso forward approximately 30 degrees, bringing the inferior border of the scapula slightly off the floor.
- Return to the staring position, maintaining the pelvic tilt at all times.
- Maintain proper kinetic chain alignment and normal breathing pattern throughout the exercise. Keep the elbows wide and do not pull the head forward.
- ⚠ **Caution:** Performing a posterior pelvic tilt while performing an abdominal crunch will increase the recruitment and activation of the rectus abdominis; however, this may also increase shear forces across the lumbar vertebrae and increase potential risk.

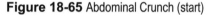

Figure 18-65 Abdominal Crunch (start)

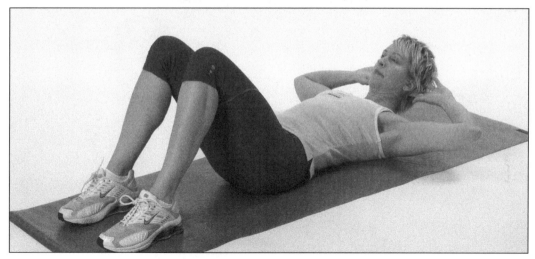

Figure 18-66 Abdominal Crunch (end)

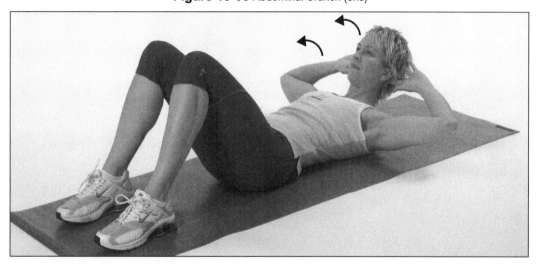

Stability Ball Abdominal Crunch

Primary Muscles:
- Rectus Abdominis
- External/Internal Obliques
- Transverse Abdominis

Joint Action:
- Spinal Flexion

Alternative Exercises:
- Floor Abdominal Crunch
- Floor Oblique Crunch
- Stability Ball Oblique Crunch
- Abdominal Machine

Exercise Execution:
- Sit on the stability ball. Walk the feet forward, rolling the ball up the body until it is resting below the lower back.
- Keeping the ball stable, flex the torso forward to approximately 30 degrees, bringing the inferior border of the scapula slightly off the ball. Do not allow the ball to roll when performing the crunch.
- Return to the starting position, maintaining the activation of the core muscles at all times.
- Maintain proper kinetic chain alignment and normal breathing pattern throughout the exercise. Do not pull the head forward.

Figure 18-67 Stability Ball Crunch (start)

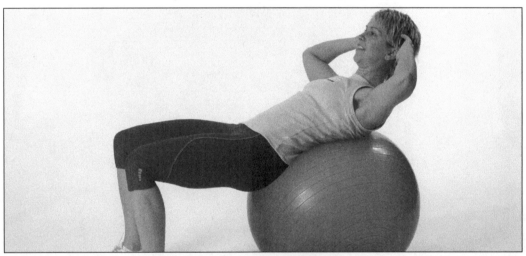

Figure 18-68 Stability Ball Crunch (end)

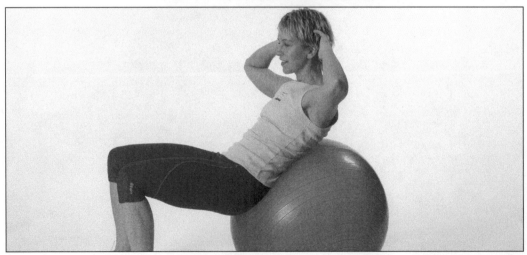

Stability Ball Bridge

Primary Muscles:
- Erector Spinae
- Gluteus Maximus
- Hamstrings

Joint Actions:
- Spinal Extension
- Hip Extension

Alternative Exercises:
- Floor Bridge
- Floor Bridge with Leg Lift Progressions
- Stability Ball Table Top
- Bird-Dog

Exercise Execution:
- Lay in the supine position with both feet positioned on the top of the stability ball.
- Elevate the hips off the floor to bring ankle, knee, hips, and shoulders into alignment.
- Hold the position for a designated amount of time.
- Maintain proper kinetic chain alignment and normal breathing pattern throughout the exercise.
- Return to the starting position.

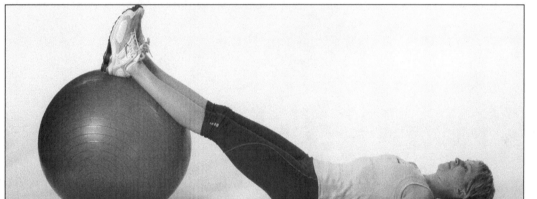

Figure 18-69 Stability Ball Bridge (start)

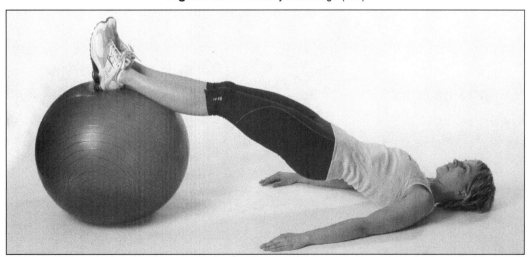

Figure 18-70 Stability Ball Bridge (end)

Bird-Dog

Primary Muscles:
- Gluteus Maximus
- Hamstrings
- Anterior Deltoid
- Erector Spinae
- Internal/External Obliques

Joint Actions:
- Hip Extension
- Shoulder Flexion
- Core Stabilization

Alternative Exercises:
- Floor Bridge
- Floor Bridge with Leg Lift Progressions
- Stability Ball Table Top
- Stability Ball Bridge

Exercise Execution:
- Position the body on hands and knees on a mat. Hands directly under shoulders and knees directly under hips.
- Engage the core musculature to maintain neutral spinal alignment.
- Extend one leg backward while simultaneously reaching the opposite arm forward.
- Hold the position for a designated amount of time. Alternate sides.
- Maintain proper kinetic chain alignment and normal breathing pattern throughout the exercise.
- Return to the starting position.

Figure 18-71 Bird-Dog (start)

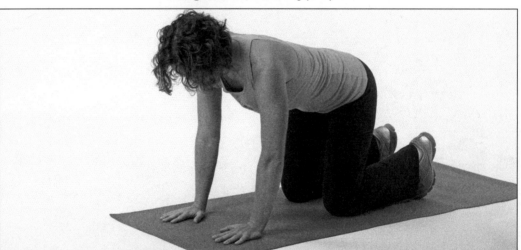

Figure 18-72 Bird-Dog (end)

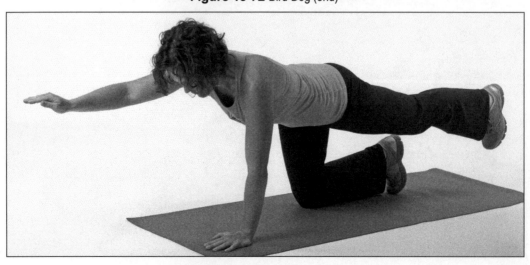

Stability Ball Back Extension

Primary Muscles:
- Erector Spinae
- Gluteus Maximus
- Hamstrings

Joint Actions:
- Spinal Extension
- Hip Extension

Alternative Exercises:
- Back Extension Machine
- Prone Cobra
- Roman Chair Back Extension

Exercise Execution:
- Position the body prone over the stability ball with anterior hips and upper thighs resting on the ball.
- Maintain legs in straight position. Secure feet at base of wall or under stable piece of equipment, if necessary.
- From the starting position, slowly lift the upper torso extending the torso/spine into a position of neutral alignment.
- Return to the starting position while maintain proper alignment of the upper torso.
- Maintain proper kinetic chain alignment throughout the exercise.
- ⚠ **Caution:** Failure to maintain a neutral spinal position may place significant stress and potentially cause injury to the lumbar spine and the intervertebral discs. Maintain neutral spinal alignment at all times. Do not flex or arch the lumbar spine

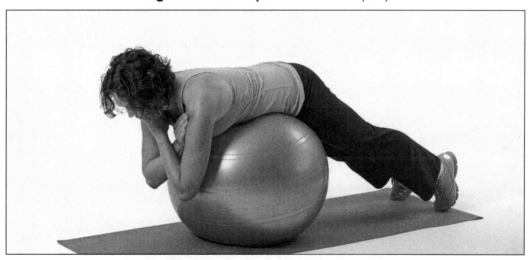

Figure 18-73 Stability Ball Back Extension (start)

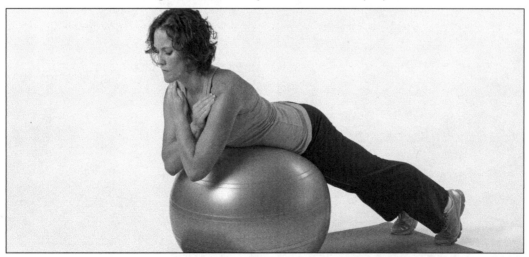

Figure 18-74 Stability Ball Back Extension (end)

Back Extension Machine

Primary Muscles:
- Erector Spinae
- Gluteus Maximus
- Hamstrings

Joint Actions:
- Spinal Extension
- Hip Extension

Alternative Exercises:
- Roman Chair Back Extension
- Prone Cobra
- Stability Ball Prone Back Extension

Exercise Execution:
- Adjust the foot plate to align the center of the hips with the axis of rotation on the machine while maintaining a slightly flexed position in the knees.
- Start with the body in a position ≤90 degrees of torso/hip flexion.
- Slowly extend the torso/hips to a straight body position with the knees, hips, shoulders, and head aligned. Do not hyperextend the lower back.
- Return to the starting position without allowing the weights to touch the weight stack.
- Maintain proper kinetic chain alignment throughout the exercise.
- ⚠ **Caution:** Failure to maintain a neutral spinal position may place significant stress and potentially cause injury to the lumbar spine and the intervertebral discs. Maintain neutral spinal alignment at all times. Do not flex or round the lumbar spine.

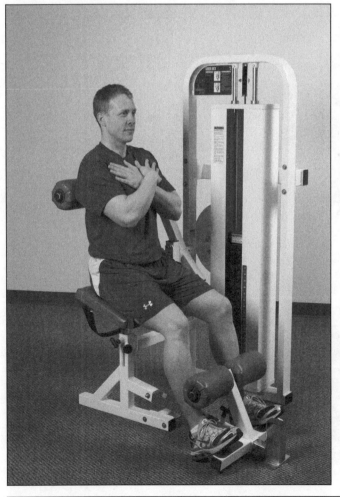

Figure 18-75 Back Extension Machine (start)

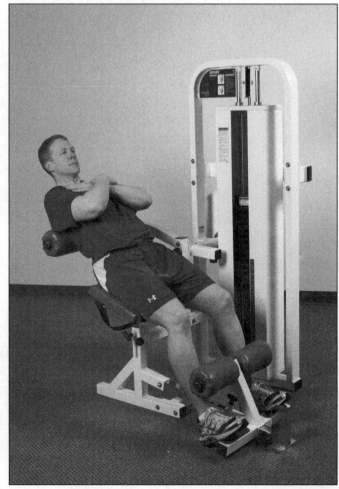

Figure 18-76 Back Extension Machine (end)

Chapter Summary

Muscular strength and endurance represent two of the health-related components of physical fitness. Various resistance training exercises may be used to build muscular fitness. These muscle-building activities provide many health and fitness benefits in addition to those derived from cardiorespiratory activity. Fitness professionals must be familiar with the guidelines for resistance training in order to create safe and effective programs for their clients. A well-designed program will include exercises representing the lower body, upper body pushing, upper body pulling, and the core. Utilizing the principles of periodization, the acute training variables should be manipulated to ensure continuous gains in muscular fitness. Rest and recovery periods should be strategically incorporated into the program to prevent training plateaus, staleness, and potential overtraining.

Chapter References

American College of Sports Medicine (2010). *ACSM's Resource Manual for Guidelines for Exercise Testing and Prescription*, 6th edition. Baltimore, MD: Lippincott, Williams, and Wilkins.

American College of Sports Medicine (2018). *ACSM's Guidelines for Exercise Testing and Prescription*, 10th edition. Philadelphia, PA: Wolters Kluwer.

Chrysant, S.G. (2010). Current evidence on the hemodynamic and blood pressure effects of isometric exercise in normotensive and hypertensive persons. *The Journal of Clinical Hypertension, 12*(9), 721-726.

Clarkson, P.M., & Hubal, M.J. (2002). Exercise-induced muscle damage in humans. *American Journal of Physical Medicine & Rehabilitation, 81*(11), S52-S69.

Fleck, S.J. (2011). Non-Linear Periodization for General Fitness & Athletes. *Journal of Human Kinetics*, (1), 41-45.

Fleck, S.J. & Kraemer, W.J. (2014). *Designing Resistance Training Programs*, 4th edition. Champaign, IL: Human Kinetics.

Folland, J.P., Hawker, K., Leach, B., Little, T., & Jones, D.A. (2005). Strength training: Isometric training at a range of joint angles versus dynamic training. *Journal of Sports Sciences, 23*(8), 817-824.

Gamble, P. (2006). Periodization of training for team sports athletes. *Strength & Conditioning Journal, 28*(5), 56-66.

Garber, C.E., Blissmer, B., Deschenes, M.R., Franklin, B.A., Lamonte, M.J., Lee, I.M., ... & Swain, D.P. (2011). American College of Sports Medicine position stand. Quantity and quality of exercise for developing and maintaining cardiorespiratory, musculoskeletal, and neuromotor fitness in apparently healthy adults: Guidance for prescribing exercise. *Medicine and Science in Sports and Exercise, 43*(7), 1334-1359.

Harries, S.K., Lubans, D.R., & Callister, R. (2015). Systematic review and meta-analysis of linear and undulating periodized resistance training programs on muscular strength. *The Journal of Strength & Conditioning Research, 29*(4), 1113-1125.

Haskell, W.L., Lee, I., Pate, R.R., Powell, K.E., Blair, S.N., Franklin, B.A., ... & Bauman, A. (2007). Physical activity and public health: Updated recommendation for adults from the American College of Sports Medicine and the American Heart Association. *Medicine and Science in Sports and Exercise, 39*(8), 1423-1434.

Lewis, P.B., Ruby, D., & Bush-Joseph, C.A. (2012). Muscle soreness and delayed-onset muscle soreness. *Clinics in Sports Medicine, 31*(2), 255-262.

Meeusen, R., Duclos, M., Foster, C., Fry, A., Gleeson, M., Nieman, D., ... & Urhausen, A. (2013). Prevention, diagnosis, and treatment of the overtraining syndrome: Joint consensus statement of the European College of Sport Science and the American College of Sports Medicine. *Medicine and Science in Sports and Exercise, 45*(1), 186-205.

Nelson, M.E., Rejeski, W.J., Blair, S.N., Duncan, P.W., Judge, J.O., King, A.C., ... & Castaneda-Sceppa, C. (2007). Physical activity and public health in older adults: Recommendation from the American College of Sports Medicine and the American Heart Association. *Medicine and Science in Sports and Exercise, 39*(8), 1435-1445.

Plisk, S.S., & Stone, M.H. (2003). Periodization strategies. *Strength & Conditioning Journal, 25*(6), 19-37.

Ratamess, N.A., Alvar, B.A., Evetoch, T.K., Housh, T.J., Kibler, W.B., & Kraemer, W.J. (2009). Progression models in resistance training for healthy adults [ACSM position stand]. *Medicine and Science in Sports and Exercise, 41*(3), 687-708.

Selye, H. (1998). A syndrome produced by diverse nocuous agents. *The Journal of Neuropsychiatry and Clinical Neurosciences, 10*(2), 230a-231.

Stone, M.H., O'Bryant, H., Garhammer, J., McMillan, J., & Rozenek, R. (1982). A theoretical model of strength training. *Strength & Conditioning Journal, 4*(4), 36-39.

Turner, A. (2011). The science and practice of periodization: A brief review. *Strength & Conditioning Journal, 33*(1), 34-46.

U.S. Department of Health and Human Services (2008). *2008 Physical Activity Guidelines for Americans*. ODPHP Publication No. U0036.

Weir, J.P., Housh, T.J., Weir, L.L., & Johnson, G.O. (1995). Effects of unilateral isometric strength training on joint angle specificity and cross-training. *European Journal of Applied Physiology and Occupational Physiology, 70*(4), 337-343.

Williams, M.A., Haskell, W.L., Ades, P.A., Amsterdam, E.A., Bittner, V., Franklin, B.A., ... & Stewart, K.J. (2007). Resistance exercise in individuals with and without cardiovascular disease: 2007 update. *Circulation, 116*(5), 572-584.

Winett, R.A., & Carpinelli, R.N. (2001). Potential health-related benefits of resistance training. *Preventive Medicine, 33*(5), 503-513.

Recommended Reading

American College of Sports Medicine (2018). Chapter 6: General Principles of Exercise Prescription. In, *ACSM's Guidelines to Exercise Testing and Prescription*, 10th edition. Philadelphia, PA: Wolters Kluwer.

Chapter 18 Review Questions

1. Microtrama inflicted upon the skeletal muscle and connective tissue during the _____ phase of resistance training is believed to be a primary factor contributing to delayed onset muscle soreness (DOMS).
    A. concentric
    B. isometric
    C. static
    D. eccentric

2. Which of the following exercises is considered to be isometric?
    A. Stability ball crunch
    B. Seated narrow row
    C. Prone plank
    D. Dumbbell biceps curl

3. According to the American College of Sports Medicine, resistance training exercise should be performed _____ days per week for each major muscle group.
    A. 3 to 5
    B. 2 to 3
    C. 1 to 4
    D. 5 to 7

4. Which of the following progressions for the squat exercise is most appropriate for a client wishing to increase muscular strength?
    A. Perform the squat on an unstable surface such as a BOSU®
    B. Increase the number of repetitions performed during each set
    C. Perform jump squats as quickly as possible
    D. Increase the workload to a higher percentage of 1-RM

5. Forcibly exhaling against a closed glottis during the concentric phase of a resistance training exercise may cause a dangerously high elevation in blood pressure. This is known as the _____.
    A. general adaptation syndrome
    B. overtraining syndrome
    C. Valsalva maneuver
    D. super compensation cycle

6. Which of the following resistance training exercises is contraindicated for a client who has had reconstructive ACL surgery and has been cleared by their health care provider to participate in a resistance training program?
    A. Stability ball leg curl
    B. Seated leg extension machine
    C. Stability ball squats
    D. Standing hip abduction with resistance tubing

Answers to Review Questions on Page 384

Note: Review questions are intended to reinforce learning and comprehension of subject matter presented in the corresponding chapter. The review questions are not intended to be representative of actual certification exam questions in terms of style, content, or difficulty.

19
Flexibility Programming

Introduction

Flexibility represents one of the components of health-related physical fitness and is defined as the ability to move a joint through a full, pain-free range of motion. **Range of motion (ROM)** is often used as the measurement of flexibility, which is typically expressed in terms of the degrees of rotary movement in a specified direction around a joint, or the inches of linear movement of a body segment (e.g., sit-and-reach test). Flexibility may be increased through stretching exercises using a variety of techniques, as well as methods of self-myofascial release utilizing foam rollers and similar exercise tools.

This chapter will present types of flexibility exercises, the potential benefits of stretching, research regarding the effects of pre-activity static stretching on athletic performance and prevention of injury, guidelines for flexibility training, and a library of recommended stretching exercises.

Sensory Receptors

Before introducing the various types of flexibility training, it is necessary to briefly review the sensory receptors that mediate the physical and physiologic responses to stretching exercises. Two important sensory receptors, also referred to as *mechanoreceptors*, include the muscle spindles and the Golgi tendon organs. The **muscle spindles** are sensory receptors located within the skeletal muscle that are sensitive to changes in length and rate of length change. When stimulated by a sudden lengthening of the muscle, the muscle spindles will cause a reflexive contraction of the muscle in an effort to prevent injury that may result from over-stretching or stretching too rapidly. This response is called the *myotatic stretch reflex*, which can be seen when a doctor uses a rubber mallet to tap the patellar tendon causing a reflexive contraction of the quadriceps. The motor unit stimulation and subsequent contraction of a muscle is accompanied by simultaneous decrease in neural drive and deactivation of the opposite muscles, causing antagonist muscle relaxation. This is known as **reciprocal inhibition**. For example, the activation and contraction of the quadriceps causes inhibition and relaxation of the hamstrings. This is the primary mechanism contributing to muscle relaxation and increased range of motion attained through active static stretching, which will be discussed in the next section.

The **Golgi tendon organs (GTO)** are sensory receptors located in the musculotendinous unit that are sensitive to changes in muscular tension and the rate of tension change. When stimulated by rapidly increasing or excessive tension, the Golgi tendon organs cause the muscle to relax, thus preventing excessive stress and potential injury. Stimulation of the Golgi tendon organs inhibits activation of the muscle spindle fibers within the same muscle, which leads to the muscle relaxation. This neural response is known as **autogenic inhibition** since the muscle's own receptors cause the relaxation. Autogenic inhibition is the primary mechanism through which passive static stretching facilitates muscle relaxation.

Types of Flexibility Exercises

A variety of flexibility exercises are used to increase joint range of motion including stretching techniques such as static, ballistic, dynamic, and proprioceptive neuromuscular facilitation (PNF), as well as self-myofascial release.

Static stretching is perhaps the most common mode of flexibility training used by fitness professionals and is generally regarded as a safe and effective method to increase range of motion. Static stretching involves moving a muscle into a lengthened position causing mild discomfort, but not pain, which is held for an extended period of time (e.g., 10-60 seconds). Static stretches may be performed either actively or passively. During an **active stretch** the targeted muscle is lengthened using internal force generated by activation of the antagonist muscles. For example, the hamstrings may be lengthened to elicit an active stretch by positioning the hip at approximately 90 degrees of flexion and then actively contracting the quadriceps to gently extend the knee. The contraction of the agonist muscle causes efferent nerve impulses to inhibit antagonist muscle activation leading to relaxation of the antagonist muscle group (i.e., reciprocal inhibition).

A **passive stretch** relies upon an external force provided by an unrelated body part, a personal trainer, or a device (e.g., stretching strap, wall, ballet barre), to position a body segment such that a stretch is applied to the targeted muscle. For example, with the client lying supine on a mat or stretching table, the personal trainer lifts the client's leg with the knee extended, moving the hip into flexion until a stretch is felt through the hamstrings. See figure 19-1. The passive lengthening of the hamstring muscles creates tension, which stimulates the GTOs and leads to relaxation of the hamstrings via autogenic inhibition. Increased range of motion attained through static stretching is also attributed to increased pain tolerance observed with regular stretching. Illustrations of recommended static stretches are provided on pages 256–259.

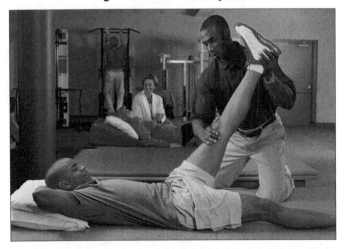

Figure 19-1 Passive Hamstring Stretch

Ballistic stretching techniques utilize rapid bouncing movements in an effort to lengthen and stretch the targeted muscle. Ballistic stretching may be counter-productive to improvements in joint range of motion since the ballistic movements may initiate the stretch reflex causing the effected muscle to contract, restricting range of motion. In addition, if ballistic stretches are performed too aggressively or are not preceded by a proper warm-up, they may cause unnecessary muscle soreness and potentially lead to musculotendinous injury. For these reasons, ballistic stretching is typically not recommended for improving range of motion among those seeking improved health and fitness. However, ballistic stretching may confer some improvements in range of motion and performance among athletes, particularly those participating in sports or activities that involve ballistic-type movements (Woolstenhulme et al., 2006).

Dynamic stretching exercises utilize slow, controlled, and rhythmic movements to actively increase joint range of motion. Dynamic stretches are typically performed during the pre-activity warm-up to replicate certain sport-specific and functional movements (Hedrick, 2000). These activities utilize body weight or light resistance (e.g., medicine ball, tubing) and involve callisthenic type movements such as body weight squats, walking and lateral lunges, and medicine ball chops and lifts. Dynamic range of motion activities may also involve single-joint movements such as shoulder circles or leg swings. The dynamic nature of these activities also function to increase tissue temperature, elasticity, and extensibility, which are likely to contribute to increased range of motion and decreased risk of injury during exercise.

Proprioceptive neuromuscular facilitation (PNF) includes several variations of stretching techniques that couple passive static stretching and muscle activation. The 'contract relax' technique typically refers to a passive stretch of the targeted muscle, followed by an isometric contraction of the targeted muscle, which is then followed by another passive stretch of the same muscle (Behm et al., 2015; Sharman et al., 2006). For example, a static stretch is passively applied to the hamstrings for 10 to 30 seconds, followed by an isometric contraction of the hamstrings for 3 to 6 seconds, which is then followed by a second passive stretch to the hamstrings held for another 10-30 seconds. An alternate PNF technique is called the 'contract relax agonist contract' (Behm et al., 2015; Sharman et al., 2006). This method follows sequence similar to the 'contract relax' technique except an antagonist muscle group contraction performed against light resistance is preceded and followed by a static stretch of the targeted muscle group (Behm et al., 2016; Sharman et al., 2006). In this case, a passive hamstring stretch is held for 10 to 30 seconds, followed by a resisted isometric contraction of the antagonist muscles (i.e., quadriceps, iliopsoas), which is then followed by another 10 to 30 second passive hamstring stretch. It has been suggested that PNF techniques may be more effective than other types of stretching to increase flexibility; however, PNF stretching may elicit muscle soreness when performed too aggressively, and it requires the assistance of an experienced trainer.

Self-myofascial release (SMR) is a technique during which an individual uses their own body weight to apply pressure to a targeted muscle using a foam roller or similar device (MacDonald et al., 2013; Paolini, 2009). SMR using foam rollers have gained popularity over the past decade and are frequently used during a pre-activity warm-up and during post-activity recovery. During SMR techniques, the participant positions the targeted muscle group on a foam roller and then performs slow rolling movements, typically starting at the proximal end of the muscle and moving distally (MacDonald et al., 2013). When an area of tightness, adhesion, or 'knot' (characterized by 'pain' and muscle spasm) is located, the individual pauses to isolate direct pressure on this area (Paolini, 2009). The focused pressure is maintained for 20 to 60 seconds or longer to allow time for the tightness and 'pain' to subside.

The increased joint range of motion obtained through self-myofascial release techniques has been attributed to three interacting mechanisms. First, the rolling and direct pressure applied to the targeted muscle through the foam roller creates friction between the *fascia* and the soft tissue. The friction causes the fascia to become warm and more viscos (fluid-like), which breaks up adhesions, increases tissue extensibility, and increases range of motion (MacDonald et al., 2013; Sefton, 2004). Second, the pressure placed on the muscle may dull the stretch sensation, which increases the stretch tolerance and further contributes to increased range of motion (MacDonald et al., 2013). Finally, the muscle tension created by the pressure on the foam roller may stimulate the Golgi tendon organs, resulting in autogenic inhibition and subsequent gains in range of motion.

Illustrations of several common self-myofascial techniques using a foam roller are provided on pages 260–261.

Benefits of Stretching

An appropriate level of flexibility is necessary for health, fitness, and in some cases performance. Proper postural alignment and neuromuscular efficiency are dependent upon a normal length-tension relationship among muscle groups. Many activities of daily living (ADLs), such as getting in and out of a car, necessitate an adequate level of flexibility. In addition, certain sports and activities (e.g., dance, gymnastics, wrestling, diving, figure skating) require a high degree of flexibility for optimal performance. Table 19-1 lists some of the potential benefits of stretching and increased flexibility.

Although most of the proposed benefits of stretching are generally accepted, in recent years some benefits have encountered a heightened level of debate among researchers. In particular, several studies have suggested that static stretching performed before or after exercise does not reduce the risk of injury or the severity of delayed onset muscle soreness (Anderson, 2005; Herbert & Gabriel, 2002; Shrier, 1999; Thacker et al., 2004). In fact, some authors have indicated that pre-activity stretching may actually contribute to higher injury rates and that the extremes of inflexibility and hyperflexibility may increase the risk of injury (Shrier, 1999; Thacker et al., 2004). In a more recent systematic review, Behm et al. (2015) concluded that pre-activity stretching may be beneficial for injury prevention in sports that include sprint running, but not in endurance-based running activities that see a preponderance of overuse injuries.

In addition, many researchers have studied the impact of static stretching on athletic performance, especially with regard to maximal force production, sprint speed, and vertical jump height (e.g., power). The results of these studies suggest that pre-activity static stretching acutely

Table 19-1 Flexibility Training Benefits

Benefits of Flexibility Training
• Restores and/or maintains muscle balance necessary for proper postural alignment
• Decreases muscular tension (i.e., hypertonicity) and musculotendinous stiffness
• Reduces joint stress
• May reduce the risk of musculoskeletal injury and delayed onset muscle soreness
• Reduces incidence of low back pain
• Facilitates physical and mental relaxation
• Increases performance in sports and activities which require a high degree of flexibility

Table 19-2 Flexibility Guidelines

	Guidelines for Flexibility Training
Frequency	• ≥2 to 3 days per week with daily being most effective
Intensity	• Stretch to the point of feeling tightness or mild discomfort, but not pain
Time	• Holding a static stretch for 10 to 30 seconds is recommended for most adults
	• In older individuals, holding a stretch for 30 to 60 seconds may provide greater benefit
	• For PNF stretching, a 3 to 6 second contraction at 20% to 75% maximum voluntary contraction followed by a 10 to 30 second assisted stretch is desirable
Type	• A series of flexibility exercises for each of the major muscle-tendon units is recommended
	• Static flexibility (i.e., active, passive), dynamic flexibility, ballistic flexibility, and PNF techniques are each effective
Repetitions	• It is recommended that each flexibility exercise is performed 2 to 4 times
Volume	• A reasonable target is to perform 60 seconds of total stretching time for each flexibility exercise
Pattern	• Flexibility exercise is most effective when the muscle is warmed through light-to-moderate aerobic activity or passively through external methods such as moist heat packs or hot baths

ACSM (2018); Garber et al. (2011)

decreases muscle strength, slows sprint speed, and reduces vertical jump height (Behm et al., 2015; Sharman et al., 2006; Magnusson & Renström, 2006; McHugh & Cosgrave, 2010; Simic et al., 2012). However, performance reductions appear to be small to moderate, and are not likely to persist into actual sports competition occurring more than 10 minutes post-stretching (Behm et al., 2015). The decrements in performance seem to be related to the total duration of static stretching such that longer durations (e.g., ≥60 seconds) are likely to have a larger negative impact on performance during explosive sport activities (Kay & Blazevich, 2012). However, it does appear that the negative effects on performance may be minimized or eliminated if pre-activity static stretching is followed by other dynamic warm-up activities prior to competition (McHugh & Cosgrave, 2010). Paradoxically, some studies have indicated that habitual stretching, excluding those performed immediately before exercise or competition, may actually improve some of these same measures of performance (Magnusson & Renström, 2006). Subsequently, athletes may be advised to avoid static stretching as the only warm-up activity prior to competition, yet to routinely perform stretching exercises at the conclusion of conditioning sessions and following competitive events (Simic et al., 2012).

Flexibility Training Guidelines

The Physical Activity Guidelines for Americans advocate for the inclusion of flexibility exercises as an appropriate component of a physical activity program (HHS, 2008). However, the time spent performing flexibility exercises is not credited toward the completion of the recommended duration of aerobic or muscle-strengthening activity (HHS, 2008). The American College of Sports Medicine has established specific guidelines for flexibility exercises (ACSM, 2018). These guidelines are summarized in table 19-2.

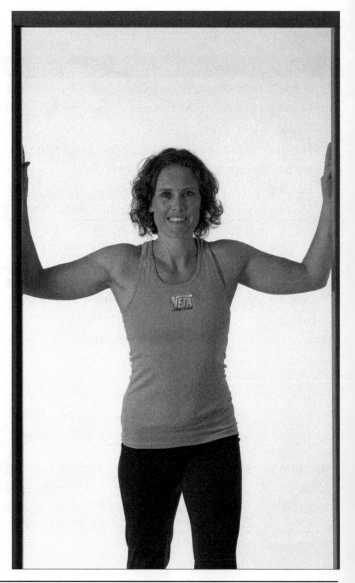

Figure 19-3 Doorway Chest

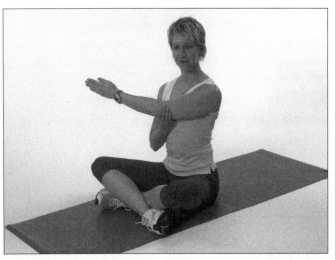

Figure 19-2 Posterior Shoulder

Figure 19-4 Active Chest Stretch

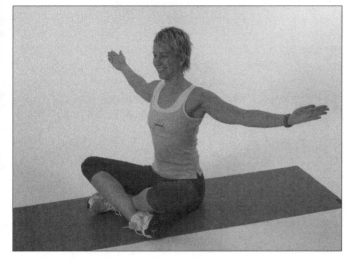

Figure 19-5 Ball Chest & Shoulder Stretch

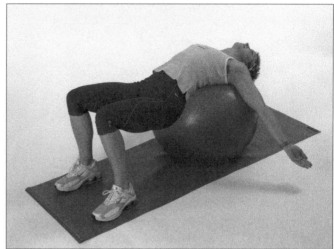

Figure 19-6 Chest & Anterior Shoulder Stretch

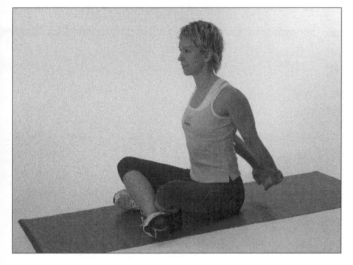

Figure 19-7 Triceps & Lats Stretch

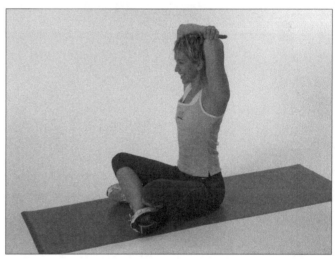

Figure 19-8 Stability Ball Latissimus Dorsi

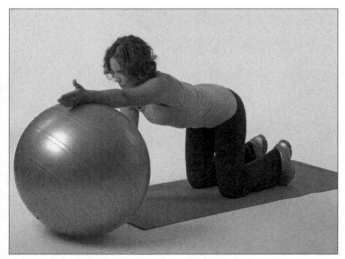

Figure 19-9 Prayer Stretch (Lats & Quadratus Lumborum)

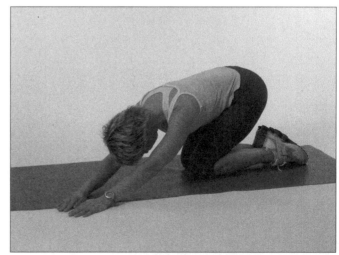

Figure 19-10 Cat Stretch (Thoracic/Lumbar Spine)

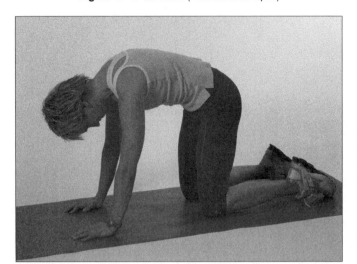

Figure 19-11 Cow Stretch (Thoracic Spine)

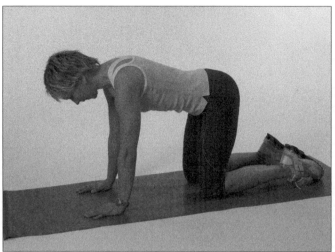

Figure 19-12 Supine Torso Rotation

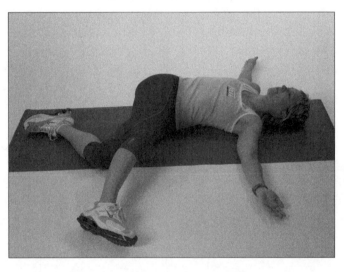

Figure 19-13 Single Knee to Chest (Gluteals)

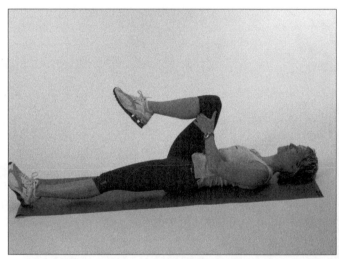

Figure 19-14 Double Knee to Chest (Glutes/Lumbar Spine)

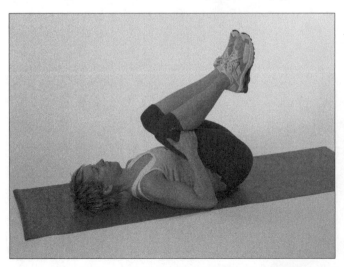

Figure 19-15 Prone Trunk Extension

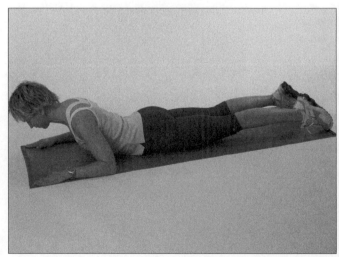

Figure 19-16 Side-Lying Quadriceps

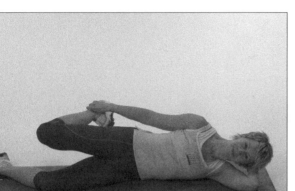

Figure 19-17 Supine Hamstrings

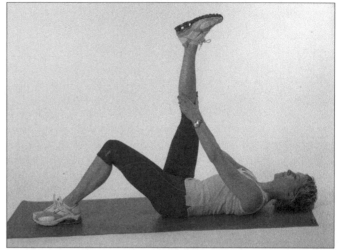

Figure 19-18 Standing Quadriceps Stretch

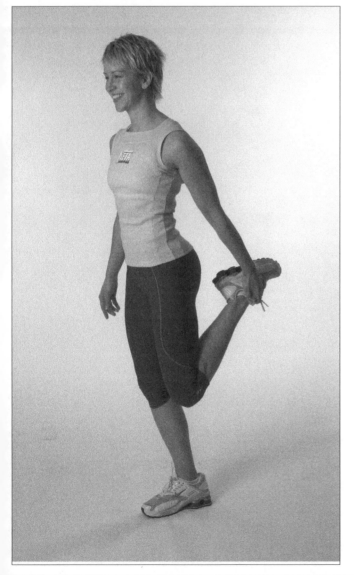

Figure 19-19 Kneeling Hip Flexor Stretch

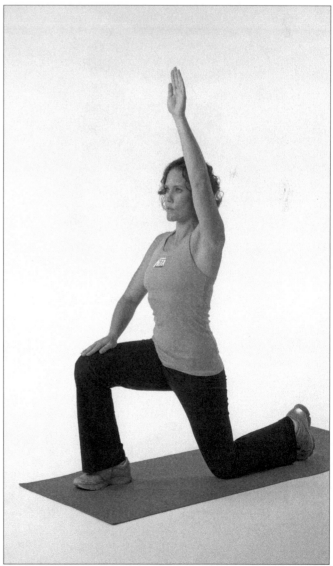

Figure 19-20 SMR Rhomboids/Mid Traps

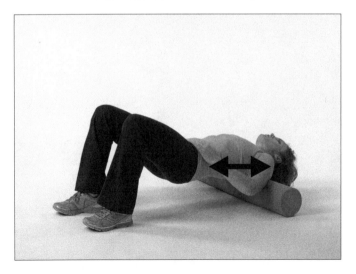

Figure 19-21 SMR Latissimus Dorsi

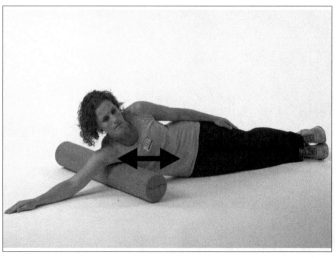

Figure 19-22 SMR Piriformis/Gluteals

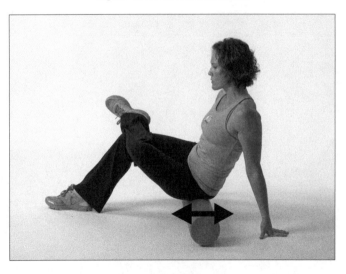

Figure 19-23 SMR Iliotibial Band

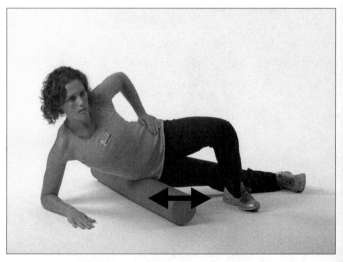

Figure 19-24 SMR Hamstrings

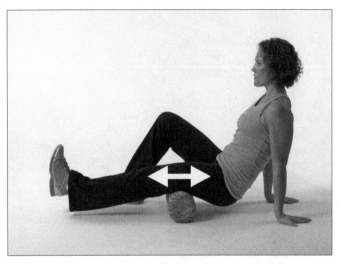

Figure 19-25 SMR Quadriceps

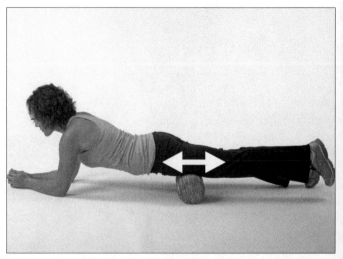

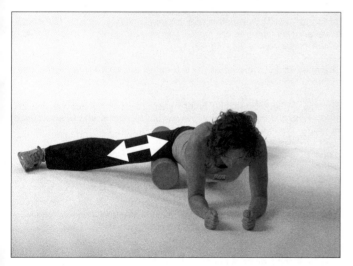

Figure 19-26 SMR Hip Adductors

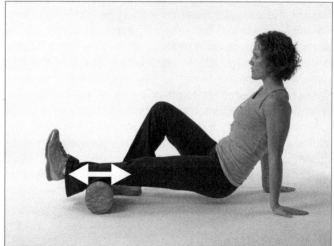

Figure 19-27 SMR Gastrocnemius/Soleus

Chapter Summary

Flexibility is the ability to move a joint through a full, pain-free range of motion. Flexibility may be increased through the use of various stretching techniques including static, dynamic, ballistic, and dynamic stretches. In addition, self-myofascial release techniques are effective at increasing range of motion. Regular flexibility training confers many health benefits. However, there is not sufficient scientific evidence to advocate for or against the use of stretching to reduce the incidence of injury or muscle soreness related to exercise and sport participation. In addition, static stretches performed immediately before strength, speed, or power activities may negatively impact performance. To maximize the safety and effectiveness of stretching, fitness professionals should observe the guidelines for flexibility training.

Chapter References

American College of Sports Medicine (2018). *ACSM's Guidelines for Exercise Testing and Prescription*, 10th edition. Philadelphia, PA: Wolters Kluwer.

Andersen, J.C. (2005). Stretching before and after exercise: Effect on muscle soreness and injury risk. *Journal of Athletic Training, 40*(3), 218-220.

Behm, D.G., Blazevich, A.J., Kay, A.D., & McHugh, M. (2015). Acute effects of muscle stretching on physical performance, range of motion, and injury incidence in healthy active individuals: A systematic review. *Applied Physiology, Nutrition, and Metabolism, 41*(1), 1-11.

Garber, C.E., Blissmer, B., Deschenes, M.R., Franklin, B.A., Lamonte, M.J., Lee, I.M., ... & Swain, D.P. (2011). American College of Sports Medicine position stand. Quantity and quality of exercise for developing and maintaining cardiorespiratory, musculoskeletal, and neuromotor fitness in apparently healthy adults: Guidance for prescribing exercise. *Medicine and Science in Sports and Exercise, 43*(7), 1334-1359.

Hedrick, A. (2000). Dynamic flexibility training. *Strength & Conditioning Journal, 22*(5), 33-38.

Herbert, R.D., & Gabriel, M. (2002). Effects of stretching before and after exercising on muscle soreness and risk of injury: Systematic review. *British Medical Journal, 325*(7362), 468-472.

Kay, A.D., & Blazevich, A.J. (2012). Effect of acute static stretch on maximal muscle performance: A systematic review. *Medicine & Science in Sports & Exercise, 44*(1), 154-64.

MacDonald, G.Z., Penney, M D., Mullaley, M E., Cuconato, A.L., Drake, C.D., Behm, D.G., & Button, D.C. (2013). An acute bout of self-myofascial release increases range of motion without a subsequent decrease in muscle activation or force. *The Journal of Strength & Conditioning Research, 27*(3), 812-821.

Magnusson, P., & Renström, P. (2006). The European College of Sports Sciences Position statement: The role of stretching exercises in sports. *European Journal of Sport Science, 6*(2), 87-91.

Mahieu, N.N., McNair, P., De Muynck, M., Stevens, V., Blanckaert, I., Smits, N., & Witvrouw, E. (2007). Effect of static and ballistic stretching on the muscle-tendon tissue properties. *Medicine and Science in Sports and Exercise, 39*(3), 494-501.

McHugh, M. P., & Cosgrave, C.H. (2010). To stretch or not to stretch: The role of stretching in injury prevention and performance. *Scandinavian Journal of Medicine & Science in Sports, 20*(2), 169-181.

Paolini, J. (2009). Therapeutic modalities-review of myofascial release as an effective massage therapy technique. *Athletic Therapy Today, 14*(5), 30-34.

Sefton, J. (2004). Alternative and complementary concepts. Myofascial release for athletic trainers, part I: Theory and session guidelines. *Athletic Therapy Today, 9*(1), 48-49.

Sharman, M.J., Cresswell, A.G., & Riek, S. (2006). Proprioceptive neuromuscular facilitation stretching. *Sports Medicine, 36*(11), 929-939.

Shrier, I. (1999). Stretching before exercise does not reduce the risk of local muscle injury: A critical review of the clinical and basic science literature. *Clinical Journal of Sport Medicine, 9*(4), 221-227.

Simic, L., Sarabon, N., & Markovic, G. (2012). Does pre-exercise static stretching inhibit maximal muscular performance? A meta-analytical review. *Scandinavian Journal of Medicine & Science in Sports, 22*(1),1-18.

Thacker, S.B., Gilchrist, J., Stroup, D.F., & Kimsey Jr, C.D. (2004). The impact of stretching on sports injury risk: A systematic review of the literature. *Medicine & Science in Sports & Exercise, 36*(3), 371-378.

U.S. Department of Health and Human Services (2008). *2008 Physical Activity Guidelines for Americans*. ODPHP Publication No. U0036.

Woolstenhulme, M.T., Griffiths, C.M., Woolstenhulme, E.M., & Parcell, A.C. (2006). Ballistic stretching increases flexibility and acute vertical jump height when combined with basketball activity. *The Journal of Strength & Conditioning Research, 20*(4), 799-803.

Recommended Reading

American College of Sports Medicine (2018). Chapter 6: General Principles of Exercise Prescription. In, *ACSM's Guidelines to Exercise Testing and Prescription*, 10th edition. Philadelphia, PA: Wolters Kluwer.

Chapter 19 Review Questions

1. According to the American College of Sports Medicine, most adults should hold a static stretch for _____.
    A. up to 10 seconds
    B. 10 to 30 seconds
    C. 3 to 6 seconds
    D. 60 to 90 seconds

2. While contracting the tibialis anterior muscle against light resistance, the gastrocnemius and soleus muscles will be stimulated to relax. This is an example of _____.
    A. autogenic inhibition
    B. synergistic dominance
    C. reciprocal inhibition
    D. neuromuscular coordination

3. What is the sensory receptor located within the musculotendinous unit that is sensitive to tension and rate of tension change?
    A. Muscle spindle
    B. Baroreceptor
    C. Purkinje fibers
    D. Golgi tendon organ

4. Which of the following is an expected benefit of a regular stretching routine?
    A. Enhanced performance during explosive activities
    B. Increased musculotendinous stiffness
    C. Reduced joint stress and muscle hypertonicity
    D. Decreased muscle tissue extensibility

5. The standing quadriceps stretch is an example of a _____ range of motion technique.
    A. active isolated
    B. passive static
    C. self-myofascial release
    D. dynamic

6. Which of the following strategies is most likely to reduce the risk of exercise-related injury?
    A. Pre-activity static stretching
    B. Ballistic stretching techniques
    C. Dynamic stretching
    D. Proprioceptive neuromuscular facilitation

Answers to Review Questions on Page 384

Note: Review questions are intended to reinforce learning and comprehension of subject matter presented in the corresponding chapter. The review questions are not intended to be representative of actual certification exam questions in terms of style, content, or difficulty.

Section VI

Fundamentals of Group Exercise

Individuals attend group exercise classes for a variety of reasons including physical transformation, cross-training, and for the social aspect of exercising in a group. To deliver a class experience that meets participant expectations, an instructor must have an understanding of class design, choreography development strategies, and cueing. Additionally, instructors also play the role of a leader, role model, and coach.

Chapter 20 defines the basic responsibilities of Group Exercise Instructors (GEIs) and outlines available career opportunities in the health and fitness industry. This chapter also provides basic information regarding screening tools and pre-class leadership responsibilities.

Chapter 21 provides basic information regarding popular group exercise class formats. In addition, it will also cover the essential components of a group exercise class: warm-up, conditioning phases, and cool-down.

Chapter 22 covers instructor attitude and leadership, and creating a positive environment for class participants. It also discusses communication and the variety of ways to give feedback. Lastly, this chapter discusses motivational readiness to change.

Chapter 23 provides the necessary base knowledge to plan and prepare to teach group exercise classes. Topics include class design, teaching techniques and strategies, music, choreography development strategies, and cueing.

20
Introduction to Group Exercise

Introduction

The NETA Group Exercise Instructor Certification

The decision to pursue a certification as a group exercise instructor (GEI) is an important step toward being recognized as a competent fitness professional. NETA's Group Exercise Instructor Certification is one of the select few in the U.S. that have earned NCCA accreditation. NETA's GEI certification exam was developed to assess candidates' competency in leading safe and effective exercise programs using a variety of leadership techniques to motivate participants, provide quality instruction, and create an inclusive exercise environment. The GEI exam will also evaluate candidates' knowledge of exercise program design for improving cardiorespiratory fitness, muscular strength and endurance, and flexibility to enhance the quality of life of exercise participants. The primary purpose of a certification is to protect the public from harm by evaluating if the fitness professional meets established levels of competence in the knowledge, skills, and abilities necessary to perform the job. For the fitness professional, a certification can separate him or her from others who have not proven themselves to be at the same level of competence.

Who is the NETA-Certified Group Exercise Instructor?

NETA-Certified Group Exercise Instructors work in a group exercise setting with apparently healthy individuals. Since the 1980s, group exercise class options have been a key component to many exercise enthusiasts engaging in physical activity. As the choreography and modalities of group exercise continue to progress, so too has the group exercise instructor. A successful group exercise instructor possesses the ability to motivate and educate participants. Instructors must also possess knowledge of exercise science and the ability to perform safe and effective exercise leadership to individuals of all skill levels and abilities.

Ideal Characteristics of a Group Exercise Instructor

A group exercise instructor's attitude, personality, and professional conduct are among the strongest motivating factors for maintaining physical activity adherence. Although group exercise instructors are responsible for developing and delivering an amazing exercise experience, those factors alone will not guarantee optimal adherence. Personal qualities of the GEI can greatly enhance one's ability to effectively motivate participants.

Some of the qualities of an effective, adherence-producing instructor are:

- Punctuality and dependability
- Professionalism
- Dedication
- Good communication skills
- Recognizing signs of instructor burnout
- Time management and planning ahead
- Willingness to take responsibility
- Commitment to life-long learning

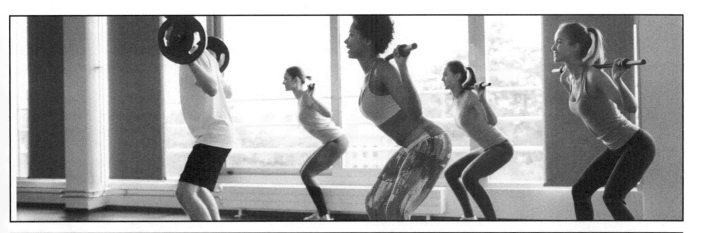

Group Exercise Employment Options

A GEI has a variety of employment options from which to choose. Most GEIs teach in a part-time capacity, but in some cases instructors work full-time managing a group fitness department and sharing the responsibility of substitute teaching when needed. Employment may fall into one of the following categories:

1. A GEI who works as an employee for a fitness facility and teaches in addition to having a full-time career.
2. A GEI who is hired by a facility to exclusively teach classes.
3. A GEI who teaches classes in a nontraditional setting such as a business, apartment complex, church, or school.

Many GEIs teach a few classes in a commercial setting and a few classes in a community setting within the same week. This provides an instructor a wide range of experience teaching to different participants of varying skills and abilities. GEIs may be employed in:

- Assisted living communities for older adults
- Commercial (for profit) health clubs and fitness facilities
- Nonprofit organizations (e.g., YMCA, YWCA, JCC)
- Corporate fitness and worksite wellness facilities
- Governmental/military base fitness facilities
- Hospital and medical fitness facilities
- Municipal community centers/parks & recreation/schools
- Self-employed fitness studios/in-home businesses
- Campus recreation/university

Group Exercise Instructor Education & Experience

Due to the large number of certification organizations, the requirements for the GEI vary greatly. The minimal requirements for a NETA Group Exercise Instructor (NETA-GEI) are:

- A high school diploma or general education diploma (GED), or
- 18 years of age, and,
- Current adult cardiopulmonary resuscitation (CPR) certification from a recognized provider including a hands-on practical skills assessment

To obtain NETA's GEI certification, a candidate must pass the certification exam. Candidates prepare for the exam through self-directed independent study. NETA highly recommends that candidates devote at least 45 days preparing prior to the certification exam. NETA offers a variety of study materials, and candidates may also attend a NETA review workshop to supplement their studies.

Group exercise instructors often get started by participating in exercise classes until they are ready to audition as instructors, and if the audition is successful, they begin teaching classes. Most employers require instructors to be certified, but some will allow instructors on the job training and a grace period to become certified. Because employment requirements vary from employer to employer, it may be helpful to contact local fitness centers or other potential employers to find out what education, background, and training they prefer.

In the long run, earning an NCCA-accredited certification, like the NETA Group Exercise Instructor certification, will provide recognition of a certification based on sound scientific principles. A recognized certification helps participants feel confident in the instructor's skills and abilities as a health and fitness leader. Starting a group exercise career with a highly respected certification is an excellent first step.

Continuing Education

Constantly learning and staying up-to-date is key to success as exercise styles, trends, and equipment in the group exercise setting evolve. Continuing education should be seen as an opportunity for the GEI to learn and grow. Instructors with new tools are those who will stand out in a competitive industry. NETA-Certified GEIs must earn 20 continuing education credits (CECs) every two years to maintain the certification with NETA.

Pre-class Leadership

As group exercise instructors, the overarching purpose for group classes is to help people live happier and healthier lives through participation in group exercise classes. For most individuals, becoming more physically active and participating in group exercise classes is a safe and effective means to improve overall health.

There are certain cases when embarking on a new physical activity program is contraindicated without a prior medical clearance. For example, a person with cardiovascular disease has an increased risk of experiencing an adverse event, such as a myocardial infarction, during exercise compared to an otherwise healthy person (Balady et al., 1998). To mitigate the risk of exercise-related medical emergencies, when necessary, participants should be advised to consult with a health care provider and obtain medical clearance prior to starting a moderate- or vigorous-intensity exercise program.

According to standards developed by the American College of Sports Medicine (ACSM), health and fitness facility operators shall offer a general pre-activity screening tool (e.g., PAR-Q) and/or a specific pre-activity screening tool to all new members and prospective users (Tharrett & Peterson, 2012). When indicated, a member or prospective user shall be advised to consult with an appropriate health care provider and obtain medical clearance prior to exercise participation (Tharrett & Peterson, 2012). Group exercise instructors should discuss pre-activity screening policies with their employer to ensure appropriate procedures are being administered.

In some instances, instructors may need to administer a pre-activity health screening tool; however, in other instances, instructors only need to be aware that screening has taken place. GEIs should review and become familiar with how to properly utilize the pre-activity health screening tools as they apply to their current place of employment. See chapter 12 for more information regarding preparticipation.

General Exercise Guidelines for Healthy Adults

Today's classes offer multiple formats and styles. One size does not fit all when it comes to group exercise classes. Class participants arrive to class with varying degrees of skills and abilities. As the fitness industry is driven by trends, programs are being continuously created by passionate and motivated fitness professionals. Therefore, it is important to be mindful of the safety and usefulness of ACSM's exercise guidelines for the apparently healthy population. The current guidelines include cardiorespiratory, muscular strength and endurance, and flexibility recommendations. These guidelines serve as a template for exercise programming and will guide the instructor with class design (ACSM, 2018). See table 20-1.

Table 20-1 General Exercise for Healthy Adults

Training Component	Frequency (days/wk)	Intensity	Time	Type
Cardiorespiratory	≥5 or ≥3 or 3–5	Moderate (40% to <60% VO2R/HRR) Vigorous (60% to <90% VO2R/HRR) Combination of moderate and vigorous	30–60 minutes 20–60 minutes 20–60 minutes	Aerobic (cardiovascular endurance) activities and weight bearing exercise
Resistance	2–3	60% to 70% of 1-RM or RPE = 5–6 (0–10 scale) for older adults	2–4 sets of 8–25 repetitions (e.g. 8–12, 10–15; depending upon goal)	8–10 exercises that include all major muscle groups (full-body or split routine); Muscular strength and endurance, calisthenics, and neuromuscular (balance and agility) exercises
Flexibility	≥2–3	Stretch to the point of slight discomfort without pain	2–4 repetitions per muscle group 10–30 seconds for most adults 10–60 seconds for older adults	All major muscle-tendon groups Static or dynamic

Key
VO2R = Oxygen Consumption Reserve
HRR = Heart Rate Reserve
1-RM = One-Repetition Maximum
RPE = Rating of Perceived Exertion

Monitoring Cardiorespiratory Intensity

Understanding target heart rate (THR), rating of perceived exertion (RPE), and the talk test is the first step in monitoring exercise intensity. There is not one method that works for all types of classes and there are no hard and fast rules for monitoring, just that it must be done. Below is a summary of how to use THR, RPE, and the talk test.

Measuring Heart Rate

Monitoring exercise intensity within the cardiorespiratory segment is key. Participants need to know the purpose of monitoring heart rate during exercise and how to obtain a pulse rate. Proper instruction on how to measure HR is the first step to monitoring exercise intensity effectively.

Heart rate may be determined by palpating the carotid artery or radial artery (figure 20-1, 20-2) and counting the number of beats. A ten-second count is multiplied by 6 or a fifteen-second count is multiplied by 4 to obtain the one-minute heart rate. There are many sites on the body to monitor heart rate. We have recommended the two below:

- **Carotid Pulse:** This pulse is taken from the carotid artery just to the side of the neck. Use light pressure from the tips of the first two fingers (not the thumb) and never palpate both carotid arteries at the same time, and always press lightly.
- **Radial Pulse:** This pulse is taken from the radial artery at the lateral wrist, in line with the thumb, using the tips of the first fingers.

Figure 20-1 Carotid Heart Rate Monitoring

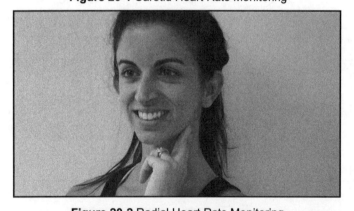

Figure 20-2 Radial Heart Rate Monitoring

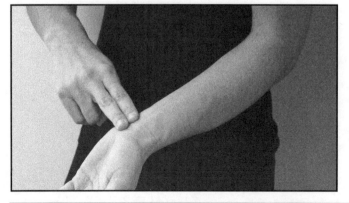

Maximal Heart Rate

One of the most common approaches to monitor exercise intensity in the fitness setting is the **maximal heart rate (MHR or HRmax) method**. This method utilizes maximal heart rate as the anchor point from which the THR is calculated as a straight percentage of the HRmax. Numerous formulas have been developed to estimate age-predicted maximum heart rate among various populations (Robergs & Landwehr, 2002). Perhaps the most frequently used equation is that proposed by Fox et al. (1971). This equation is:

$$\text{Estimated HRmax} = 220 - \text{age}$$

The simplicity of this prediction equation has likely contributed to its widespread use among fitness professionals despite the many research studies that have noted a significant margin of error among HRmax values derived from this formula (Cleary et al., 2011; Gellish et al., 2007; Robergs & Landwehr, 2002; Tanaka et al., 2001). It has been reported that the "220 – age" formula tends to overestimate HRmax in adults younger than 40 years old and underestimates HRmax with increasing age over 40 (Tanaka et al., 2001). See table 20-2.

Another approach to determine the target heart rate is known as the **heart rate reserve (HRR) method**. This method was first introduced by the physiologist, Dr. M.J. Karvonen and has therefore come to be known as the **Karvonen Formula** (Karvonen et al., 1957). The calculation of target heart rate begins with the standard "220 – age" to estimate maximum heart rate. The next step is to calculate the heart rate reserve, which is the difference between the maximum heart rate and the resting heart rate (HRR = HRmax – RHR). The heart rate reserve is multiplied by the desired training percentage, and then the resting heart rate is added back in to obtain the target heart rate.

Rating of Perceived Exertion

The use of **rating of perceived exertion (RPE)** was first introduced by Gunnar Borg and has since become widely used in a variety of fitness and clinical exercise settings (Borg, 1982). The rating of perceived exertion provides a subjective indication regarding the difficulty of the exercise being performed by the participant. The original RPE scale, known as the category scale, includes a 15-point range of values from 6 to 20, which was intended to loosely correspond to heart rates ranging from 60 to 200 beats per minute (Borg, 1982).

The original rating of perceived exertion scale is provided in table 20-3. Using the original RPE scale, a rating of 12 to 13 is considered to be moderate-intensity and a rating of 14 to 17 is considered vigorous-intensity. A revised rating of perceived exertion scale, known as the category-ratio scale, was introduced (Borg, 1982). This revised scale provides a range of values from 0 to 10 (see table 20-4).

Using the revised scale, a rating of 5 to 6 represents moderate-intensity exercise and a rating of 7 to 8 represents vigorous-intensity. The category-ratio scale has gained popularity due to its relative simplicity, which allows for ease of use and understanding by lay populations and fitness professionals. Similar 10-point scales have subsequently been developed for a variety of subjective measures, such as pain and stress.

Talk Test

In addition to target heart rate and rating of perceived exertion, the 'Talk Test' is another technique that takes into account an exerciser's ability to breathe and talk during a workout. If a person can comfortably answer a question while exercising, it is likely that the activity being performed is appropriate for cardiorespiratory conditioning. The talk test is especially useful for those who are beginners, and are learning to monitor their bodies and exercise intensity.

A GEI can conduct the talk test by simply asking class participants questions and listening for responses during the cardiorespiratory conditioning segment of class. Preferably, the responses of the participants should be in the form of sentences, rather than one-word statements, such as "good" or "okay." The GEI could ask a participant to describe how he or she is feeling and the participants may say, "I'm working pretty hard." If the class participants can string several words together in a sentence without gasping for air, he or she is working at an appropriate intensity.

Table 20-3 Original RPE Scale

Original RPE Scale	
6	
7	Very, very light
8	
9	Very light
10	
11	Fairly light
12	
13	Somewhat hard
14	
15	Hard
16	
17	Very hard
18	
19	Very, very hard
20	

Borg, (1982)

Table 20-2 Sample Calculation

Sample Calculation Using HRR to Determine Target HR	
A 40-year-old participant with a resting HR of 60 bpm wants to exercise at 50% to 75% of her HR Reserve. What is the range of her target heart rate?	
Step 1	Estimate HRmax (220 – age)
• 220 – age • 220 – 40 = 180 bpm (HRmax)	
Step 2	Find HR Reserve
• HRmax – RHR = HRR • 180 – 60 = 120 HRR	
Step 3	Find Target HR Range (50% to 75%)
• HRR x Desired Intensity % + RHR = Target Heart Rate (THR) • 120 x 50% (.50) intensity = 60 + 60 (RHR) = 120 Target Heart Rate • 120 x 75% (.75) intensity = 90 + 60 (RHR) = 150 Target Heart Rate	

Target HR Range (50%-75%)
- 120–150bpm Target Heart Rate

Table 20-4 Revised RPE Scale

Revised RPE Scale	
0	Nothing at all
0.5	Very, very weak
1	Very weak
2	Weak
3	Moderate
4	Somewhat strong
5	Strong
6	
7	Very strong
8	
9	
10	Very, very strong

Borg, (1982)

Group exercise instructors should teach class participants how to monitor their exercise intensity. Of course, a GEI must be able to recognize warning signs that indicate participants are in distress due to overexertion, but ultimately the responsibility for exercising at an appropriate intensity rests with the participant. This concept should be explained by the instructor at the beginning of each class. It is important for class participants to understand that while the GEI will provide safe and effective exercises for all, each individual participant should gage their own exercise intensity and adjust accordingly.

It is helpful to explain to class participants that there are physical sensations and feelings that are normal with various levels of intensity and how to adjust performance, if necessary. For example, a GEI could announce, *"We will check intensity efforts at different points throughout class. I will ask you to think about how hard you are working. You should reflect on how fast you are breathing and how fatigued you feel at that moment. If you feel like you're working too hard (at an intensity that cannot be maintained for the reminder of class), I will provide you modifications so your exercise intensity can be reduced or adjusted."*

It is advisable to monitor exercise intensity and perform checks several times throughout class. An intensity check can be as simple as the talk test or using the RPE scale. At the very least, an intensity check should be performed during the highest point of the cardiorespiratory conditioning segment of class.

It is up to the GEI to choose an exercise intensity method that works best for the skills, abilities, and fitness level of the class participants attending class. Whether using target heart rate, RPE, or the talk test, a GEI must feel comfortable with the method so that participants understand how to apply it to their exercise session.

Signs of Fatigue
Occasionally, even while monitoring exercise intensity, participants can overexert themselves during a group exercise class. A competent GEI will be able to recognize clues or warning signs of fatigue that require exercise options for the entire class to lower intensity levels.

The first warning sign often seen when a participant is working too vigorously is a breakdown in proper form and technique during exercise execution. For example, an individual who is beginning to fatigue during a step training class might not be able to set his or her foot completely on the step. Failing to place the entire foot on the step increases the risk of injury to the participants and those around them. Another example may be seen while performing a standing climb on an indoor cycling bike during which a participant has placed all of his or her weight on the handle bars indicating that he or she is fatigued.

In either situation, it would be appropriate for the GEI to recommend exercise options for each movement, thereby reducing the intensity of the exercise. In most cases, it is best to make a general statement to the entire class about proper execution of the exercise or movement, and how to reduce the intensity through options that were just suggested if they find that they cannot maintain proper form and technique. However, it might be necessary for the GEI to approach an individual participant and use specific, direct feedback if the exerciser continues with poor form and is at risk for injury. A non-intimidating way of doing this in class would be for the GEI to walk over to the participant, mute the microphone, and give the participant a few cues to help correct from.

Other key warning signs that could indicate a need for reducing exercise intensity include labored breathing, excessive sweating, and dizziness. When a GEI sees these clues and signs, he or she is should encourage participants to reduce the intensity and lightly march in place or stop exercise all together until the symptoms subside. As heart rate lowers and breathing is controlled, the participant can resume activity at a lower exercise intensity.

Chapter Summary
Group exercise instructors play an important role within the fitness industry in that they are responsible for leading safe and effective classes to new and experienced participants. Exposing groups of individuals to the fun, challenging, and social elements of exercise increases motivation and the likelihood that they will make regular exercise part of their lifestyle. It is common for a GEI to have participants of various skills and abilities in class, so the GEI must have the knowledge of the health screening process and how to properly monitor participants' intensity level.

Chapter References
American College of Sports Medicine (2018). *ACSM's Guidelines for Exercise Testing and Prescription,* 10th edition. Philadelphia, PA: Wolters Kluwer.

Borg, G.A.V. (1982). Psychophysical bases of perceived exertion. *Medicine and Science in Sports and Exercise*, 14(5), 377-381.

Balady, G. J., Chaitman, B., Driscoll, D., Foster, C., Froelicher, E., Gordon, N., & Bazzarre, T. (1998). Recommendations for cardiovascular screening, staffing, and emergency policies at health/fitness facilities. *Circulation*, 97(22), 2283-2293.

Cleary, M.A., Hetzler, R.K., Wages, J.J., Lentz, M.A., Stickley, C.D., & Kimura, I.F. (2011). Comparisons of age-predicted maximum heart rate equations in college-aged subjects. *The Journal of Strength & Conditioning Research*, 25(9), 2591-2597.

Fox, S.M., Naughton, J.P., & Haskell, W.L. (1971). Physical activity and the prevention of coronary heart disease. *Annals of Clinical Research*, 3(6), 404-432.

Gellish, R.L., Goslin, B.R., Olson, R.E., McDonald, A., Russi, G.D., & Moudgil, V.K. (2007). Longitudinal modeling of the relationship between age and maximal heart rate. *Medicine and Science in Sports and Exercise*, 39 (5), 822-829.

Karvonen, M., Kentala, E., & Mustala, O. (1957). The effects of training on heart rate: A longitudinal study. *Annals Medicinae Experimentalis et Biologiae Fenniae*, 35(3), 307-315.

Robergs, R.A., & Landwehr, R. (2002). The surprising history of the "HRmax= 220-age" equation. *Journal of Exercise Physiology*, 5(2), 1-10.

Tanaka, H., Monahan, K.D., & Seals, D.R. (2001). Age-predicted maximal heart rate revisited. *Journal of the American College of Cardiology*, 37(1), 153-156.

Tharrett, S.J. & Peterson, J.A. (Eds.) (2012). *ACSM's Health/Fitness Facility Standards and Guidelines*, 4th edition. Champaign, IL: Human Kinetics.

United States Department of Health and Human Services (2008). *2008 Physical Activity Guidelines for Americans*. www.health.gov/paguideliens.

Chapter 20 Review Questions

1. In order to maintain the NETA Group Exercise Instructor certification in good standing, how many continuing education credits (CECs) must be earned every two years?
    A. 10
    B. 15
    C. 20
    D. 25

2. Which of the following is likely to be a sign of fatigue for a class participant?
    A. RPE of 4 on the category ratio scale
    B. Responding to a question using full sentences
    C. Reduced range of motion during body weight squats
    D. Heart rate at 60% of the HRR during peak of cardiorespiratory segment of class

3. Using the revised Borg scale, a rating of 5 to 6 represents _____.
    A. moderate-intensity
    B. vigorous-intensity
    C. maximum-intensity
    D. low-intensity

4. Which of the following is a general pre-activity screening tool that may be utilized with group exercise class participants?
    A. Karvonen Formula
    B. Rating of Perceived Exertion
    C. Talk Test
    D. PAR-Q

5. American College of Sports Medicine's exercise guidelines for healthy adults include _____, muscular strength and endurance, and _____ which serve as a template for exercise programming and will guide the instructor with class design.
    A. cardiorespiratory, flexibility
    B. cardiorespiratory, dynamic stretching
    C. cardiorespiratory, balance
    D. cardiorespiratory, PNF

6. What is the target heart rate (THR) at 80% of the heart rate reserve (HRR) for a 53-year-old class participant with a resting heart rate (RHR) of 70 bpm?
    A. 134 bpm
    B. 148 bpm
    C. 167 bpm
    D. 180 bpm

Answers to Review Questions on Page 384

Note: Review questions are intended to reinforce learning and comprehension of subject matter presented in the corresponding chapter. The review questions are not intended to be representative of actual certification exam questions in terms of style, content, or difficulty.

21
Group Exercise Formats and Components

Introduction
Group exercise program design has come a long way from the early days of aerobic dance-based classes developed by Jackie Sorenson in 1969. Today, group exercise classes include traditional step, indoor cycling, kickboxing, dance, boot camp, water exercise, strength conditioning, and mind-body classes. Other growing trends include group exercise classes performed outdoors and branded pre-choreographed programs such as Les Mills and MOSSA.

Now is the time to explore the options as a group exercise instructor by learning a few of the many formats in the industry today. It's important for a group exercise instructor to select a class format that suits his or her abilities, interest, and style.

Group Exercise Class Formats
Cardio Dance
Cardio dance can range from traditional hi/lo aerobics (e.g., jazzercise®) to Latin or hip-hop dance formats (e.g., Zumba™). Dance classes may contain choreography designed for each song that includes specific movement sequences, while others may be taught with more of an add-on style of teaching. It is highly recommended that cardio dance instructors have knowledge of the 32-count structure of music and are well versed in the genre of dance they are teaching. Understanding basic dance vocabulary, movement transitions, and teaching progressions is also important. A new instructor may find it helpful to seek out a cardio dance format for which pre-choreographed material is provided. However, there is usually a licensing fee associated with this type of programming, and it is still the responsibility of the instructor to master and seamlessly deliver the class content.

Step Training
Step training was extremely popular in the 1990s, and while overall interest has declined, many step enthusiasts still request and attend step classes. The step is versatile in that it can be used to perform a variety of basic speed drills to increase intensity level, or it can be used to create challenging choreography via step patterns and combinations.

Stepping involves utilizing a platform (i.e., step, bench) and risers to create a base that can vary in height. Increasing the step height will increase intensity, but will also increase the risk of injuries. Therefore, it is recommended that only advanced exercisers, or those with long legs, use step heights greater than 8 inches (i.e., step and 2 or more risers on each side) (Kennedy et al., 2009). Another safety precaution includes playing step music more slowly when compared to most other cardiovascular group exercise classes. It is recommended that step music be played between 118 to 128 beats per minute depending on the complexity of choreography and the participants' ability level.

Kickboxing
Kickboxing classes can include a wide variety of martial arts based movements and can be completely pre-choreographed to music or taught with less planned structure. The majority of participants attend these classes for overall health and fitness benefits, while only a minority of individuals seek out classes that are more marital arts or boxing based to practice and perfect their form. Kickboxing classes typically include a variety of punches (e.g., jab, cross-jab, hook, uppercut), kicks (e.g., front, back, side, roundhouse), stances (e.g., ready, staggered), and jumping rope. If available, classes can include the use of gloves, kicking shields/pads, and punching bags.

Instruction regarding safe execution of punches and kicks is vital to prevent injuries in all kickboxing formats. Similar to all fitness formats, kickboxing classes should include a gradual increase in intensity and the warm-up should include rehearsal moves specific to kickboxing. To assist participants in performing the movements with appropriate biomechanics, it is recommended that kickboxing music be played at 125 to 135 beats per minute (Kennedy-Armbruster & Yoke, 2014).

Indoor Group Cycling
Indoor group cycling classes were first introduced in the 1990s and they continue to be highly attended. This class format can focus on either cardiorespiratory endurance or anaerobic power utilizing slow and steady workouts, heart rate training, or interval and high intensity interval training (H.I.I.T.). Individuals participate in class on a specialized

stationary bicycle that includes multiple adjustment options so the cycle can be fitted to the rider's body. It is extremely important that a knowledgeable instructor fits each participant to his or her cycle to avoid injuries, especially knee and low back injuries. NETA's Bike Fit home study is highly recommended for more in-depth information regarding appropriate bike adjustment. Instructors should also teach proper hand placement, riding positions, and alignment of the upper body.

A typical indoor group cycling class involves an instructor leading the participants through a routine that can involve simulated terrain, hill climbs, sprints, or races. To create the best possible experience for their students, instructors should utilize music, visualization, and motivational coaching to inspire their participants. An advantage of indoor cycling is each participant can control his or her own speed and intensity while remaining part of the group. The intensity of the workout can be manually manipulated by each rider by increasing or decreasing the resistance on the flywheel or by adjusting cadence (i.e., rate of pedaling). To assist participants in assessing their work rate, the use of a heart rate monitor is highly encouraged in group cycling classes.

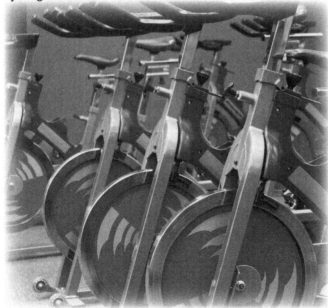

Boot Camp
Although boot camp has been around for decades, this format has been an emerging trend showing substantial growth over the last several years. The workout was based off of the Army's 8-week basic training program used to get new recruits into shape and included exercises such as push-ups, squat thrusts, and other body weight exercise. Today, most fitness facilities offer some sort of boot camp format since this style of class offers participants a workout that is challenging and offers a variety of training techniques and equipment. Boot camp style classes can include various forms of cardiorespiratory exercise (e.g., running, interval training, obstacle courses, and relay races) as well as resistance training, calisthenics, plyometrics, speed, and agility training. Conducting a class outside allows for stairs, benches or picnic tables, hills, and playground equipment to also be incorporated into the workout.

Interval Training
Interval training includes alternating work and recovery periods. One of the most common forms of interval training is high intensity interval training (H.I.I.T.). This form of interval training involves a series of short vigorous-intensity bouts of exercise well above the anaerobic threshold, followed by low-intensity active recovery intervals. While H.I.I.T. was originally intended for performance enhancement among athletes, it has been modified for use by nearly all fitness levels and populations. H.I.I.T. is designed to improve metabolic and cardiorespiratory conditioning; therefore, the selected movements during the work interval should be compound, yet simple movements that deliver an immediate heart rate response versus exercises that are complex or focus on resistance or strength training (a bicep curl, plank, or similar exercises are not ideal to include in H.I.I.T classes). Options, or progressions and regressions, for all chosen exercises should be demonstrated to accommodate all fitness levels. Fitness professionals also need to be able to modify the work-to-recovery interval length of their H.I.I.T. workout to fit the needs and ability levels of all their clients or participants.

Group Resistance Training
Group resistance training includes all fitness classes during which the focus is on creating muscular strength or muscular endurance using body weight or equipment. Some classes are equipment-based including kettlebell, suspension training (e.g., TRX®) and balance trainers (e.g., BOSU®, Step 360™). However, most widely available group exercise equipment (e.g., resistance tubing, light weight dumbbells, and body weight) is conducive to creating a muscular endurance training effect. Since resistance equipment is often limited in a group exercise format, an instructor should encourage participants to use adequate resistance levels so that muscle fatigue is reached by 15-20 repetitions to facilitate muscular endurance gains. With regard to the order of exercises in a class setting, it is recommended that the same guidelines be followed as those found in Chapter 18, table 18-3 for general resistance training. These include performing large muscle group exercises before small muscle group exercises, performing multiple-joint exercises before single-joint exercises, and performing higher-intensity exercises before lower-intensity exercises. In order to utilize the entire class time, it is advisable to perform exercises that alternate between upper and lower body, or that alternate between muscle groups that oppose one another (e.g., biceps and triceps, chest and back). This provides a built-in recovery period before conducting another set for the same muscle group.

Circuit Training

Circuit training is a time efficient form of resistance training that is used to elicit strength, endurance, and metabolic training effects. Classes utilizing this format of training usually involve several stations of exercises that are performed with minimal rest between exercises. Most circuit training classes are focused on muscular endurance as the exercises are often performed for a pre-determined amount of time (e.g., 30-45 seconds). Circuits usually include approximately 6-15 exercises, and may consist of all resistance training exercises, or may consist of both resistance and cardiorespiratory exercises. See chapter 18, figure 18-4 and 18-5 for sample circuit training formats. It is advisable that instructors demonstrate the exercises at the beginning of class and use signs or pictures at each station as a nonverbal cue to assist participants in recalling the exercise designated for each station. There are many mobile device applications available for download that can be set to pre-determined work and rest ratios. This allows the instructor to focus on participant form and cueing instead of a stopwatch; therefore, enhancing the students' experience. Benefits of circuit training include adding variety to a workout routine and reducing the risk of injury, which may result from continuously performing the same workout program.

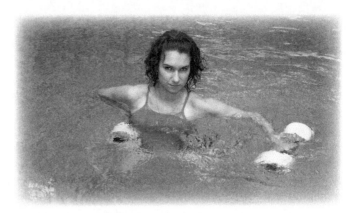

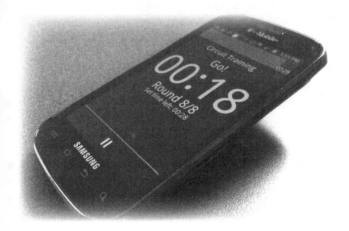

Water Exercise

Water-based exercise or aqua aerobics classes, became more prevalent in mainstream fitness in the 1990s, and remains a very effective form of exercise that everyone can participate in regardless of ability level. The resistance created by the water provides an ideal environment for a full body workout, while also reducing joint stress. However, water fitness is not simply a land aerobics class performed in the pool. Instructors must be able to appropriately adapt typical land-based movements to the unique characteristics (e.g., buoyancy, drag, turbulence) of the aquatic environment. In addition, instructors must understand the physical laws of movement in the water, the effective use of water resistance, and the unique properties of water and how they affect exercise intensity. A review article by Graef and Kruel (2006) has shown that exercise heart rate in water can be anywhere from 5-16 beats less per minute compared to that on land. Therefore, calculated target heart rate ranges for water classes need to be decreased, or rate of perceived exertion may be used to determine exercise intensity instead. Although heart rate may be lower in water exercise classes than in land classes, research shows that metabolic and cardiovascular benefits are comparable.

Specialty Classes

Specialty classes such as Pilates, yoga, and barre require specialized training and certifications. Instructor training programs and certifications vary from 8-hour workshops to significant hours of course work and extensive practice teaching.

Pilates

Pilates is a method that was developed by Joseph H. Pilates. As a child, he suffered from rickets, asthma, and rheumatic fever. These ailments prompted him to study the human body and develop a system of exercises to restore physical health. They are designed to promote a balanced musculoskeletal system resulting in core strength, flexibility, good posture, and improved body awareness. For decades, Joseph Pilates worked with dancers in New York and passed his body of knowledge onto his students, which has since found its way into mainstream fitness. The exercises can be performed on the floor (i.e., mat Pilates) or on specialized Pilates equipment (e.g., reformer, chair, barrel). Fitness professionals wishing to teach Pilates classes are highly encouraged to receive specialized training before instructing the exercises to others.

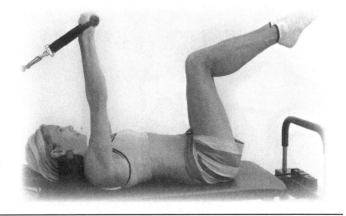

Yoga

Yoga was developed in ancient India and was practiced by monks to help their body prepare to sit for long periods of time in meditation. The word yoga means 'to join or yoke together' as in bringing the mind, body, and spirit together. While there are many types of yoga, Hatha yoga is the most widely practiced form in the U.S. This form of yoga includes nearly 200 physical postures, breathing techniques, and often meditation to promote physical health and mental well-being. Practicing yoga helps to improve flexibility and alleviate stress, and allows the mind to become more focused and centered. Specialized yoga training is recommended for fitness professionals interested in teaching yoga postures or classes.

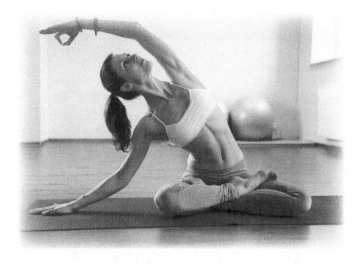

Class Components

A properly designed class includes the following components: warm-up, cardiorespiratory, muscular strength and endurance, and flexibility/cool-down. There is no single class format that fits every type of group exercise class. For example, in a step class, it is very fitting to warm up using a step. However, in a kickboxing class, preforming boxing movements during the warm-up is more fitting than using a step.

Instructors who understand the class components will be able to apply this knowledge to various class formats, which may result in the ability to teach numerous classes. Teaching multiple formats may increase the fitness professional's employment opportunities and his or her ability to positively impact a wide variety of participants.

Warm-up

The purpose of a warm-up is to prepare the body for more rigorous demands of the cardiorespiratory and/or muscle conditioning segment by raising the internal body temperature. It is recommended that the first 5-10 minutes of a class be devoted to the warm-up. The warm-up includes light-to-moderate intensity aerobic activity utilizing rehearsal moves (i.e., movements similar to those the students will perform in class, using only body weight). The movements in a warm-up should begin with smaller movements and gradually increase in range of motion and intensity and can include dynamic stretching. Dynamic stretching will be discussed next.

Here are a few guidelines for a warm-up:
- Include dynamic movements
- Focus on rehearsal movements
- Include all major muscle groups (if appropriate)
- Ensure clear verbal instructions, volume, tempo, and atmosphere are created

The potential physiological benefits of a warm-up include:
- Increased metabolic rate
- Gradual redistribution of blood flow to the working muscles
- Increased speed and force of muscle contractions
- Increased tendon, ligament, and muscle elasticity
- Gradual increase in energy production which minimizes metabolic acidosis
- Reduced risk of abnormal heart rhythms

Many of these physiological effects may reduce the risk of injury because they have the potential to increase neuromuscular coordination, delay fatigue, and make the tissues less susceptible to damage (Alter, 2004).

Dynamic Stretches

Dynamic stretching exercises utilize slow, controlled, and rhythmic movements to actively increase joint range of motion. It's recommended that instructors include dynamic stretches during their warm-up and that static stretching be performed at the end during the cool-down phase (Hedrick, 2000). These activities utilize body weight or light resistance (e.g., medicine ball, tubing) and involve calisthenic type movements such as body weight squats, walking and lateral lunges, and medicine ball chops and lifts. Dynamic range of motion activities may also involve single joint movements such as shoulder circles or leg swings. The dynamic nature of this activity also functions to increase tissue temperature, elasticity, and extensibility, which are likely to contribute to increased range of motion and decreased risk of injury during exercise.

Cardiorespiratory Segment

The cardiorespiratory conditioning segment (i.e., component) of the class primarily consists of aerobic-type exercise meant to increase endurance. This portion of the class is typically 20-60 minutes, depending on the class format and duration. The cardiorespiratory segment of the class should follow the F.I.T.T. guidelines (i.e., frequency, intensity, time, type) presented in chapter 17 on pages 196-197. Classes should begin with light-to-moderate levels of activity and then continue to gradually increase in complexity and intensity.

Gradually Increase Intensity

The human body adapts to exercise very efficiently. Gradually increasing intensity is necessary for the following physiological reasons:

- It allows blood flow to be redistributed from the internal organs to the working muscles.
- It allows the heart time to adapt to the change from a resting to a working level.
- It allows for an appropriate increase in respiratory rate.

For example, to gradually increase intensity during a boot camp class, begin the class with a light jog around the room, progress to performing drills such as skipping, butt kicks, and then progress to drills that incorporate ladders, hurdles, or cones. Gradually adding intensity and complexity will allow participants to warm-up physiologically, neurologically, and psychologically, better preparing them for the overall exercise experience.

Intensity Options

As discussed in chapter 20, instructors should promote self-responsibility and encourage class participants to work at their own pace and an intensity level that works for them. The group exercise instructor should be sure to demonstrate heart rate (HR) monitoring, rating of perceived exertion (RPE), or the talk test, and use verbal cues and descriptors to inform participants how they should feel. For example, during the peak portion of the cardiorespiratory segment, tell participants that they should feel out of breath, but should still be able to speak a few sentences. Be as descriptive as possible when checking RPE. Offer progressions and regressions as necessary. A regression offers an exerciser a way to decrease intensity or complexity, while a progression increases one or both. Offering "level 1" and "level 3" options while teaching to the intermediate intensity or "level 2" for a majority of the time provides participants with options making them feel successful. An example of a progression and regression for a jumping jack would be a side tap (level 1) while encouraging those who want more intensity to perform a regular jumping jack (level 2), and those who want even more intensity to perform an air jack (level 3). Help participants achieve the level of effort they need to reach, and continually encourage them that reaching that point is their responsibility.

Building Sequences

Building sequences involves taking complex moves and breaking them down into smaller blocks of work so that participants are able to learn the movements and are set up for success. In a kickboxing class, for example, building sequences logically would include teaching class participants how to perform a jab with a side kick for the first time by breaking down the movement. First, have class participants perform a front jab slowly by teaching them to extend the arm and retract the arm back to the starting position without locking the elbow. Once the front jab has been mastered, add a side kick with the opposite leg. Again, breaking down the side kick step by step, ensuring proper kicking technique and form. When movements or choreography are complex, it will be necessary to break down movements into smaller blocks of eight counts and then addon until a series of four groups of eight counts is completed. If combinations are logical and progressively put together, participants will be able to learn and follow the exercises, which also leaves them feeling successful and likely to return to class.

Muscular Conditioning Segment

The muscle-conditioning segment (i.e., component) of a class may occur immediately after the warm-up or after the cardiorespiratory conditioning phase of class depending on the format. The muscle conditioning portion of a class may focus on muscular strength, muscular endurance, or a combination of both. However, due to the often limited equipment available for muscular strength training, most classes focus on muscular endurance using standard group exercise equipment (e.g., resistance tubing, light-weight dumbbells). The basic principles and guidelines of resistance training discussed in chapter 18 should be applied to the muscle conditioning portion of group exercise classes.

Here are a few common principles for the muscular strength and endurance segment of most group exercises classes. It is suggested that group exercise instructors:

- Promote muscular balance, functional fitness, and proper progression,
- Maintain proper form, observe participants' form, and suggest modification for injuries and special needs,
- Give verbal, visual, and physical cues on posture/alignment and body mechanics,
- Use equipment safely and effectively, and
- Create a motivational atmosphere.

Muscle Balance

During activities of daily living such as walking and climbing stairs we primarily use the quadriceps and hip flexor muscles. Group exercise class design often includes movements that also include the use of those same muscle groups; however, continuing to use the quadriceps and hip flexors repeatedly during exercise classes is unnecessary. Striving to balance daily flexion, which takes place in the sagittal plane, with movements in other planes (e.g. hip abduction and adduction in the frontal plane) is critical to prevent injury. Understanding how the body functions in daily movements can help GEIs determine which muscles need to be strengthened and stretched during classes. For example, marching works the hip flexors. Focusing on exercise selection that utilizes the gluteus maximus (the opposing muscle group to the hip flexors) would help with muscle balance. The strategy for dealing with muscle imbalances is to strengthen the weak and stretch the tight muscles. For example, the abdominals typically are weak; therefore, it makes sense to include strengthening exercises into the class. See table 21-1.

Proper Form and Technique

As an instructor, it is essential to have good alignment while demonstrating all exercises, to understand participants' needs and abilities, and find ways to help them achieve ideal form, technique, and posture. When asking participants to focus on form and technique, coaching skills are very useful. Hence, a group exercise 'coach' will utilize various cues and demonstrations and provide feedback to help participants achieve optimal form.

It's important for group exercise instructors to make their way around the studio to observe and assist their class participants. Instructors should demonstrate the movement, perform a few repetitions, and then move around the studio to observe participants movements checking for proper form and technique. By staying at the front of the room, the group exercise instructor provides class participants with only one frame of reference.

Giving appropriate verbal, visual, and physical cues is one of the most important aspects of instructing the muscular strength and endurance segment of class. Verbal cues include cueing movements with appropriate terminology and instruction. For example, when performing a standing lateral leg lift to strengthen the gluteus medius, the following verbal cues are recommended:

- Instruct participants to contract the stabilizer muscles
- Give appropriate postural cues
- Remind participants the appropriate range of motion
- Keep the movement slow and controlled, and promote muscle balance

Visual cues include the instructor's form. It is imperative that when verbal cues are given the instructor also performs the movement effectively because participants tend to 'do as you do.' For example, when performing the standing lateral leg lift, if the instructor says, "Lift the leg 45-degrees," but is lifting the leg higher than instructed, this may cause confusion among participants.

It is also important to note which style of learning works best for participants – auditory (verbal cueing), visual (demonstration), or kinesthetic (physical feelings). Observing the group and being prepared to demonstrate and modify teaching techniques for different learning styles is an important skill for the GEI. Providing and getting feedback from class participants is another important key to learning and growing as an instructor. Fitness professionals who give and ask for feedback on a regular basis are providing good customer service, which ensures participants come back to class. Cueing will be discussed in more detail in chapter 23.

Cool-down

The cool-down follows the conditioning (i.e., cardiorespiratory or muscle conditioning) phase of the class and should last 5-10 minutes. The cool-down is often a combination of light- to moderate-intensity aerobic activity, standing and/or seated stretches, and optional core exercises. The movements of the cool-down are opposite of the warm-up as they begin larger and decrease in intensity, range of motion, and speed. Flexibility training is an important part of any exercise program and is ideal to include during the cool-down when muscles are warm and more easily stretched. After several minutes of the aerobic component of the cool-down, standing static stretches can be conducted to allow more time for the participants heart rates to decrease and to prevent blood from pool-

Table 21-1 Common Muscle Imbalances

Muscle	Problem	Typical Cause	Correction
Pectoralis Major	Tight	Poor posture when sitting and standing	Stretch
Posterior deltoid, middle trapezius, rhomboids	Weak, overstretched	Poor posture when sitting and standing	Strengthen
Shoulder internal rotators	Tight	Poor posture, carrying and holding objects close to body	Stretch
Shoulder external rotators	Weak	Poor posture	Strengthen
Abdominals	Weak	Poor posture, obesity	Strengthen
Erector spinae	Tight & weak	Poor posture, obesity	Stretch & strengthen
Hip flexors	Tight	Poor posture, sedentary lifestyle, prolonged sitting	Stretch
Hamstrings	Tight	Sedentary lifestyle, prolonged sitting	Stretch
Calves	Tight	Wearing high heels	Stretch
Tibialis anterior	Weak	Not enough use in activities of daily living	Strengthen

ing in the lower extremities. To avoid the aforementioned, a proper cool-down is highly recommended before transitioning to stretches or core work in a prone or supine position. Planning class segments and exercises carefully is important to allow all class components to be included during the allotted time. Incomplete planning can lead to limited time focused on the cool-down and flexibility training, even though both are important components for participant safety.

Flexibility Segment

It is important to stretch all the major muscle groups, giving special attention to those muscles that are commonly tight. For example, after an indoor cycling class, stretching the hip flexors, quadriceps, hamstrings, and calves is important since these are major muscles used during an indoor cycling class and are often tight.

ACSM (2018) suggests performing static stretches for 10 to 30 seconds for most adults, two to four repetitions per muscle group, a minimum of two to three days per week. However, it's not always possible to perform four repetitions in a group exercise setting; therefore, participants should be encouraged to perform additional stretching on their own.

Benefits of Flexibility Training:
- Enhanced performance of activities of daily living
- Decreased low-back pain
- Decreased risk of injury
- Reduced muscle tension
- Increased relaxation
- Increased ROM
- Decreased stress and tension
- Increased mind-body connection
- Improved posture

Table 21-2 Group Exercise Class Components

The group exercise instructor pre-class preparation:
- ✓ Is available before class; welcomes and orients new participants
- ✓ Discusses and models appropriate attire and footwear, and brings water to class
- ✓ Has music cued and equipment ready before class begins
- ✓ Give the class INTRO (introduces him or herself, name of class, type of class, reassures new participants and organizes equipment)

Warm-up Segment
- ✓ Includes an appropriate amount of dynamic movements
- ✓ Includes rehearsal moves and dynamic movements
- ✓ Offers clear verbal direction and ensures that volume, temp, and environment created by the music are all appropriate

Cardiorespiratory Segment
- ✓ Gradually increases exercise intensity
- ✓ Provides intensity options (progression/regression)
- ✓ Builds sequences progressively and logically
- ✓ Uses music to create a motivational atmosphere
- ✓ Monitors intensity using HR, RPE, or talk test

Muscular Conditioning Segment
- ✓ Encourages muscle balance
- ✓ Observes participants' form and technique, and suggests modifications for injuries or special needs
- ✓ Offers appropriate verbal, visual, and physical cues on form and technique
- ✓ Utilizes equipment safely and effectively
- ✓ Creates a motivational atmosphere

Flexibility Segment
- ✓ Performs stretching of major muscle groups in a safe and effective manner
- ✓ Concludes with relaxation and visualization

Chapter Summary

The fundamental components of a group exercise class discussed in this chapter are important for participant safety. Successful fitness classes require both proper planning and preparation, and each component should be thoughtfully designed by the instructor. Every group exercise format will involve different activities and movements; however, the basic structure of each class format should remain similar to one another. Fitness professionals are highly encouraged to gain additional knowledge and training for all class formats they intend to instruct. The fitness industry is constantly changing and evolving, therefore it is in the best interest of group exercise instructors to stay informed regarding emerging trends related to equipment and class formats. Instructors who are knowledgeable and are able to teach multiple formats are a great asset to both their fitness facility and participants.

Chapter References:

Alter, M.J. (2004). *Science of flexibility*. Champaign, IL: Human Kinetics.

American College of Sports Medicine (2018). *ACSM's Guidelines for Exercise Testing and Prescription,* 9th edition. Philadelphia, PA: Wolters Kluwer.

Graef, F.I., & Kruel, L.F.M. (2006). Heart rate and perceived exertion at aquatic environment: Differences in relation to land environment and applications for exercise prescription-A review. *Revista Brasileira de Medicina do Esporte*, 12(4), 221-228.

Hedrick, A. (2000). Dynamic flexibility training. *Strength & Conditioning Journal*, 22(5), 33-38.

Kennedy-Armbruster, C., & Yoke, M. (2014). *Methods of Group Exercise Instruction*. Champaign, IL. Human Kinetics.

Chapter 21 Review Questions

1. Which of the following is the most accurate regarding the cardiorespiratory segment?
    A. Include an appropriate amount of dynamic movements
    B. Static stretching should be performed
    C. Rehearsal moves should be performed
    D. Monitors intensity using HR, RPE, or Talk Test

2. Which class format has the greatest need for an experienced instructor to assist the participant with equipment set up?
    A. Kickboxing
    B. Indoor Group Cycling
    C. Step
    D. High Intensity Interval Training

3. Which of the following class formats was originally created for use by athletes?
    A. Kickboxing
    B. Indoor Group Cycling
    C. Boot Camp
    D. High Intensity Interval Training

4. Increased speed and force of muscle contractions and increased tendon, ligament, and muscle elasticity are all potential physiological benefits of a _____.
    A. warm-up
    B. cardiorespiratory phase
    C. muscle conditioning phase
    D. cool-down

5. A group exercise instructor's demonstration of proper exercise form and technique provides _____ cue.
    A. a visual
    B. a verbal
    C. an auditory
    D. a kinesthetic

6. During which class component is it most appropriate to perform dynamic stretching?
    A. Warm-up
    B. Cardiorespiratory phase
    C. Muscle conditioning phase
    D. Cool-down

Answers to Review Questions on Page 384

Note: Review questions are intended to reinforce learning and comprehension of subject matter presented in the corresponding chapter.
The review questions are not intended to be representative of actual certification exam questions in terms of style, content, or difficulty.

22
Leadership, Communication, & Motivation

Introduction
An effective class begins with the right attitude, professionalism, and pre-class leadership demonstrated by the instructor. A welcoming environment builds a sense of community and is often what brings individuals to a group exercise setting. The environment created can be influenced by a wide range of factors such as the quality of instruction, communication skills, and ability to motivate class participants. Each factor is influenced by the GEI's attitude and professionalism.

Pre-class Leadership
Preparing to teach a group exercise class involves more than choosing the choreography, designing the class, and selecting fun music. Pre-class leadership should also include an evaluation of the room and equipment available prior to class. Equipment also includes audio equipment (e.g., sound system and microphone). The GEI should be familiar with where the sound system is located, how to operate the equipment, and where additional batteries are located.

Evaluating the Space and Equipment
A GEI should evaluate the size of the room and equipment availability prior to designing a class. If the room is small, has support columns in the center, or has carpet, the format and design of the class should reflect these factors. The type of equipment available to the instructor will also dictate the class format. Instructors should not only ask what equipment is available, but where it is located. It is not uncommon for fitness facilities to store their group exercise equipment in multiple studios, so knowing when and what equipment is available at a particular class time is important. Any group exercise equipment that does not appear to be functioning properly should be removed from storage and turned-in to the facility manager or made inaccessible to participants. An evaluation of audio equipment (e.g., volume and bass) should also be completed to ensure a pleasant sound experience for all.

Creating the Class Environment
Successful group exercise instructors understand the importance of creating an energetic and welcoming environment to set the tone of the class. Begin with an inspiring introduction that creates a feeling of inclusion and acceptance for individuals of all skill levels and abilities. This can be achieved through an introduction, greeting participants by name, facing the students as often as possible, making eye contact, and establishing rapport. GEIs should always make a brief statement at the beginning of each class that includes an introduction or "INTRO." Even if participants are not new to the class, this type of opening statement is a good practice and reminder to the attendees that the GEI is ready to start class.

- **I:** **Introduce** yourself
- **N:** Tell participants the **Name** of the class
- **T:** Tell participants what **Type** of group exercise class they are attending
- **R:** **Reassure** new participants
- **O:** Tell participant what equipment they will need and how to **Organize** it

An **INTRO** may sound something like this, *"Welcome, my name is Samantha (introduction) and I will be teaching All Strength (name of class) today. This strength class includes a total body strength conditioning workout (type of class). If you're working on building strength, I can assure you there will be exercise options and you can always use a lighter set of dumbbells, if needed (reassure those who are new). Time to get your equipment. I'd like everyone to get a mat and two sets of dumbbells, one light set and one heavy set (tell participants to get and organize their equipment)."*

Communication Skills
Teaching group exercise classes is about establishing and maintaining relationships. The more group exercise instructors understand how to communicate with class participants, the more effective an instructor will be. Good communication is the foundation of successful relationships, and success in the health and fitness industry is dependent on the ability to establish positive relationships. Group exercise instructors often place a great deal of value on the process of providing information and instruction; however, the challenge for many fitness professionals is to become proficient at listening. The concept of giving and receiving information is a form of communication referred to as feedback.

Verbal and Nonverbal Communication Skills

The basis of how people communicate can be described by "what we say" (verbal communication), "how we say it" (paraverbal communication), and how we look when we deliver a message (nonverbal communication). Understanding the importance and proper application of each can significantly impact the success of a GEI. For example, the actual delivery of the message is more than simply what you say, as explained by the 7% - 38% - 55% rule. When we deliver a message, 7% is the content of words, 38% is tone of voice, and 55% is body language. If body language, tone of voice, and words disagree, then body language and tone of voice will carry more weight than the words. See figure 22-1.

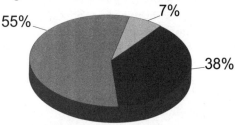

Figure 22-1 Verbal and Nonverbal Communication Skills

- What you say. Actual Words.
- How you say it. Tone of voice.
- How you look. Body Language.

Verbal communication is often referred to by GEIs as "feedback" and is a critical component and the success of any instructor. Tone of voice and the rhythm of speech are also critical components of verbal communication (both factors are directly related to the potential of motivating the class). Tone of voice refers to inflection and shows excitement of the instructor. Rhythm of speech impacts the ability of participants to understand directions. Open hand gestures (figure 22-2) displays trust. Closed or hand facing down commands authority.

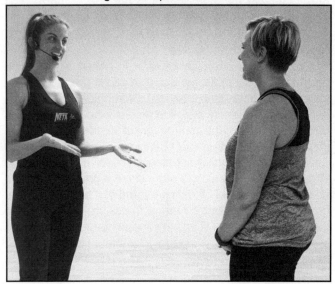

Figure 22-2 *Open Hand Gesture*

Understanding the importance of nonverbal communication skills is critical for GEIs. The body language of an instructor can have a major impact of the perception of the participants. Participants will be evaluating the body language of the instructor from the moment he or she enters the room, which plays a large role in setting the tone for the class. A closed posture with arms crossed (figure 22-3) can display disinterest or being closed off. A GEI should keep their body open and relaxed.

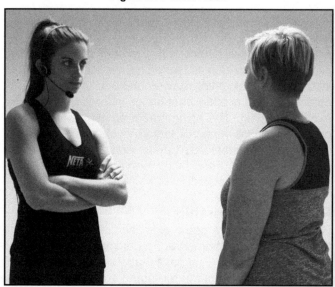

Figure 22-3 Closed Posture

Check your nonverbal communication skills:

Facial Expressions and Eye Contact
- ✓ Does your face express enthusiasm?
- ✓ Are you able to make eye contact with participants?

Tone of Voice
- ✓ Does your tone of voice include appropriate inflections?
- ✓ Does your tone of voice express enthusiasm?

Posture and Gestures
- ✓ Does your body convey enthusiasm?
- ✓ Does your body appear to be relaxed and stress free?

Touch
- ✓ Are you comfortable using touch as a cue?
- ✓ Can you read the body language of a participant before using touch as a cue?

Keys to Successful Feedback

Feedback serves two main purposes. From the viewpoint of the instructor, appropriate feedback is a means to provide corrections that will either reinforce or improve the performance of each participant. From the viewpoint of the participant, appropriate feedback includes following verbal and/or visual cues and ensuring that the instructor knows whether or not the participants understand his or her directions. The key to providing appropriate feedback is to constantly watch the participants and provide information based upon their responses. GEIs should provide participants with information that will enhance their opportunities for success while maintaining a safe and effective exercise environment. Instructors can enhance the motivation of the participants by providing feedback that is growth-oriented and positive, so that participants understand the correct way to preform movements. For example, when performing a plank, ask class participants to maintain a flat back position and to engage the core. For those individuals who are not able to maintain the flat back position, it is helpful to provide immediate feedback that is specific and that they can relate to. Immediately point out that the back should be flat as a board, so the participant could balance a glass of water (analogy) on it. In addition, the instructor could emphasize that having a strong core may reduce back pain.

The Keys to Feedback:
- Provide feedback immediately (once the instructor observes the need for a correction)
- Be specific with comments
- Make comments growth-oriented and positive
- Use analogies participants understand

Transtheoretical Model and Readiness to Change

One role of a GEI is to appropriately motivate class participants. Motivation is linked to behavior change and explained in the model, known as the transtheoretical model (TTM) of behavior change developed by Prochaska and DiClemente in the late 1970s. The model identifies five specific stages that individuals progress through as they adopt and maintain a new habit or behavior. See table 22-1. Researchers have since adapted the original model to apply specifically to physical activity (Marcus et al., 1992). Group exercise class participants will be at the preparation, action, or maintenance stage. It is the role of instructors to aid all participants to progress towards and remain in the maintenance stage. There are numerous strategies that instructors can apply during classes to help participants increase and maintain overall physical activity levels throughout their lifespan. Some of those strategies include influencing attitudes and assisting an individual as he or she thinks through a situation. See chapter 3 to learn more about behavior change and the TTM. The next section discusses strategies to promote motivation and exercise adherence.

Motivation

Motivation is the degree of determination, drive, or desire with which an individual approaches (or avoids) a behavior. Motivation is said to be intrinsic or extrinsic.

Intrinsic motivation involves participation in an activity for the experience, self-satisfaction, personal gratification, or sense of accomplishment. People who are intrinsically motivated report being physically active because they truly enjoy it. Such participation in an activity is associated with positive attitudes and emotions (e.g., happiness and relaxation) when faced with barriers.

The reality is that most adults depend on some amount of extrinsic motivation. Extrinsic motivation involves the engagement in an activity for benefits and reinforcement from outside of the self, such as tangible rewards or recognition by others.

Group exercise instructors can help create an optimal environment for building the intrinsic motivation of participants by striving to enhance the feelings of enjoyment and accomplishment that come with participating in classes. This can be done by providing clear and consistent feedback, taking into account participant's feedback regarding class design, and create a welcoming environment which was discussed earlier in this chapter. All of these factors will increase the degree of motivation during class.

Table 22-1 Transtheoretical Model

Stages of Change	
Precontemplation	inactive and not thinking about becoming active
Contemplation	inactive but thinking about becoming active
Preparation	physically active but not at the recommended levels (30 min or more of moderate-intensity physical activity on most, preferably all days of the week)
Action	physically active at the recommended levels and have been active for <6 months
Maintenance	physically active at the recommended levels and have been for 6 or more months

The following is a list of strategies to promote motivation and exercise adherence:

- **Enjoyable Activities** – if participants enjoy it, they are more likely to continue (intrinsic motivation)
- **Availability and Convenience** – consider time, equipment needs, portability of program, and access to facilities.
- **Health Benefits vs. Appearance** – research has demonstrated that emphasis on physical appearance as an outcome 'measure' decreases self-esteem, reduces positive affect, increases negative perceptions of body image, increases social anxiety, and increases depression (Lox et al., 2016).
- **Social Support** – those with support are better able to overcome lapses and retain motivation, especially when supporting individuals are adopting or maintaining the same lifestyle behaviors. Group exercise classes can be an opportunity to create social support and accountability.

Types of Learning

The process of learning is actually a process of self-discovery and therefore will occur differently among class participants. Nicholl (1997) describes the preferences as three styles of learning: visual, verbal/auditory, and kinesthetic. Research also indicates that most individuals do not only use one learning style; they often occur together. However, there is always a preferred style for various activities.

The visual learner prefers to learn through sight. This type of learning is often very social and responds favorably to the use of charts, videos, and articles. They can learn specifics by watching demonstrations and taking notes for review at a later time.

The verbal/auditory learner prefers to learn through hearing or listening. This type of learner is often analytical and responds to verbal directions, so the instructor's tone of voice and pace of speech are major factors that influence learning.

Kinesthetic learner prefers to learn by doing the skill or exercise introduced. They also benefit from physical assistance from the instructor, so it may be helpful for the instructor to be more 'hands-on' by actually assisting the participant in order to ensure proper execution of the skill or exercise. The GEI should always ask for and receive permission prior to assisting or physically touching any participant in class.

A common mistake many GEIs make is to teach using predominately their personally preferred style. Keep in mind that the majority of the population prefer visual learning and athletes tend to be kinesthetic, so apply various teaching styles to address all learning preferences.

Chapter Summary

Providing a positive exercise environment requires the application of many different skills and strategies by the GEI. An instructor should ensure that participants feel welcome, learn effectively, and are working towards their goals. It is important that instructors move beyond emphasizing the magnitude of fitness gains and future outcomes and understand that the real power of exercise lies in the experience itself. Understanding and applying the principles of pre-class leadership, communication, and motivation described in this chapter will help the GEI become a more effective instructor and fitness professional.

Chapter References:

Dunn, A.L., Marcus, B.H., Kampert, J.B., Garcia, M.E., Kohl III, H.W., & Blair, S.N. (1999). Project Active—A 24-month randomized trial to compare lifestyle and structured physical activity interventions. *Journal of the American Medical Association*, 281, 327-334.

Lox, C.L., Martin Ginis, K.A., & Petruzzello, S.J., (2016) *The Psychology of Exercise: Integrating Theory and Practice*, 3rd edition. Scottsdale, AZ: Holcomb Hathaway, Publishers, Inc.

Marcus, B.H., Rossi, J.S., Selby, V.C., Niaura, R.S., & Abrams, D.B. (1992). The stages and processes of exercise adoption and maintenance in a worksite sample. *Health Psychology*, 11(6), 386-95.

Nicholl, M.J. (1997). *Accelerated Learning For The 21st Century*. New York, NY: Dell Publishing.

Prochaska, J.O., & DiClemente, C.C. (1994). *The Transtheoretical Approach: Crossing Traditional Boundaries of Therapy*, Reprint edition. Malabar, FL: Krieger Publishing Company.

Chapter 22 Review Questions

1. Voice inflection, rate of speech, and tonality are all referred to as which component of a message?
   A. Verbal Communication
   B. Paraverbal Communication
   C. Nonverbal Communication
   D. Kinesthetic Communication

2. Which of the following reflects the most pure form of intrinsic motivation?
   A. "I exercise because I enjoy it."
   B. "I exercise to look better."
   C. "I exercise because my doctor says I should."
   D. "I exercise to get a health insurance discount."

3. Eye contact and facial expressions are both forms of _____ skills.
   A. verbal communication
   B. paraverbal communication
   C. nonverbal communication
   D. Kinesthetic communication

4. A class participant mentions that she catches on best to new moves by watching the instructor's demonstration. What is most likely to be the participant's preferred learning style?
   A. Visual
   B. Auditory
   C. Olfactory
   D. Kinesthetic

5. Group exercise instructors can help create an optimal environment for building the _____ of participants by striving to enhance the feelings of enjoyment and accomplishment.
   A. intrinsic motivation
   B. extrinsic motivation
   C. amotivation
   D. promotivation

6. During a pre-class inspection of equipment to be used during a group exercise class, the instructor notices several pieces of resistance tubing are worn and close to snapping in two. Which of the following is the most appropriate course of action?
   A. Instruct the class participants to be especially careful when using the worn resistance tubing.
   B. Remove the worn resistance tubing from the studio and inform the group exercise manager.
   C. Return the worn resistance tubing to the equipment storage room and select different tubing.
   D. Allow only experienced class participants to use the worn tubing and replace when it snaps.

Answers to Review Questions on Page 384

Note: Review questions are intended to reinforce learning and comprehension of subject matter presented in the corresponding chapter. The review questions are not intended to be representative of actual certification exam questions in terms of style, content, or difficulty.

23
Teaching a Group Exercise Class

Introduction

Establishing class objectives are key to group exercise instruction. Setting a class objective defines what the instructor expects the participants to learn or gain from that particular class.

Select the objectives for a class based on the format, and participants' skills and abilities. For example, in a circuit training class, the objective could be to alternate cardio, strength, and core movements for 30 to 40 minutes to improve cardiorespiratory fitness, muscular strength, and build core stability.

Exercise selection then becomes easy because it fits into class goals and objectives. Coaching tips are purposeful and lead participants towards reaching that class goal. When classes are designed with clear goals and objectives, the participants gain more focus and have a purpose.

Class Design

The best group exercise classes are well-planned to balance as many different variables as possible. However, there are always aspects of the group experience that cannot be controlled, like participants coming in late or their energy level, but GEIs can control most aspects of the group exercise class design. Novice instructors can benefit from a "class design planning sheet." A class template helps the instructor prepare for, plan, and practice various components of the class.

The group exercise planning sheet (table 23-1) has a list of considerations at the top followed by three major sections: "warm-up," "conditioning phase," and "cool-down." These three phases merit equal planning and preparation, while keeping the objectives or "purpose" of each section in knowing why specific movements were chosen. In the choreography delivery method section, an instructor might design a freestyle class using a linear progression. For each of the three sections of class, the instructor can plan the timeframe and the moves they wish to include, being sure to create enough familiarity with these moves to be able to offer progressions and regressions, in terms of both intensity and complexity. The final column, "purpose," helps instructors see that their movements have purpose, ensuring they fit into the goals and objectives.

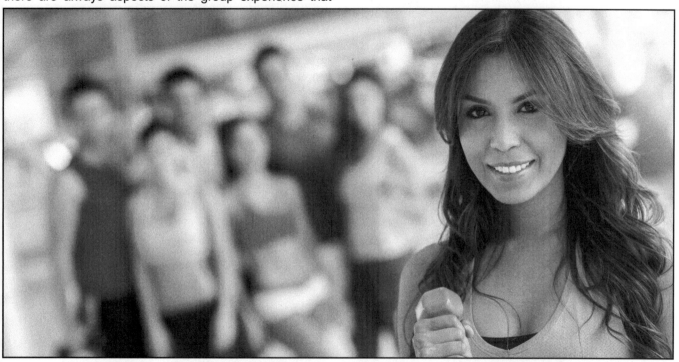

Table 23-1 Class Design Planning Sheet

| Format: |
| Total Time: |
| Class Goals/Objectives: |
| Equipment Needed: |
| Music: |

Warm-up

Duration	Exercise (progression/regression)	Purpose

Class Body

Duration	Exercise (progression/regression)	Purpose

Cool-down

Duration	Exercise (progression/regression)	Purpose

Class Configuration

Class configuration refers to the physical layout used by instructors to provide their participants with maximum opportunities for learning throughout class. All group exercise classes should be arranged to ensure the safety of participants. Be mindful of appropriate space per group exercise participants. The *American College of Sports Medicine Health/Fitness Facility Standards and Guidelines* (2012) recommends 40 - 60 square feet per participant at any given time in a group exercise room. The safety of participants also includes the ability to hear the instructor over the music, not only for safety, but also for other factors including crowd control and motivation. In the most typical group exercise class configuration, the instructor stands at the front of the room either facing a mirror or the participants. Typically, the most experienced participants naturally stand in the front of the room while the less experienced participants tend to 'hide in the back of the studio.' Therefore, instructors should become accustomed to teaching to the participants in the front and back of the studio at all times, providing equal attention and instruction to all. The GEI must be mindful to avoid unknowingly embarrassing a participants or making someone feel uncomfortable through unwanted attention.

Class Duration

Group exercise classes can range from 30-minutes ("express") to 60-minutes, and even 90-minutes in length. The class duration depends on the class goals and objectives, and the format presented. For example, a high intensity interval training (H.I.I.T) class would typically be designed with a 2:1 ratio, where participants are working harder for a short duration providing a time-efficient class option of 30 minutes. Regardless of the class duration, it is important to address all class components (e.g., warm-up, cardiorespiratory, muscle strength, flexibility, and cool-down). Adjust those components based on class duration, ensuring that none of the critical class components, such as the warm-up or cool-down, are omitted.

Pre-class Leadership and Preparation

Group exercise instructors should arrive early to class for several reasons. First, the instructor should set up their equipment and check to ensure that the equipment they will use that day is in good condition. Next, music should be cued and ready, and instructors may want to check volume, bass, and that the microphone is in working condition. Finally, they can establish rapport with participants even before the class starts, creating a welcome environment as discussed in chapter 20.

Exercise Selection

One of the most important tasks performed by the GEI is learning how to select appropriate exercises that will meet the goals and objective of the class and are safe and effective for all participants. Having both an understanding of exercise science and the purpose of each exercise is key. In addition, the GEI may have participants inquire about exercises they have seen on the internet or on TV, so a good understanding of exercise science is a must.

Using the exercise selection criteria below helps instructors get into the habit of analyzing exercises to identify joint actions, proper biomechanics, and appropriate progressions or regressions. Working through the exercise selection criteria requires time and practice.

Exercise Class Selection Criteria
To ensure effectiveness, promote safety, good posture, proper alignment, and balanced biomechanics, it is crucial that an instructor consider the following when selecting exercises for their class.

When designing a class it is important for an instructor to ask the following questions:

1. What is the goal and objective of this class?
   - Is the purpose muscular strength, cardiorespiratory endurance, to challenge both the anaerobic and aerobic energy systems (i.e., metabolic conditioning) or enhance flexibility?
2. Which joint actions (and other movements) achieve that goal and objective safely?
   - When using bodyweight as resistance, is the muscle action opposing gravity?
   - When using equipment, is the appropriate muscle being worked safely?
3. What exercise will be conducted to balance this exercise?
   - Conducting exercises for both upper back and chest, or both low back and abdominals.
4. What is the primary muscle group targeted in this exercise? What are the secondary muscle groups being utilized in this exercise? What is the movement pattern?
   - Does the class provide a balance of exercises including movements that push, pull, rotate, and squat?
5. Who is this class appropriate for?
   - What are appropriate exercise progressions and/or regressions for the success of all participants (beginner- level 1, intermediate- level 2, or advanced- level 3)?

Fundamental Choreography
Group exercise instructors should prepare objectives for all classes and then develop a plan to reach those objectives. When instructors design their plan for class it becomes choreography. Developing and delivering choreography can take many forms, repetition reduction, to add-on, from freestyle to various types of repeating choreography.

Base Moves
Base moves involve basic steps such as marching, heel taps, step touches, knee lifts, jumping jacks, and many others. When creating choreography, it is important to understand the base movements and how many counts (i.e., beats) each movement requires. This knowledge will assist an instructor in creating 4- and 8-count phrases of base moves that can be combined to create a 32-count phrase of choreography. See table 23-2 for base move.

Note: Starting position for all base moves is standing with feet hip-width apart.

Building a Basic 32-Count
Here are a few steps used when creating a basic 32-count of choreography:
1. Start with four lower-body moves that flow together. Select exercises that fill 8 counts for a total of 32 counts.
2. Find upper-body movements that go with the lower-body combination.
3. Check the combination:
   - Is the combination balanced (i.e., balance muscles groups)?
   - Can the movements be progressions/regressions (intensity options)?
   - Does the combination flow and do the movements have smooth transitions?
4. Repeat this process to create another 32-count combination or block of work.

Table 23-2 Summary of Base Movements

Base Move	Count(s)	Movement Description
March (R/L)	2 counts	Lift the right knee and return to starting position
Lunge	2 counts	Step right foot backwards into a lunge, and return right foot to starting position
Heel Taps	2 counts	Extend right leg from the hip and gently press right heel into the floor in front of body, return right foot back to starting position
Step Knee (Knee Lifts)	2 counts	Step right foot into floor, lift left knee up
Jack	2 counts	Jump both feet out wide, jump feet back together to meet in starting position
Step Touch	2 counts	Step right foot out to the right, step left foot to the right to meet the right foot
2 Step Touches (Grapevine)	4 counts	Step right foot out to the right, step left foot to the right to meet the right foot (or left foot crosses behind the right foot for grapevine), step right foot out to the right again, step left foot to the right to meet the right foot
V-Step	4 counts	Step right foot forward and out wide to the right, step left foot forward and out wide to the left, step right foot back to center, step left foot back to center

32-Count Example	
Count	Combination
8	Step Touch
8	Double Step Touch
8	Grapevine
8	Hamstring Curls
32 Count Phase	

Movement Variation

Movement variations can help you extend the life of your choreography, reduce overuse injuries, and boredom. Variations give the illusion of new choreography, when in fact GEIs are only tweaking the movements that participants are already familiar with. The primary elements of variation are the lever, plane, direction, and intensity.

Performing a lever variation means moving from a movement with a short lever to a movement with a long lever, or vice versa. For example, changing from a side knee lift to a side kick is a lever change. However, this element does not work for all movements. A plane variation is changing the plane of motion in which the movement takes place. For example, changing from a side kick to a front kick, changes the plane of motion from frontal to sagittal. A directional variation means changing the direction of the movement. If you are facing the back of the room, perform the same movement facing the front or side of the room. Directional variations can also mean traveling forward, backward, or diagonally. Lastly, intensity variations are movements that can be made more challenging by increasing the impact or intensity. For example, take a squat and performing a power squat, or a jumping jack to an air jack.

Transitions

When movements flow seamlessly from one to the next, choreography is easier, which leaves participants feeling successful. Creating smooth transitions can be simple, but it is best to change only one element at a time (e.g., lever, direction).

Some movements naturally transition smoothly from one to the next. Performing a plane change from a side kick to a front kick is an example of a smooth transition. Notice that each of the movements has the same starting and ending points. The smoothest transitions connect movements that have these points in common. Likewise, both the front raise and lateral raise begin and end with the arms in the same position at the sides of the body. These two movements flow together well because they share a common starting point: arms down. Thus, it is easy to transition back and forth between the two movements (Kennedy & Yoke, 2014).

One last factor for creating smooth transitions and easy-to-follow choreography is to select and maintain a lead foot throughout class. For example, when starting a march with the right foot (right foot leads on the first count or downbeat), then start your next movement (e.g., step touch) with the right lead. It is always wise to perform a combination with the right leg lead and then perform the same movement with the left leg lead to balance the body's neuromuscular system.

Choreography Delivery Strategies

Here are a few of many different choreography delivery strategies an instructor may use to help participants understand the movements by breaking down or building up a move or exercise routine:

Pyramid/Repetition Reduction

The pyramid/repetition reduction strategy involves reducing the number of repetitions that make up a sequence. An instructor may have participants execute eight alternating grapevines followed by four hamstring curls. This could be reduced to four alternating grapevines and two hamstring curls, eventually reduced to single repetitions.

Add-On or Part-to-Whole

A group exercise instructor, using the add-on or part-to-whole teaching strategy breaks down a movement in their simplest form. For example, when teaching burpees, an instructor might show proper push-up form and proper squat jump form before having participants perform a full burpee. Once participants have mastered each component, the instructor then demonstrates how to combine the movements to become more functional and challenging.

Simple-to-Complex

When using the simple-to-complex strategy, which is an advanced teaching strategy, instead of separating movement patterns into segments, the instructor will reduce all complexity options to the least common denominator and engage the class in movement. Next, the instructor adds layers of complexity onto these movements. For example, consider the performance of a grapevine and two alternating step-touches for a total of eight counts. The instructor engages all participants in this pattern from the start. While engaging everyone in repetition for mastery, the instructor offers additional options, which could include leaping to the side twice instead of the grapevine and a full 360-degree pivot with hamstring curls in place of the step-touches. Generally, additional complexity involves changes in lever, plane, and direction.

Freestyle

The freestyle strategy of choreography, also known as linear progression, requires the instructor to teach a movement or skill, and then changes to a new movement or skill. Instructors rarely return participants to previously taught movements to "add on" to them. For example, if a class starts with squats, then the class would not repeat squats again during that class period. Advantages of the freestyle method include varying exercises and movements that reduce boredom. A disadvantage of this delivery strategy is that participants are unable to sequence combinations of movements and repeat them as their proficiency improves because they cannot predict the next movement.

Repeating Choreography

Another choreography delivery strategy is repeating choreography. Repeating choreography has two forms: scripted and pre-planned. Instructors follow scripted with written music, cues, and movements all outlined from start to finish. The intent is a performance-like consistency of delivery, discouraging variations among instructors. Les Mills- BODY-PUMP™ is an example of a scripted choreography. An advantage from the perspective of participants includes the predictability of being able to gauge their intensity more effectively, since they know the format and movements, and can measure their improvements over time. A disadvantage of this type is that, because instructors must follow a script, there is often little room for customizing specific progressions and regressions as appropriate for the individuals in each class.

Pre-Planned

Lastly, pre-planned is another type of repeating choreography delivery strategy. Instructors receive guidelines and suggestions of what a class should include and as long as instructors follows these guidelines, they can make their own choices on things like, song selection, sequence, and movements. Examples of this type of choreography format include programs like Pi-Yo® and Zumba®. An advantage to the pre-planned choreography method from an instructor's perspective include receiving a class "in a box," but the freedom to add their own music, cues, and movements based on their class participants skill levels and abilities.

Integrating Music

Music is a vital part of almost all group exercise classes and is used as a way to motivate class participants and enhance the enjoyment of the class. Latin and hip-hop are common in dance-oriented classes. Pilates and yoga favor new age, smooth, jazz, and trance. Cardio and high-intensity classes gravitate toward club and top 40 music with strong rhythms. There typically is a mixture of music styles for indoor cycling and water classes. Ultimately, all music chosen should contribute to, rather than distract from, the overall class experience. It's always best to purchase music that is legally licensed and specifically prepared for fitness professionals and group exercise classes, because its phrases and beats are consistently developed according to industry-standardized beats-per-minute guidelines.

Music Volume

The United States Occupational Safety and Health Administration (OSHA) has established safety standards for noise levels for workers, states that ear protection must be provided for workers if noise level on the job average 90 decibels (dB) over an eight-hour period (Griest et al., 2007). Chronic exposure to loud noise can impair or damage hearing. It is generally recommended that music volume during a group exercise class should not exceed 90 decibels (ACSM, 2012; DeSimone, 2015). When in doubt, a group exercise instructor should play the music volume at a level that allows participants to hear the instructor's voice and cues clearly at all times.

Beat, Measure, and Phrase

Understanding the components of music is essential for any GEI. The beat is made up of a regular pulsations that usually have an even rhythm and occur in a continuous pattern of strong and weak pulsations. Strong pulsations collectively form the **downbeat**, while the weaker pulsations form the **upbeat**. A **measure** is comprised of a series of downbeats and upbeats that are organized into a pattern. Most popular music includes measures that contain 4 beats per measure and is said to be in 4/4 metered time, which indicates there are four beats and four quarter notes in each measure. When measures are placed together, a phrase is created. A **phrase** consists of 2 measures or more, and when combined, can create an 8-count phrase (2 measures), a 16-count phrase (4 measures) or a 32-count phrase (8 measures). A 32-count phrase is ideal for creating choreography for exercise classes. Table 23-3 provides a graphic of music structure.

Table 23-3 Music Structure

	Music Structure			
Downbeat	★★★★★★★★	★★★★★★★★	★★★★★★★★	★★★★★★★★
Numerical Value of Downbeat	1 2 3 4 5 6 7 8	1 2 3 4 5 6 7 8	1 2 3 4 5 6 7 8	1 2 3 4 5 6 7 8
Measures	[- - - -][- - - -]	[- - - -][- - - -]	[- - - -][- - - -]	[- - - -][- - - -]
8-Count Phrase	[- - - - - - - -]	[- - - - - - - -]	[- - - - - - - -]	[- - - - - - - -]
32-Count Phrase	[- -]			

When choosing music for a particular class, the first consideration is whether the music's role will be in the foreground or background. When music is in the foreground, instructors will incorporate its **tempo** in the class. Examples of using music in the foreground include stepping to the downbeat, used when performing step and choreography formats. When music is in the background, tempo is not a factor. Music if often used in the background in yoga, boot camp, and some types of circuit training classes where music is a motivator, but not a key player in determining speed of movement. However, not all class formats fall clearly into these two roles of music. Indoor cycling classes and water classes include both foreground and background music.

The two main considerations when choosing music are purpose and participants. Understanding the music's purpose helps the group exercise instructor understand what types of music would be most appropriate for the goals and objectives of class. For example, if the purpose is cardiorespiratory training, such as in step or water conditioning classes, choosing music with a consistent tempo would be wise. Knowing the class participants and their musical preferences also helps enhance the class experiences for everyone.

Tempo should be carefully considered as it can dictate the energy level of the class, the speed of movement, and the intensity of an exercise. Tempo is determined by selecting music with the appropriate beat per minute (BPM) based on the class format and participants' ability level.

Please note that tempo recommendations vary among different organizations in the fitness industry, but table 23-4 summarizes generally-accepted guidelines. Instructors should use their best judgment when selecting music tempo based on the general ability and fitness level of their class participants.

When creating music specifically for group exercise, most music companies make it easy for instructors to find the start of the musical phrases. Adding special elements like distinct chorus, drum rolls, and vocal cues all help the seasoned ear pick up the start of a 32-count phrase. In addition, seasoned instructors are able to cue in advance of the start of each musical phrase so that their participants can begin a 32-count combination at the start, or "top," of the musical phrase.

The following companies have music CDs or music apps formatted for various fitness classes.
- AeroBeats www.aerobeats.com
- Dynamix www.dynamixmusic.com
- Muscle Mixes www.musclemixes.com
- Power Music www.workoutmusic.com

Music Mastery
Steps to practice music mastery:
- Find the downbeat and march in place. Next, locate the 32-count phrase. At the top of each musical phrase, practice cueing "8-7-6-5-4-3-2-1" with the music.
- Practice cueing "8-7-6-5" for the first four counts of music and then substituting the four words "tell (4) – them (3) – what (2) - to/do (1)" for the last four counts of music.
- When ready, practice cueing "8-7-6-5" for the first four counts of music and then substituting specific verbal movement cues for the last four counts, such as "8-7-6-5, grapevine to the left."

As a GEI becomes skillful at cueing movements at least four counts before the movement is to happen, they can then give meaningful cues in place of the four counts of "8-7-6-5." These cues could be for direction, form, alignment, and motivation. As an example of the total mastery in this case would be "grapevine left and right and shoulders down and back."

Warm-Up Cueing Sample

Step 1. "Let's start marching." The instructor makes sure that everyone finds the beat and chats with the class while waiting for the last few beats of the phrase, at which point he or she can start cueing the rest of the movements at the top of the phrase.

Step 2. "8-7-6-5, alternating grapevine left and right" (4 counts each so a total of 8 counts of music).

Step 3. "Shoulders down and back, two grapevines lefts and right" (for a total of 8 counts of music).

Table 23-4 Recommended Beats Per Minute (Tempo)

Group Exercise Format	General BPM Guidelines
Indoor Cycling	60-110
Yoga/Pilates	<110-120
Step	118-128
Low Impact Cardiorespiratory Training	120-140
Resistance Training/Muscle Toning	122-129
High Impact Cardiorespiratory Training	135-155

The GEI should continue to cue this movement until the majority of the class demonstrates mastery of the combination with minimal dependence on the cueing. When the instructor is ready to add more movement, such as step touches, he or she could cue:

Step 4. "8-7-6-5, step-touches left and right" (for a total of 8 counts of music). When the class demonstrates mastery of the new move, the instructor can provide additional cues.

Step 5. "8-7-6-5, four alternating knee lifts moving forward" (for a total of eight counts of music). Again, when mastery is demonstrated, add additional cues.

Step 6. "8-7-6-5, hamstring curls moving backward, with single, single, double" (for a total of 8 counts of music).

Notice how the warm-up cueing sample (table 23-5) provides verbal cues ("two grapevines left and right"), numerical cues ("four"), and directional cues ("moving forward or backward"), but only in small increments, each taking up between four and eight counts of music. Below is the combination in its whole.

Music Copyright Laws and Licensing

Purchasing music specifically designed for fitness professionals is ideal as the beats and phrases are consistent, the music is blended into continuous 32-count phrases, the BPM are based on the class format and industry standards, and the music has a strong, easy-to-hear beat. Furthermore, it is illegal to use copyrighted music in group fitness classes without obtaining the necessary licensures. Without these licensures, it can place instructors and fitness centers in jeopardy of violating copyright laws and facing potential fines and penalties.

The 1976 U.S. Copyright Law allows original artists to copyright their media (e.g., music, video, choreography) and states that copyright owners have the right to charge a fee for the use of their music in a public performance. All fitness classes fall into the category of public performance; therefore, instructors cannot legally copy or play copyrighted music in their classes without paying for the right to do so.

Some companies (e.g., Power Music, Muscle Mixes) have paid for the license and rights to legally obtain a master recording for group exercise music (e.g., CD, digital format), and are able to duplicate that recording for public sale. It is important to note that the license fees paid by these companies protect the company and not the instructor. Therefore, it is important that fitness clubs and studios ob-

Counts or Beats?

When you instruct your class to do 8 counts of squats, does it mean to squat for 8 music beats or to do 8 repetitions of squats? If 8 counts refers to music beats, you have to decide the exercise execution speed to know how many repetitions to perform. For example, you can squat down in 1 beat, come up in 1 beat stopping after you hit the 8th beat, resulting in 4 repetitions. Alternatively, taking 2 beats to squat down and 2 beats to come up would result in 2 repetitions. On the other hand, use 4 beats down and 4 beats to come up for 1 completed repetition.

If 8 counts refers to 8 repetitions, you use 16 music beats when you preform the exercise at a pace of 1 beat down and 1 beat up. If your pace is 2 beats down and 2 beats up, it takes 32 music beats. If the pace is 4 beats down and 4 beats up, it takes 64 counts to complete the same tasks.

Every count is always a music beat, but every music beat is not always a count. To avoid confusion whenever you give a numerical cue, clearly communicate if you are cueing music beats, music counts (may or may not be the same as a beat), or repetition.

Table 23-5 Warm-up Cueing Sample

Warm-up Sample Combination		
#	Movement	Counts
1	LLL: Two alternating grapevines	1-8
2	LLL: Four alternating step-touched in place	9-16
3	LLL: Four alternating knee lifts moving forward	17-24
4	LLL: Hamstring curls moving backward (SSD)	25-32
Repeat the 32- count combo with the right leg lead (RRL)		
Notes: LLL = Left Leg Lead; RLL = Right Leg Lead; SSD = Single, Single, Double		

tain a music license to avoid copyright infringement. If an instructor teaches in a home studio or as an independent contractor, the instructor is responsible for paying these fees.

For more information about licensing fees and requirements, contact the agencies listed in table 23-6.

Table 23-6 Music Licensing Resources

The American Society of Composers, Authors and Publishers (ASCAP)
1900 Broadway New York, NY 10023
1-800-952-7227
www.ascap.com

Broadcast Music, Inc. (BMI)
7 World Trade Center
250 Greenwich Street
New York, NY 10007-0030
(212) 220-3000
www.bmi.com

SESAC, Inc. (formerly the Society of European Stage Authors and Composers)
55 Music Square East
Nashville, TN 37203
(615) 320-0055
www.sesac.com

Cueing

Fitness professionals utilize cueing techniques to communicate class movements, correct biomechanics, and provide motivation and education to their participants. Proper cueing is one of the most difficult tasks an instructor can undertake. It can lead to participant's frustration if done poorly or success if done well. Therefore, it is important for a group exercise instructor to have knowledge of the different types of cueing, as well as the ability to communicate cues effectively. Here are three general cueing categories: verbal/visual, technique/safety, and motivational.

Movement Cues

There are several types of cues that GEIs should use, movement (verbal and visual), safety, and motivational cues. Movement cues are verbal instructions on what to do and when to do it. Describe the exercise or movement and give signals, or cues, to indicate when the exercise will start, stop, or change. Verbal cues include the name of the exercise (e.g., grapevine), directions (e.g., to the right), and when it will happen (e.g., 5-4-3-grapevine-here).

It is important to allow for reaction time by cueing on counts 5 of the 8-count phrase, which allows counts 4 – 1 for participants to react to the indicated change. For example, practice cueing "8-7-6-5" for the first four counts of music and then substituting the four words "tell (4) – them (3) – what (2) - to/do (1)" for the last four counts of music. Providing cues too early or too late can cause participants to move too quickly or not to move on time and become frustrated.

It is recommended that verbal cues be positive, concise, and consistent. Positive cueing assists participants in developing a sense of success and accomplishment. Cues should also be short in duration since lengthy explanations can be confusing and most participants will only hear the first few words spoken. Additionally, counting every repetition or move can become monotonous and eliminates the instructor's opportunity to utilize other beneficial cues. These include offering progressions or regressions to accommodate the ability level of each individual. Also, it is advisable to keep the names of movements consistent to enable participants to transition easily into the next movement without spending unnecessary time contemplating which movement is being cued.

Another important aspect of verbal cueing is an instructor's voice as it can be used to help set the tone of the class and create the desired experience for participants (e.g., peaceful for yoga or authoritative for boot camp). The use of voice variations can engage participants' interest and signal that a change in movement is going to occur. The use of a microphone is recommended for most class formats to help protect the instructor's vocal chords.

Visual cueing uses the body, hand gestures, signage, or pictures to convey a message. Pointing right will help your class see which way to move. Holding your hand up can signal to hold or stop. Fingers can designate the number of repetitions left to perform. A visual preview is a demonstration of the next movement or exercise to come. Instructors can have class continue with an exercise while demonstrating the next movement. Visual previews are advantageous when introducing an exercise for the first time and for teaching complex movements. See figures 23-1 to 23-8 for common visual group exercise cues.

Technique and Safety Cueing

Technique and safety cues are imperative to providing safe and effective classes for all. These cues, both verbal and visual, focus on appropriate technique while performing exercises, alignment, and breathing. For example, the movement cue for a squat is to bend at the hips, knees, and ankles. A technique cue might be, "keep the chest lifted during the squat." The same cue could be given visually by demonstrating the squat and tapping on the chest. When delivering technique and safety cues, it's important that you provide the class participants feedback. Here are five methods to deliver feedback to the class as a whole:

1. **General feedback.** Providing general feedback addresses the entire group at once. This is the first method of feedback for those making mistakes to remain

anonymous and can potentially correct the problem without drawing unnecessary attention to one specific individual. For example, the GEI may say , "I'd like you to keep your chest up and weight in your heels during the next four squats."

2. **Indirect feedback**. Adding body language to safety cues allows you to be a bit more specific with the participants without verbally identifying that individual. Through eye contact and gestures, try to gain the participant's attention and then give general feedback. With the same cue above, turn toward the participant, lock eyes with him or her, tap on your chest and point to the heels, and restate the same cue.

3. **Direct feedback.** Direct feedback involves addressing the participant by name or walking over to that individual. While sometimes it's the easiest method it should be used as a last resort. Be sure to keep the direct feedback and cues light hearted so that it's not seen as criticism or intimidation.

4. **Tactile feedback.** This method if often use in yoga, Pilates, and small group training classes. Using a hand-on approach, passively place the participant's limb in a precise position or guide a body part through a specific movement. Lightly touch the area of focus to clearly identify the muscle groups to engage or move, see figure 23-9. While also explaining where the movement should be felt, how it should feel, and what to do if they cannot feel it. While some learn well with this method it's not for all participants, and the GEI should be sure to gain permission to touch any participant.

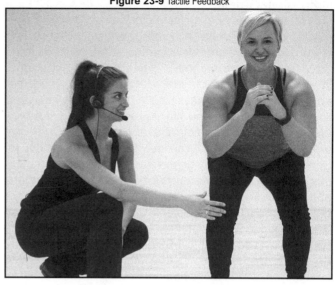

Figure 23-9 Tactile Feedback

5. **Delayed feedback.** If all other methods fail, delayed feedback can be used. Inform the participant who needs correction that you would like to see him or her after class for a few moments. Once the class is over, discuss the exercise, offer more instruction, and safety tips. Without other class participants around, avoid embarrassment to the individual and make that one on one connection.

Figure 23-1 Time Out

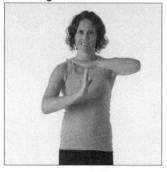

Figure 23-2 Hold/Stay

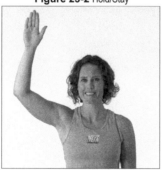

Figure 23-3 From the Top

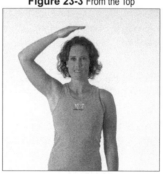

Figure 23-4 Number of Reps

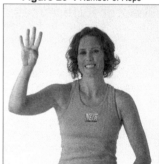

Figure 23-5 Forward

Figure 23-6 Backward

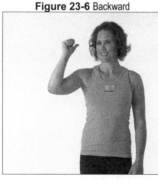

Figure 23-7 Thumbs Up

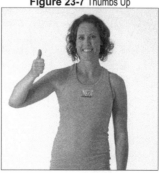

Figure 23-8 Direction

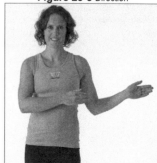

Motivational Cueing

Motivational cues help an instructor provide positive feedback to build confidence and energy within their class, and also encourages a greater work ethic within the class (e.g., "You are doing a great job!", "Feel how strong you are!", "You are athletic and can make it to the end!"). These examples are just a few ways for a group exercise instructor to integrate verbal cueing into classes. Over time, it is beneficial to listen to the motivational cues given. Cues that are used too frequently eventually lose their effectiveness. Some cues may simply be misplaced and sound ambiguous, or they lose their authenticity. While being energetic and upbeat is an expectation in a group class, it is not necessary to fill every moment with a "good job," or "way to go!" Choose words carefully. Keep in mind, participants can detect artificial enthusiasm and overhyped comments. Be sincere and genuine as to when the class could most benefit from words of inspiration.

Chapter Summary

A group exercise instructor must possess a variety of skills to be effective and successful. This chapter addressed some of the most challenging teaching skills including understanding music and the 32-count phrase, the intricacies of cueing, and the complexity of creating class choreography. Regardless of the exercise format or whether the class is choreographed to a 32-count phrase, instructors need to be knowledgeable regarding music structure, cueing techniques, adult learning styles, as well as the legal issues involved with playing copyrighted music. While not all classes involve choreography, all movements incorporated into a class should be planned, undergo an exercise analysis, and be cued properly for both participant and instructor success.

Chapter References

American College of Sports Medicine. (2012). ACSM's *Health/Fitness Facility Standards and Guidelines,* 4th edition. Champaign, IL: Human Kinetics.

DeSimone, G. (2015). *ACSM's Resources for the Group Exercise Instructor*. Philadelphia, PA: Wolters Kluwer Health/Lippincott Williams & Wilkins.

Griest, S.E., Folmer, R.L., & Martin, W.H. (2007). Effectiveness of "Dangerous Decibels," A school-based hearing loss prevention program. *American Journal of Audiology*, 16(2), S165-S181.

Kennedy-Armbruster, C., & Yoke, M. (2014). *Methods of Group Exercise Instruction*. Champaign, IL: Human Kinetics.

Mosston, Muska (2001). *Teaching Physical Education,* 5th edition. San Francisco, CA: Benjamin Cummings.

Chapter 23 Review Questions

1. Group exercise music tempo can influence both the energy level and exercise progression of a class and is determined by the _____.
    A. downbeat
    B. phrase
    C. measure
    D. beats per minute

2. Playing copyrighted music in a group exercise class is legal when _____.
    A. the instructor purchased the music legally (e.g., iTunes®)
    B. the instructor purchased aerobic music specifically designed for use by fitness professionals
    C. the facility where the instructor teaches has purchased a licensing fee to play the music specifically designed for use by fitness professionals
    D. the instructor teaches in their own home studio

3. Holding up fingers to indicate how many repetitions of a movement are remaining would be an example of what kind of cue?
    A. Verbal
    B. Visual
    C. Auditory
    D. Kinesthetic

4. Performing 4 step touches, 2 jumping jacks, and 1 grapevine equals how many counts?
    A. 8 counts
    B. 16 counts
    C. 24 counts
    D. 32 counts

5. Lever, plane, direction, and intensity are all _____.
    A. transitions
    B. types of feedback
    C. elements of variation
    D. choreography development strategies

6. Which of the following teaching strategies would be the best option to reduce boredom?
    A. Repeating
    B. Add-on
    C. Pyramid/repetition reduction
    D. Freestyle

Answers to Review Questions on Page 384

Note: Review questions are intended to reinforce learning and comprehension of subject matter presented in the corresponding chapter. The review questions are not intended to be representative of actual certification exam questions in terms of style, content, or difficulty.

Section VII

**Injury Management, Emergency Response,
Medical Considerations & Special Populations**

Although the benefits of regular physical activity and exercise far outweigh the potential risks, occasionally unexpected, yet foreseeable, emergencies and medical conditions will arise. Fitness professionals must be able to recognize the signs and symptoms of injury and cardiovascular events, respond to medical emergencies, and modify exercise to the needs of special populations.

Chapter 24 discusses strategies to prevent and manage common exercise-related injuries. This chapter also provides a review of appropriate emergency response, preventative strategies, and basic care for those suffering from adverse cardiovascular events and heat-related disorders. It is important to keep in mind that fitness professionals are not qualified to treat injuries beyond basic first aid and emergency assistance. Although clients may ask questions about an injury or medical condition, fitness professionals must not attempt to provide a diagnosis and should refrain from offering information that may be interpreted as medical advice.

Chapter 25 discusses medical conditions and chronic diseases often present among clients and class participants. Information and programming recommendations are provided with regard to asthma, arthritis, diabetes, hypertension, and osteoporosis. In addition, this chapter covers general considerations with regard to exercise programming for special population groups including pregnant women, older adults, and youth and adolescents.

24
Injury Management & Emergency Response

Introduction
Fitness professionals must know how to prevent, recognize, and respond to exercise-related injuries. Of course the best strategy is to take every measure possible to prevent injuries and adverse health events. However, even in the presence of a thorough risk management plan, unexpected, yet foreseeable, injuries and medical emergencies do occur. Fitness professionals must be prepared to recognize the signs and symptoms of these medical emergencies, implement the appropriate steps within an emergency response plan, and provide basic care until the arrival of advanced medical personnel.

Occurrence of Exercise-Related Injuries
High rates of injury among exercisers cost time, money, and enthusiasm. According to an epidemiological study conducted by Kerr et al. (2010), 25,335 injuries related to resistance training were treated in a sample of 100 emergency rooms in the United States from 1990 to 2007. This translates to an estimation of approximately 970,800 injuries associated with resistance training nationwide (Kerr et al., 2010). The most common type of injury was sprains and strains, accounting for 46.1% of the reported injuries (Kerr et al., 2010). In addition, other soft tissue injuries, fractures, dislocations, lacerations, and concussions were also reported (Kerr et al., 2010). The most commonly affected sites include the lower back, shoulder, and hand. Exercise-related injuries are not limited to resistance training. For example, from the years 2000 to 2001, an estimated 4.3 million sports- and recreation-related injuries were treated in U.S. hospital emergency rooms (Gotsch et al., 2002). Sprains and strains again represented the largest proportion of injuries (29.1%), followed by fractures, contusions, and lacerations (Gotsch et al., 2002). The incidence of injury is also high in the group exercise setting. According to cross-sectional studies, an estimated 45% of group exercise participants and 75% of instructors report injuries; however, the injuries do tend to be less severe and most frequently affect the lower leg (Dishman et al., 2013). Best prevented by applying knowledge and precaution, this section provides essential information for preventing and identifying exercise-related injuries.

An exercise-related injury represents trauma to tissue sufficient to cause disability, pain, swelling, and sometimes weakness. As noted earlier, exercise participants may suffer sprains, strains, fractures, dislocations, lacerations, contusions, and concussions. In addition, excessive muscle soreness resulting from overexertion may also result in limited function.

An **acute injury** occurs as a single and instantaneous incident of physical trauma to the body. Although often preventable, acute injuries are typically unpredictable and accidental in nature. Chronic is an important term in medicine that comes from the Greek word 'chronos', meaning time or lasting a long time. A **chronic injury** develops more gradually and may not be associated with a single incident. Chronic injuries result in response to overuse, repetitive motions, inappropriate exercise intensity, insufficient rest, poor body mechanics and postural alignment, or improper use of equipment. Symptoms of a chronic injury typically have a more gradual onset and are often associated with inflammation of soft tissue (e.g., ligament, tendon, bursa sac). Although chronic injuries may initially be less debilitating, if not treated appropriately these injuries may result in significant disability and time lost from activity participation. **Chronic pain** differs from chronic injury in that chronic pain persists for a long, continuous period of time; whereas, a chronic injury may be recurring, but not necessarily continuous. The U.S. National Center for Health Statistics defines a chronic condition as one lasting 3 months or more.

It is important to understand the psychological toll that both chronic injury and chronic pain may take on an individual. Chronic pain can lead to sleep deprivation, the restriction of normal activities, and major changes in daily routine. Depression and anxiety may also be a compounding factor in many people with chronic pain.

The **injury cycle** begins with trauma to a joint, muscle, or other tissue. Ruptured blood vessels hemorrhage, leaking blood into tissue, causing inflammation and pain. Occasionally a person may have muscle spasms in the injured area. Muscle spasms serve to limit muscle use, thereby protecting the injured area while increasing the amount of pain. All injuries require a period of immobilization and non-use. Unfortunately, prolonged immobilization allows muscle to atrophy resulting in loss of muscular strength.

Furthermore, the tissue's healing process generates inelastic and weak scar tissue that can rupture more easily than healthy tissue. To prevent further injury, a person must strengthen muscles and related structures slowly before engaging in activities at the pre-injury exercise intensity. Without proper treatment, a single injury can lead to a prolonged episode of disability and pain. If any participant experiences pain, swelling, or reduced range of motion for more than three days, he or she should cease exercise and consult with a health care provider.

Important warning signs of injury include:
- Point-specific or radiating pain
- Prolonged swelling in a joint or muscle
- Reduced or painful range of motion
- Muscle weakness
- Numbness or tingling

Common Exercise-Related Injuries
Exercise participants may suffer from a wide variety of exercise-related injuries. Therefore, fitness professionals must be familiar with common injuries and prepared to respond to in a manner that is safe, responsible, and within the legal scope of practice. This section defines the most common exercise-related injuries that fitness professionals are likely to encounter.

Strains
A **strain** occurs when a muscle or tendon tears as the result of a forceful contraction or overstretching. If the musculotendinous unit is subjected to forces (internal or external) that exceed the tensile strength, then the tissue will tear, causing pain and inflammation. Health care providers and athletic trainers grade muscle injuries based on the degree of tissue damage. A Grade 1 injury is classified as a strain, which involves tearing of just a few muscle fibers (Chan et al., 2012). This type of injury involves mild swelling and discomfort, some strength deficits, and only minimal loss of function (Chan et al., 2012). Since a strained muscle is still functional, people may often overlook the injury and attempt to work through the pain. However, a strain does weaken the muscle and tendon, making them more susceptible to further injury until properly healed and reconditioned. A Grade 2 injury involves a partial tear of up to two-thirds of the full muscle or tendon thickness. Increased swelling, hemorrhage, pain, and tissue deformity are evident at the site of the injury (Chan et al., 2012). There is moderate strength deficits and significant loss of function in the affected muscle. A Grade 3 muscle injury is the most severe and is characterized by a complete tear, retraction of the muscle ends, a complete loss of muscle function (i.e., ability to contract), and extreme pain (Chan et al., 2012). Complete muscle tears require medical treatment and surgical repair. Factors that may increase the risk of strains include poor flexibility, muscle imbalances, an inadequate warm-up, postural misalignments, muscle fatigue, and improper training.

Sprains
An injury that damages a ligament is called a **sprain**. Sprains often occur when a joint undergoes a forceful or sudden motion that exceeds the joint's normal range of motion such as hyperextension, hyperflexion, or twisting. A ligament sprain is characterized by pain, swelling, discoloration, joint instability, and loss of range of motion. In more severe cases, there may also be dislocation or deformity of the affected joint. Similar to musculotendinous injuries, sprains are classified based on the severity of the injury ranging from mild sprains involving minimal tearing (Grade 1), to a partial tear (Grade 2), and to a complete tear (Grade 3).

Ankle sprains are the most common injury among athletic populations accounting for up to 30% of all injuries (Waterman et al., 2010). The rate of ankle injuries is likely to be even higher considering that many mild sprains go unreported. Lateral ankle sprains account for the majority of ankle injuries. A lateral ankle sprain occurs when the individual lands on an inverted and plantar-flexed foot, which results in damage to the lateral ankle ligaments (e.g., anterior talofibular, calcaneofibular, posterior talofibular). Once pain and swelling have subsided, and the individual is cleared to return to activity, the fitness professional may focus on activities to restore proprioception, range of motion, and strength to the affected ankle.

Anterior Cruciate Ligament
The **anterior cruciate ligament (ACL)** is the primary structure stabilizing the knee by providing restraint to anterior translation (i.e., movement) of the tibia under the femur (Cimino et al., 2010). See figure 24-1. ACL injuries are among the most common sports-related knee injury, leading to significant disability and high health care expenditures. Research indicates that women are 1.4 to 9.5 times more likely to suffer from an ACL injury compared to men (Cimino et al., 2010). Approximately 70 percent of ACL tears are non-contact injuries, which occur during deceleration, such as a sudden stop or cutting motion, combined with a twisting or pivoting change of direction maneuver (Cimino et al., 2010; Renstrom et al., 2008). Individuals sustaining an ACL tear often report a 'popping' sound immediately followed by pain and swelling of the knee (Renstrom et al., 2008). ACL injuries often require reconstructive surgery followed by a long period of rehabilitation. Once the individual has been cleared for return to activity, exercises that focus on continued restoration of strength, range of motion, and neuromuscular control should be emphasized. Closed kinetic chain resistance training exercises produce less pain, less joint laxity, and provide superior outcomes with regard to gains in functional strength (Nyland et al., 2010). In contrast, open chain quadriceps strengthening (i.e., seated leg extension) may

increase ACL strain, tibiofemoral shear forces, and patellofemoral joint compression near the end range of knee extension; therefore, exercises of this nature should be avoided (Nyland et al., 2010).

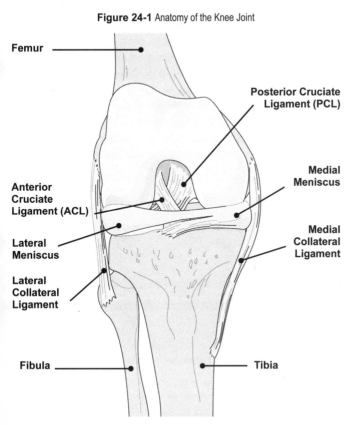

Figure 24-1 Anatomy of the Knee Joint

Labels: Femur, Posterior Cruciate Ligament (PCL), Medial Meniscus, Medial Collateral Ligament, Tibia, Fibula, Lateral Collateral Ligament, Lateral Meniscus, Anterior Cruciate Ligament (ACL)

Chondromalacia Patellae

Articular (hyaline) cartilage lines the bone surfaces at joint articulations and provides a smooth surface for movement and shock absorption within the joint. Deterioration of cartilage leads to a damaged articular surface, joint pain, and dysfunction. **Chondromalacia patellae** is a condition in which the cartilage lining the posterior surface of the patella becomes softened and swollen, progressing to fragmentation and flaking, and eventually to erosion of the cartilage down to the bone (Outerbridge & Outerbridge, 2001). Many factors are suggested to contribute to the development of chondromalacia patella including overuse from stair climbing, frequent kneeling, high-impact activities on hard surfaces, and extreme knee flexion.

Poor alignment of the femur and tibia may also accelerate cartilage damage. As such, contraction of the quadriceps moves the patella slightly out of its intended tracking trajectory. Muscular imbalance in the quadriceps and weakness or tightness in the hamstrings can increase the risk of chondromalacia patellae. Since the extremes of knee flexion place considerable pressure and friction on the undersurface of the patella, it is suggested that knee flexion is limited to no more than 90 degrees while performing squats or lunges. Maintaining balanced strength between the vastus medialis and vastus lateralis will minimize the tendency to pull the patella laterally, out of alignment. Balanced leg strength will also help participants maintain proper alignment in the knees and hips during exercise. If dynamic movements are uncomfortable or contraindicated, isometric strengthening is an effective alternative for the major muscles surrounding the knee joint.

If cartilage damage is suspected, a qualified health care provider should design and supervise a rehabilitation program. Serious cartilage damage may lead to degenerative arthritis later in life. If a person intends to lead an active lifestyle, precaution must be taken to limit damage to the hips and knees. As cartilage damage advances, participation in many activities may eventually be limited.

Meniscus Tears

Meniscus is a small pad of fibrocartilage tissue resting on the medial and lateral aspects of the tibia in the knee joint. See figure 24-1. The medial and lateral menisci provide joint stability, absorb shock transmitted between the femoral condyles and the tibia, and distribute weight evenly with each step or turn (Cimino et al., 2010). Meniscal tissue can tear if the knee twists forcefully or if the knee straightens or flexes with great momentum. Meniscus tears cause pain, swelling, joint locking, popping, or clicking during flexion and extension. Severe meniscus damage may require surgery to remove damaged tissue and realign structures in the knee joint. Like cartilage damage, meniscus damage can contribute to accelerated and permanent deterioration of the knee joint.

Patellofemoral Pain Syndrome

Patellofemoral pain syndrome (PFPS), also referred to as 'anterior knee pain' or 'runner's knee,' is one of the most common knee conditions experienced by active populations (Dixit et al., 2007). Patellofemoral pain syndrome is characterized by complaints of pain behind and around the patella that is increased with running and other activities that involve knee flexion such as squatting, stair climbing, biking, and prolonged sitting. The suspected cause of PFPS is abnormal tracking of the patella during knee flexion and extension that leads to increased patellofemoral joint forces (Bolgla & Boling, 2011; Dixit et al., 2007). The faulty patellar tracking may be attributed to quadriceps weakness, quadriceps imbalances (i.e., overactive vastus medialis, underactive vastus lateralis), tight lateral structures (i.e., iliotibial band, lateral retinaculum), weak hip muscles, and altered foot kinematics (Bolgla & Boling, 2011; Dixit et al., 2007). Clients or class participants noting persistent and worsening anterior knee pain should be encouraged to visit a medical professional for evaluation and diagnosis. The most common exercise intervention for PFPS is quadriceps strengthening (Bolgla & Boling, 2011). In addition, the exercise program should include strengthening of the hip abductors and external rotators, stretching for the hamstrings and calves, and self-myofascial release using a foam roller for the iliotibial band.

Tendonitis

As noted in chapter 5, a tendon is a tough, yet flexible band of fibrous tissue that connects muscle to bone. The force generated by the contracting skeletal muscle is transmitted through the tendon to the bone, thus enabling movement.

Occasionally, an overuse injury known as **tendonitis** ('-itis' = inflammation) may occur when the normally smooth gliding motion of the tendon is impaired. Coupled with repetitive movement, this impairment causes irritation, inflammation, pain, and reduced range of motion. Many factors may contribute to the onset of tendonitis including improper mechanics and joint alignment, and poor training strategies such as inadequate rest, aggressive program progression, and lack of program variation. In addition, age-related changes to the tendon tissue and structural anomalies may play a role in the development of tendonitis. Achilles tendonitis, patellar tendonitis (i.e., 'jumper's knee'), and rotator cuff tendonitis are common exercise and sports-related overuse injuries.

Management of and recovery from tendonitis requires a period of reduced activity or full rest of the affected body part. Initially, the goal is to manage and control the inflammation and pain through the application of ice and use of nonsteroidal anti-inflammatory drugs (NSAIDs) as directed by a health care provider. Once inflammation and pain have been reduced, appropriate stretching, strengthening, and corrective exercises may be prescribed by a physical therapist or athletic trainer. The fitness professional should communicate closely with these allied health care professionals to ensure appropriate exercise selection and to avoid activities that may cause increased pain.

Shoulder Impingement Syndrome

Shoulder impingement syndrome (SIS) is often associated with sports and activities that involve repetitive overhead motions. In a properly functioning shoulder, the rotator cuff muscles are able to move smoothly under the acromion process of the scapula in the area known as the subacromial space. Shoulder impingement occurs when the rotator cuff tendons (typically the supraspinatus) and the subacromial bursa sac (a small fluid filled sac) get pinched or impinged between the acromion process and the greater tubercle of the humerus. See figure 24-2. Over time, the tendons and bursa get inflamed resulting in pain, especially during shoulder abduction. Shoulder impingement syndrome may result from several, often interrelated factors. In some cases, structural abnormalities create a reduction in the subacromial space, which predisposes the development of SIS. Secondary factors that contribute to SIS include underlying instability of the glenohumeral joint and dysfunctional movement of the scapulothoracic joint (Ellenbecker & Cools, 2010). This instability and dysfunction result from weakness of the rotator cuff and muscle imbalances that contribute to faulty movement of the shoulder complex. Additionally, these underlying factors are compounded by irritation and fatigue from repetitive overhead motions. Individuals complaining of pain during shoulder abduction and overhead movements should be referred to the appropriate health care provider for evaluation and diagnosis. Once pain and inflammation are reduced, treatment of shoulder impingement often involves exercises to restore normal flexibility and strength to the shoulder complex, including strengthening both the rotator cuff muscles and the muscles responsible for stabilization and movement of the scapula. In severe cases, a cortisone injection or surgery may be necessary.

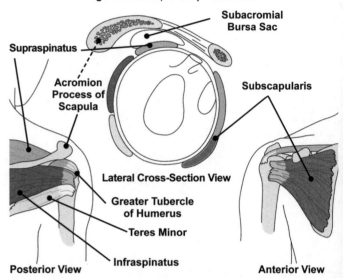

Figure 24-2 Deep Anatomy of the Shoulder

Fitness professionals working with individuals recovering from shoulder impingement should avoid overhead movements. Placing the shoulder in 90 degrees of abduction and 90 degrees of external rotation (known as the 'closed-pack' position) causes the tendons of the supraspinatus and infraspinatus to rotate posteriorly increasing compression and impingement (Ellenbecker & Cools, 2010). Therefore, exercises that place the shoulder in this position (e.g., lat pulldown, shoulder press, military press) should be avoided. In addition, exercises that internally rotate the arm cause the rotator cuff tendons to be pinched between the greater tubercle of the humerus and the acromion process (Durall et al., 2001). The upright row, involving shoulder internal rotation coupled with abduction, has been implicated as an exercise that may lead to shoulder impingement and should be avoided (Durall et al., 2001).

Plantar Fasciitis

Another '-itis' overuse injury is **plantar fasciitis**, a painful inflammatory condition affecting the plantar fascia. The plantar fascia is a thick fibrous band of connective tissue originating on the bottom surface of the calcaneus (heel bone) and extending toward the toes, providing support to the arch of the foot. It has been reported that 10% of the American population will suffer from plantar fasciitis in their lifetime. A common symptom of plantar fasciitis is heel and arch pain upon first standing in the morning or after prolonged periods of sitting (Goff & Crawford, 2011). Risk factors for plantar fasciitis include excessive foot pronation, excessive running and jumping, high arches, obesity, occupations involving prolonged standing and walking, sedentary lifestyle, and tightness of the calf muscles and Achilles tendon (Goff & Crawford, 2011). Immediate management of plantar fasciitis includes rest, ice, activity modification to minimize weight bearing, and NSAIDs as recommended by a health care provider (Goff & Crawford, 2011). In addition, pain symptoms may improve with stretching exercises for the plantar fascia, intrinsic foot muscles, and the gastrocnemius and soleus.

Shin Splints

Shin splints (also called *medial tibial stress syndrome*) is a condition characterized by pain through the anterior and medial aspects of the lower leg, which increases during activity and persists as a dull ache following activity. Originally, shin splints was attributed to irritation of the posterior tibialis muscle; however, it is now believed to be related more so to irritation of the deep fascial origin of the medial soleus muscle (Tolbert & Binkley, 2009). In addition, other structures may also be affected including the tibialis anterior and the periosteum (i.e., connective tissue covering the bone of the tibia). Some of the probable causes of shin splints include unforgiving (i.e., hard) training surfaces, rapid progression to high-intensity exercise, sudden increases in running mileage, high or low arches, muscle imbalances (i.e., tight gastrocnemius and soleus, weak tibialis anterior), foot pronation, and improper or worn-out footwear (Tolbert & Binkley, 2009). Management of shin splints involves rest, ice, and cross-training to non-weight-bearing activities. The exercise program should also include static stretches for the hamstrings, gastrocnemius, and soleus, as well as strengthening exercises involving ankle dorsiflexion, inversion, and eversion using light-to-moderate resistance tubing (Tolbert & Binkley, 2009). If pain persists, the individual should consult with a health care provider to rule out more serious injuries such as a stress fracture, exercise-induced compartment syndrome, or popliteal artery entrapment (Tolbert & Brinkley, 2009).

Bone Fractures

Bone fractures may be the result of trauma or be pathological in nature. A traumatic fracture is the result of an accident such as a fall, a collision, or being struck by an object. Pathological fractures are related to underlying infection or disease including cancer, osteoporosis, and osteogenesis imperfecta (i.e., 'brittle bone disease'). A *simple fracture* (i.e., closed fracture) does not cause the broken bone to puncture the surface of the skin; whereas, a *compound fracture* (i.e., open fracture) does puncture through the skin exposing the broken bone. A *complete fracture* involves complete separation of the broken bone and an *incomplete fracture* involves only a partial separation.

When an individual is suspected of having an acute fracture, the emergency medical service (i.e., 911) should be called immediately and the victim should not move the affected body part unless necessary. If the individual must be moved for safety, then immobilize the injured site to prevent further damage. Additional care for a fracture includes dressing any open tissue with sterile gauze to protect from exposure and infection, and monitor the individual for signs and symptoms of shock (e.g., cool and clammy skin, pale or grey color, weak yet rapid pulse rate, low blood pressure, altered respiration, nausea) or other life-threatening conditions.

Stress Fractures

A stress fracture is an overuse injury that may occur when unusual or repetitive forces are chronically exerted upon a bone in excess of the bone's rate of remodeling, which leads to weakening of the bone and subsequent micro-fracture (Conte et al., 2011). Stress fractures typically affect the tibia, tarsals, metatarsals, pelvis, and vertebrae. Stress fractures are characterized by a sharp, radiating pain and tenderness that worsens with weight-bearing activity. Risk factors for the development of stress fractures include high-volume weight-bearing training, uneven and unforgiving (i.e., hard) training surfaces, anatomic anomalies, and nutritional factors such as inadequate intake of calcium, vitamin D, or protein (Conte et al., 2011). Women are at increased risk for stress factors compared to men. This may be attributed to hormonal factors (i.e., low estrogen), amenorrhea, and eating disorders.

Table 24-1 Prevention of Stress Fractures

Guidelines to Prevent Stress Fractures
• Maintain a healthful diet, including foods rich in calcium and vitamin D, to help build bone strength.
• Use proper sports equipment, avoiding old or worn-out running shoes.
• Alternate your activities (i.e., cross-training); for example substituting jogging with swimming or cycling.
• Start any new sports activity slowly, with a gradual progression (e.g., 10% per week in time, speed, or distance).
• Resistance training can help prevent early muscle fatigue and prevent the loss of bone density associated with aging.
• If pain or swelling occurs, stop the activity and rest for a few days; if pain continues, see a health care provider.

Conte et al. (2011)

Management of a stress fracture includes a reduction in activity level below the threshold of symptoms or complete cessation of activity, depending on the pain levels and progression of the stress fracture (Conte et al., 2011). Non-weight-bearing activities such as rowing machines, stationary bicycles, swimming, and aquatic jogging are recommended. Successful management of a stress fracture generally requires an extended period (e.g., up to 12 weeks) of rest or activity restriction (Conte et al., 2011). Table 24-1 provides guidelines to prevent stress fractures from the American Academy of Orthopedic Surgeons.

Low Back Pain

The low back region consists of the five lumbar vertebrae, intervertebral discs, intervertebral ligaments, and several muscles. Weak core muscles (e.g., rectus abdominis, obliques, transverse abdominis) and tightness through the erector spinae, hamstrings, and iliopsoas muscle groups are all typical of those with low back pain. In addition, poor posture, congenital conditions, obesity, improper body mechanics, and disease may also contribute to the onset of low back pain. A wide variety of conditions affecting the lower back can result in pain and disability. Among these conditions are lower back sprains and strains, disc herniation, spinal stenosis, spondylolisthesis, spondylitis, and degenerative disc disease. A comprehensive review of these conditions is beyond the scope of this manual. As with any orthopedic injury, fitness professionals should not diagnose or attempt to treat conditions of the low back. Individuals with significant and persistent lower back pain should be referred to the appropriate health care provider for evaluation and treatment.

To prevent the onset of lower back pain, fitness professionals should educate clients and class participants regarding proper postural alignment, body mechanics, and lifting techniques. In addition, preventative exercises should be included in a well-designed exercise program including core stabilization and strength, appropriate flexibility (e.g., hamstrings, iliopsoas, erector spinae), cardiorespiratory conditioning, and balanced resistance training. Participants should also avoid exercises involving unsupported spinal flexion, isolated twisting movements of the spine, and extreme hyperextension.

Wounds and Lacerations

A **closed-wound**, such as a *contusion* or *bruise*, is caused by a direct impact force that results in bleeding within the underlying tissues. Common symptoms include discoloration, which may not appear immediately, swelling, and localized tenderness. More severe closed-wounds may also result in decreased muscle function and range of motion. Immediate care for closed-wounds includes rest, ice, and gentle stretching when tolerated.

An **open-wound**, such as a *laceration*, is a jagged-edge cut or tearing of the skin resulting in external bleeding. An incision is a cut with smooth edges (such as those made by a surgeon), and a puncture is a penetration of the skin with a pointed object. An *abrasion* is the scraping or removal of the outermost layers of skin leaving nerve endings and capillaries exposed. Immediate care for open-wounds includes protecting the exposed subcutaneous tissue from infection by immediately covering the wound with a sterile gauze dressing. This will also help control any bleeding until the wound can be cleaned and bandaged. A health care provider should clean a deep wound and provide more extensive treatments, which may include stitches and/or a tetanus shot.

Overtraining

As discussed in chapter 18, **overtraining** may occur when there is an imbalance between training and recovery time. Fitness professionals need to continually emphasize the importance of adequate rest as an essential factor contributing to and maintaining a high level of physical fitness. Overtraining due to exercise usually occurs because of increases in exercise frequency, duration, or intensity without adequate recovery time between workouts. When high-intensity exercise is performed without proper rest and recovery, the muscles and connective tissue cannot repair damage or respond well to further exercise demands. Unfortunately, overtraining typically afflicts the most motivated individuals, who may enter a cycle of injury and re-injury. As such, the most active and motivated participants should understand the indicators and repercussions of overtraining.

Overtraining alters the body's chemistry producing several identifiable physiologic and behavioral changes. An overtrained individual's heart rate will remain elevated long after exercise, even perhaps throughout the day. An exercise-induced imbalance of hormones, fluids, and electrolytes will often disturb sleep patterns causing insomnia or prolonged non-exercise fatigue and exhaustion. Other indicators of overtraining include reduced appetite, decreased sexual desire, feelings of restlessness or depression, and more frequent occurrences of minor illnesses. Overtrained participants may experience excessive training fatigue, prolonged performance impairment lasting several weeks to months, and greater incidence of injuries. Avoidance of overtraining is a primary prevention strategy for exercise-related injuries (Bullock et al., 2010).

In many cases, group exercise instructors have limited class scheduling options because they must teach on certain days. The body typically recovers from aerobic activity within 24 hours, but recovery can take more time after a difficult or rigorous exercise schedule. Group exercise instructors should consider reducing their personal intensity level of the classes they lead and develop teaching skills that do not require continuous active participation. The best way to prevent injury is to listen carefully to the body. Do not disregard pain or the body's need for rest, proper recovery time, adequate carbohydrates, and fluids. Fitness professionals may find that scheduled rest days will increase performance, reduce overall fatigue, and allow exercise participation as a lifetime activity. The fitness professional's teaching and training schedules should promote a well-balanced fitness program that maximizes long-term fitness participation.

Care for Exercise-Related Injuries

The recommended treatment for most exercise-related injuries includes P.R.I.C.E.: protection, rest, ice, compression, and elevation. After an acute injury, there may be sudden swelling due to broken blood vessels and/or fluid leaking into surrounding tissue. The amount of swelling often reflects the injury's severity. If swelling is controlled and minimized, the injured area is less painful and rehabilitation can begin sooner. An injured person should conduct all five aspects of P.R.I.C.E.

> **Good to Know**
> **P**rotection
> **R**est
> **I**ce
> **C**ompression
> **E**levation

The injured muscle, joint, or structure should be protected from further injury for a minimum of 24 hours. Rest may include a decrease in activity or a complete cessation of activity. Many health care provider recommend gentle range of motion of an injured joint rather than complete immobilization following the acute phase of injury to improve healing and expedite rehabilitation. Chronic injuries may require a much longer rest period. Sometimes alternative exercise modalities can help the individual maintain general fitness levels without stressing the injured area. Participants should not ignore injuries and should be discouraged from exercising through pain.

Ice causes vasoconstriction of blood vessels limiting the infiltration of fluid and blood into the injured site and the adjacent tissue. Ice also numbs nerve endings to reduce pain sensations. Ice should be applied as soon as possible after an injury by using a thin cloth barrier to protect the skin. Failure to protect the skin can cause frostbite. The ice should stay on for no longer than 20 minutes (no longer than 10 minutes if the injury is superficial). The injury should remain uncovered for an hour before ice is reapplied. Repeated ice applications reduce the duration and severity of internal bleeding and swelling in most injuries. Ice and compression work most effectively together. Compression can be as simple as leaving the shoe on an injured ankle or wrapping a towel tightly around an injured limb. Compression should be applied to reduce the swelling response, but to otherwise allow normal blood circulation.

Elevation of the injury above the heart reduces swelling to the area as gravity impedes the blood flow. A person should keep the injured area above the level of the nearest joint and preferably above the heart. For example, a sprained ankle should be elevated above the knee.

Injury Prevention Strategies

Fitness professionals and exercise participants can prevent injuries by following principles of proper muscle conditioning, biomechanics, exercise program design, environmental factors, and proper use of equipment. These recommendations might seem obvious; however, all participants are likely to benefit from regular reminders.

1. Thorough Warm-Up
All exercise activity requires a minimum of 5 to 10 minutes warm-up time to prepare the muscles and cardiovascular system for exercise. A proper warm-up may include both light cardiorespiratory activity and dynamic flexibility exercises. Fitness professionals should encourage a full warm-up with gentle, large, rhythmic movements to gradually increase heart rate, respiratory rate, blood flow, muscle oxygenation, and mental focus.

2. Correct Biomechanics
Use controlled movements with proper biomechanics. The fitness professional should demonstrate how to perform movements within a safe range of motion, particularly avoiding hyperextension of knees, elbows, shoulders, neck, and back. During all varieties of cardiovascular exercise, participants can reduce the risk of injury by maintaining the spine in neutral alignment and keeping the toes, knees, and hips aligned. If a person cannot maintain alignment, he or she should modify the movement intensity, speed, position, or cease the activity to prevent injury.

3. Listen to Your Body
If participants experience pain in a joint, muscle, or structure, they should modify the exercise intensity, range of motion, plane of motion, body alignment, or stop the activity all together. A person acquires physical fitness by gradually increasing exercise intensity or duration, not by sudden or painful increases. Fitness professionals should remind participants to reduce exercise intensity, frequency, or duration if pain develops.

4. Proper Program Design
When performing a resistance workout, one should increase the resistance gradually. A safe program starts with low workloads and allows the person to perform exercises in a pain-free range of motion. A person trying to increase muscle strength should gradually increase the number of repetitions before increasing the exercise resistance load. The body requires time to adapt to these small increases in exertion by repairing and building muscle tissue. Sufficient repetitions and sets of muscle conditioning exercises, with appropriate levels of resistance, should be done to achieve muscular fatigue. However, participants should not be encouraged to work if pain or a persistent burning

sensation is present. Participants should work at a resistance level appropriate for their own strength and training capabilities. Fitness professionals should encourage participants to recognize muscle fatigue and to rest when the muscle reaches fatigue to prevent torn muscle fibers and/or recruiting inappropriate muscles or structures to support the joints. Such compensations may be observed by a change of posture or technique to facilitate additional repetitions when the targeted muscles fail due to pain or weakness. Safe and effective program design includes appropriate overload, gradual progression, adequate rest and recovery, and periodization.

5. Maintain Muscular Balance

Muscles work in opposing pairs (i.e., agonist, antagonist) so that activation of one muscle group facilitates relaxation in the other. For example, the rectus abdominis works in opposition to the erector spinae muscles. A strong agonist muscle can overpower its inflexible or weak counterpart. Conversely, balanced muscles exert approximately equal force on a joint and do not overstress each other. Because muscles help support many intricate joints such as the knee, hip, shoulders, and back, joints that are surrounded and supported by balanced muscles suffer fewer injuries. A properly designed program includes flexibility training and muscle conditioning strategically designed to maintain balance between opposing muscle groups.

6. Correct Use of Equipment

New exercise equipment is effective in motivating participants to adhere to an exercise program and should be introduced gradually. Proper technique is critical to avoid injury and to obtain the desired training effects. Inspect equipment before every use for potential breakage that may cause injury. Misuse of exercise equipment, both intentionally and unintentionally, is a significant factor contributing to exercise-related injuries.

7. Appropriate Footwear

Shoes that are specifically developed for a particular activity are preferable, but a cross-training shoe is adequate for most group exercise classes and fitness activities. Fitness professionals should encourage all exercise participants to wear shoes during an exercise session. Shoes should be supportive and cushioned appropriately for the activity. Most shoes worn only during exercise sessions last less than approximately six months if a person exercises several times a week. Fitness professionals and participants should invest in good shoes that provide shock absorption, arch support, and flexibility in the forefoot, and that prevent excessive foot pronation or supination.

8. Flooring

The exercise surface should be even and provide impact absorption. All cardiorespiratory activities should be conducted on a yielding surface versus cement or pavement. A yielding surface absorbs some of the shock created by the foot landing on the surface. Carpeting may provide yielding surface; however, it may be laid over concrete decreasing the cushioning effect or may be so thick that it allows for too much ankle movement causing ankle injuries. Improper shoes and exercise surfaces may contribute to nerve and joint cartilage irritation, particularly in the feet, and can result in foot conditions such as a neuroma (i.e., inflammation and enlargement of an intermetatarsal nerve causing a burning pain) or metatarsalgia (i.e., pain in the forefoot that is associated with increased stress and inflammation of the metatarsal heads).

9. Workout Pace

Conducting exercises at the appropriate pace allows participants to perform exercises using good biomechanics, full range of motion, controlled movement, and proper body alignment. Participants in a group exercise class will achieve better results if they can execute the moves safely and effectively while keeping pace with the tempo of the music. During resistance training, slower is better when the objective is to increase muscular strength.

10. Maintain Adequate Flexibility

If stretching is a scheduled part of the training program, it should follow the cool-down. Proper stretching involves elongation of the muscle to a point of tension, without pain. The proper stretching technique needs to be applied for safe and effective results. Although pre-activity static stretching does not appear to protect against exercise-related injuries, regular stretching does promote muscle balance, reduced joint stress, and a lower incidence of lower back pain.

Heat-Related Disorders

Heat-related disorders include exertional heat cramps, heat exhaustion, and exertional heatstroke. Environmental factors, such as high ambient air temperature, high relative humidity, low wind speed, and solar radiant heat contribute to excessive fluid loss (i.e., dehydration) and elevate core body temperature (i.e., hyperthermia). These conditions may lead to the development of heat-related disorders. Preventative strategies are crucial for reducing the onset of heat-related disorders.

Exertional Heat Cramps

Exertional heat cramps are painful involuntary muscle spasms, often affecting the lower extremities and abdomen, that may occur during or after prolonged strenuous exercise in the heat (ACSM, 2018; Armstrong et al., 2007). The factors that contribute to the onset of heat cramps include exercise-induced muscle fatigue, dehydration, and electrolyte imbalance resulting from significant losses of sodium via sweat (Armstrong et al., 2007; Binkley et al., 2002). Immediate care for exertional heat cramps includes rest, static stretching of the affected muscle groups, and consumption of fluids and foods containing sodium chloride (i.e., table salt) (Armstrong et al., 2007). Heat cramps may be prevented by maintaining proper fluid and salt balance during exercise.

Heat Exhaustion

Heat exhaustion is the most common type of serious heat-related disorders. The signs and symptoms of heat exhaustion include low blood pressure, elevated heart rate and respiratory rate, profuse sweating, slightly elevated core body temperature, headache, weakness, nausea, irritability, and decreased muscle coordination (Armstrong et al., 2007). In addition, the skin appears ashen or pale, clammy, and often with 'goose bumps' (Armstrong et al., 2007). An individual suspected of suffering from heat exhaustion should be moved into a shaded or air conditioned area, excess clothing should be removed, and fluids (e.g., water and/or sports drink) should be consumed if the individual is able to swallow and is not vomiting (Armstrong et al., 2007). The individual should lay in a supine position with the legs elevated and monitored closely during recovery. Most individuals will respond favorably to prompt care; however, if symptoms do not improve or worsen, the individual should receive advanced emergency treatment from the appropriate personnel (Armstrong et al., 2007).

Exertional Heatstroke

Exertional heatstroke (EHS) is a life-threatening medical emergency. EHS is defined as hyperthermia (i.e., core body temperature >40°C or >104°F), central nervous system dysfunction, and multiple organ system failure (ACSM, 2018; Armstrong et al., 2007). It is often difficult to discern severe heat exhaustion from heatstroke as many of the signs and symptoms are similar. Although the skin may initially appear sweaty and pale, classic heatstroke is characterized by dry, hot, and red skin (Armstrong et al., 2007). Symptoms of exertional heatstroke related to central nervous system dysfunction include dizziness, confusion, disorientation, irrational behavior, impaired balance and coordination, seizures, loss of consciousness, and coma (Armstrong et al., 2007; Binkley et al., 2002). In addition, victims of heatstroke are likely to be severely dehydrated and may have symptoms such as tachycardia (i.e., heart rate >100 beats/min), hyperventilation, low blood pressure, vomiting, and diarrhea (Armstrong et al., 2007; Binkley et al., 2002).

When exertional heatstroke is suspected, the emergency medical system should be activated immediately (i.e., call 911). Successful treatment and survival from EHS requires immediate, whole-body cooling using cold water or ice water immersion (ACSM, 2018; Armstrong et al., 2007). If whole-body immersion is not possible, then ice water towels should be applied on the head, torso, and extremities and ice packs applied to the neck, axillary region, and groin (Armstrong et al., 2007).

The greatest risk for exertional heatstroke, as well as other heat-related disorders, is present when the *wet-bulb globe temperature (WBGT)* is greater than 28°C (82°F) (Armstrong et al., 2007). Table 24-2 provides a summary of heatstroke risk associated with increasing WBGT. Additional risk factors for EHS include obesity, low cardiorespiratory fitness, lack of heat acclimatization, dehydration, history of heatstroke, prolonged strenuous exercise, sweat gland dysfunction, sunburn, viral illness, diarrhea, and certain medications (Armstrong et al., 2007).

In order to prevent the possible onset of serious heat-related disorders, the following strategies should be implemented (Armstrong et al., 2007; Binkley et al., 2002):

- Schedule activity during the cooler times of day or within a climate controlled environment.
- Allow a minimum of 10 to 14 days for acclimatization to hot and humid environments. Gradually increase exercise intensity and duration during the period of acclimatization.
- Monitor the environment for conditions that may increase the incidence of heat-related disorders.
- Conduct a preparticipation screening to identify those with a history of heat-related disorders. Monitor all individuals during exercise for signs and symptoms of heat stress.
- Educate participants regarding proper fluid intake. Ensure adequate fluids are available during activity. Enforce fluid intake recommendations. Monitor pre- and post-activity body weight to ensure adequate hydration and rehydration.
- Reduce exercise intensity and duration in high risk environmental conditions. Plan for frequent breaks and rest periods.
- Dress appropriately for the weather conditions. Wear light weight, light colored, moisture-wicking clothing. Avoid clothing, materials, and equipment that create a vapor barrier inhibiting the evaporative cooling effect of sweat.

Table 24-2 WBGT and Heatstroke Risk

Risk of Exertional Heatstroke Related to WBGT		
WBGT	Level of Risk	Action
<18° C (<65°F)	Low	Risk is low, but still exists among those with pre-existing risk factors.
18 - 23°C (65 - 73°F)	Moderate	Risk level increases as activity progresses through the day. Allow for longer rest periods and enforce fluid intake recommendations.
23 - 28°C (73 - 82°F)	High	Everyone should be aware of potential for heat-related disorders. Individuals at high risk should not participate.
>28°C (> 2°F)	Extreme	Consider cancelling or rescheduling activity until safer conditions prevail.

Binkley et al. (2002)

Cardiovascular Events

According to National Vital Statistics Reports, 611,105 deaths occurred in 2013 as the result of heart disease (Heron, 2016). The American Heart Association (AHA) reports that the 2011 overall rate of death attributable to **cardiovascular disease (CVD)** was 229.6 per 100,000 people (Mozaffarian et al., 2015). Based on this data, every day in the United States more than 2,150 Americans die of cardiovascular disease, an average of 1 CVD death every 40 seconds (Mozaffarian et al., 2015). Although it is well-established that regular physical activity reduces the risk of coronary heart disease, strenuous physical exertion does act as a strong trigger for a heart attack (i.e., myocardial infarction), especially among those who do not exercise regularly (Nawrot et al., 2011; Willich et al., 1993). Therefore, fitness professionals must be aware of the signs and symptoms of a heart attack and prepared to provide emergency care during these adverse events.

Myocardial Infarction

Coronary heart disease is caused in part by atherosclerosis (ath-er-o-sklear-osis), which refers to the general hardening, thickening, and narrowing of arterial blood vessels. The word atherosclerosis is derived from the Greek words *athero* (meaning gruel or paste) and *sclerosis* (meaning harden or hardness). See figure 24-3. Atherosclerosis is a process during which fatty substances such as cholesterol, calcium, and fibrin (i.e., a clotting agent in blood) accumulate as a plaque within the inner linings of the arterial wall. This build-up of plaque can rupture, causing blood to clot and the formation of a thrombosis at the damaged rupture site. As this thrombosis grows larger it begins to restrict blood flow through the artery and may eventually create a complete blockage or occlusion, which prevents vital oxygen and nutrients from reaching the tissue or organ supplied by the artery. The restricted or insufficient supply of blood to a tissue is called *ischemia*, and in the case of the heart it is known as a heart attack or myocardial infarction.

Figure 24-3 Atherosclerosis

Normal Artery   Artery Narrowed by Plaque

Blood Flow   Atherosclerotic Plaque

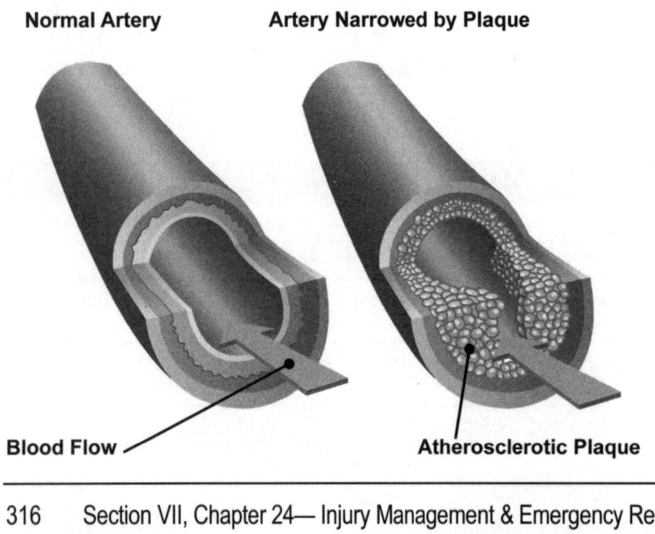

Recognizing the symptoms of a heart attack, prompt emergency care, and advanced life support is critical for survival. Although sometimes the onset of symptoms may be very sudden and intense, oftentimes heart attacks start slowly with only mild symptoms and discomforts. If a participant seems to be having a heart attack, the emergency medical service should be called immediately. The warning signs and symptoms of a heart attack may include:

- Prolonged or intermittent squeezing, pressure or pain in the chest (angina pectoris). These sensations may spread to the arms, shoulders, jaw, upper back, or upper abdomen (may feel like indigestion)
- Shortness of breath or difficulty breathing
- Feelings of restlessness, apprehension, dizziness, or extreme weakness
- Nausea or vomiting
- Loss of consciousness
- Cold or clammy skin
- Bluish skin tone
- Absence of pulse
- Dilated pupils

The immediate care provided to a victim of a heart attack is critical to the outcome and survival from this adverse event. For each minute that emergency care (i.e., CPR, AED) is delayed, the individual's chance for survival reduces by approximately 10 percent (ARC, 2011). The American Red Cross has outlined four steps in the "cardiac chain of survival" (ARC, 2011). These four steps include:

1. Early recognition of an adverse cardiovascular event and early activation of the **emergency medical system (EMS)** by calling 9-1-1.
2. Early administration of **cardiopulmonary resuscitation (CPR)**, a life support method using both chest compressions and mouth-to-mouth ventilation. CPR helps to supply oxygen to the brain and other vital organs until advanced care arrives.
3. Early use of an automated external defibrillator (AED). An AED delivers a small electrical shock to the heart that may be effective to restore normal heart rhythm.
4. Early arrival of advanced medical care. Trained EMS professionals are able to provide more advanced care and transportation of the victim to local emergency facilities.

When approaching an emergency situation or an individual suspected of suffering a heart attack, the first responder should begin by sizing up the scene to determine if the area is safe for themselves, the victim, and other bystanders. Next, check the victim for responsiveness. If the victim is unresponsive, then appoint a bystander to call 9-1-1. Next, perform a primary assessment of the victim guided by C-A-B: chest compressions, airway, breathing. In 2010, the American Heart Association (AHA) changed the sequence of basic life support steps from A-B-C (airway, breathing, circulation) to C-A-B (chest compressions, airway, breathing) (Field et al., 2010; Neumar et al., 2015).

C = Chest Compressions: Check for a pulse. If there is no pulse, begin chest compressions. Chest compressions help circulate the oxygen-rich blood throughout the body.

A = Airway: Open the victim's airway and check for signs of breathing. Look to see if the chest rises and falls. Listen near the mouth for breath sounds. Feel for air passing through the nose and mouth.

B = Breathing: If the signs of breathing are absent, then begin rescue breathing. The purpose of rescue breathing is to supply oxygen via the cardiorespiratory system to the brain and vital organs.

The acronym C.A.B. may also be expanded to include a 'D' for defibrillation. An **automated external defibrillator (AED)** is a relatively small portable electronic device used to analyze the heart's rhythm and provide defibrillation (when necessary) through the delivery of a small electrical shock. This electrical shock can re-establish normal heart rhythm and when administered promptly can significantly increase the victim's chance for survival. All fitness facilities should have at least one AED on site and staff trained to use this device during emergency situations. At the present time, a relatively small number of states and municipalities mandate the presence of an AED in fitness facilities. However, similar requirements may become more common as the standard of care regarding AEDs continue to evolve. Liability issues have also been raised in cases of ill-equipped fitness facilities unable to appropriately respond to foreseeable cardiac emergencies (Abbott, 2012a). The ACSM and AHA recommend that an AED is available in all fitness facilities: (1) having more than 2,500 members, (2) offer programs and services for the elderly or those with medical conditions, and (3) are located where the response time of EMS care is anticipated to be greater than 5 minutes (ACSM, 2012; Abbott, 2012a; Balady et al., 2002).

NETA-certified fitness professionals must hold an appropriate emergency cardiovascular care certification (e.g., CPR, CPR/AED) granted by a reputable provider such as the American Red Cross, the American Heart Association, the American Safety and Health Institute, or the National Safety Council. At minimum, NETA-certified Group Exercise Instructors must hold adult CPR certification, and NETA-certified Personal Trainers must hold adult CPR/AED certification. Acceptable emergency cardiovascular care certifications must include a live hands-on practical skills evaluation.

Stroke

A **stroke** is a condition that affects the arteries supplying oxygen-rich blood to and within the brain. Each year, approximately 795,000 strokes occur in the United States (Mozaffarian et al., 2015). In 2013, nearly 129,000 deaths in the U.S. were attributable to stroke (i.e., cerebrovascular disease), making stroke the fifth leading cause of death among Americans (Heron, 2016). A stroke occurs when an artery supplying the brain is either blocked (i.e., ischemic stroke) or ruptures (i.e., hemorrhagic stroke). In either case, the part of the brain supplied by the affected artery cannot receive the vital oxygen and nutrients needed to survive, resulting in death of brain cells. The outcome of a stroke may include paralysis, physical disabilities, visual or speech impairments, memory loss, altered cognition, and even death.

> **Good to Know**
> **Recognizing a Stroke**
>
> **F**ace Drooping
> **A**rm Weakness
> **S**peech Difficulty
> **T**ime to call 911

An individual suspected of having a stroke requires immediate medical attention. Early recognition and prompt activation of the EMS is critical. The American Stroke Association has developed an acronym, F.A.S.T., to help identify a stroke.

F = Face Drooping: Does one side of the face droop or is it numb? Ask the person to smile. Is the person's smile uneven?

A = Arm Weakness: Is one arm weak or numb? Ask the person to raise both arms. Does one arm drift downward?

S = Speech Difficulty: Is speech slurred? Is the person unable to speak or hard to understand? Ask the person to repeat a simple sentence, like "The sky is blue." Is the sentence repeated correctly?

T = Time to call 911: If someone shows any of these symptoms, even if the symptoms go away, call 9-1-1 and get the person to the hospital immediately. Check the time to note when the first symptoms appeared.

There are many factors that may contribute to stroke among which hypertension is the leading cause and perhaps the most important controllable risk factor. As indicated in chapter 7, systolic blood pressure (SBP) will increase during cardiorespiratory exercise in proportion to the exercise intensity, typically rising 8 to 12 mmHg per MET of activity (Pescatello et al., 2004). However, the diastolic pressure (DBP) will remain unchanged or may decrease slightly during cardiorespiratory exercise. The effects on blood pressure during aerobic exercise are attributed to the 'volume load' placed on the heart and cardiovascular system, which is characterized by an increase in cardiac output (i.e., increased heart rate and stroke volume) and a decrease in peripheral vascular resistance (i.e., increased arterial vasodilation) (Sorace et al., 2012).

During the performance of resistance training exercises, both the systolic and diastolic blood pressures may be expected to increase. This acute blood pressure response is related to a 'pressure load' (also known as the 'pressor response') during which the total arterial peripheral resistance increases in conjunction with only a slight elevation in cardiac output (Sorace et al., 2012). The magnitude of this 'pressure load' is influenced by the relative intensity of the resistance training (i.e., % of 1-RM), the size of the muscles being utilized, and the duration of muscular contraction in proportion to the rest periods between sets (Sorace et al., 2012). The blood pressure response is also exaggerated during isometric contractions and when the exerciser performs the Valsalva maneuver.

It has been suggested that extreme blood pressure elevations experienced during high-intensity resistance training performed with the Valsalva maneuver, may contribute to the onset of hemorrhagic stroke (Haykowsky et al., 1996). As such, fitness professionals should advise their clients regarding proper breathing techniques during resistance training. In addition, high risk populations (e.g., older adults, hypertensive individuals, those with a history of CVD or stroke) should avoid high-intensity (i.e., ≥85% 1-RM) resistance training. Individuals with uncontrolled high blood pressure (i.e., SBP ≥160 mmHg and/or DBP ≥100 mmHg) should work with their health care provider to bring hypertension under control before starting an exercise program (Braith & Stewart, 2006). It has also been recommended that cardiorespiratory exercise tests should be terminated if the systolic blood pressure is greater than 250 mmHg or the diastolic blood pressure is greater than 115 mmHg (ACSM, 2018; Pescatello et al., 2004).

Emergency Response Plan

Injuries and cardiovascular events are foreseeable in fitness settings when people are challenging their physical capabilities. Therefore, every fitness facility must have a written **emergency response plan (ERP)** outlining policies and procedures related to emergency response (ACSM, 2012; Abbott, 2012b; ACSM & AHA, 1998). The ERP should be reviewed periodically including the rehearsal of probable emergency scenarios. Fitness professionals should be familiar with the ERP for each of their work environments. Recognizing signs and symptoms of medical distress will help the fitness professional react appropriately to possible emergency situations. The first response to a life-threatening incident can determine the eventual outcome.

There are several steps for pre-crisis preparation:
- Be prepared before an emergency occurs.
  - Post the name of the facility, address, and phone number near the phone.
  - Know where the fire exits, extinguishers, and severe weather shelters are located.
  - Maintain a well-stocked first aid kit.
  - Equip your facility with an automated external defibrillator. Inspect the AED regularly to ensure proper function. Replace battery as needed.
  - Maintain CPR, AED, and other safety certifications such as standard first aid and emergency oxygen administration.
- Do not move a victim unless there is clear and present danger to that person or yourself.
- Don't panic. Stay calm and take control of the situation.
- Don't hesitate to activate the emergency medical system. Call 9-1-1.
- Provide the EMS personnel with any known information about the victim.

Chapter Summary

Although exercise-related injuries, heat illnesses, and adverse cardiovascular events are unfortunate, these incidents are foreseeable and in many cases preventable. Fitness professionals must implement strategies to reduce the occurrence of accidents, injuries, and potentially life-threatening events. In addition, fitness professionals must recognize the signs and symptoms of these events and must respond appropriately as emergency situations do arise.

Chapter References

Abbott, A.A. (2012a). Code blue: Member down. *ACSM's Health & Fitness Journal, 16*(3), 31-34.

Abbott, A.A. (2012b). Emergency response plan. *ACSM's Health & Fitness Journal, 16*(5), 33-36.

American College of Sports Medicine (2012). *ACSM's Health/Fitness Facility Standards and Guidelines*, 4th edition. Tharrett, S.J., & Peterson, J.A. (Eds.). Champaign, IL: Human Kinetics.

American College of Sports Medicine (2018). *ACSM's Guidelines for Exercise Testing and Prescription*, 10th edition. Philadelphia, PA: Wolters Kluwer.

American College of Sports Medicine and American Heart Association (1998). Position Stand: Recommendations for cardiovascular screening, staffing, and emergency policies at heath/fitness facilities. *Medicine & Science in Sports & Exercise, 30*(6),1009-18.

American Red Cross (2011). *CPR/AED for Professional Rescuers and Health Care Providers Handbook*. StayWell Health & Safety Solutions.

Armstrong, L.E., Casa, D.J., Millard-Stafford, M., Moran, D.S., Pyne, S.W., & Roberts, W.O. (2007). American College of Sports Medicine position stand. Exertional heat illness during training and competition. *Medicine and Science in Sports and Exercise, 39*(3), 556-572.

Balady, G.J., Chaitman, B., Foster, C., Froelicher, E., Gordon, N., & Van Camp, S. (2002). Automated external defibrillators in health/fitness facilities supplement to the AHA/ACSM recommendations for cardiovascular screening, staffing, and emergency policies at health/fitness facilities. *Circulation, 105*(9), 1147-1150.

Binkley, H.M., Beckett, J., Casa, D.J., Kleiner, D.M., & Plummer, P.E. (2002). National Athletic Trainers Association position statement: Exertional heat illnesses. *Journal of Athletic Training,* 37(3), 329-343.

Bolgla, L.A., & Boling, M.C. (2011). An update for the conservative management of patellofemoral pain syndrome: A systematic review of the literature from 2000 to 2010. *International Journal of Sports Physical Therapy, 6*(2), 112-125.

Braith, R.W., & Stewart, K.J. (2006). Resistance exercise training its role in the prevention of cardiovascular disease. *Circulation, 113*(22), 2642-2650.

Bullock, S.H., Jones, B.H., Gilchrist, J., & Marshall, S.W. (2010). Prevention of physical training–related injuries: Recommendations for the military and other active populations based on expedited systematic reviews. *American Journal of Preventive Medicine, 38*(1), S156-S181.

Chan, O., Del Buono, A., Best, T.M., & Maffulli, N. (2012). Acute muscle strain injuries: A proposed new classification system. *Knee Surgery, Sports Traumatology, Arthroscopy, 20*(11), 2356-2362.

Cimino, F., Volk, B.S., & Setter, D. (2010). Anterior cruciate ligament injury: Diagnosis, management, and prevention. *American Family Physician, 82*(8), 917-922.

Conte, M., Caputo, F., Piu, G., Sechi, S., Isoni, F., & Salvi, M. (2011). Stress Fractures. In *Orthopedic Sports Medicine* (pp. 73-87). Springer Milan.

Dishman, R.K., Heath, G.W., & I-Min, L. (2013). *Physical Activity Epidemiology*, 2nd edition. Champaign, IL: Human Kinetics.

Dixit, S., Difiori, J.P., Burton, M., & Mines, B. (2007). Management of patellofemoral pain syndrome. *American Family Physician, 75*(2), 194-202.

Durall, C.J., Manske, R.C., & Davies, G.J. (2001). Avoiding shoulder injury from resistance training. *Strength & Conditioning Journal, 23*(5), 10-18.

Ellenbecker, T.S., & Cools, A. (2010). Rehabilitation of shoulder impingement syndrome and rotator cuff injuries: An evidence-based review. *British Journal of Sports Medicine, 44*(5), 319-327.

Field, J.M., Hazinski, M.F., Sayre, M.R., Chameides, L., Schexnayder, S.M., Hemphill, R., ... & Cave, D.M. (2010). Part 1: Executive summary 2010 American Heart Association guidelines for cardiopulmonary resuscitation and emergency cardiovascular care. *Circulation,* 122(18 suppl 3), S640-S656.

Goff, J.D., & Crawford, R. (2011). Diagnosis and treatment of plantar fasciitis. *American Family Physician, 84*(6), 676-82.

Gotsch, K., Annest, J.L., Holmgreen, P., & Gilchrist, J. (2002). Nonfatal sports- and recreation-related injuries treated in emergency departments-United States, July 2000-June 2001. *Morbidity and Mortality Weekly Report, 51*(33), 736-740.

Haykowsky, M.J., Findlay, J.M., & Ignaszewski, A.P. (1996). Aneurysmal subarachnoid hemorrhage associated with weight training: Three case reports. *Clinical Journal of Sport Medicine, 6*(1), 52-55.

Heron, M. (2016). *Deaths: Leading Causes for 2013*. National vital statistics reports: from the Centers for Disease Control and Prevention, National Center for Health Statistics, National Vital Statistics System, 65(2), 1-14.

Kerr, Z.Y., Collins, C.L., & Comstock, R.D. (2010). Epidemiology of weight training-related injuries presenting to United States emergency departments, 1990 to 2007. *The American Journal of Sports Medicine, 38*(4), 765-771.

Mozaffarian, D., Benjamin, E.J., Go, A.S., Arnett, D.K., Blaha, M.J., Cushman, M., ... & Huffman, M.D. (2015). Executive Summary: Heart disease and stroke statistics—2015 update a report from the American Heart Association. *Circulation*, 131(4), 434-441.

Nawrot, T.S., Perez, L., Künzli, N., Munters, E., & Nemery, B. (2011). Public health importance of triggers of myocardial infarction: A comparative risk assessment. *The Lancet, 377*(9767), 732-740.

Neumar, R.W., Shuster, M., Callaway, C.W., Gent, L.M., Atkins, D.L., Bhanji, F., ... & Kleinman, M.E. (2015). Part 1: Executive summary 2015 American Heart Association guidelines update for cardiopulmonary resuscitation and emergency cardiovascular care. *Circulation*, 132(18 suppl 2), S315-S367.

Nyland, J., Brand, E., & Fisher, B. (2010). Update on rehabilitation following ACL reconstruction. *Open Access Journal of Sports Medicine, 1*, 153-160.

Outerbridge, R.E., & Outerbridge, H.K. (2001). The etiology of chondromalacia patellae. *Clinical Orthopaedics and Related Research, 389*, 5-8.

Pescatello, L.S., Franklin, B.A., Fagard, R., Farquhar, W.B., Kelley, G.A., & Ray, C.A. (2004). American College of Sports Medicine position stand. Exercise and hypertension. *Medicine and Science in Sports and Exercise, 36*(3), 533-553.

Renstrom, P., Ljungqvist, A., Arendt, E., Beynnon, B., Fukubayashi, T., Garrett, W., ... & Engebretsen, L. (2008). Non-contact ACL injuries in female athletes: An International Olympic Committee current concepts statement. *British Journal of Sports Medicine, 42*(6), 394-412.

Sorace, P., Churilla, J. R., & Magyari, P. M. (2012). Resistance training for hypertension: Design safe and effective programs. *ACSM's Health & Fitness Journal, 16*(1), 13-18.

Tolbert, T.A., & Binkley, H.M. (2009). Treatment and prevention of shin splints. *Strength & Conditioning Journal, 31*(5), 69-72.

Waterman, B R., Owens, B.D., Davey, S., Zacchilli, M.A., & Belmont, P.J. (2010). The epidemiology of ankle sprains in the United States. *The Journal of Bone & Joint Surgery, 92*(13), 2279-2284.

Willich, S.N., Lewis, M., Lowel, H., Arntz, H.R., Schubert, F., & Schroder, R. (1993). Physical exertion as a trigger of acute myocardial infarction. *New England Journal of Medicine, 329*(23), 1684-1690.

Chapter 24 Review Questions

1. Your new client underwent an ACL reconstruction surgery ten months ago. She has been discharged from physical therapy and is planning to continue her post-rehabilitative fitness program working with you as her personal trainer. She has received clearance from her orthopedic doctor to participate in a fitness program. Which of the following exercises is considered to be contraindicated for this client?
    A. Seated leg curl machine
    B. Leg press machine
    C. Stability ball squat
    D. Leg extension machine

2. You are conducting a 45-minute lunchtime outdoor boot camp class on a relatively hot summer day. As you near the end of the class, a participant reports feelings of dizziness, headache, and nausea. He is sweating profusely and his skin feels cold and clammy. Based on these signs and symptoms, the participant is most likely to be suffering from which of the following?
    A. Exertional heat cramps
    B. Heat exhaustion
    C. Hyponatremia
    D. Heatstroke

3. Which of the following is the most appropriate first aid care to be provided for a muscle strain or a ligament sprain?
    A. FAST
    B. DOMS
    C. PRICE
    D. CABD

4. A 58-year-old male has recently joined your health club. He has just completed a fairly vigorous 30-minute workout on the treadmill. As you enter the locker room, you find this member sitting in a slumped-over position on the bench near his locker. He is sweating profusely, seems restless, is having difficulty breathing, and is massaging what appears to be soreness in his left shoulder. You approach the member to inquire about his well-being. He indicates that he has not been feeling well since he finished his workout and is feeling somewhat nauseous. Which of the following life-threatening conditions is this member likely to be experiencing?
    A. Hemorrhagic stroke
    B. Myocardial Infarction
    C. Shoulder impingement syndrome
    D. Exertional heatstroke

5. Shoulder impingement syndrome often involves a pinching of the _____ muscle during _____ of the humerus.
    A. infraspinatus, internal rotation
    B. teres major, horizontal abduction
    C. subscapularis, flexion
    D. supraspinatus, abduction

6. In an effort to prepare for accidents and adverse events, and to minimize unnecessary liability exposure, fitness professionals must be familiar with the fitness facility's _____.
    A. informed consent form
    B. emergency response plan
    C. emergency medical services
    D. employee assistance program

Answers to Review Questions on Page 384

Note: Review questions are intended to reinforce learning and comprehension of subject matter presented in the corresponding chapter.
The review questions are not intended to be representative of actual certification exam questions in terms of style, content, or difficulty.

25
Medical Conditions & Special Populations

Introduction

Fitness professionals will often work with clients that have special health concerns. This chapter outlines several common medical conditions facing the American population today. These conditions include asthma, arthritis, diabetes, hypertension, and osteoporosis. Each medical condition is briefly described including statistical data, programming considerations, and recommended exercise guidelines. These conditions should be identified through the preparticipation screening process conducted prior to starting an exercise program. When indicated, clients and class participants should consult with their health care provider and obtain medical clearance to participate along with exercise guidelines and potential limitations. Fitness professionals should observe any parameters that have been established and maintain open lines of communication with the individual's health care providers, when necessary. In addition, this chapter will also review exercise programming guidelines for special population groups including pregnant women, older adults, and youth and adolescents.

Asthma

Asthma is a chronic inflammatory disease that affects the lining of the airways (i.e., bronchi, bronchioles) within the lungs. The inflammation causes the smooth muscles surrounding the airways to contract. The narrowing of the airways is called *bronchospasm* or *bronchoconstriction*, which restricts airflow to the lungs and reduces delivery of oxygen to the rest of the body. See figure 25-1. The cells lining the airways also overproduce mucus, a thick sticky fluid that causes further airway restriction. The bronchospasm and airway restriction cause symptoms such as recurrent episodes of wheezing (i.e., a whistling sound when breathing), chest tightness, shortness of breath (i.e., dyspnea), and coughing, which often occurs at night or early in the morning.

In 2010, an estimated 25.7 million Americans had asthma including 18.7 million adults and 7.0 million youth (Moorman et al., 2012). There is no known cure for asthma and it is currently unclear how to prevent asthma from developing. However, there are many known environmental factors that may contribute to the onset of asthma attacks among those with the disease. Exposure to allergens

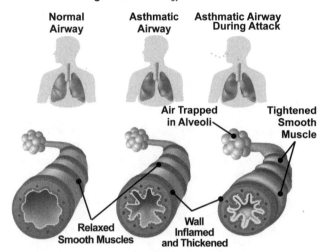

Figure 25-1 Pathology of Asthma

(e.g., pollen, dust mites, pet dander), air pollution, tobacco smoke, chemicals, and dry or cold air are all known triggers of asthma attacks. Limiting exposure to these environmental factors may help to minimize the occurrence of asthmatic episodes.

Physical activity may also trigger bronchospasm among individuals with or without chronic asthma. For those with underlying asthma, the bronchospasm occurring during or immediately after exercise is referred to as *exercise-induced asthma (EIA)*; whereas, among those without asthma it is referred to as *exercise-induced bronchospasm (EIB)* (Billen & Dupont, 2008). The common symptoms of EIA and EIB include coughing, wheezing, chest tightness, and dyspnea; however, other less-common symptoms may also include headache, abdominal pain, muscle cramps, dizziness and fatigue (Billen & Dupont, 2008). The bronchospasm and related symptoms typically begin within 6 to 8 minutes after the start of exercise and may peak 5 to 15 minutes after exercise has been ended (Billen & Dupont, 2008). Bronchospasm induced by exercise may be controlled or prevented through the use of short-acting inhaled beta-agonist medications (e.g., albuterol, levalbuterol) taken 15 minutes before exercise (Naguwa et al., 2012). Those with chronic asthma are also typically treated with inhaled corticosteroids, which may play an additional role in the management of EIA and EIB (Naguwa et al., 2012).

Individuals with asthma, exercise-induced asthma, or

exercise-induced bronchospasm may generally follow the cardiorespiratory, resistance training, and flexibility training guidelines advocated for healthy populations. As with any individual, the initial frequency, duration, and intensity should be appropriate based on the participant's level of conditioning, physical limitations, and tolerance to exercise. The fitness professional should be particularly conservative in the selection of exercise intensity and duration since higher intensity and longer duration exercise can trigger bronchoconstriction. In addition, the following special considerations are advised in the design and implementation of exercise programs for those with asthma (ACSM, 2018, Billen & Dupont, 2008; Naguwa et al., 2012).

- Individuals experiencing an asthmatic episode should not exercise until symptoms and airway function have improved.
- Use of short-acting bronchodilators, as prescribed by a health care provider, may be necessary before or after exercise to prevent or manage exercise-induced bronchoconstriction.
- A prolonged warm-up period of at least 15 minutes, during which heart rate reaches 50% to 60% of HR_{max} may help to reduce incidence of EIA or EIB.
- A cool-down period of 10 to 15 minutes is advised to prevent rapid rewarming of the airway lining (i.e., epithelium).
- Limit or avoid exercise in environments that expose the individual to pollen, pollution, or cold air. Wearing a face mask during exercise in cold, dry air allows the air to be warmed and humidified to minimize onset of bronchoconstriction.
- Swimming and aquatic exercise tend to be better tolerated by asthmatic populations; however, pools with a high chlorine concentration may trigger asthmatic events.

Arthritis

Arthritis affects the lives of the young and old alike. Although arthritis is often referred to as if it were a single disease, it is actually a collection of over 100 rheumatic diseases. This family of diseases affects the musculoskeletal system and specifically the joints. Arthritis-related symptoms include muscle and joint pain, stiffness, inflammation, and damage to articular cartilage and joint structures. Such damage can lead to joint weakness, instability, and visible deformities. Arthritis and rheumatic diseases continue to be the leading cause of pain and disability in the United States, collectively affecting 52.5 million Americans (CDC, 2013). Arthritis decreases functional capacity, the ability to perform daily tasks, and the overall quality of life. The two most prevalent forms of arthritis are osteoarthritis followed by rheumatoid arthritis.

Osteoarthritis (OA) is a degenerative joint disease in which the cartilage that covers the ends of bones deteriorates, causing pain and loss of movement as bone begins to rub against bone. Osteoarthritis can affect one or multiple joints, most commonly including the knees, hips, spine, and ankles. OA can also lead to the development of bone spurs that irritate soft tissue surrounding a joint. In most cases, arthritis-related pain is exacerbated when a person overuses an arthritic joint or dramatically changes their activity level. Arthritis often develops in a joint that has been injured, subjected to prolonged stress, or overused through repetitive motion. The prevalence of osteoarthritis is expected to grow since older age and excess body weight are both well-established risk factors for the development of OA, especially of the knee (Golightly et al., 2012). Osteoarthritis also contributes to the rising number of knee and hip replacement surgeries. Conservative treatment often involves the use of nonsteroidal anti-inflammatory drugs (NSAIDs) under the direction of a health care provider. There is strong evidence to support the use of both cardiorespiratory (e.g., land-based, water-based) and resistance training exercise programs to improve pain and function for those with mild-to-moderate osteoarthritis (Golightly et al., 2012). In addition, there is growing evidence to support the use of other exercise modalities such as Tai Chi, balance training, and proprioceptive training as effective approaches to manage and improve symptoms associated with osteoarthritis (Golightly et al., 2012).

Rheumatoid Arthritis (RA) is an autoimmune disease in which the body's immune system mistakenly attacks the tissues of the joints. Unlike the degenerative nature of OA, rheumatoid arthritis is a chronic inflammatory condition affecting the synovial lining of joints causing painful swelling, which progresses to erosion of bone tissue and joint deformity. Rheumatoid arthritis is one of the most serious and disabling types of arthritis. RA affects approximately 1% of the population with a prevalence rate about 5 times higher among women and a typical onset between the ages of 40 and 60 (Plasqui, 2008). RA most often affects the small joints of the hands and feet, leading to restricted mobility, loss of function, and decreased quality of life. As the result of joint pain, decreased mobility, fatigue, and reduced physical capacity, it is likely that those with RA are generally less active and may be apprehensive to engage in physical activity or exercise for fear of exacerbation of symptoms. However, research has indicated that those engaging in appropriate physical activity and exercise programs do benefit from increased cardiorespiratory and muscular fitness leading to improved functional capacity and quality of life (Plasqui, 2008). In addition, there is no evidence that appropriate levels of exercise progress disease activity or cause increased pain and joint damage (Pasqui, 2008).

With the guidance of a health care provider, regular physical activity and exercise should be encouraged for all individuals with arthritis. In addition to managing the physical symptoms of arthritis, physical activity may also promote overall health and fitness, increase energy levels, improve quality of sleep, maintain a healthy body weight, decreasing feelings of depression and anxiety, and increase self-esteem and self-efficacy. The following special considerations are advised in the design and implementation of exercise programs for those with arthritic conditions (ACSM, 2018).

- Most individuals with arthritis should strive toward a goal of ≥150 minutes of moderate-intensity aerobic exercise per week. Initially, shorter bouts of exercise are better tolerated since long continuous bouts may be difficult for some with regard to arthritic symptoms and physical conditioning.
- Guidelines used for healthy populations with regard to cardiorespiratory, resistance, and flexibility training are applicable to those with arthritis; however, an emphasis on lower intensity exercise is recommended.
- Progression of activity should be gradual and individualized based on the participant's pain and other symptoms.
- Low-impact aerobic activities such as walking, biking, and swimming are most appropriate. High-impact activities such as running, stair climbing, and those with stop and go actions or quick directional changes are not recommended.
- Avoid vigorous-intensity exercise during acute symptom flare ups and increased inflammation. Gentle range of motion activities are most appropriate during these times.
- Adequate warm-up and cool-down periods of at least 5 to 10 minutes are essential to minimize pain.
- Encourage exercise during the time of day when pain and other arthritic symptoms are least severe or plan exercise in conjunction with periods of peak pain relief provided by medication.
- Incorporate functional activities as tolerated such as rising from a chair and step-ups to improve neuromuscular control, balance, and improved ability to perform activities of daily living (ADLs).
- For aquatic exercise, water temperature should be 83° to 88°F (28° to 31°C) since warm water helps to relax muscles and reduce pain.
- Inform participants with arthritis that a small amount of discomfort in the muscles and joints immediately following exercise is common and is not necessarily an indication of further joint damage. However, if pain ratings 2 hours after exercise are higher than pre-exercise levels, then exercise intensity and/or duration should be reduced appropriately for future sessions.

Diabetes

Diabetes mellitus (DM) is a group of metabolic diseases characterized by elevated blood glucose (i.e., sugar) levels, a condition known as *hyperglycemia*. The elevated blood glucose levels are the result of insufficient insulin production and/or an inability of the muscle cells to properly utilize insulin (ACSM, 2018). Diabetes is a significant cause of morbidity and premature death related to atherosclerosis, cardiovascular disease, stroke, kidney and nerve damage, blindness, organ failure, and lower limb amputation (CDC, 2012; Colberg et al., 2010). In 2013, diabetes was the seventh leading cause of death in the U.S. (Heron, 2016). According to the Centers for Disease Control and Prevention, approximately 29.1 million Americans (9.3% of the U.S. population) had diabetes of which 27.8% were undiagnosed (CDC, 2015). In addition, an estimated 86 million American adults are at a very high risk of developing diabetes due to a condition called prediabetes (CDC, 2015). *Prediabetes* is a condition characterized by high blood glucose (e.g., *impaired fasting glucose, impaired glucose tolerance*) or elevated hemoglobin A1c levels, either of which are higher than normal, but not high enough to be diagnosed as diabetes (ACSM, 2018; CDC, 2015). Another condition known as metabolic syndrome is also associated with an increased risk of diabetes as well as cardiovascular disease and stroke. *Metabolic syndrome (MetSyn)* encompasses a number of disorders including central (i.e., abdominal) obesity, hypertension, impaired fasting glucose, elevated triglycerides, and low HDLs (ACSM, 2018). The incidence and prevalence of diabetes, prediabetes, and metabolic syndrome in the United States have grown steadily over the previous decades. If these trends continue, it has been estimated that by the year 2050 one of three Americans could have diabetes (Boyle et al., 2010). The two most common types of diabetes are type 1 diabetes (previously called juvenile diabetes or insulin dependent diabetes mellitus) and type 2 diabetes (previously called adult-onset diabetes or non-insulin dependent diabetes mellitus).

Type 1 diabetes represents about 5% to 10% of all diabetic cases. Type 1 diabetes is an autoimmune disorder characterized by the destruction of insulin-producing beta-cells of the pancreas causing an absolute deficiency of *insulin*, which leads to an inability to properly regulate blood sugar levels (ACSM, 2018; Colberg et al., 2010). Type 1 diabetes is typically first diagnosed in youth and adolescents, although it can occur at any age. Individuals with type 1 diabetes must receive insulin from an injection or a pump to regulate blood glucose to survive.

Type 2 diabetes represents 90% to 95% of the cases of diabetes. Type 2 diabetes results from both the skeletal muscle's inability to properly utilize insulin (i.e., *insulin resistance*) and a gradual loss in the ability of the pancreas to produce insulin (CDC, 2015; Colberg et al., 2010). Type 2 diabetes is associated with risk factors such as older age, family history of diabetes, history of gestational diabetes, impaired glucose metabolism, and race or ethnicity (CDC, 2015). In addition, type 2 diabetes is highly correlated to controllable factors such as obesity and physical inactivity. Prevention and management of type 2 diabetes is dependent upon maintenance of a healthy body weight through regular physical activity and a healthy diet within caloric needs. Many individuals with type 2 diabetes will also require oral medications to control blood sugar levels and without proper treatment and lifestyle modification may also require exogenous insulin (ACSM, 2018; CDC, 2015).

Regular cardiorespiratory exercise is essential to those with diabetes given the many positive effects related to physical activity. First of all, glucose uptake and insulin sensitivity within active skeletal muscles are increased during and following physical activity (Colberg et al., 2010). Many diabetics who exercise regularly may find that their need for oral medications or insulin may decrease over time as directed by their physician. Regular physical activity and exercise also help to reduce overweight and obesity, leading to a healthier body weight. In addition, exercise plays an important role to achieve and maintain healthy blood pressure, to reduce blood cholesterol and triglycerides, and subsequently to decrease the risk of cardiovascular disease and stroke.

To ensure safe participation in physical activity and exercise programs, the following considerations are recommended for those with diabetes (ACSM, 2018; Colberg et al., 2010).

- Frequency of physical activity should be emphasized for those with diabetes, striving for 3 to 7 days of aerobic exercise per week with no more than 2 consecutive days of inactivity allowed.
- Intensity of aerobic exercise should be at least moderate, corresponding to 40% to 60% of VO_2max or an RPE of 5 to 6 on the category-ratio scale (i.e., 0 to 10).
- Diabetics should be encouraged to engage in a minimum of 150 minutes per week of moderate-intensity physical activity and work toward an increase to ≥300 minutes per week of moderate-to-vigorous activity to maximize caloric expenditure and to facilitate weight management.
- *Hypoglycemia* (i.e., low blood sugar <70 mg/dL) is a serious problem for diabetics and may occur during or up to 12 hours following exercise. Monitor for signs and symptoms of hypoglycemia including shakiness, weakness, abnormal sweating, nervousness, anxiety, hunger, headache, confusion, and tingling of the mouth or fingers. Left untreated, hypoglycemia can lead to seizures and coma.

- As a precaution, diabetics should carry sugar or glucose with them at all times. Fitness professionals should also have access to a readily available carbohydrate source in the event an exercise participant is suspected of experiencing a hypoglycemic reaction.
- Hyperglycemia is a concern for those with type 1 diabetes, particularly those who do not appropriately control blood sugar levels. Monitor for symptoms including frequent or excessive urination, fatigue, weakness, increased thirst, and acetone breath.
- Do not perform exercise if blood sugar is greater than 250 mg/dL (milligrams per deciliter) and ketones are positive. This is an indication that there already may be a lack of insulin and exercise will only cause a greater rise in blood sugar. Hydrate well and adjust insulin as necessary. Contact their health care provider, if necessary.
- Use caution when exercising if blood sugar is greater than 300 mg/dL without evidence of ketones. Exercise may help decrease sugars, but it is possible they will increase instead. Hydrate well prior to and after exercise and keep track of sugars and ketones.
- Blood glucose should be monitored before and for several hours following exercise. Adjust carbohydrate intake and/or medications before or after exercise based on blood glucose levels and exercise intensity. Avoid exercise during periods of peak insulin or medication activity.
- Persons with diabetes should not work out alone, but rather ideally with someone who knows what to do if a low blood-sugar reaction occurs.
- For individuals with peripheral neuropathy, take proper care of the feet to prevent blisters and foot ulcers.
- Given the likelihood of impaired thermoregulation, additional precautions should be taken when exercising in hot and cold environments. Drink plenty of fluids to maintain proper hydration.
- Consult with a health care provider regarding additional limitations or precautions, and to determine what types of exercise might be most appropriate. Complications of diabetes such as severe eye disease and nerve damage may make some forms of exercise dangerous.

Hypertension

Hypertension is defined as a systolic blood pressure of ≥140 mmHg or a diastolic blood pressure of ≥90 mmHg confirmed on two separate occasions, or those taking antihypertensive medications (ACSM, 2018). The overall prevalence of hypertension among U.S. adults aged 18 years and older is approximately 30.4% or an estimated 66.9 million (Valderrama et al., 2012). Among those with hypertension, an estimated 35.8 million (53.5%) do not have their hypertension controlled (Valderrama et al.

2012). Hypertension contributes to an increased risk of cardiovascular disease, stroke, heart failure, peripheral artery disease, and chronic kidney disease (Pescatello et al., 2004). Hypertension is a leading contributor to cardiovascular mortality and premature death from all other causes. Hypertension is known as the 'silent killer' because it does not manifest itself in readily identifiable indicators (Sorace et al., 2012).

Hypertension can occur as the result of many factors including smoking, obesity, excessive dietary sodium, excessive alcohol consumption, genetic predisposition, ethnicity, vascular disease, and age. As such, hypertension can be effectively controlled through lifestyle modifications such as smoking cessation, weight management, reduced sodium intake, moderation of alcohol consumption, adoption of the DASH dietary pattern, and regular physical activity (ACSM, 2018). In addition, hypertension may also be treated through the use of prescribed antihypertensive medications such as beta-blockers, calcium channel blockers, and diuretics.

Higher levels of regular physical activity and greater cardiorespiratory fitness are both associated with a reduced incidence of hypertension (Pescatello et al., 2004). Regular aerobic exercise leads to reductions in resting blood pressure of 5 to 7 mmHg in individuals with normal and high blood pressure, and reduces blood pressure at a fixed submaximal intensity (Pescatello et al., 2004). Resistance training performed at the recommended level also contributes to reductions in blood pressure (Pescatello et al., 2004). In order to maximize the safety and effectiveness of exercise to manage hypertension, the following considerations are recommended (ACSM, 2018; Pescatello et al., 2004; Sorace et al., 2012).

- Individuals with severe or uncontrolled blood pressure (i.e., resting SBP ≥180 mmHg and/or DBP ≥110 mmHg) should begin exercise only after evaluation and clearance by a health care provider and initiation of antihypertensive medication.
- Antihypertensive medications (e.g., beta-blockers, diuretics) may impair thermoregulation in hot and humid environments and may increase the predisposition for hypoglycemia. Educate participants regarding the signs and symptoms of heat illnesses and hypoglycemia, and observe normal precautions to avoid these adverse events.
- Antihypertensive medications (e.g., alpha-blockers, calcium channel blockers, vasodilators) may lead to sudden excessive reductions in blood pressure following exercise (i.e., post-exercise hypotension). An extended cool-down period is recommended for these individuals.
- Heart rate response to exercise may be reduced or limited by certain antihypertensive medications (e.g., beta-blockers). Therefore, rate of perceived exertion (RPE) may be necessary to monitor exercise intensity.
- Cardiorespiratory and resistance training guidelines used for healthy populations are appropriate for those with hypertension, placing an emphasis on low- to moderate-intensity levels to maximize safety and effectiveness.
- The primary focus of an exercise program should be placed on aerobic exercise, striving toward a minimum of 150 minutes of moderate-intensity activity per week. Resistance training exercise may be used as a supplement to aerobic training.
- Since many individuals with hypertension are also overweight or obese, a focus should be placed on maximizing caloric expenditure through regular physical activity and reduced caloric intake.
- It is imperative that individuals with hypertension are educated regarding proper breathing technique to prevent excessive elevations of blood pressure during resistance training. Avoid the Valsalva maneuver during resistance training.

Osteoporosis

Osteoporosis (meaning 'porous bones') is a disease affecting the skeletal system in which low bone mineral density and changes in the microstructure of the bone increases the risk of fracture (ACMS, 2018). See figure 25-2. *Osteoporosis* is defined as a *bone mineral density (BMD)* value greater than 2.5 standard deviations below the young adult mean value (Korhrt et al., 2004; Levine, 2011). Osteoporotic fractures occur most often at the wrist (e.g., distal radius), spine, and hip (Kohrt et al., 2004). Fractures related to osteoporosis can significantly reduce functional abilities and quality of life, and are a significant cause of mortality (due to secondary factors and complications related to fractures) among the elderly (Kohrt et al., 2004). According to the National Health and Nutrition Examination Survey, 2005–2008, 9% of U.S. adults 50 years and older had osteoporosis, with the prevalence being greater among women (Looker et al., 2012). An additional 49% of these adults have low bone mass or *osteopenia*, defined as a BMD between 1.0 and 2.5 standard deviations below the mean for young adults (Levine, 2011; Looker et al., 2012). A low peak bone mass developed during adolescence is a primary factor associated with the risk of osteoporosis (Korhrt et al., 2004). The effect of amenorrhea on the bone density of young female athletes is of great concern due to the significantly elevated risk of developing osteoporosis later in life (Nattiv et al., 2007). In addition, declining bone mineral density after the age of 40 may be attributed to endocrine changes (e.g., lower estrogen levels), the aging process, calcium and vitamin D insufficiency, and low levels of physical activity (Korhrt et al., 2004).

Figure 25-2 Osteoporosis

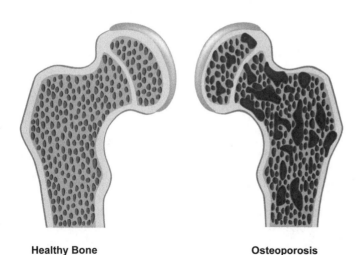

Healthy Bone   Osteoporosis

Physical activity plays an important role in maximizing bone mass attained during adolescence, maintaining bone mineral density through the fifth decade of life, slowing the rate of bone loss with aging, and reducing falls and fractures among the elderly (ACSM, 2018; Korhrt et al., 2004). Weight-bearing exercise and resistance training are particularly important for the prevention of osteoporosis since the overload forces applied to the bone stimulate an adaptive remodeling of the skeletal tissue. In addition, balance training is an important component of exercise programs for older adults to reduce the risk of falling (Korhrt et al., 2004). Although the exercise program guidelines for healthy individuals generally apply to those with osteoporosis, the following recommendations should also be considered (ACSM, 2018).

- Select weight-bearing cardiorespiratory exercises such as walking with intermittent jogging, stair climbing, or others as tolerated.
- Perform resistance training 2 to 3 days per week at a moderate intensity corresponding to 60% to 80% of 1-RM or 8 to 12 repetitions per set. Some individuals may be able to tolerate more intense workloads.
- For older adults, include appropriate neuromuscular exercises that improve balance and proprioception to reduce the risk of falling.
- Exercises that involve explosive movements or high-impact loading should be avoided. Activities that cause twisting, bending, or compression of the spine should also be avoided.
- Results of a bone density test (e.g., dual-energy x-ray absorptiometry) provide valuable information regarding risk for osteoporosis and fracture, and to guide appropriate exercise selection and intensity.

- High-risk populations (e.g., post-menopausal women, older age, Caucasian or Asian descent, family history of osteoporosis, small body frame, low calcium intake, history of eating disorders, past or present cancer treatments) should consult with their health care provider regarding the need for a bone density test.
- Individuals with indications of or confirmed diagnosis of osteoporosis should consult with a health care provider before beginning a resistance training program or impact activities.

Pregnancy

For many years it was believed that exercise during pregnancy could harm the developing baby and cause complications during the gestational period and delivery. However, in the absence of medical or obstetric complications, pregnant women should be encouraged to participate in moderate-intensity physical activity and appropriate exercise programs according to their symptoms, discomforts, and abilities throughout pregnancy (ACOG, 2002; ACSM, 2018). In addition to maintenance of physical fitness and management of healthy weight gain, regular exercise may also reduce the risk of developing pregnancy-related conditions such as gestational diabetes and pregnancy-induced hypertension (ACOG, 2002; ACSM, 2018). In order to safely advise women with regard to appropriate exercise during pregnancy, fitness professionals should have knowledge of the basic physical and physiologic adaptations associated with pregnancy, warning signs and contraindications to exercise, and exercise program considerations during pregnancy and the post-partum period.

Several musculoskeletal changes occur during pregnancy. The increased body weight during pregnancy may significantly increase the force across joints (e.g., knees, hips), especially during weight bearing activities, which may cause discomfort or perhaps increase damage to joints with underlying arthritis (Artal & O'Toole, 2003). Weight gain and anatomical changes also alter the woman's center of gravity, which may lead to loss of balance and falls. These anatomical alterations also contribute to the development of lumbar lordosis and a high prevalence of low back pain among pregnant women (Artal & O'Toole, 2003). Increasing levels of the hormones estrogen and relaxin lead to increased ligamentous laxity, causing joint instability and increased risk of strains and sprains (Artal & O'Toole, 2003). Pregnant women may also experience **diastasis recti**, a vertical separation of the linea alba caused by stretching and thinning of the tissue as the result of the expanding abdomen (Bowman, 2013).

Many changes also occur throughout the cardiorespiratory system in pregnant women. The heart enlarges, the heart walls thicken, and blood volume increases. Resting and submaximal heart rate may rise by as much as 20% during the second and third trimesters (Artal & O'Toole, 2003). Stroke volume and cardiac output increase 30%

to 50% by mid-pregnancy (Artal & O'Toole, 2003). Additionally, systemic vascular resistance decreases and mean arterial pressure decreases by 5 to 10 mmHg (Artal & O'Toole, 2003). Cardiac reserves (i.e., the ability of the heart to meet the body's demands) diminish causing quicker fatigue levels. After the first trimester, lying in the supine position restricts or obstructs venous return of blood to the heart causing decreased cardiac output and orthostatic hypotension (ACOG, 2002; Artal & O'Toole, 2003). Significant respiratory changes are also associated with pregnancy including an increase in tidal volume and an increase in respiratory rate, each contributing to an increase in minute ventilation of almost 50% (Artal & O'Toole, 2003). However, as the diaphragm moves upward in response to the increasing size of the uterus, mild breathing difficulties may arise. This may cause a tendency to hyperventilate. Oxygen consumption increases by 10% to 20%, but the available oxygen reserves stored in the blood and the muscles decrease.

Although most pregnant women can safely exercise, it is recommended that women consult with their health care provider throughout pregnancy. In particular, women who are extremely obese, have gestational diabetes, or hypertension should consult with their health care provider before engaging in an exercise program (ACSM, 2018). Fitness professionals may use the *PARmed-X for Pregnancy* as a preparticipation health screening tool for pregnant women (Wolfe & Davies, 2003). The PARmed-X for Pregnancy was created to facilitate communication between the pregnant woman, her health care provider, and the fitness professional (Wolfe & Davies, 2003). A copy of the PARmed-X for Pregnancy can be found in the appendix on pages 362–365. The relative and absolute contraindications to exercise during pregnancy are listed in table 25-1. In addition, fitness professionals must be aware of the warning signs to terminate exercise while pregnant as listed in table 25-2.

During pregnancy, most women can safely participate in a variety of exercise programs; however, as with any individual, the program should be tailored to the health status, fitness level, goals, and limitations of the participant. With some exceptions, the guidelines for exercise observed for healthy populations are applicable to pregnant women with the following additional considerations (ACOG, 2002; ACSM, 2018; Artal & O'Toole, 2003).

- To reduce the risk of having a low birth weight baby, research suggests an ideal frequency of 3 to 4 days per week of cardiorespiratory exercise.
- For women with a pre-pregnancy body mass index less than 25 kg/m², moderate-intensity aerobic exercise is recommended; whereas, for those with a pre-pregnancy BMI ≥s25 kg/m², light-intensity exercise is recommended.

Table 25-1 Exercise Contraindications

Contraindications for Exercise During Pregnancy
Relative Contraindications
• Severe anemia
• Unevaluated maternal cardiac arrhythmia
• Chronic bronchitis
• Poorly controlled type I diabetes
• Extreme morbid obesity
• Extreme underweight (body mass index <12)
• History of extremely sedentary lifestyle
• Intrauterine growth restriction in current pregnancy
• Poorly controlled hypertension
• Orthopedic limitations
• Poorly controlled seizure disorder
• Poorly controlled hyperthyroidism
• Heavy smoker
Absolute Contraindications
• Hemodynamically significant heart disease
• Restrictive lung disease
• Incompetent cervix/cerclage
• Multiple gestation at risk for premature labor
• Persistent second or third trimester bleeding
• Placenta previa after 26 weeks gestation
• Premature labor during the current pregnancy
• Ruptured membranes
• Preeclampsia/pregnancy-induced hypertension

ACOG (2002); ACSM (2018); Artal & O'Toole (2003)

Table 25-2 Warning Signs

Warning Signs to Terminate Exercise While Pregnant
• Vaginal bleeding
• Dyspnea before exertion
• Dizziness or feeling faint
• Headache
• Chest pain
• Muscle weakness
• Calf pain or swelling (need to rule out thrombophlebitis)
• Preterm labor
• Decreased fetal movement
• Amniotic fluid leakage

ACOG (2002); Artal & O'Toole (2003)

- Women who exercised regularly before pregnancy and have an uncomplicated, healthy pregnancy should be able to engage in high-intensity exercise without adverse effects.
- Rating of perceived exertion is useful during pregnancy in conjunction with or as an alternate to heart rate monitoring.
- Avoid exercise performed in the supine position after the first trimester to avoid obstructed venous return of blood to the heart.
- Limit any repetitive isometric or high-intensity resistance training as well as exercises that may elicit a significant pressor response. Avoid performing the Valsalva maneuver during resistance training.
- Avoid contact sports, activities with a high risk of abdominal trauma, and activities with a high risk of falling or loss of balance.
- Avoid exercising in hot and humid environments, stay well-hydrated, and dress appropriately to avoid heat-related disorders.
- Scuba diving should be avoided during pregnancy since it places the fetus at increased risk for decompression sickness. However, swimming and aquatic exercise are recommended and well-tolerated due to increased buoyancy and reduced joint stress.
- Metabolic needs increase by approximately 300 calories per day after the 13th week of pregnancy. Caloric intake should be increased appropriately to meet the caloric cost of pregnancy and exercise.
- Women with a history of or at risk for preterm labor or fetal growth restriction should be advised to reduce activity levels during the second and third trimesters.

Exercise may be resumed as soon as physically and medically safe following birth. Many of the physiological and morphological changes of pregnancy last for four to six weeks into the post-partum period (ACOG, 2002; Artal & O'Toole, 2003). Generally, exercise may begin approximately 4 to 6 weeks after normal vaginal delivery or about 8 to 10 weeks after cesarean section delivery with medical clearance (ACSM, 2018). However, return to exercise varies greatly among individuals and some women are able to safely resume exercise within days of delivery (ACOG, 2002). Physical activity and exercise after pregnancy have been associated with deceased post-partum depression, provided the exercise is stress relieving and not provoking (ACOG, 2002; Artal & O'Toole, 2003).

Youth and Adolescents

Regular physical activity among youth and adolescents (i.e., 6 to 17 years old) is essential to promote health and fitness. As with adults, lack of regular physical activity and poor dietary habits contribute to childhood obesity. In 2009-2010, the prevalence of obesity in U.S. children and adolescents was 16.9% (Ogden et al., 2012). Childhood obesity predisposes youth to obesity in adulthood and increases the risk of developing obesity-related chronic diseases at an early age and throughout the lifespan. In comparison to the physical activity guidelines established for youth and adolescence, it has been found that among a nationally representative sample of U.S. adolescents in 1999–2006, less than 20% reported meeting both aerobic and muscle-strengthening guidelines, and approximately 50% reported meeting neither the aerobic nor the muscle-strengthening guideline (Song et al., 2013). Fitness professionals have an opportunity to positively influence youth and adolescents to improve their exercise and dietary habits.

In the past, there have been some concerns regarding the safety of resistance training among youth and adolescence. Although there are inherent risks associated with physical activity and resistance training, in general, the risk of injury is similar for youth and adults. In fact, the risk of musculoskeletal injury is no greater than that which is seen with many other sporting and recreational activities frequently performed by youth and adolescents (Faigenbaum et al., 2009). The risk of injury related to resistance training may be minimized by providing adult supervision, qualified instruction, appropriate program design and progression, and careful selection of resistance training equipment (Faigenbaum et al., 2009).

Similar to adults, youth obtain a wide variety of health and fitness benefits from regular physical activity. The *Physical Activity Guidelines for Americans* and the American College of Sports Medicine recommend that children and adolescents aged 6 to 17 engage in 60 minutes or more of physical activity each day, including aerobic, muscle-strengthening, and bone-strengthening exercises (ACSM, 2018; DHH, 2008). These physical activity guidelines are provided in table 25-3 and specific guidelines for resistance training are outlined in table 25-4.

In addition to the physical activity and resistance training guidelines, fitness professionals should also consider the following points when designing exercise programs for youth and adolescents (ACSM, 2018; Faigenbaum et al., 2009; Kohrt et al., 2004).

- Youth must be both mentally and physically ready to comply with instructions and to withstand the stress of an appropriately-designed exercise training program.
- Supervision and instruction should be provided by adults having an understanding of youth training guidelines and knowledge of the unique physical and psychosocial characteristics of youth.
- Youth must receive thorough instruction regarding proper resistance training technique, safety precautions, and appropriate program progression.

Table 25-3 Youth Exercise Guidelines

Youth & Adolescent Exercise Guidelines

Cardiorespiratory Exercise

Frequency	• Daily
Intensity	• Most should be moderate- to vigorous-intensity aerobic exercise and should include vigorous-intensity exercise at least 3 days per week. Moderate-intensity corresponds to noticeable increases in heart rate and breathing. Vigorous-intensity corresponds to substantial increases in heart rate and breathing.
Time	• ≥60 minutes per day
Type	• Enjoyable and developmentally appropriate aerobic physical activities, including running, brisk walking, swimming, dancing, and bicycling.

Muscle Strengthening Exercise

Frequency	• ≥3 days per week
Time	• As part of their 60 minutes per day or more of exercise
Type	• Muscle strengthening physical activities can be unstructured (e.g., playing on playground equipment, climbing trees, tug-of-war) or structured (e.g., lifting weights, working with resistance bands).

Bone Strengthening Exercise

Frequency	• ≥3 days per week
Time	• As part of their 60 minutes per day or more of exercise
Type	• Bone strengthening activities include running, jumping rope, basketball, tennis, resistance training, and hopscotch.

ACSM (2018); HHS (2008)

Table 25-4 Youth Resistance Training Guidelines

Youth Resistance Training Guidelines

- Provide qualified instruction and supervision
- Ensure the exercise environment is safe and free of hazards
- Start each training session with a 5- to 10-minute dynamic warm-up period
- Begin with relatively light loads and always focus on the correct exercise technique
- Perform 1–3 sets of 6–15 repetitions on a variety of upper- and lower-body strength exercises
- Include specific exercises that strengthen the abdominal and lower back region
- Focus on symmetrical muscular development and appropriate muscle balance around joints
- Perform 1–3 sets of 3–6 repetitions on a variety of upper- and lower-body power exercises
- Sensibly progress the training program depending on needs, goals, and abilities
- Increase the resistance gradually (5–10%) as strength improves
- Cool-down with less intense calisthenics and static stretching
- Listen to individual needs and concerns throughout each session
- Perform resistance training 2–3 times per week on nonconsecutive days
- Use individualized workout logs to monitor progress
- Keep the program fresh and challenging by systematically varying the training program
- Optimize performance and recovery with healthy nutrition, proper hydration, and adequate sleep
- Support and encouragement from instructors and parents will help maintain interest

Faigenbaum et al. (2009)

- Enjoyment and self-improvement should be emphasized over competition.
- Activities that generate relatively high, yet appropriate loading forces (e.g., plyometrics, jumping, skipping, running, gymnastics, resistance training) should be included to stimulate increased bone mineral density.
- Due to their immature thermoregulatory system, youth and adolescents are at a greater risk of heat-related disorders. The lower output of heat-activated sweat glands, lower ratio of body mass to surface area to help dissipate heat, and lower skin blood flow rates greatly affect a child's ability to maintain a core temperature within acceptable ranges during exercise. It is extremely important to stress proper hydration and to minimize prolonged exposure to hot and humid environments during exercise.
- The stage of neurological development will determine a child's ability to participate in organized activities requiring complex, coordinated movements.
- Although the exercise guidelines for adults are generally applicable, it's important that youth and adolescents are not treated like miniature adults.
- Discourage time spent in sedentary activities such as watching television, playing video games, and 'surfing' the Internet. Encourage activities such as walking and biking to promote lifelong fitness.

Older Adults

Although the population of older adults is extremely varied in terms of health status, functional capacity, and physiological age, this broad group of people is defined as those adults with a chronological age ≥65 years and adults age 50 to 64 years with clinically significant chronic conditions and/or functional limitations (ACSM, 2018; Nelson et al., 2007). In addition to the countless health and fitness benefits gained by younger individuals, older adults also attain several positive outcomes as the result of regular exercise. Among active older adults, exercise slows the physiologic changes associated with aging, improves psychologic and cognitive well-being, manages chronic disease, reduces the incidence of falls and injuries from falls, decreases the risk of physical disability, facilitates independent living, and increases longevity and quality of life (ACSM, 2018). Unfortunately, the older adult population remains the least active among all age groups across the lifespan (Nelson et al., 2007). According to the U.S. Census Bureau, the population of American adults age 65 years and older is expected to grow from approximately 40 million in 2010 to an estimated 72 million in 2030 (Vincent & Velkoff, 2010). Programming for older adults has ranked among the top twenty worldwide fitness trends identified by ACSM every year since 2008, ranking eleventh overall for 2017 (Thompson, 2016). In consideration of these trends, fitness professionals must be prepared to design and deliver safe and effective exercise programs for older adults.

There are many musculoskeletal, cardiorespiratory, neurologic, and cognitive changes that occur with aging. Many of these changes may be attributed to the combination of the natural aging process and the increasing physical inactivity that often accompanies aging. Muscular strength decreases by approximately 25% from age 40 to 65, with a more rapid decline thereafter (Jones & Rose, 2005). Body composition (i.e., % body fat) increases due to a decline of 2% to 3% in lean body mass per decade from age 30 to 70 years and an increase in adipose tissue (Chodzko-Zajko et al., 2009). Bone mineral density also decreases and bone matrix deteriorates beginning at age 25 and accelerates more rapidly among postmenopausal women (Jones & Rose, 2005). Muscle and tendon elasticity decreases resulting in a 7% decrease in flexibility per decade during adulthood (Jones & Rose, 2005). Stroke volume and cardiac output decrease contributing to a 9% decline per decade in maximal oxygen consumption among healthy sedentary adults (Chodzko-Zajko et al., 2009). Blood pressure increases at rest and during submaximal exercise (Chodzko-Zajko et al., 2009). Neuromotor function also declines as seen through a decrease in balance and proprioception, slowed reaction time, and decreased muscular coordination (Jones & Rose, 2005). Aging is also associated with declining cognitive and neurologic functions such as memory impairment, decreased attention, slowed information processing, and deterioration of senses (e.g., vision, hearing, smell, taste) (Jones & Rose, 2005). The ACSM position stand titled, "Exercise and Physical Activity for Older Adults," provides a detailed summary of the physiological and physical changes that accompany aging (Chodzko-Zajko et al., 2009).

The physical activity recommendations and exercise guidelines for older adults are largely similar to those advocated for younger adults; however, as with any special population group some unique considerations do exist (ACSM, 2018, Nelson et al., 2007).

- Older adults should strive toward performing the equivalent of 150 minutes of moderate-intensity physical activity per week. When chronic conditions or limitations prevent them from attaining this minimum goal, they should engage in physical activity as allowed by their abilities and conditions to avoid a sedentary lifestyle.
- Older adults should exceed the minimum recommended amounts of physical activity provided they do not have conditions that would preclude higher amounts of activity.
- Exercise modalities that do not impose excessive orthopedic stress, such as walking aquatic exercise, and stationary cycling, are preferable for those with limited tolerance to weight-bearing activity.
- Whereas exercise intensity for younger adults is classified in absolute terms (i.e., METs), exercise and

physical activity for older adults should be defined relative to the individual's level of fitness using a 10-point scale of perceived physical exertion, where 0 is considered sitting quietly and 10 is considered an 'all-out' effort. Moderate-intensity corresponds to a 5 or 6 and produces noticeable increases in heart rate and respiration; vigorous-intensity corresponds to a 7 or 8 and produces large increases in heart rate and respiration.

- To maximize strength development, resistance training should be performed on at least 2 nonconsecutive days per week, consisting of 8 to 10 exercises representing the major muscle groups, performed for 10 to 15 repetitions for each of one or more sets.

- For more deconditioned or frail older adults a lighter-intensity (i.e., 40-50% of 1-RM) may be more appropriate and muscle strengthening activities may need to precede cardiorespiratory training.

- To maintain flexibility necessary for activities of daily living and an active lifestyle, older adults should perform stretching exercises at least 2 days per week for at least 10 minutes each day following flexibility training guidelines similar to younger adults.

- To reduce the risk of falling and injuries from falls, older adults should perform neuromotor exercises to improve balance, agility, and proprioception. These activities may include gradual reductions to base of support, training on progressively unstable surfaces, dynamic movement to disrupt center of gravity, or decreasing sensory input (e.g., closed eyes).

- In consideration of the fact that older adults are more likely to have chronic disease and other medical conditions, the special considerations and programming guidelines specific to these situations will be applicable.

Chapter Summary

Nearly all individuals, regardless of health status, age, or special considerations, derive health and fitness benefits from an active lifestyle and regular exercise. This chapter provided a brief overview regarding physical activity and exercise programming for special population groups and those with medical considerations. Fitness professionals are encouraged to pursue additional knowledge and information regarding these subgroups as well as others (e.g., cancer survivors, Parkinson's disease, multiple sclerosis, intellectual disabilities, etc.) not presented in this chapter.

Chapter References

American College of Obstetricians and Gynecologists, Committee on Obstetric Practice (2002). Committee Opinion # 267: Exercise during pregnancy and the postpartum period. *Obstetrics and Gynecology*, 99(1), 171-173.

American College of Sports Medicine (2018). *ACSM's Guidelines for Exercise Testing and Prescription*, 10th edition. Philadelphia, PA: Wolters Kluwer.

Artal, R., & O'Toole, M. (2003). Guidelines of the American College of Obstetricians and Gynecologists for exercise during pregnancy and the postpartum period. *British Journal of Sports Medicine*, 37(1), 6-12.

Billen, A., & Dupont, L. (2008). Exercise induced bronchoconstriction and sports. *Postgraduate Medical Journal*, 84(996), 512-517.

Bowman, K. (2013) Diastasis recti: When the abs don't come together. *IDEA Fitness Journal*, 10(5), 28-31.

Boyle, J.P., Thompson, T.J., Gregg, E.W., Barker, L.E., & Williamson, D.F. (2010). Projection of the year 2050 burden of diabetes in the US adult population: Dynamic modeling of incidence, mortality, and prediabetes prevalence. *Population Health Metrics*, 8(1), 29-40.

Centers for Disease Control and Prevention (2013). Prevalence of doctor-diagnosed arthritis and arthritis-attributable activity limitation: United States, 2010-2012. *Morbidity and Mortality Weekly Report*, 62(44), 869-873.

Centers for Disease Control and Prevention (20115. *National Diabetes Statistics Report: Estimates Of Diabetes And Its Burden In The United States, 2014*. Atlanta, GA: U.S. Department of Health and Human Services, Centers for Disease Control and Prevention.

Centers for Disease Control and Prevention (2012). *Diabetes Report Card 2012*. Atlanta, GA: Centers for Disease Control and Prevention, US Department of Health and Human Services.

Chodzko-Zajko, W., Proctor, D., Singh, M., Minson, C.T., Nigg, C.R., Salem, G.J., & Skinner, J.S. (2009). Exercise and physical activity for older adults: Position stand. *Medicine and Science in Sports and Exercise*, 41(7), 1510-1530.

Colberg, S.R., Sigal, R.J., Fernhall, B., Regensteiner, J.G., Blissmer, B.J., Rubin, R.R., ... & Braun, B. (2010). Exercise and type 2 diabetes. The American College of Sports Medicine and the American Diabetes Association: Joint position statement. *Diabetes Care*, 33(12), e147-e167.

Faigenbaum, A.D., Kraemer, W.J., Blimkie, C.J., Jeffreys, I., Micheli, L.J., Nitka, M., & Rowland, T.W. (2009). Youth resistance training: Updated position statement paper from the national strength and conditioning association. *The Journal of Strength & Conditioning Research*, 23(5), S60-S79.

Golightly, Y.M., Allen, K.D., & Caine, D.J. (2012). A comprehensive review of the effectiveness of different exercise programs for patients with osteoarthritis. *The Physician and Sportsmedicine*, 40(4), 52-65.

Heron, M. (2016). *Deaths: Leading Causes for 2013*. National vital statistics reports: from the Centers for Disease Control and Prevention, National Center for Health Statistics, National Vital Statistics System, 65(2), 1-14.

Jone, C.J., & Rose, D.J. (Eds.). (2005). *Physical Activity Instruction of Older Adults*. Champaign, IL: Human Kinetics.

Kohrt, W.M., Bloomfield, S.A., Little, K.D., Nelson, M.E., & Yingling, V.R. (2004). American College of Sports Medicine Position Stand: Physical activity and bone health. *Medicine and Science in Sports and Exercise*, 36(11), 1985-1996.

Levine, J.P. (2011). Identification, diagnosis, and prevention of osteoporosis. *American Journal of Managed Care*, 17(6), S170-S176.

Looker, A.C., Borrud, L.G., Dawson-Hughes, B., Shepherd, J.A., Wright, N.C. (2012). Osteoporosis or low bone mass at the femur neck or lumbar spine in older adults: United States, 2005–2008. *NCHS Data Brief No. 93*. Hyattsville, MD: National Center for Health Statistics.

Moorman, J.E., Bailey, C., Zahran, H.S., King, M., Johnson, C.A., & Liu, X. (2012). *Trends in asthma prevalence, health care use, and mortality in the United States, 2001-2010*. US Department of Health and Human Services, Centers for Disease Control and Prevention, National Center for Health Statistics.

Naguwa, S., Afrasiabi, R., & Chang, C. (2012). Exercise-induced asthma. In *Bronchial Asthma* (pp. 251-266). New York, NY: Springer.

Nattiv, A., Loucks, A.B., Manore, M.M., Sanborn, C.F., Sundgot-Borgen, J., & Warren, M.P. (2007). American College of Sports Medicine position stand. The female athlete triad. *Medicine and Science in Sports and Exercise, 39*(10), 1867-1882.

Nelson, M.E., Rejeski, W.J., Blair, S.N., Duncan, P.W., Judge, J.O., King, A.C., ... & Castaneda-Sceppa, C. (2007). Physical activity and public health in older adults: Recommendation from the American College of Sports Medicine and the American Heart Association. *Medicine and Science in Sports and Exercise, 39*(8), 1435-1445.

Ogden, C.L., Carroll, M.D., Kit, B.K., & Flegal, K.M. (2012). Prevalence of obesity and trends in body mass index among US children and adolescents, 1999-2010. *The Journal of the American Medical Association, 307*(5), 483-490.

Pescatello, L.S., Franklin, B.A., Fagard, R., Farquhar, W.B., Kelley, G.A., & Ray, C.A. (2004). American College of Sports Medicine position stand. Exercise and hypertension. *Medicine and Science in Sports and Exercise, 36*(3), 533-553.

Plasqui, G. (2008). The role of physical activity in rheumatoid arthritis. *Physiology & Behavior, 94*(2), 270-275.

Song, M., Carroll, D.D., & Fulton, J.E. (2013). Meeting the 2008 Physical Activity Guidelines for Americans among US youth. *American Journal of Preventive Medicine*, 44(3), 216-222.

Sorace, P., Churilla, J.R., & Magyari, P.M. (2012). Resistance training for hypertension: Design safe and effective programs. *ACSM's Health & Fitness Journal, 16*(1), 13-18.

Subbarao, P., Mandhane, P.J., & Sears, M.R. (2009). Asthma: Epidemiology, etiology and risk factors. *Canadian Medical Association Journal, 181*(9), E181-E190.

Thompson, W.R. (2016). Worldwide survey of fitness trends for 2017. *ACSM's Health & Fitness Journal*, 20(6), 8-17.

U.S. Department of Health and Human Services (2008). *2008 Physical Activity Guidelines for Americans*. ODPHP Publication No. U0036.

Valderrama, A.L., Gillespie, C., King, S.C., George, M.G., Hong, Y., & Gregg, E. (2012). Vital Signs: Awareness and treatment of uncontrolled hypertension among adults- United States, 2003-2010. *Morbidity and Mortality Weekly Report, 61*(35), 703–709.

Vincent, G.K. & Velkoff, V.A. (2010) *THE NEXT FOUR DECADES, The Older Population in the United States: 2010 to 2050*, Current Population Reports, P25-1138, U.S. Census Bureau, Washington, DC.

Wolfe, L.A., & Davies, A.L.G. (2003). Canadian guidelines for exercise in pregnancy. *Clinical Obstetrics and Gynecology, 46*(2), 488-495.

Recommended Reading

American College of Sports Medicine (2018). Chapters 7,9,10, and 11. In, *ACSM's Guidelines to Exercise Testing and Prescription*, 10th edition. Philadelphia, PA: Wolters Kluwer.

Chapter 25 Review Questions

1. Which of following activities is likely to be tolerated best by an individual with asthma?
    A. Skating on an indoor ice rink
    B. Jogging outdoors in a highly urbanized area
    C. Swimming in a body of open water
    D. Interval training in a humid group exercise studio

2. Which of the following exercises should be avoided by a woman who is in her 24th week of pregnancy?
    A. Dumbbell chest press on a flat bench
    B. Stability ball squat performed to 90 degrees of knee flexion
    C. Seated wide row using an adjustable cable column
    D. Standing hip abduction using a resistance band

3. Which of the following statements is true with regard to exercise programming for youth and adolescents?
    A. Jumping, bounding, and hopping activities should be avoided due to increased loading of the skeletal system.
    B. A low body mass to surface area ratio predisposes youth to heat exhaustion and heatstroke.
    C. Youth and adolescents should perform a minimum of 30 minutes of physical activity on most days of the week.
    D. Youth and adolescents may safely perform unsupervised resistance training as long as their parent or guardian signs a waiver form.

4. Your new 58-year-old client is being treated for hypertension with beta-blockers prescribed by his health care provider. Using a straight percentage of his age-predicted maximum heart rate, you calculate the client's target heart rate to be 122 beats per minute at 75% of HRmax. Considering the antihypertensive medication, this client's actual heart rate during exercise is likely to be _____ his calculated target heart rate.
    A. higher than
    B. the same as
    C. equivalent to
    D. lower than

5. Your 25-year-old female client has type 1 diabetes. Which of the following conditions is most likely to occur when performing moderate- to vigorous-intensity cardiorespiratory exercise shortly after a self-administered injection of insulin?
    A. Hyperglycemia
    B. Hyperthermia
    C. Hyponatremia
    D. Hypoglycemia

6. A 74-year-old male client has a recent history of falling several times at home. He has not sustained any significant injuries, but has become more fearful of falling. Which of the following activities may be an important addition to this client's exercise program?
    A. Moderate-intensity plyometric exercises to increase bone density and decrease risk of fractures due to falling.
    B. Resistance training exercise consisting of 6 to 8 repetitions-maximum lifts on selectorized machines to increase musculoskeletal resiliency.
    C. Standing balance exercises that gradually reduce base of support and/or introduce dynamic movements to alter center of gravity for improved proprioception.
    D. Ballistic stretching exercises to increase musculotendinous elasticity and reduce the risk of strains and sprains.

Answers to Review Questions on Page 384

Note: Review questions are intended to reinforce learning and comprehension of subject matter presented in the corresponding chapter. The review questions are not intended to be representative of actual certification exam questions in terms of style, content, or difficulty.

Section VIII
Administrative & Legal Considerations

Fitness professionals have a responsibility to ensure the safety of all participants under their supervision and direction. Unfortunately, accidents do happen and fitness professionals occasionally make an error in judgment. As a result, serious injuries and even catastrophic events do occur. Fitness professionals with knowledge of common liability exposures, legal considerations, and administrative responsibilities may avert these foreseeable events and minimize the risk of litigation.

Chapter 26 reviews legal considerations and risk management strategies for fitness professionals. Topics covered include sources of liability, scope of practice, and liability insurance. In addition, several case studies will be presented regarding lawsuits that have been brought forth against fitness professionals.

Chapter 27 continues the topic of risk management with a review of documentation and record keeping associated with the delivery of fitness services. Important documentation includes informed consent, preparticipation screening questionnaires, liability waivers, fitness assessment data, exercise training logs, and incident reports, each of which will be briefly addressed.

26
Risk Management for Fitness Professionals

Introduction
Our society has become increasingly litigious and unfortunately, fitness professionals have not been immune to this trend. As the fitness industry continues to evolve, the role of the fitness professional has expanded in both depth and breadth. Additionally, the use of fitness services continue to grow steadily, which in combination with the poor health status of many participants, elevates the risk of injury, adverse medical events, and subsequent litigation. Fitness professionals are particularly exposed to lawsuits due to the inherent risks associated with exercise and the lack of standardized regulation over the fitness industry (Riley, 2005a). It is of little surprise that the number of lawsuits against fitness professionals and fitness facilities has increased significantly in recent years. Nevertheless, proactive fitness professionals may minimize this threat through familiarization with recognized standards of care, education regarding common liability exposures, and implementation of a comprehensive risk management plan. This chapter addresses legal terminology and liability considerations that are applicable to fitness professionals. The information is intended to be educational and does not take the place of legal advice.

Standard of Care
A **standard of care** represents the manner with which professional services should be delivered in order to provide reasonable assurance that the expected outcome is attained without unnecessary risk of harm to the participant (Ehrman, 2010; Eickhoff-Shemek et al., 2009). The standards of care represent the duties that are required of a reasonably prudent fitness professional acting in the same or similar circumstances (Eickhoff-Shemek et al., 2009). A *duty* is an obligation or responsibility that arises as a result of the special relationship between the fitness professional and a participant such that the fitness professional must protect the participant from unreasonable risks that may result in harm (Eickhoff-Shemek et al., 2009).

Since fitness professionals, including personal trainers, are not licensed professionals, the standards of care within the fitness industry are not regulated by states or the federal government (Riley, 2005a). Subsequently, several industry organizations have established professional *standards* and *guidelines* including the American College of Sports Medicine (ACSM, 2012; ACSM, 2018), the National Strength and Conditioning Association (Waller et al., 2009), and the Medical Fitness Association (MFA, 2013). Unfortunately, it appears that many fitness facilities are not fully compliant with these standards (Eickhoff-Shemek & Deja, 2002; Riley, 2005a). Furthermore, it is likely that many fitness professionals fail to keep up to date or are even aware of the most current standards, guidelines, and consensus statements published by fitness industry associations. Since jurors in a lawsuit will not be familiar with fitness industry standards and guidelines, the plaintiff's attorney will call upon expert witness testimony to educate the court regarding the standards applicable to a particular case (Eickhoff-Shemek et al., 2009).

Negligence
The majority of the lawsuits filed against fitness professionals are civil lawsuits related to claims of negligence. **Negligence** may be defined as failure to act according to a generally accepted standard of care consistent with the manner in which a reasonable, prudent person would have acted under similar or identical circumstances (Eickhoff-Shemek et al., 2009). Negligence may be the result of an *act of commission*, which is inappropriately or incorrectly performing a duty or doing something that a knowledgeable and prudent professional would not have done (Eickhoff-Shemek et al., 2009). Negligence may also be the result of an *act of omission*, which is failing to perform a duty that a professional would have performed in a similar situation (Eickhoff-Shemek et al., 2009).

In order for a fitness professional to be found negligent, four elements must be demonstrated (ACSM, 2012; Eickhoff-Shemek et al., 2009; Waller et al., 2009). The four elements of negligence include: (1) a legal duty owed to the participant, (2) a breach of this duty, (3) proximate cause, and (4) damages sustained (ACSM, 2012; Eickhoff-Shemek et al., 2009, Waller et al., 2009). In a lawsuit filed against a fitness professional and/or a fitness facility, the court or the judge presiding over the case will determine if a legal duty was owed to the participant (i.e., the plaintiff). A breach of duty (i.e., act of commission, act of omission) will be determined based on adherence to the standards of care that are deemed applicable to the circumstances surrounding the incident in question. If a breach of duty plays a substantial role or directly results in an event (i.e., damages), then this breach of duty is said to be the proximate cause of the damages. Finally, in order for negligence to exist, there must be an indication of subsequent damages, which may include physical injury, emotional distress, property losses, or even death. If the defendant (i.e., fitness professional) is found to be negligent, then they will be liable or legally responsible for compensation of damages as determined by the court.

Liability Exposures

A **liability exposure** is any situation that increases the risk of an injury, a medical emergency, or the severity of medical emergencies that do occur (Eickhoff-Shemek, 2010; Eickhoff-Shemek et al., 2009; Waller et al., 2009). Liability exposures also increase the possibility of litigation against a fitness professional and/or a fitness facility. The following is a list of common liability exposures often seen in the fitness industry (Eickhoff-Shemek, 2010; Waller et al., 2009).

- Failure to conduct an appropriate preparticipation screening and failure to refer for medical evaluation, diagnosis, and clearance to participate in exercise programming, when indicated.
- Failure to administer proper evaluation (i.e., fitness assessment) of participants' physical capacities for the purpose of appropriate, safe, and effective program design, and failure to identify limitations or possible exercise contraindications.
- Failure to recommend appropriate exercise intensity related to the participant's level of conditioning in terms of metabolic and cardiovascular demand.
- Failure to adequately or competently supervise and/or instruct participants regarding the safe performance of recommended exercises and proper use of exercise equipment.
- Delivery of services or making statements outside the scope of practice for a fitness professional.
- Failure to terminate exercise testing and/or exercise participation when 'warning signs' (e.g., signs or symptoms of abnormal cardiovascular, physiological, or physical responses) are present, or if the participant requests to stop.
- Failure to maintain proper documentation and record keeping such as, but not limited to, preparticipation screening, informed consent, liability waivers, health/fitness assessment data, progress notes, injury/incident reports, and exercises logs including the relevant acute training variables.
- Failure to obtain or maintain appropriate credentials (i.e., professional certification(s), safety certifications) as identified in published standards, guidelines, and industry recommendations for fitness professionals.
- Failure to provide and maintain a safe environment (e.g., facility) including appropriate equipment set-up, inspection, maintenance, repair, and signage.
- Failure to execute an emergency response plan and provide emergency care (e.g., standard first aid, CPR, AED) when the situation arises.

Scope of Practice

A **scope of practice** defines the specific boundaries within which an individual (i.e., fitness professional) may perform the tasks associated with their profession (Berger, 2013; Eickhoff-Shemek et al., 2009; Janot, 2004). In other words, a scope of practice designates what a fitness professional can and cannot do (Abbott, 2012). At the present time, fitness professionals are not licensed health care providers; therefore, their scope of practice is restricted from and indirectly defined by the service parameters reserved for licensed health care professionals (e.g., physician, physical therapist, chiropractor, registered dietitian, licensed psychologist). Fitness professionals must know and abide by the scope of practice limitations based on their education, credentials, knowledge, and skill. Failure to do so may lead to accusations of practicing medicine or dietetics without a license. Violation of a state licensure law is a criminal offense, which may be subject to misdemeanor or felony penalties ranging in severity from a 'cease and desist' order to fines or imprisonment (Kruskall et al., 2017; Riley 2005b; Sass et al., 2007). Unlike charges of negligence, the criminal charges for violating a state licensure law can occur despite the fact that no harm may have been inflicted upon a participant.

To avoid crossing the line into the unlawful practice of medicine, fitness professionals should observe the following recommendations (Abbott, 2012; Janot, 2004; Riley, 2005b):

- Do not diagnose illness, chronic disease, medical conditions, or injuries. Do not make statements or offer opinions that may be misinterpreted as a diagnosis or medical advice.
- Do not attempt to rehabilitate or treat injuries, diseases, or medical conditions. Do not counsel individuals with psychological disorders. Fitness professionals do not 'prescribe' corrective exercises, but they do design exercise programs intended to improve one or more components of health-related physical fitness.
- Do not provide hands-on manipulation (e.g., massage, myofascial release) of soft tissue or musculoskeletal adjustments such as 'cracking' an individual's spine to realign vertebrae and relieve stiffness.
- Do not misrepresent health screening protocols or fitness assessments as a medical evaluation. The purpose of a health history questionnaire, a health risk appraisal, health screening measurements (e.g.,

resting blood pressure, resting heart rate, body mass index), and the fitness assessments administered by the fitness professional are, in part, to identify those who may require further medical evaluation and possible diagnosis by a qualified health care provider.

- Do not make recommendations for an individual to alter their treatment plan, including medications prescribed by a physician, or other licensed health care providers.
- When indicated, refer clients and participants to the appropriate health care provider for medical evaluation and diagnosis.

In the United States, the practice of dietetics is regulated in most states either through licensure or the statutory certification of dietetic professionals (e.g., registered dieticians) (Kruskall et al., 2017; Sass et al., 2007). As of March 2017, 46 states, the District of Columbia, and Puerto Rico have enacted statutory provisions regulating the practice of nutrition and/or dietetics through either state licensure or statutory certification (Kruskall et al., 2017). Arizona, Colorado, New Jersey, and Michigan are the only states that do not presently regulate the practice of nutrition/dietetics (Kruskall et al., 2017). In order to avoid straying into the scope of practice reserved for dietetic professionals, fitness professionals should observe the following recommendations with regard to nutrition and dietetics (Kruskall et al., 2017; Meyers, 2009; Sass et al., 2007):

- Do not perform nutritional assessments to determine specific nutrient needs, excesses, deficiencies, or to recommend appropriate nutritional intake.
- Do not design or prescribe specific meal plans or diets.
- Do not provide or prescribe dietary recommendations intended to treat or manage illness, chronic disease, or other special medical considerations.
- Do not recommend, encourage, provide, or sell dietary supplements or other ergogenic aids.
- Do not promote or misrepresent yourself as a 'dietitian,' 'registered dietitian,' 'nutritionist,' 'certified nutritionist,' 'nutrition specialist', or any other occupational title using the word 'dietitian' or 'nutritionist'.
- Do not attempt to counsel individuals with known or suspected eating disorders. Refer these individuals to a licensed psychologist and/or registered dietitian for professional treatment.
- Become familiar with the regulations regarding the practice of dietetics in your state. The State Licensure Agency List, maintained by the Commission on Dietetic Registration, provides a state-by-state list of links to agencies that regulate dietetics throughout the United States. http://cdrnet.org/state-licensure-agency-list

> "Those who provide advice as to the use of vitamins, minerals or other supplements or those who may even sell, recommend or 'prescribe' such products, also face the potential for claim and suit in the event that such supplements cause harm to clients."
> —Herbert & Herbert (2002)

Given the importance of proper nutrition with regard to optimal health, fitness, and athletic performance, fitness professionals do play an important role in guiding individuals to make healthy dietary choices. As non-licensed professionals, fitness professionals are permitted to provide general non-medical nutrition information including (Kruskall et al., 2017; Meyers, 2009; Sass et al., 2007):

- Information regarding principles of good nutrition and food preparation,
- Recommendations regarding nutrient-dense foods to be included in the normal daily diet as identified by food guidance systems such as the USDA's *MyPlate* graphic and the *Dietary Guidelines for Americans*,
- Information on the essential nutrients needed by the body and the recommended amounts of the essential nutrients for healthy populations,
- Education regarding appropriate portion and serving sizes,
- Information regarding the purpose and actions of essential nutrients in the body,
- Information on the effects of deficiencies or excesses of nutrients,
- Recommendations regarding foods that are good sources of essential nutrients, and
- Education regarding how to read and interpret Nutrition Facts labels.

The scope of practice for the fitness professional may be inferred from a job task analysis, also known as a role delineation or practice analysis. A job task analysis identifies the tasks performed by the fitness professional, and the knowledge and skill one must possess to safely and effectively perform these tasks (Berger, 2013). The job task analyses for NETA's NCCA-accredited certifications are available at www.netafit.org.

Risk Management Plan

Risk management is defined as "a proactive administrative process that will help minimize liability losses for fitness professionals and the organizations they represent" (Eickhoff-Shemek et al., 2009). Fitness professionals and fitness facilities should attempt to maximize participant safety and minimize potential litigation through the adoption of a comprehensive risk management plan, which includes assessment of potential liability exposures, development of risk management strategies, implementation of the plan, and evaluation of plan effectiveness (Eickhoff-Shemek et al., 2009). The following list includes some key strategies for fitness professionals to manage liability and risk exposures (Ehrman, 2010; Abbott, 2011).

- Be familiar with and abide by the most current industry standards and guidelines applicable to the nature of your specific services, participants, and facilities.
- Maintain appropriate professional credentials (e.g., NCCA-accredited certification) and safety certifications (e.g., standard first aid, CPR, AED).
- Utilize appropriate informed consent and liability waiver forms with all participants.
- Complete a thorough preparticipation screening, initial health and fitness assessments, and obtain medical clearance prior to participation (when indicated).
- Design exercise programs appropriate to the participant's health status, level of conditioning, physical capabilities, limitations, goals, and needs.
- Provide proper instruction and supervision regarding the use of exercise equipment, performance of recommended exercises, and appropriate program progression.
- Modify or terminate exercise when adverse signs and symptoms are observed or if the participant requests to discontinue exercise.
- Provide a safe exercise environment including proper installation, spacing, and function of exercise equipment in accordance with industry standards and guidelines, and manufacturer specifications.
- Do not provide services or act in a manner that may be considered outside the scope of practice for the fitness professional.
- Develop and regularly practice an emergency response plan.
- Maintain appropriate documentation and record keeping. See chapter 27.
- Obtain professional liability insurance coverage.

Professional Liability Insurance

Professional liability insurance provides financial protection with regard to expenses incurred in the defense of a lawsuit and payment of damages that may be awarded to plaintiffs as the result of a negligence verdict against the fitness professional. Although liability insurance does not release the fitness professional from liability, it may help defray the high cost of legal actions taken against them. Fitness professionals, especially those who are self-employed or work as independent contractors, are strongly encouraged to purchase professional liability insurance. Liability insurance is available through many reputable insurance companies offering coverage to fitness professionals and fitness facilities. NETA has partnered with FitnessPak to offer professional liability insurance to NETA-certified fitness professionals. For more information, please visit: http://fitnesspak.com/fitness-instructors/neta/.

Case Studies

Lawsuits that have been brought forth against fitness professionals can serve as an invaluable learning opportunity for all. The following section provides some selected case studies of actual lawsuits that have been filed against fitness professionals.

Capati v. Crunch Fitness International et al.
In the case of *Capati v. Crunch Fitness*, a personal trainer allegedly recommended that his 37-year-old client, Anne Marie Capati, take a variety of over-the-counter dietary supplements including some that contained ephedra. Capati had previously informed the personal trainer that she was taking prescribed medications for hypertension. In October 1998, while performing squats at the club, Capati became ill, lost consciousness, and several hours later passed away at the hospital from a hemorrhagic stroke. Her death was alleged to be the result of the lethal combination of antihypertensive medications and ephedra-containing supplements. The decedent's family filed a wrongful death lawsuit seeking $320 million in damages, naming the personal trainer, the club, as well as other defendants in the claim. The case was settled before going to trial for a total aggregate payment of over 4 million dollars, of which Crunch Fitness and the personal trainer were liable for $1,750,000 of the total settlement (Eickhoff-Shemek, 2010; Eickhoff-Shemek et al., 2009; Sass et al., 2007).

Corrigan v. Musclemakers, Inc.
In the case of *Corrigan v. Musclemakers, Inc.*, the plaintiff, a 49-year-old woman, purchased a membership at a Gold's Gym in April 1996. She had never belonged to a health club and had never used a treadmill. During the first of three personal training sessions included with her membership, a personal trainer placed her on a treadmill set at 3.5 mph for 20 minutes and then left her unattended. The trainer did not provide any instruction regarding how to operate or stop the treadmill. Shortly into the walk, the plaintiff drifted toward the back of the belt and, despite trying to walk faster, she was thrown from the treadmill sustaining a fractured ankle. The plaintiff filed a negligence lawsuit claiming that the personal trainer failed to provide instruction regarding how to use the treadmill and it's control panel, and failed to provide appropriate supervision. The appellate court upheld the trial court's ruling to dismiss the defendant's motion for summary judgment. The defendant's assumption of risk defense was ineffective because of the negligent conduct of the personal trainer (Eickhoff-Shemek, 2010; Eickhoff-Shemek et al., 2009).

Proffitt v. Global Fitness Holdings, LLC et al.
In the case of *Proffitt v. Global Fitness Holdings*, the plaintiff, Vince Proffitt, joined the Urban Active health club in

Kentucky. In early February 2011, Mr. Proffitt arrived for his first session with a personal trainer, which he believed would entail a fitness evaluation and instruction regarding various pieces of equipment. During this first session, the personal trainer had him perform several bouts of strenuous exercise and directed him to continue the exercises even after signs and symptoms of overexertion and requests by Proffitt to stop. For many hours after the session, Proffitt experienced extreme pain and fatigue and after 38 hours he noticed his urine was dark brown. He went to the emergency room where he was diagnosed with rhabdomyolysis resulting in 8 days of hospitalization and permanent injuries including a 30% loss of muscle tissue in both quadriceps muscles. The plaintiff filed a negligence lawsuit against the trainer and the facility claiming the personal trainer failed to assess his health and fitness status, failed to provide an exercise program safely within his fitness capacity, and failed to respond to his complaints of fatigue and requests to stop during the training session. Based upon lost wages and medical expenses, this case was settled for $75,000 in damages. Similar lawsuits related to incidents of rhabdomyolysis have also been filed against fitness professionals including *Guthrie v. Crouser* and *Pineda v. Town Sports International, Inc.*

Makris v. Scandinavian Health Spa, Inc.
In the case of *Makris v. Scandinavian Health Spa*, while using the leg press machine during her first of two complimentary personal training sessions, the plaintiff, Caliope Makris, informed her trainer that she felt a sharp pain in her neck that radiated down her arm. The trainer told her the pain was due to upper body weakness. Makris experienced the same pain during several subsequent training sessions when using the leg press and believed the trainer who assured her that the pain would subside as she became stronger. However, the pain became increasingly intense and constant. Several months later an MRI revealed Makris had suffered three herniated cervical discs. Approximately two years later, after a former employee of the Spa informed Makris that her injury was likely to be caused by the conduct of the personal trainer, Makris filed a personal injury lawsuit against the defendants alleging they "rendered negligent training, monitoring, instruction, supervision, and advice." The trial court granted the defendants motion for summary judgment claiming that the lawsuit was not filed within the statute of limitations. The appellate court reversed the trial court's decision and sent the case back to the trial court for further proceedings (Eickhoff-Shemek et al., 2009).

Bain v. Woodson YMCA et al.
In the case of *Bain v. Woodson YMCA*, the plaintiff, Dorothy Bain, was performing resistance training exercises during a supervised personal training session at the Woodson YMCA. The plaintiff began to feel ill shortly after the session and later went to the hospital for treatment. Ms. Bain had suffered a hemorrhagic stroke resulting in life-long disability, which she alleges to be the result of the weight lifting activities performed during the personal training session. A lawsuit was filed claiming that the personal trainer acted negligently by failing to provide proper instruction regarding appropriate breathing technique and avoidance of the Valsalva maneuver during resistance training, as well as failure to provide warning regarding the possible consequences of not observing proper breathing technique. The plaintiff also claimed that the YMCA failed to provide appropriate training to its employees regarding proper weightlifting techniques. This case reached a confidential settlement shortly before going to a scheduled trial.

Zihlman and Zihlman v. Wichita Falls YMCA
In the case of *Zihlman and Zihlman v. Wichita Falls YMCA*, Elaine Thomas, a 56-year-old female was exercising at the YMCA in September of 2007 when she suffered a sudden cardiac arrest. The YMCA had an AED and staff certified in both the use of an AED and CPR. However, contrary to published industry standards and requirements outlined in the YMCA's Emergency Procedures, YMCA employees did not begin CPR and, although the AED was retrieved, the unit was not opened or used. EMS was contacted and arrived on scene approximately 10 minutes after the call to 911. Although EMS detected a shockable heart rhythm, due to the passage of time between her collapse and delivery of defibrillation shocks, Thomas died despite efforts by EMS personnel to resuscitate her. The surviving daughters of Thomas filed a wrongful death lawsuit claiming the defendants failed to utilize the AED and as a consequence their mother died; failed to provide reasonable care for the safety, protection, and first aid in the event of a medical emergency; and failed to have accessible AEDs and properly trained staff. This case was still pending at the printing of this manual.

The case studies provided represent just a very small sample of the countless lawsuits that have been filed against fitness professionals. Each of these cases illustrates one or more of the liability exposures discussed in this chapter. Fitness professionals are encouraged to stay informed of past and present lawsuits in an effort to expand their knowledge and adopt risk management strategies to minimize their personal liability exposures and potential litigation.

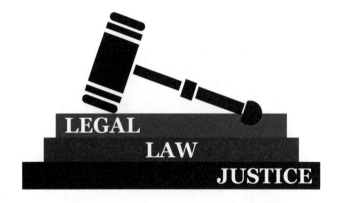

Chapter Summary

This chapter presented an overview of important legal considerations, liability exposures, and risk management strategies to ensure the safety of participants and to minimize the possibility of litigation against fitness professionals. The information provided in this chapter is intended to be educational and to increase the legal awareness of fitness professionals. The information contained within this manual should not take the place of legal advice from a qualified attorney. Fitness professionals and fitness facilities should consult with their risk management team and legal counsel to develop a customized risk management plan meeting the unique circumstances of their situation.

Chapter References

Abbott, A.A. (2011). The legal aspects: Personal training – litigation insulation. *ACSM's Health & Fitness Journal, 15*(5), 40-44.

Abbott, A.A. (2012). The legal aspects: Scope of practice. *ACSM's Health & Fitness Journal, 16*(1), 31-34.

American College of Sports Medicine (2012). *ACSM's Health/Fitness Facility Standards and Guidelines*, 4th edition. Tharrett, S.J., & Peterson, J.A. (Eds.). Champaign, IL: Human Kinetics.

American College of Sports Medicine (2018). *ACSM's Guidelines for Exercise Testing and Prescription*, 10th edition. Philadelphia, PA: Wolters Kluwer.

Bain v. Woodson YMCA. In: Herbert, D.L. (2009). Weightlifting injuries result in suit against personal trainer and facility. *The Exercise Standards and Malpractice Reporter*. 23(6), 81-85.

Berger, C.G. (2013). Scope of practice in the health sciences: A tutorial and call to action for fitness professionals. *The Exercise, Sports, and Sports Medicine Standards & Malpractice Reporter*, 2(4), 49-54.

Capati v. Crunch Fitness International, Inc., 295 A.D.2d 181, 743 N.Y.S.2d 474 (App. Div. 2002).

Corrigan v. Musclemakers, Inc., 258 A.D.2d 861, 686 N.Y.S.2d 143 (App. Div. 1999).

Ehrman, J.K. (Ed.). (2010). *ACSM's Resource Manual for Guidelines for Exercise Testing and Prescription*, 6th edition. Baltimore, MD: Lippincott Williams & Wilkins.

Eickhoff-Shemek, J.M. (2010). The legal aspects: An analysis of 8 negligence lawsuits against personal fitness trainers. *ACSM's Health & Fitness Journal*, 14(5), 34-37.

Eickhoff-Shemek, J.M., & Deja, K. (2002). Are health/fitness facilities complying with ACSM standards? Part 2. *ACSM's Health & Fitness Journal*, 6(3), 19-24.

Eickhoff-Shemek, J.M., Herbert, D.L., & Connaughton, D.P. (2009). *Risk Management for Health/Fitness Professionals: Legal Issues and Strategies*. Baltimore, MD: Lippincott, Williams & Wilkins.

Guthrie v. Crouser. In: Herbert, D.L. (2008). Qualifications/certification of personal trainers again in the news. *The Exercise Standards and Malpractice Reporter*, 22(3), 36-38.

Herbert, D.L., & Eickhoff-Shemek, J.M. (2010). The legal aspects: New standards statements legal considerations for the fitness industry. *ACSM's Health & Fitness Journal*, 14(3), 31-33.

Herbert, D.L., & Herbert, W.G. (2002). *Legal Aspects of Preventative Rehabilitation and Recreational Exercise Programs*. 4th edition. Canton, OH: PRC Publishing.

Janot, J.M. (2004). Do you know your scope of practice? *IDEA Fitness Journal*, 1(1).

Makris v. Scandinavian Health Spa, Inc., 1999 Ohio App. LEXIS 4416. In: Herbert, D.L. (2000) Another suit over personal trainer's alleged advice, *The Exercise Standards and Malpractice Reporter*, 14(6), 95.

Medical Fitness Association (2013). *Standards and Guidelines for Medical Fitness Center Facilities, 2nd edition*. Monterey, CA: Healthy Learning.

Meyers, C. (2009). [Your name], certified personal trainer and...nutritionist?. *ACE Certified News*, 15(6), 12-13.

Pineda v. Town Sports International, Inc. In: Herbert, D.L. (2010). Clubs members lawsuit for rhabdomyolysis. *The Exercise Standards and Malpractice Reporter*, 24(1), 5-7.

Proffitt v. Global Fitness Holdings, LLC, et al. In: Herbert, D.L. (2013). New lawsuit against personal trainer and facility in Kentucky – Rhabdomyolysis alleged. *The Exercise, Sports and Medicine Standards & Malpractice Reporter*, 2(1), 1, 3-10.

Riley, S. (2005a). Why you need a legal education. *IDEA Trainer Success*, 2(1), 1-2.

Riley, S. (2005b). Legal & risk management: Respecting your boundaries. *IDEA Trainer Success*, 2(4).

Sass, C., Eickhoff-Shemek, J.M., Manore, M.M., & Kruskall, L.J. (2007). Crossing the line: Understanding the scope of practice between registered dietitians and health/fitness professionals. *ACSM's Health & Fitness Journal*, 11(3), 12-19.

Waller, M., Piper, T., & Miller, J. (2009). National Strength and Conditioning Association: Strength and conditioning professional standards and guidelines. *Strength and Conditioning Journal*, 31(5), 14-38.

Zihlman and Zihlman v. Wichita Falls YMCA, In: Herbert, D.L. (2010). New AED case filed against YMCA in Texas. *The Exercise Standards and Malpractice Reporter*, 24(5), 74-79.

Chapter 26 Review Questions

1. Which of the following would be considered within the scope of practice of the fitness professional?
   A. Visiting a local nutrition store with your client to help them select the right dietary supplements.
   B. Performing a dietary assessment to identify nutrient deficiencies for a client suspected of having an eating disorder.
   C. Planning a meal with a low glycemic index for your diabetic client.
   D. Teaching your client how to calculate the percent of fat in a food item using data found on a Nutrition Facts label.

2. The manner in which personal training services should be appropriately delivered to a client as outlined by authoritative fitness industry associations represents the _____.
   A. standards of care
   B. risk management plan
   C. scope of practice
   D. acts of commission

3. You are meeting with a 34-year-old male client for his first personal training session. The client appears to be fit and indicates that he is in good health. He seems eager to get started with exercise, so you decide to forgo the preparticipation screening and immediately challenge him with a high intensity interval training workout. Midway through the session, the client complains of dizziness, nausea, and a headache. You later learn that this client has recently been diagnosed with hypertension and frequently forgets to take his medication. This scenario represents an _____ by the personal trainer.
   A. act of correlation
   B. act of incompetence
   C. act of omission
   D. act of noncompliance

4. Which of the following must be present for a verdict of negligence in a civil lawsuit against a personal trainer?
   A. The personal trainer must have liability insurance.
   B. The personal trainer must have collected payment for services provided.
   C. The personal trainer must have a signed liability waiver on file.
   D. The personal trainer must have a responsibility or obligation to protect the client from foreseeable harm.

5. While performing the preparticipation screening with a new male client, you discover his resting blood pressure to be 148/96 mmHg. After having the client sit quietly for 5 minutes, you re-measure his blood pressure and find it to be 142/94 mmHg. Which of the following statements represents the most appropriate action to be taken by the personal trainer?
   A. Advise the client that he has hypertension and should contact his health care provider to get a prescription for medication
   B. Explain to the client that you are concerned about his elevated blood pressure and recommend he visit his health care provider for further evaluation.
   C. Recommend that the client reduce his sodium intake to less than 1,500 mg per day.
   D. Request that the client sign a release of liability waiver before you proceed with additional fitness assessments.

6. Failure to act according to a generally accepted standard of care consistent with the manner in which a reasonable, prudent person would have acted under similar or identical circumstances is known as _____.
   A. negligence
   B. liability
   C. a breach of contract
   D. a liability exposure

Answers to Review Questions on Page 384

Note: Review questions are intended to reinforce learning and comprehension of subject matter presented in the corresponding chapter. The review questions are not intended to be representative of actual certification exam questions in terms of style, content, or difficulty.

27
Documentation & Record Keeping

Introduction
One component of a comprehensive risk management plan is the maintenance of appropriate documentation and record keeping related to the delivery of fitness services. Documentation provides evidence of the fitness professional's supervision to ensure safe and effective exercise programming, reflects the standard of care provided to the participant, and may serve an important function in the defense of a lawsuit. This chapter provides an overview of the minimal documentation that should be maintained by the fitness professional. In addition, the appendix of this manual provides sample forms; however, fitness professionals should consult with their employer, risk management team, and legal counsel to identify and adopt the forms best suited for their specific needs.

Participant Files

Confidentiality
The fitness professional (e.g., personal trainer, wellness coach) should maintain an individual file for each client utilizing their services. The files should be handled and stored with great care to ensure the security and confidentiality of clients' personal information. Participant files should be stored in a locked file cabinet, in a secured office space, with access limited to only authorized individuals. Participant files should not be left unattended in common areas in which unauthorized individuals may access and review file contents. Electronic records must be stored in a secure and password provided database. As stated in NETA's Professional Code of Ethics, NETA-certified fitness professionals must, "respect and maintain the confidentiality of all client information."

HIPAA
The Health Insurance Portability and Accountability Act of 1996 (HIPAA) became effective in April of 2003. HIPAA's privacy regulations mandate that health care providers protect the privacy of their patients, maintain the confidentiality of *personal health information*, and discipline individuals who violate privacy and confidentiality requirements (Blair, 2003; Ehrman, 2010). HIPAA applies to any entity that is a health care provider conducting certain transactions in electronic form, a medical claims clearinghouse, or health insurance carriers (Ehrman, 2010). Fitness professionals who interact with health care providers and other 'covered entities', and who access a participant's medical records in conjunction with the delivery of fitness services are also affected by HIPAA regulations (Ehrman, 2010). The applicability of HIPAA rules to fitness professionals should be addressed through consultation with your risk management team and legal counsel. HIPAA regulations may be accessed by visiting http://www.hhs.gov/ocr/privacy/.

Waiver and Release of Liability
A *waiver and release of liability* is a document through which the participant knowingly releases the fitness professional from responsibility and agrees to give up their rights to seek legal recourse and damages in the event of an injury sustained in conjunction with fitness programming (Ehrman, 2010; Eickhoff-Shemek et al., 2009). Waivers and releases are generally recognized in most states for the release of ordinary negligence, but not for extreme forms of negligence such as gross negligence, reckless behavior, willful and wanton conduct, and criminal conduct (Eickhoff-Shemek et al., 2009; Eickhoff-Shemek & Forbes, 1999). The effectiveness of waivers has been debated. A signed waiver and release of liability form may or may not be upheld in a court of law (see case studies). However, it is still prudent to have participants sign a liability waiver form. Since not all states uphold waiver forms, and laws regarding waivers vary from state to state, it is recommended to seek the advice of an attorney to construct a legally-defensible waiver form. Below is an example of language that may be included in a waiver and release of liability. This should serve only as an example and is not intended to be legally defensible.

I, _____ (participant's name) have enrolled in a fitness program consisting of, but not limited to, cardiorespiratory exercise, resistance training, and flexibility activities with _____ (your name or company name). I hereby attest to being in good physical condition and do not suffer from any disability that would prevent or limit my participation in the above mentioned exercise program.

I understand there are inherent risks involved in my participation in this exercise program. My participation in this program is voluntary and I have full knowledge of the risks involved.

I, _____ (participant's name) my heirs, and my estate release _____ (your name or company name), including the owner and any employees, instructors or trainers, from any liability for injury, death, or losses suffered in conjunction with my participation in this exercise program.

_____   _____
(signature of participant)   (date)

Case Studies

Hussein v. L.A. Fitness International, LLC.

In the case of *Hussein v. L.A. Fitness*, the plaintiff, Sahal Hussein, was exercising independently (i.e., unsupervised) at a L.A. Fitness club in Chicago, IL. While utilizing the assisted dip/chin machine, Hussein fell, struck his head and body, and was rendered a quadriplegic. The plaintiff filed a lawsuit claiming that L.A. Fitness breached its duty of ordinary care by failing to inspect and maintain the equipment; and failing to appropriately and properly monitor, supervise, or instruct members on the proper use of equipment. The appellate court upheld the trial court's ruling that the membership agreement signed by Hussein, which contained clear and prominent language regarding the 'release and waiver of liability and indemnity' was properly worded and executed, thereby barring Hussein's personal injury claim against the defendant. Properly written and executed waiver and release of liability agreements have also successfully barred lawsuits in *Hazelwood v. L.A. Fitness International, LLC.*; *Quintana v. CrossFit Dallas, LLC.*; and many other cases.

Brooten v. Hickok Rehabilitation Services, LLC et al.

In the case of *Brooten v. Hickok Rehabilitation*, the plaintiff, Robert Brooten, was injured at Chetek Fitness while using an adjustable bench. The bench was adjustable to decline, flat, or inclined positions. As Brooten performed the bench press exercise, the bench collapsed from a flat to a declined position because the T-bar used to secure the bench position was loose and shifted laterally allowing the back rest to fall. Since the club required all members to sign a waiver of liability before use of the facility, Brooten had signed the waiver. Nevertheless, the plaintiff filed a common law negligence, safe place, and strict liability claim against Chetek Fitness. The circuit court granted summary judgment in favor of the defendant, determining the waiver was enforceable and barred Brooten's claims. Upon appeal, the appellant court ruled that Chetek Fitness's liability waiver was contrary to public policy regarding the language of enforceable waivers and, therefore, void and unenforceable. Subsequently the case was returned to the trial court.

Informed Consent

Prior to fitness testing and participation in an exercise program, it is important both legally and ethically to obtain the client's informed consent. The informed consent document is used to communicate important information to the participant prior to beginning exercise testing or training. The exact language contained within the informed consent document may vary based on the exercise setting and the type of assessments being administered. However, the fitness professional must ensure that the participant clearly understands the inherent risks and potential discomforts associated with the planned fitness assessments and subsequent exercise program. When developing an informed consent document, the following information must be included:

- Explanation of the purpose and procedures
- Explanation of the inherent risks and potential discomforts
- Expected benefits and outcomes
- Responsibilities of the participant
- Confidentiality and use of information
- Questions and inquiries from the participant
- Assumption of risk/freedom of consent

After the participant has reviewed the informed consent and all questions have been answered, it should be signed, dated, and maintained in the participant's permanent file. Additional information regarding the informed consent document and procedures can be found in chapter 12.

> **Good to Know**
> **Contents of a Personal Training Client File**
> - Waiver/Release of Liability
> - Informed Consent
> - Health & Lifestyle Questionnaire
> - PAR-Q
> - Medical Clearance (if necessary)
> - Fitness Assessment Data Tracking Sheet
> - Exercise & Training Logs
> - Progress (SOAP) Notes

Preparticipation Screening Questionnaires

In conjunction with the preparticipation screening procedures, several questionnaires may be used to gather important health information from the participant. These questionnaires may include a health and lifestyle questionnaire, the Physical Activity Readiness Questionnaire (PAR-Q), and other previously validated versions of the PAR-Q (e.g., P*AR-Q+, PARmed-X for Pregnancy*). Additional information regarding these preparticipation screening questionnaires can be found in chapter 12. Samples of these questionnaires may also be found in the appendix of this manual. Completed preparticipation questionnaires should be maintained in the participant's permanent file.

Medical Clearance for Exercise Participation

Although most individuals can safely participate in exercise testing and programming, it is highly recommended that all individuals consult with their health care provider prior to participation. Based on the information gathered through preparticipation screening questionnaires and subsequent risk stratification, individuals classified as being 'high risk' must be advised to consult with their health care provider and obtain written medical clearance prior to exercise participation. A completed and signed medical clearance form should be obtained from the participant's health care provider. On this form, the health care provider may also indicate recommendations or limitations to be observed in the design and implementation of the individual's exercise program. A sample medical clearance for exercise participation form may be found in the appendix of this manual. Refer to chapter 12 for more information regarding medical clearance.

Fitness Assessment Data Tracking

The data obtained during both initial fitness assessments and reassessments should be documented and tracked in the participant's file. The tracking sheet should include documentation of the specific assessment protocols utilized, assessment results, notation of relevant observations, and any other pertinent details. This information may be documented on a 'paper and pencil' assessment sheet or may be organized into an electronic spreadsheet (e.g., Microsoft Excel), which is then printed and placed in the participant's file. A sample Fitness Assessment Data Sheet can be found in the appendix of this manual.

Exercise and Training Logs

Fitness professionals must maintain a detailed record of the exercises and activities performed during each session with a participant. The exercise and training logs should include appropriate documentation regarding the acute training variables (e.g., workload, repetitions, sets, intensity, etc.) associated with each exercise as well as response and outcome measurements (e.g., average heart rate, caloric expenditure, distance, rate of perceived exertion, METs, etc.). An endless number of exercise training logs have been created to accommodate the preferences, needs, and situations of each fitness professional or facility. Sample exercise training logs can be found in the appendix of this manual.

Progress (SOAP) Notes

Fitness professionals should document pertinent information related to training sessions with their clients. One method of maintaining such documentation is known as SOAP notes. SOAP is an acronym that stands for subjective, objective, assessment, and plan (Ball & Murphy, 2008; Kettenbach, 2004). Health care providers have used the SOAP format to document progress notes for many decades and in recent years a similar approach has been adopted by many fitness professionals. Documenting sessions and client progress using SOAP notes serves many purposes and provides several benefits as outlined in table 27-1.

The first component of a SOAP note contains subjective information, which includes any pertinent information, verbal or written, that is provided to the fitness professional by the participant (Kettenbach, 2004). During the initial sessions of a personal training relationship, this may include a summary of key information gathered from health history and preparticipation screening questionnaires. On an ongoing basis, this subjective information may include responses to questions posed to the participant such as, "How are you feeling today?", "What activities have you completed since our last session?", or "Tell me about your diet over the last couple days." (Ball & Murphy, 2008). The fitness professional may directly quote or paraphrase the participant's responses to capture the relevant thoughts and information in the SOAP note.

Table 27-1 SOAP Notes

Purposes and Benefits of SOAP Notes
SOAP Notes:
• Facilitate communication with other fitness professionals and health care providers who may share responsibilities in managing a client's exercise program.
• Provide tracking to compile relevant information and observations related to positive and negative behavioral patterns in a client.
• Offer evidence of progress toward desired goals and outcomes.
• Help the fitness professional to organize decision making related to developing, implementing, and maintaining continuity of an exercise program.
• Maintain a written record of the activities performed during a training session and the client's response to these activities.
• Provide a written record of any unusual events, outcomes, or problems associated with the exercise program or that may have been reported from outside of supervised training sessions.
• Demonstrate professionalism, compliance with standards of care, and may provide important documentation in defense of lawsuits.

Ball & Murphy (2008); Kettenbach (2004)

The second section of the SOAP note represents objective information that may include measurements obtained, exercises performed, or data collected with regard to the exercises and activities completed during the session (Ball & Murphy, 2008; Kettenbach, 2004). In most cases, much of this objective information will be documented on the assessment data sheet or the exercise training log, in which case the fitness professional may simply refer to these sources of documentation in the SOAP note. However, if there is noteworthy information (e.g., a new exercise, a significant program change), this may also be stated concisely in the SOAP note.

The next section of the SOAP note is the assessment. This is not to be confused with a fitness assessment, but rather this represents the fitness professional's interpretations and observations of the client's performance, tolerance, progress, and outcomes. This section of the SOAP note may also be used to document statements made by the client during the course of a session that relate to their feelings and responses to the activities performed.

> **Good to Know**
> **Components of a Progress Note**
> **S**ubjective
> **O**bjective
> **A**ssessment
> **P**lan

The final component of the SOAP note is the plan. The plan represents statements looking forward such as expected outcomes, program progression or modification, new activities, and participant 'homework' assignments. This section may be particularly helpful in maintaining the continuity of an exercise program when there are extended gaps between supervised training sessions.

When writing SOAP notes, fitness professionals should observe the following recommendations and guidelines (Ball & Murphy, 2008; Kettenbach, 2004).

Do's:
- Write progress notes in a timely fashion, immediately following the session if possible, to ensure accurate and complete recall of important information.
- Be concise. Use clear, short sentences. Avoid long-winded statements.
- Use common industry abbreviations (e.g., HR, RPE, reps) whenever possible.
- Always write legibly. The purpose of writing the progress note is defeated if the note cannot be easily read.
- Document information that you receive from the client or other health care providers, information regarding your direct observations, and information that is pertinent to the design, implementation, and outcome of the exercise program.
- Note factors from outside supervised training sessions that are self-reported by the client and are pertinent to the activities and outcomes associated with the exercise program.
- Stay within your scope of practice as a fitness professional.
- Sign and date each progress note.

Do not's:
- Never knowingly document false or inaccurate information.
- Never document or verbally communicate information that may directly or indirectly imply you are attempting to make a medical diagnosis, prescribe treatment or rehabilitation, or provide dietary assessment or nutritional advice considered to be outside the scope of practice of a fitness professional.
- Do not use correction fluid (e.g., White-out®) or correction tape to edit information in the progress note. The proper method of correcting a mistake is to put a single line through the error, rewrite the corrected statement, initial, and indicate the date of the correction.
- Do not include criticisms of other staff members, complaints about the working conditions, or personal judgments regarding the client's character or behavior.

The following examples are representative of SOAP notes that may be written by a personal trainer following a session.

"Bill reports that he is feeling well today with no complaints to report. Indicates that he has been consistent with his CRE, having completed 150 min last wk. Began today's session w/ 10 min on the TM x 0.65 mi. Completed RTEs per training log. Concluded with static stretches to HS, pecs, gast/sol, and HF. Bill tolerated today's session w/o any problems. Appears to be making good progress with both his RTEs and wkly CRE. Cont' with the current program progressing RT workloads as able and maintaining a minimum of 150 min/wk of CRE."

"Lisa reports that she is feeling tired today. Work has been stressful lately and she has not been sleeping well. Also has not been able to keep up with her independent ex. Began session w/ 10 min on elliptical @ avg. HR ~115 b/min. Completed full-body RTE routine, 1 set per ex. @ workloads < normal and reps at 12-15/set. See training log for details. Concluded with add'l 20 min CRE at HR ~130-135 b/min. Tolerated session fairly well, although overall intensity decreased due to feeling tired. Motivation seemed down today compared to previous sessions. Encouraged to set aside some time for PA in order to help with fitness and stress mgmt. Next session scheduled for 8/15 @ 6 PM. Cont' w/ current program as able."

Additional Forms and Record Keeping

In addition to the forms and documentation previously discussed, personal training and wellness coaching client files may also include a service agreement or contract. This agreement typically outlines the nature of services to be provided as well as terms and conditions such as the late cancellation or no show policy, fees, and payment options.

Fitness professionals should also develop a system to track their professional certifications and safety certifications to ensure all credentials are maintained and renewed prior to expiration. The tracking system should include a record of specific continuing education courses completed and continuing education credits (CECs) earned.

Situations may also arise that warrant the completion of an accident or incident report. This report should document important information related to the accident or incident such as the date and time of the incident, the location, persons involved including contact information, witnesses to the incident including contact information, details of the incident, actions taken in response to the incident, signature of the individual completing the report, and details related to any follow-up with the person(s) involved or their families (Ehrman, 2010).

Fitness professionals and fitness facilities should also maintain documentation with regard to preventative maintenance, service, and repair of exercise equipment (ACSM, 2012). In addition, the emergency response plan should be documented including a record of emergency scenario rehearsals, AED inspections, and first aid kit inventory (ACSM, 2012).

Chapter Summary

This chapter presented important information regarding common documentation and record keeping maintained by fitness professionals. Appropriate documentation is a key component of the risk management plan for both the fitness professional and a fitness facility. This chapter is not intended to be all-inclusive of the documentation and record keeping that may be required of the fitness professional. It is highly recommended that fitness professionals consult with their risk management team and become familiar with the documentation requirements specific to their work environment.

Chapter References

American College of Sports Medicine (2012). *ACSM's Health/Fitness Facility Standards and Guidelines*, 4th edition. Tharrett, S.J., & Peterson, J.A. (Eds.). Champaign, IL: Human Kinetics.

Ball, D., & Murphy, B. (2008). Taking SOAP notes: Clean up your client documentation using a system favored by the medical community. *IDEA Fitness Journal, 5*(4), 32-35.

Blair, S.A. (2003). The legal aspects: Implementing HIPAA. *ACSM's Health & Fitness Journal, 7*(5), 25-27.

Brooten v. Hickok Rehabilitation Services, LLC et al. In: Herbert, D.L. (2013). *Waiver does not protect club in Wisconsin. The Exercise, Sports and Medicine Standards & Malpractice Reporter, 2*(4), 61-63.

Eickhoff-Shemek, J.M., & Forbes, F.S. (1999). Waivers: Are usually well worth the effort. *ACSM's Health & Fitness Journal, 3*(4), 24-30.

Eickhoff-Shemek, J.M., Herbert, D.L., & Connaughton, D.P. (2009). *Risk Management for Health/Fitness Professionals: Legal Issues and Strategies*. Baltimore, MD: Lippincott, Williams & Wilkins.

Ehrman, J.K. (Ed.). (2010). *ACSM's Resource Manual for Guidelines for Exercise Testing and Prescription*, 6th edition. Baltimore, MD: Lippincott Williams & Wilkins.

Hazelwood v. L.A. Fitness International, LLC. In: Herbert. D.L. (2012). Another release upheld in California. *The Exercise, Sports and Medicine Standards & Malpractice Reporter, 1*(1), 5-6.

Hussein v. L.A. Fitness International, LLC. In: Herbert, D.L. (2013). Release bars personal injury claim against fitness club. *The Exercise, Sports and Medicine Standards & Malpractice Reporter, 2*(3), 45-47.

Kettenbach, G. (2004). *Writing SOAP Notes: With Patient/Client Management Formats*, 3rd edition. Philadelphia, PA: F.A. Davis Company.

Quintana v. CrossFit Dallas, LLC. In: Herbert, D.L. (2012). Suit against personal trainer and fitness facility results in defense judgment. *The Exercise, Sports and Medicine Standards & Malpractice Reporter, 1*(3), 37-39.

Chapter 27 Review Questions

1. Prior to a training session, your client reports that she believes her shoulder was strained while playing tennis over the weekend. In which section of the SOAP note would it be most appropriate to document this information?
    A. Subjective
    B. Objective
    C. Assessment
    D. Plan

2. Which of the following documents is used to communicate the inherent risks and dangers associated with participation in an exercise program?
    A. Physical Activity Readiness Questionnaire
    B. Informed Consent
    C. Personal Training Service Agreement
    D. Physician Release for Exercise Participation

3. In most states, a properly written and executed Waiver and Release of Liability form is likely to be enforceable in which of the following circumstances?
    A. Gross negligence
    B. Criminal conduct
    C. Reckless behavior
    D. Ordinary negligence

4. In which section of a SOAP note would the following statement be documented? "The client's resting blood pressure was measured as 118/82 mmHg before today's personal training session."
    A. Subjective
    B. Objective
    C. Assessment
    D. Plan

5. The late cancellation policy related to personal training sessions is typically communicated to a client through which document?
    A. An informed consent form
    B. An exercise training log
    C. A waiver and release of liability form
    D. A service agreement or contract

6. Which of the following statements is most appropriately included in the 'assessment' component of a SOAP note following a personal training session?
    A. "The client tolerated the session well today. Appeared highly motivated and gave a great effort with all exercises."
    B. "I think the client is really lazy since he never follows through with his exercise plan between our sessions and won't ever reach his weight loss goal."
    C. "The client appears to have suffered a third degree talofibular sprain as the result of a loss of balance during BOSU® squats."
    D. "We began today's session with a 10-minute warm-up on the treadmill followed by resistance training exercises as indicated on the training log."

Answers to Review Questions on Page 384

Note: Review questions are intended to reinforce learning and comprehension of subject matter presented in the corresponding chapter.
The review questions are not intended to be representative of actual certification exam questions in terms of style, content, or difficulty.

Appendix

Physical Activity Readiness
Questionnaire - PAR-Q
(revised 2002)

PAR-Q & YOU

(A Questionnaire for People Aged 15 to 69)

Regular physical activity is fun and healthy, and increasingly more people are starting to become more active every day. Being more active is very safe for most people. However, some people should check with their doctor before they start becoming much more physically active.

If you are planning to become much more physically active than you are now, start by answering the seven questions in the box below. If you are between the ages of 15 and 69, the PAR-Q will tell you if you should check with your doctor before you start. If you are over 69 years of age, and you are not used to being very active, check with your doctor.

Common sense is your best guide when you answer these questions. Please read the questions carefully and answer each one honestly: check YES or NO.

YES	NO		
☐	☐	1.	Has your doctor ever said that you have a heart condition <u>and</u> that you should only do physical activity recommended by a doctor?
☐	☐	2.	Do you feel pain in your chest when you do physical activity?
☐	☐	3.	In the past month, have you had chest pain when you were not doing physical activity?
☐	☐	4.	Do you lose your balance because of dizziness or do you ever lose consciousness?
☐	☐	5.	Do you have a bone or joint problem (for example, back, knee or hip) that could be made worse by a change in your physical activity?
☐	☐	6.	Is your doctor currently prescribing drugs (for example, water pills) for your blood pressure or heart condition?
☐	☐	7.	Do you know of <u>any other reason</u> why you should not do physical activity?

If you answered

YES to one or more questions

Talk with your doctor by phone or in person BEFORE you start becoming much more physically active or BEFORE you have a fitness appraisal. Tell your doctor about the PAR-Q and which questions you answered YES.

- You may be able to do any activity you want — as long as you start slowly and build up gradually. Or, you may need to restrict your activities to those which are safe for you. Talk with your doctor about the kinds of activities you wish to participate in and follow his/her advice.
- Find out which community programs are safe and helpful for you.

NO to all questions

If you answered NO honestly to <u>all</u> PAR-Q questions, you can be reasonably sure that you can:
- start becoming much more physically active – begin slowly and build up gradually. This is the safest and easiest way to go.
- take part in a fitness appraisal – this is an excellent way to determine your basic fitness so that you can plan the best way for you to live actively. It is also highly recommended that you have your blood pressure evaluated. If your reading is over 144/94, talk with your doctor before you start becoming much more physically active.

DELAY BECOMING MUCH MORE ACTIVE:
- if you are not feeling well because of a temporary illness such as a cold or a fever — wait until you feel better; or
- if you are or may be pregnant — talk to your doctor before you start becoming more active.

PLEASE NOTE: If your health changes so that you then answer YES to any of the above questions, tell your fitness or health professional. Ask whether you should change your physical activity plan.

<u>Informed Use of the PAR-Q</u>: The Canadian Society for Exercise Physiology, Health Canada, and their agents assume no liability for persons who undertake physical activity, and if in doubt after completing this questionnaire, consult your doctor prior to physical activity.

No changes permitted. You are encouraged to photocopy the PAR-Q but only if you use the entire form.

NOTE: If the PAR-Q is being given to a person before he or she participates in a physical activity program or a fitness appraisal, this section may be used for legal or administrative purposes.

"I have read, understood and completed this questionnaire. Any questions I had were answered to my full satisfaction."

NAME _____

SIGNATURE _____ DATE _____

SIGNATURE OF PARENT _____ WITNESS _____
or GUARDIAN (for participants under the age of majority)

Note: This physical activity clearance is valid for a maximum of 12 months from the date it is completed and becomes invalid if your condition changes so that you would answer YES to any of the seven questions.

© Canadian Society for Exercise Physiology   www.csep.ca/forms

2017 PAR-Q+

The Physical Activity Readiness Questionnaire for Everyone

The health benefits of regular physical activity are clear; more people should engage in physical activity every day of the week. Participating in physical activity is very safe for MOST people. This questionnaire will tell you whether it is necessary for you to seek further advice from your doctor OR a qualified exercise professional before becoming more physically active.

GENERAL HEALTH QUESTIONS

Please read the 7 questions below carefully and answer each one honestly: check YES or NO.	YES	NO
1) Has your doctor ever said that you have a heart condition ☐ OR high blood pressure ☐?	☐	☐
2) Do you feel pain in your chest at rest, during your daily activities of living, **OR** when you do physical activity?	☐	☐
3) Do you lose balance because of dizziness **OR** have you lost consciousness in the last 12 months? Please answer **NO** if your dizziness was associated with over-breathing (including during vigorous exercise).	☐	☐
4) Have you ever been diagnosed with another chronic medical condition (other than heart disease or high blood pressure)? **PLEASE LIST CONDITION(S) HERE:** _____	☐	☐
5) Are you currently taking prescribed medications for a chronic medical condition? **PLEASE LIST CONDITION(S) AND MEDICATIONS HERE:** _____	☐	☐
6) Do you currently have (or have had within the past 12 months) a bone, joint, or soft tissue (muscle, ligament, or tendon) problem that could be made worse by becoming more physically active? Please answer **NO** if you had a problem in the past, but it *does not limit your current ability* to be physically active. **PLEASE LIST CONDITION(S) HERE:** _____	☐	☐
7) Has your doctor ever said that you should only do medically supervised physical activity?	☐	☐

☑ **If you answered NO to all of the questions above, you are cleared for physical activity.**
Go to Page 4 to sign the PARTICIPANT DECLARATION. You do not need to complete Pages 2 and 3.

- ▶ Start becoming much more physically active – start slowly and build up gradually.
- ▶ Follow International Physical Activity Guidelines for your age (www.who.int/dietphysicalactivity/en/).
- ▶ You may take part in a health and fitness appraisal.
- ▶ If you are over the age of 45 yr and **NOT** accustomed to regular vigorous to maximal effort exercise, consult a qualified exercise professional before engaging in this intensity of exercise.
- ▶ If you have any further questions, contact a qualified exercise professional.

⬤ **If you answered YES to one or more of the questions above, COMPLETE PAGES 2 AND 3.**

⚠ **Delay becoming more active if:**
- ✓ You have a temporary illness such as a cold or fever; it is best to wait until you feel better.
- ✓ You are pregnant - talk to your health care practitioner, your physician, a qualified exercise professional, and/or complete the ePARmed-X+ at **www.eparmedx.com** before becoming more physically active.
- ✓ Your health changes - answer the questions on Pages 2 and 3 of this document and/or talk to your doctor or a qualified exercise professional before continuing with any physical activity program.

OSHF
Ontario Society for Health and Fitness

Copyright © 2017 PAR-Q+ Collaboration
01-01-2017

2017 PAR-Q+

FOLLOW-UP QUESTIONS ABOUT YOUR MEDICAL CONDITION(S)

1.	**Do you have Arthritis, Osteoporosis, or Back Problems?**		
	If the above condition(s) is/are present, answer questions 1a-1c	If **NO** ☐ go to question 2	
1a.	Do you have difficulty controlling your condition with medications or other physician-prescribed therapies? (Answer **NO** if you are not currently taking medications or other treatments)	YES ☐	NO ☐
1b.	Do you have joint problems causing pain, a recent fracture or fracture caused by osteoporosis or cancer, displaced vertebra (e.g., spondylolisthesis), and/or spondylolysis/pars defect (a crack in the bony ring on the back of the spinal column)?	YES ☐	NO ☐
1c.	Have you had steroid injections or taken steroid tablets regularly for more than 3 months?	YES ☐	NO ☐
2.	**Do you currently have Cancer of any kind?**		
	If the above condition(s) is/are present, answer questions 2a-2b	If **NO** ☐ go to question 3	
2a.	Does your cancer diagnosis include any of the following types: lung/bronchogenic, multiple myeloma (cancer of plasma cells), head, and/or neck?	YES ☐	NO ☐
2b.	Are you currently receiving cancer therapy (such as chemotherapy or radiotherapy)?	YES ☐	NO ☐
3.	**Do you have a Heart or Cardiovascular Condition?** *This includes Coronary Artery Disease, Heart Failure, Diagnosed Abnormality of Heart Rhythm*		
	If the above condition(s) is/are present, answer questions 3a-3d	If **NO** ☐ go to question 4	
3a.	Do you have difficulty controlling your condition with medications or other physician-prescribed therapies? (Answer **NO** if you are not currently taking medications or other treatments)	YES ☐	NO ☐
3b.	Do you have an irregular heart beat that requires medical management? (e.g., atrial fibrillation, premature ventricular contraction)	YES ☐	NO ☐
3c.	Do you have chronic heart failure?	YES ☐	NO ☐
3d.	Do you have diagnosed coronary artery (cardiovascular) disease and have not participated in regular physical activity in the last 2 months?	YES ☐	NO ☐
4.	**Do you have High Blood Pressure?**		
	If the above condition(s) is/are present, answer questions 4a-4b	If **NO** ☐ go to question 5	
4a.	Do you have difficulty controlling your condition with medications or other physician-prescribed therapies? (Answer **NO** if you are not currently taking medications or other treatments)	YES ☐	NO ☐
4b.	Do you have a resting blood pressure equal to or greater than 160/90 mmHg with or without medication? (Answer **YES** if you do not know your resting blood pressure)	YES ☐	NO ☐
5.	**Do you have any Metabolic Conditions?** *This includes Type 1 Diabetes, Type 2 Diabetes, Pre-Diabetes*		
	If the above condition(s) is/are present, answer questions 5a-5e	If **NO** ☐ go to question 6	
5a.	Do you often have difficulty controlling your blood sugar levels with foods, medications, or other physician-prescribed therapies?	YES ☐	NO ☐
5b.	Do you often suffer from signs and symptoms of low blood sugar (hypoglycemia) following exercise and/or during activities of daily living? Signs of hypoglycemia may include shakiness, nervousness, unusual irritability, abnormal sweating, dizziness or light-headedness, mental confusion, difficulty speaking, weakness, or sleepiness.	YES ☐	NO ☐
5c.	Do you have any signs or symptoms of diabetes complications such as heart or vascular disease and/or complications affecting your eyes, kidneys, **OR** the sensation in your toes and feet?	YES ☐	NO ☐
5d.	Do you have other metabolic conditions (such as current pregnancy-related diabetes, chronic kidney disease, or liver problems)?	YES ☐	NO ☐
5e.	Are you planning to engage in what for you is unusually high (or vigorous) intensity exercise in the near future?	YES ☐	NO ☐

2017 PAR-Q+

6.	**Do you have any Mental Health Problems or Learning Difficulties?** *This includes Alzheimer's, Dementia, Depression, Anxiety Disorder, Eating Disorder, Psychotic Disorder, Intellectual Disability, Down Syndrome*	
	If the above condition(s) is/are present, answer questions 6a-6b If **NO** ☐ go to question 7	
6a.	Do you have difficulty controlling your condition with medications or other physician-prescribed therapies? (Answer **NO** if you are not currently taking medications or other treatments)	YES ☐ NO ☐
6b.	Do you have Down Syndrome **AND** back problems affecting nerves or muscles?	YES ☐ NO ☐
7.	**Do you have a Respiratory Disease?** *This includes Chronic Obstructive Pulmonary Disease, Asthma, Pulmonary High Blood Pressure*	
	If the above condition(s) is/are present, answer questions 7a-7d If **NO** ☐ go to question 8	
7a.	Do you have difficulty controlling your condition with medications or other physician-prescribed therapies? (Answer **NO** if you are not currently taking medications or other treatments)	YES ☐ NO ☐
7b.	Has your doctor ever said your blood oxygen level is low at rest or during exercise and/or that you require supplemental oxygen therapy?	YES ☐ NO ☐
7c.	If asthmatic, do you currently have symptoms of chest tightness, wheezing, laboured breathing, consistent cough (more than 2 days/week), or have you used your rescue medication more than twice in the last week?	YES ☐ NO ☐
7d.	Has your doctor ever said you have high blood pressure in the blood vessels of your lungs?	YES ☐ NO ☐
8.	**Do you have a Spinal Cord Injury?** *This includes Tetraplegia and Paraplegia*	
	If the above condition(s) is/are present, answer questions 8a-8c If **NO** ☐ go to question 9	
8a.	Do you have difficulty controlling your condition with medications or other physician-prescribed therapies? (Answer **NO** if you are not currently taking medications or other treatments)	YES ☐ NO ☐
8b.	Do you commonly exhibit low resting blood pressure significant enough to cause dizziness, light-headedness, and/or fainting?	YES ☐ NO ☐
8c.	Has your physician indicated that you exhibit sudden bouts of high blood pressure (known as Autonomic Dysreflexia)?	YES ☐ NO ☐
9.	**Have you had a Stroke?** *This includes Transient Ischemic Attack (TIA) or Cerebrovascular Event*	
	If the above condition(s) is/are present, answer questions 9a-9c If **NO** ☐ go to question 10	
9a.	Do you have difficulty controlling your condition with medications or other physician-prescribed therapies? (Answer **NO** if you are not currently taking medications or other treatments)	YES ☐ NO ☐
9b.	Do you have any impairment in walking or mobility?	YES ☐ NO ☐
9c.	Have you experienced a stroke or impairment in nerves or muscles in the past 6 months?	YES ☐ NO ☐
10.	**Do you have any other medical condition not listed above or do you have two or more medical conditions?**	
	If you have other medical conditions, answer questions 10a-10c If **NO** ☐ read the Page 4 recommendations	
10a.	Have you experienced a blackout, fainted, or lost consciousness as a result of a head injury within the last 12 months **OR** have you had a diagnosed concussion within the last 12 months?	YES ☐ NO ☐
10b.	Do you have a medical condition that is not listed (such as epilepsy, neurological conditions, kidney problems)?	YES ☐ NO ☐
10c.	Do you currently live with two or more medical conditions?	YES ☐ NO ☐
	PLEASE LIST YOUR MEDICAL CONDITION(S) AND ANY RELATED MEDICATIONS HERE: _____	

> **GO to Page 4 for recommendations about your current medical condition(s) and sign the PARTICIPANT DECLARATION.**

2017 PAR-Q+

☑ **If you answered NO to all of the follow-up questions about your medical condition, you are ready to become more physically active - sign the PARTICIPANT DECLARATION below:**

▶ It is advised that you consult a qualified exercise professional to help you develop a safe and effective physical activity plan to meet your health needs.

▶ You are encouraged to start slowly and build up gradually - 20 to 60 minutes of low to moderate intensity exercise, 3-5 days per week including aerobic and muscle strengthening exercises.

▶ As you progress, you should aim to accumulate 150 minutes or more of moderate intensity physical activity per week.

▶ If you are over the age of 45 yr and **NOT** accustomed to regular vigorous to maximal effort exercise, consult a qualified exercise professional before engaging in this intensity of exercise.

○ **If you answered YES to one or more of the follow-up questions** about your medical condition:
You should seek further information before becoming more physically active or engaging in a fitness appraisal. You should complete the specially designed online screening and exercise recommendations program - the **ePARmed-X+ at www.eparmedx.com** and/or visit a qualified exercise professional to work through the ePARmed-X+ and for further information.

⚠ **Delay becoming more active if:**

✓ You have a temporary illness such as a cold or fever; it is best to wait until you feel better.

✓ You are pregnant - talk to your health care practitioner, your physician, a qualified exercise professional, and/or complete the ePARmed-X+ **at www.eparmedx.com** before becoming more physically active.

✓ Your health changes - talk to your doctor or qualified exercise professional before continuing with any physical activity program.

- You are encouraged to photocopy the PAR-Q+. You must use the entire questionnaire and NO changes are permitted.
- The authors, the PAR-Q+ Collaboration, partner organizations, and their agents assume no liability for persons who undertake physical activity and/or make use of the PAR-Q+ or ePARmed-X+. If in doubt after completing the questionnaire, consult your doctor prior to physical activity.

PARTICIPANT DECLARATION

- All persons who have completed the PAR-Q+ please read and sign the declaration below.
- If you are less than the legal age required for consent or require the assent of a care provider, your parent, guardian or care provider must also sign this form.

I, the undersigned, have read, understood to my full satisfaction and completed this questionnaire. I acknowledge that this physical activity clearance is valid for a maximum of 12 months from the date it is completed and becomes invalid if my condition changes. I also acknowledge that a Trustee (such as my employer, community/fitness centre, health care provider, or other designate) may retain a copy of this form for their records. In these instances, the Trustee will be required to adhere to local, national, and international guidelines regarding the storage of personal health information ensuring that the Trustee maintains the privacy of the information and does not misuse or wrongfully disclose such information.

NAME _____   DATE _____

SIGNATURE _____   WITNESS _____

SIGNATURE OF PARENT/GUARDIAN/CARE PROVIDER _____

For more information, please contact
www.eparmedx.com
Email: eparmedx@gmail.com

Citation for PAR-Q+
Warburton DER, Jamnik VK, Bredin SSD, and Gledhill N on behalf of the PAR-Q+ Collaboration. The Physical Activity Readiness Questionnaire for Everyone (PAR-Q+) and Electronic Physical Activity Readiness Medical Examination (ePARmed-X+). Health & Fitness Journal of Canada 4(2):3-23, 2011.

Key References
1. Jamnik VK, Warburton DER, Makarski J, McKenzie DC, Shephard RJ, Stone J, and Gledhill N. Enhancing the effectiveness of clearance for physical activity participation; background and overall process. APNM 36(S1):S3-S13, 2011.
2. Warburton DER, Gledhill N, Jamnik VK, Bredin SSD, McKenzie DC, Stone J, Charlesworth S, and Shephard RJ. Evidence-based risk assessment and recommendations for physical activity clearance; Consensus Document. APNM 36(S1):S266-s298, 2011.
3. Chisholm DM, Collis ML, Kulak LL, Davenport W, and Gruber N. Physical activity readiness. British Columbia Medical Journal. 1975;17:375-378.
4. Thomas S, Reading J, and Shephard RJ. Revision of the Physical Activity Readiness Questionnaire (PAR-Q). Canadian Journal of Sport Science 1992;17:4 338-345.

The PAR-Q+ was created using the evidence-based AGREE process (1) by the PAR-Q+ Collaboration chaired by Dr. Darren E. R. Warburton with Dr. Norman Gledhill, Dr. Veronica Jamnik, and Dr. Donald C. McKenzie (2). Production of this document has been made possible through financial contributions from the Public Health Agency of Canada and the BC Ministry of Health Services. The views expressed herein do not necessarily represent the views of the Public Health Agency of Canada or the BC Ministry of Health Services.

Physical Activity Readiness
Medical Examination for
Pregnancy (2002)

PARmed-X for PREGNANCY — PHYSICAL ACTIVITY READINESS MEDICAL EXAMINATION

PARmed-X for PREGNANCY is a guideline for health screening prior to participation in a prenatal fitness class or other exercise.

Healthy women with uncomplicated pregnancies can integrate physical activity into their daily living and can participate without significant risks either to themselves or to their unborn child. Postulated benefits of such programs include improved aerobic and muscular fitness, promotion of appropriate weight gain, and facilitation of labour. Regular exercise may also help to prevent gestational glucose intolerance and pregnancy-induced hypertension.

The safety of prenatal exercise programs depends on an adequate level of maternal-fetal physiological reserve. PARmed-X for PREGNANCY is a convenient checklist and prescription for use by health care providers to evaluate pregnant patients who want to enter a prenatal fitness program and for ongoing medical surveillance of exercising pregnant patients.

Instructions for use of the 4-page PARmed-X for PREGNANCY are the following:

1. The patient should fill out the section on PATIENT INFORMATION and the PRE-EXERCISE HEALTH CHECKLIST (PART 1, 2, 3, and 4 on p. 1) and give the form to the health care provider monitoring her pregnancy.
2. The health care provider should check the information provided by the patient for accuracy and fill out SECTION C on CONTRAINDICATIONS (p. 2) based on current medical information.
3. If no exercise contraindications exist, the HEALTH EVALUATION FORM (p. 3) should be completed, signed by the health care provider, and given by the patient to her prenatal fitness professional.

In addition to prudent medical care, participation in appropriate types, intensities and amounts of exercise is recommended to increase the likelihood of a beneficial pregnancy outcome. PARmed-X for PREGNANCY provides recommendations for individualized exercise prescription (p. 3) and program safety (p. 4).

NOTE: Sections A and B should be completed by the patient before the appointment with the health care provider.

A PATIENT INFORMATION

NAME _____

ADDRESS _____

TELEPHONE _____ BIRTHDATE _____ HEALTH INSURANCE No. _____

NAME OF
PRENATAL FITNESS PROFESSIONAL _____ PRENATAL FITNESS PROFESSIONAL'S PHONE NUMBER _____

B PRE-EXERCISE HEALTH CHECKLIST

PART 1: GENERAL HEALTH STATUS

In the past, have you experienced (check YES or NO):

	YES	NO
1. Miscarriage in an earlier pregnancy?	❏	❏
2. Other pregnancy complications?	❏	❏
3. I have completed a PAR-Q within the last 30 days.	❏	❏

If you answered YES to question 1 or 2, please explain:

_____

Number of previous pregnancies? _____

PART 2: STATUS OF CURRENT PREGNANCY

Due Date: _____

During this pregnancy, have you experienced:

	YES	NO
1. Marked fatigue?	❏	❏
2. Bleeding from the vagina ("spotting")?	❏	❏
3. Unexplained faintness or dizziness?	❏	❏
4. Unexplained abdominal pain?	❏	❏
5. Sudden swelling of ankles, hands or face?	❏	❏
6. Persistent headaches or problems with headaches?	❏	❏
7. Swelling, pain or redness in the calf of one leg?	❏	❏
8. Absence of fetal movement after 6th month?	❏	❏
9. Failure to gain weight after 5th month?	❏	❏

If you answered YES to any of the above questions, please explain:

_____

PART 3: ACTIVITY HABITS DURING THE PAST MONTH

1. List only regular fitness/recreational activities:

_____
_____

INTENSITY	FREQUENCY (times/week)			TIME (minutes/day)		
	1-2	2-4	4+	<20	20-40	40+
Heavy	___	___	___	___	___	___
Medium	___	___	___	___	___	___
Light	___	___	___	___	___	___

2. Does your regular occupation (job/home) activity involve:

	YES	NO
Heavy Lifting?	❏	❏
Frequent walking/stair climbing?	❏	❏
Occasional walking (>once/hr)?	❏	❏
Prolonged standing?	❏	❏
Mainly sitting?	❏	❏
Normal daily activity?	❏	❏
3. Do you currently smoke tobacco?*	❏	❏
4. Do you consume alcohol?*	❏	❏

PART 4: PHYSICAL ACTIVITY INTENTIONS

What physical activity do you intend to do?

_____

Is this a change from what you currently do?   ❏ YES   ❏ NO

*NOTE: PREGNANT WOMEN ARE STRONGLY ADVISED NOT TO SMOKE OR CONSUME ALCOHOL DURING PREGNANCY AND DURING LACTATION.

© Canadian Society for Exercise Physiology
Société canadienne de physiologie de l'exercice

Supported by: Health Canada / Santé Canada

Physical Activity Readiness
Medical Examination for
Pregnancy (2002)

PARmed-X for PREGNANCY — PHYSICAL ACTIVITY READINESS MEDICAL EXAMINATION

C CONTRAINDICATIONS TO EXERCISE: to be completed by your health care provider

Absolute Contraindications
Does the patient have: YES NO

1. Ruptured membranes, premature labour? ❏ ❏
2. Persistent second or third trimester bleeding/placenta previa? ❏ ❏
3. Pregnancy-induced hypertension or pre-eclampsia? ❏ ❏
4. Incompetent cervix? ❏ ❏
5. Evidence of intrauterine growth restriction? ❏ ❏
6. High-order pregnancy (e.g., triplets)? ❏ ❏
7. Uncontrolled Type I diabetes, hypertension or thyroid disease, other serious cardiovascular, respiratory or systemic disorder? ❏ ❏

Relative Contraindications
Does the patient have: YES NO

1. History of spontaneous abortion or premature labour in previous pregnancies? ❏ ❏
2. Mild/moderate cardiovascular or respiratory disease (e.g., chronic hypertension, asthma)? ❏ ❏
3. Anemia or iron deficiency? (Hb < 100 g/L)? ❏ ❏
4. Malnutrition or eating disorder (anorexia, bulimia)? ❏ ❏
5. Twin pregnancy after 28th week? ❏ ❏
6. Other significant medical condition? ❏ ❏

Please specify: _____

NOTE: Risk may exceed benefits of regular physical activity. The decision to be physically active or not should be made with qualified medical advice.

PHYSICAL ACTIVITY RECOMMENDATION: ❏ Recommended/Approved ❏ Contraindicated

Prescription for Aerobic Activity

RATE OF PROGRESSION: The best time to progress is during the second trimester since risks and discomforts of pregnancy are lowest at that time. Aerobic exercise should be increased gradually during the second trimester from a minimum of 15 minutes per session, 3 times per week (at the appropriate target heart rate or RPE) to a maximum of approximately 30 minutes per session, 4 times per week (at the appropriate target heart rate or RPE).

WARM-UP/COOL-DOWN: Aerobic activity should be preceded by a brief (10-15 min.) warm-up and followed by a short (10-15 min.) cool-down. Low intensity calesthenics, stretching and relaxation exercises should be included in the warm-up/cool-down.

PRESCRIPTION/MONITORING OF INTENSITY: The best way to prescribe and monitor exercise is by combining the heart rate and rating of perceived exertion (RPE) methods.

TARGET HEART RATE ZONES

The heart rate zones shown below are appropriate for most pregnant women. Work during the lower end of the HR range at the start of a new exercise program and in late pregnancy.

Age	Heart Rate Range
< 20	140-155
20-29	135-150
30-39	130-145

RATING OF PERCEIVED EXERTION (RPE)

Check the accuracy of your heart rate target zone by comparing it to the scale below. A range of about 12-14 (somewhat hard) is appropriate for most pregnant women.

6	
7	Very, very light
8	
9	Somewhat light
10	
11	Fairly light
12	
13	Somewhat hard
14	
15	Hard
16	
17	Very hard
18	
19	Very, very hard
20	

F I T T

FREQUENCY	INTENSITY	TIME	TYPE
Begin at 3 times per week and progress to four times per week	Exercise within an appropriate RPE range and/or target heart rate zone	Attempt 15 minutes, even if it means reducing the intensity. Rest intervals may be helpful	Non weight-bearing or low-impact endurance exercise using large muscle groups (e.g., walking, stationary cycling, swimming, aquatic exercises, low impact aerobics)

"TALK TEST" - A final check to avoid overexertion is to use the "talk test". The exercise intensity is excessive if you cannot carry on a verbal conversation while exercising.

The original PARmed-X for PREGNANCY was developed by L.A. Wolfe, Ph.D., Queen's University. The muscular conditioning component was developed by M.F. Mottola, Ph.D., University of Western Ontario. The document has been revised based on advice from an Expert Advisory Committee of the Canadian Society for Exercise Physiology chaired by Dr. N. Gledhill, with additonal input from Drs. Wolfe and Mottola, and Gregory A.L. Davies, M.D., FRCS(C) Department of Obstetrics and Gynaecology, Queen's University, 2002.

No changes permitted. Translation and reproduction in its entirety is encouraged.

Disponible en français sous le titre «Examination medicale sur l'aptitude à l'activité physique pour les femmes enceintes (X-AAP pour les femmes enceintes)»

Additional copies of the PARmed-X for PREGNANCY, the PARmed-X and/or the PAR-Q can be downloaded from: www.csep.ca/publications
For more information contact the:

Canadian Society for Exercise Physiology
18 Louisa Street, Suite 370, Ottawa, Ontario CANADA K1R 6Y6
tel.: 1-877-651-3755   www.csep.ca

Physical Activity Readiness
Medical Examination for
Pregnancy (2002)

PARmed-X for PREGNANCY
PHYSICAL ACTIVITY READINESS MEDICAL EXAMINATION

Prescription for Muscular Conditioning

It is important to condition all major muscle groups during both prenatal and postnatal periods.

WARM-UPS & COOL DOWN:
Range of Motion: neck, shoulder girdle, back, arms, hips, knees, ankles, etc.

Static Stretching: all major muscle groups

(DO NOT OVER STRETCH!)

EXAMPLES OF MUSCULAR STRENGTHENING EXERCISES

CATEGORY	PURPOSE	EXAMPLE
Upper back	Promotion of good posture	Shoulder shrugs, shoulder blade pinch
Lower back	Promotion of good posture	Modified standing opposite leg & arm lifts
Abdomen	Promotion of good posture, prevent low-back pain, prevent diastasis recti, strengthen muscles of labour	Abdominal tightening, abdominal curl-ups, head raises lying on side or standing position
Pelvic floor ("Kegels")	Promotion of good bladder control, prevention of urinary incontinence	"Wave", "elevator"
Upper body	Improve muscular support for breasts	Shoulder rotations, modified push-ups against a wall
Buttocks, lower limbs	Facilitation of weight-bearing, prevention of varicose veins	Buttocks squeeze, standing leg lifts, heel raises

PRECAUTIONS FOR MUSCULAR CONDITIONING DURING PREGNANCY

VARIABLE	EFFECTS OF PREGNANCY	EXERCISE MODIFICATIONS
Body Position	• in the supine position (lying on the back), the enlarged uterus may either decrease the flow of blood returning from the lower half of the body as it presses on a major vein (inferior vena cava) or it may decrease flow to a major artery (abdominal aorta)	• past 4 months of gestation, exercises normally done in the supine position should be altered • such exercises should be done side lying or standing
Joint Laxity	• ligaments become relaxed due to increasing hormone levels • joints may be prone to injury	• avoid rapid changes in direction and bouncing during exercises • stretching should be performed with controlled movements
Abdominal Muscles	• presence of a rippling (bulging) of connective tissue along the midline of the pregnant abdomen (diastasis recti) may be seen during abdominal exercise	• abdominal exercises are not recommended if diastasis recti develops
Posture	• increasing weight of enlarged breasts and uterus may cause a forward shift in the centre of gravity and may increase the arch in the lower back • this may also cause shoulders to slump forward	• emphasis on correct posture and neutral pelvic alignment. Neutral pelvic alignment is found by bending the knees, feet shoulder width apart, and aligning the pelvis between accentuated lordosis and the posterior pelvic tilt position.
Precautions for Resistance Exercise	• emphasis must be placed on continuous breathing throughout exercise • exhale on exertion, inhale on relaxation using high repetitions and low weights • Valsalva Manoevre (holding breath while working against a resistance) causes a change in blood pressure and therefore should be avoided • avoid exercise in supine position past 4 months gestation	

PARmed-X for Pregnancy - Health Evaluation Form
(to be completed by patient and given to the prenatal fitness professional after obtaining medical clearance to exercise)

I, _____ PLEASE PRINT (patient's name), have discussed my plans to participate in physical activity during my current pregnancy with my health care provider and I have obtained his/her approval to begin participation.

Signed: _____ Date: _____
(patient's signature)

HEALTH CARE PROVIDER'S COMMENTS:

Name of health care provider: _____

Address: _____

_____

Telephone: _____

_____
(health care provider's signature)

3

Medical Examination for Pregnancy (2002)

Advice for Active Living During Pregnancy

Pregnancy is a time when women can make beneficial changes in their health habits to protect and promote the healthy development of their unborn babies. These changes include adopting improved eating habits, abstinence from smoking and alcohol intake, and participating in regular moderate physical activity. Since all of these changes can be carried over into the postnatal period and beyond, pregnancy is a very good time to adopt healthy lifestyle habits that are permanent by integrating physical activity with enjoyable healthy eating and a positive self and body image.

Active Living:
- see your doctor before increasing your activity level during pregnancy
- exercise regularly but don't overexert
- exercise with a pregnant friend or join a prenatal exercise program
- follow FITT principles modified for pregnant women
- know safety considerations for exercise in pregnancy

Healthy Eating:
- the need for calories is higher (about 300 more per day) than before pregnancy
- follow Canada's Food Guide to Healthy Eating and choose healthy foods from the following groups: whole grain or enriched bread or cereal, fruits and vegetables, milk and milk products, meat, fish, poultry and alternatives
- drink 6-8 glasses of fluid, including water, each day
- salt intake should not be restricted
- limit caffeine intake i.e., coffee, tea, chocolate, and cola drinks
- dieting to lose weight is not recommended during pregnancy

Positive Self and Body Image:
- remember that it is normal to gain weight during pregnancy
- accept that your body shape will change during pregnancy
- enjoy your pregnancy as a unique and meaningful experience

For more detailed information and advice about pre- and postnatal exercise, you may wish to obtain a copy of a booklet entitled *Active Living During Pregnancy: Physical Activity Guidelines for Mother and Baby* © 1999. Available from the Canadian Society for Exercise Physiology, 185 Somerset St. West, Suite 202, Ottawa, Ontario Canada K2P 0J2 Tel. 1-877-651-3755 Fax: (613) 234-3565 Email: info@csep.ca (online: www.csep.ca). Cost: $11.95

For more detailed information about the safety of exercise in pregnancy you may wish to obtain a copy of the Clinical Practice Guidelines of the Society of Obstetricians and Gynaecologists of Canada and Canadian Society for Exercise Physiology entitled *Exercise in Pregnancy and Postpartum* © 2003. Available from the Society of Obstetricians and Gynaecologists of Canada online at www.sogc.org

For more detailed information about pregnancy and childbirth you may wish to obtain a copy of *Healthy Beginnings: Your Handbook for Pregnancy and Birth* © 1998. Available from the Society of Obstetricians and Gynaecologists of Canada at 1-877-519-7999 (also available online at www.sogc.org) Cost $12.95.

For more detailed information on healthy eating during pregnancy, you may wish to obtain a copy of *Nutrition for a Healthy Pregnancy: National Guidelines for the Childbearing Years* © 1999. Available from Health Canada, Minister of Public Works and Government Services, Ottawa, Ontario Canada (also available online at www.hc-sc.gc.ca).

SAFETY CONSIDERATIONS

- Avoid exercise in warm/humid environments, especially during the 1st trimester
- Avoid isometric exercise or straining while holding your breath
- Maintain adequate nutrition and hydration — drink liquids before and after exercise
- Avoid exercise while lying on your back past the 4th month of pregnancy
- Avoid activities which involve physical contact or danger of falling
- Know your limits — pregnancy is not a good time to train for athletic competition
- Know the reasons to stop exercise and consult a qualified health care provider immediately if they occur

REASONS TO STOP EXERCISE AND CONSULT YOUR HEALTH CARE PROVIDER

- Excessive shortness of breath
- Chest pain
- Painful uterine contractions (more than 6-8 per hour)
- Vaginal bleeding
- Any "gush" of fluid from vagina (suggesting premature rupture of the membranes)
- Dizziness or faintness

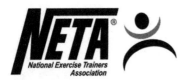

Health & Lifestyle Questionnaire

Instructions: Please complete the entire questionnaire, responding to all requested information and providing as much detail as possible. Indicate "N/A" for those items that are not applicable.

Name: _____ Date: _____

Home Phone: _____ Work Phone: _____ DOB: _____

Address: _____ Age: _____

E-mail Address: _____

Employer/Occupation: _____

How many hours do you work per week?   < 35 ☐   35-40 ☐   40-45 ☐   45-50 ☐   > 50 ☐

What are the primary physical requirements of your job?

Phone/computer ☐   Sitting ☐   Standing ☐   Lifting ☐   Travel ☐

Please rate your level of stress on the following scale (circle one)

Home:	Low Stress	1	2	3	4	5	High Stress
Work:	Low Stress	1	2	3	4	5	High Stress

Please list a relative whom we may contact in case of an emergency.

Name: _____ Relation: _____

Home Phone: _____ Work Phone: _____

Please complete the information for your personal health care provider.

Name of Provider: _____

Clinic Name: _____

Address: _____

Office Phone: _____ Office Fax: _____

Page 1

Family Health History

Please indicate if you have any *primary relatives* who have any of the following conditions. (check all that apply)

Asthma ☐	Cancer ☐	Hypertension ☐	High Cholesterol ☐
Arthritis ☐	Diabetes ☐	Heart Disease ☐	Osteoporosis ☐
Obesity ☐	Stroke ☐	Other:	_____

Please provide a brief explanation for any of the above that have been checked.

_____
_____
_____

Personal Health History

Please indicate if *you* have any of the following conditions. (check all that apply).

Asthma ☐	Cancer ☐	Hypertension ☐	High Cholesterol ☐
Arthritis ☐	Diabetes ☐	Heart Disease ☐	Osteoporosis ☐
Obesity ☐	Stroke ☐	Other:	_____

Please provide a brief explanation for any of the above that have been checked.

_____
_____
_____

Please indicate if you have had any joint injuries or surgeries that may limit or effect your ability to exercise.

Neck ☐	Hip ☐	Wrist/Hand ☐
Shoulder ☐	Knee ☐	Ankle/Foot ☐
Elbow ☐	Low Back ☐	Other ☐

Please provide a brief explanation for any of the above that have been checked.

_____
_____
_____

Please indicate any medications currently used.

Type of Medication	Purpose
_____	_____
_____	_____
_____	_____

Do you smoke cigarettes?   Yes ☐   No ☐   If yes, how often? _____

Are you a past smoker?   Yes ☐   No ☐   If yes, when did you quit? _____

Do you drink alcoholic beverages?   Yes ☐   No ☐   If yes, how much, often? _____

Are you presently dieting or on a weight control program?   Yes ☐   No ☐

If yes, please provide a brief explanation. _____

_____

_____

Do you have any past or present medical conditions, not already addressed, which may influence your ability to safely participate in an exercise program? If yes, please explain.

_____

_____

_____

Please provide a brief explanation of your current exercise program. Include types of activity and frequency.

_____

_____

_____

What are your current health and fitness goals? Please be as specific as possible.

_____

_____

Do you foresee any barriers that may prevent you from adhering to a regular exercise program?

_____

_____

How do you rate your level of motivation and commitment to achieving your goals? (circle one)

Low   1   2   3   4   5   High

Have you worked with a personal trainer in the past?   Yes ☐   No ☐

When are you available to meet with a trainer?

Morning ☐   Day ☐   Evening ☐   Other: _____

Do you prefer to work with a male or female trainer?   Male ☐   Female ☐   No preference ☐

How did you hear about our Personal Training services?

Brochure/Flyer ☐   Referral from friend ☐   Staff ☐

Promotional offer ☐   Website ☐   Other: _____

Health Risk Appraisal

Major Signs and Symptoms Suggestive of Cardiovascular, Pulmonary, or Metabolic Disease

	Yes	No
Do you experience pain or discomfort (tightness, constriction, squeezing, burning) in the chest, neck, jaw, arm and other areas that may result from lack of adequate blood supply?		
Do you experience shortness of breath at rest or with mild exertion?		
Do you experience shortness of breath while at rest in a reclined position that is relieved promptly by sitting upright or standing?		
Do you experience shortness of breath beginning usually 2-5 hours after onset of sleep, which may be relieved by sitting upright on the side of the bed or getting out of bed?		
Do you have regular swelling of the ankles?		
Do you experience heart palpitations (an unpleasant awareness of the forceful or rapid beating of the heart) or the sensation of a "racing" heart?		
Do you experience muscle pain when walking that goes away after 1-2 minutes after stopping exercise?		
Has your doctor ever said that you have a heart murmur?		
Do you experience unusual fatigue or shortness of breath with usual daily activities?		
Do you ever experience unexplained dizziness or loss of consciousness?		

Risk Factors for CVD

Positive Risk Factors (+1 for each "Yes")		Yes	No
Age	Men ≥45 years; Women ≥55 years		
Family History	Myocardial infarction, coronary revascularization, or sudden death before 55 years of age in father or other male first-degree relative, or before 65 years of age in mother or other female first-degree relative.		
Cigarette Smoking	Current cigarette smoker or those who quit within the previous six months, or exposure to environmental tobacco smoke		
Hypertension	Systolic blood pressure ≥140 mmHg and/or diastolic pressure ≥90mHg, confirmed by measurements on at least two separate occasions, or on antihypertensive medication.		
High Cholesterol	LDL-C ≥130 mg/dL or HDL-C ≤40 mg/dL, or on lipid-lowering medication. If total serum cholesterol is all that is available, use ≥200 mg/dL.		
Diabetes	Fasting plasma glucose ≥126 mg/dL or 2-hour plasma glucose values in oral glucose tolerance test (OGTT) ≥200 mg/dL or HbA1c ≥6.5%.		
Obesity	BMI ≥30 kg/m^2 or waist circumference >102 cm (40 inches) for men and >88 cm (35 inches) for women.		
Sedentary Lifestyle	Not participating in at least 30 minutes of moderate intensity physical activity on at least three days per week for at least three months.		
Negative Risk Factor (-1 for "Yes")			
HDL Cholesterol	HDL-C ≥60 mg/dL		

Net Total Number of Risk Factors = _____

The information I have provided in this questionnaire (pages 1-4) is true and accurate to the best of my knowledge. I understand that this information is necessary for the purpose of developing and implementing a safe and effective exercise program. The information I have provided is to remain confidential. I agree to provide updated health information when it is relevant to the ongoing safety and effectiveness of my personal exercise program.

_____   _____   _____
Signature   **Printed Name**   **Date**

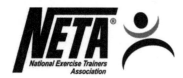

Medical Clearance for Exercise Participation

To:
Name: _____
Clinic: _____
Address: _____
_____
Phone: _____
Fax: _____

Date: _____

From:
Name: _____
Title: _____
Facility: _____
Address: _____
_____
Phone: _____
Fax: _____
Email: _____

Dear, _____
(Health Care Provider's Name)

Your patient, _____ (DOB)_____, has applied for enrollment in the health/fitness testing and/or exercise programs at _____. The health/fitness testing involves a submaximal test for cardiorespiratory fitness, body composition analysis, flexibility tests, and a muscular strength and endurance tests. The exercise programs are designed to start easy and become progressively more difficult over a period of time. A more detailed description of the fitness testing protocols and exercise programs is available upon request. All health/fitness assessments and exercise programs will be guided by a qualified fitness professional holding a nationally-accredited personal training certification as well as certifications in cardiopulmonary resuscitation (CPR) and the use of an automated external defibrillator (AED).

By completing the box below, however, you are not assuming any responsibility for our administration of the health/fitness testing and/or exercise programs. If you know of any medical or other reasons why participation in the fitness testing and/or exercise programs by this applicant would be unwise, please indicate so on this form.

If you have any questions, please feel free to call me at _____.

Report of Health Care Provider

❑ I know of no reason why the applicant may not participate in the fitness testing and/or exercise program.

❑ I believe the applicant may participate, but I recommend the following guidelines and precautions are observed:
- _____
- _____

❑ The applicant should not engage in the following activities:
- _____
- _____

❑ I recommend that the applicant NOT participate at this time.

Signature: _____   Date: _____

I hereby consent to the release of pertinent health information to _____ for the purpose of designing a safe and effective exercise program. I understand that this information will be kept confidential and only persons involved in the design and implementation of my exercise program will be viewing this information.

_____
Signature   Date

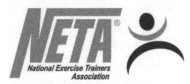

Exercise and Training Log

Name:	Date:														
Cardiorespiratory Exercise (CRE)	T	D	T	D	T	D	T	D	T	D	T	D	T	D

Resistance Training Exercise (RTE)	W	S	R	W	S	R	W	S	R	W	S	R	W	S	R	W	S	R	W	S	R
Lower Body Exercises																					
Upper Body Push																					
Upper Body Pull																					
Core																					
Other																					

Flexibility Training Exercises (FTE)	S	T	S	T	S	T	S	T	S	T	S	T	S	T

T = Time; S = Sets; D = Distance; W = Weight/Workload; R = Repetitions

Exercise Program Log

When card is finished, please see a Trainer for program revisions.

Name: _____
Date: _____
Trainer: _____

Resistance Training Exercise	Seat Adj.	Date: Wt x Reps	Wt x Reps	Wt x Reps	Wt x Reps	Wt x Reps	Wt x Reps	Wt x Reps	Wt x Reps	Wt x Reps

Cardiorespiratory Exercise	Seat Adj.	Time / Dist.	Time / Dist.	Time / Dist.	Time / Dist.	Time / Dist.	Time / Dist.	Time / Dist.	Time / Dist.	Time / Dist.

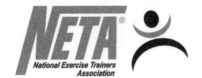

Fitness Assessment (Male)

NAME: _____

AGE: _____ **DOB:** _____ **HEIGHT:** _____

MEASUREMENTS

Date:				
Neck	cm	cm	cm	cm
Upper Arm (L/R)	cm	cm	cm	cm
Chest	cm	cm	cm	cm
Waist	cm	cm	cm	cm
Abdominal	cm	cm	cm	cm
Hips	cm	cm	cm	cm
Thigh (L/R)	cm	cm	cm	cm
Calf (L/R)	cm	cm	cm	cm
Waist-to-Hip Ratio				
Blood Pressure	/	/	/	/

BODY COMPOSITION

Date:								
Weight	lbs.		lbs.		lbs.		lbs.	
Body Mass Index (BMI)	kg/m^2		kg/m^2		kg/m^2		kg/m^2	
Body Fat % (*calipers*)	Chest	mm	Chest	mm	Chest	mm	Chest	mm
	Abdominal	mm	Abdominal	mm	Abdominal	mm	Abdominal	mm
	Thigh	mm	Thigh	mm	Thigh	mm	Thigh	mm
	Sum	mm	Sum	mm	Sum	mm	Sum	mm
	Est. % BF	%	Est. % BF	%	Est. % BF	%	Est. % BF	%

FITNESS ASSEMENT

Date:				
Cardiovascular Fitness	RHR:		RHR:	
Protocol:	Time:	HR:	Time:	HR:
	Est. VO_2max:		Est. VO_2max:	
	Rating:		Rating:	
Muscular Fitness				
Full-Body Push-up Test	#:	Rating:	#:	Rating:
Partial Curl-up Test	#:	Rating:	#:	Rating:
Other:				
Other:				
Flexibility				
Sit and Reach Test	Inches:	Rating:	Inches:	Rating:
Shoulder Flexibility	Good Fair Poor		Good Fair Poor	
Other:				
Other:				

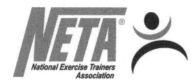

Fitness Assessment (Female)

NAME: _____

AGE: _____ **DOB:** _____ **HEIGHT:** _____

MEASUREMENTS				
Date:				
Neck	cm	cm	cm	cm
Upper Arm (L/R)	cm	cm	cm	cm
Chest	cm	cm	cm	cm
Waist	cm	cm	cm	cm
Abdominal	cm	cm	cm	cm
Hips	cm	cm	cm	cm
Thigh (L/R)	cm	cm	cm	cm
Calf (L/R)	cm	cm	cm	cm
Waist-to-Hip Ratio				
Blood Pressure	/	/	/	/

BODY COMPOSITION									
Date:									
Weight		lbs.		lbs.		lbs.		lbs.	
Body Mass Index (BMI)		kg/m²		kg/m²		kg/m²		kg/m²	
Body Fat % (calipers)	Triceps	mm	Triceps	mm	Triceps	mm	Triceps	mm	
	Suprailiac	mm	Suprailiac	mm	Suprailiac	mm	Suprailiac	mm	
	Thigh	mm	Thigh	mm	Thigh	mm	Thigh	mm	
	Sum	mm	Sum	mm	Sum	mm	Sum	mm	
	Est. % BF	%	Est. % BF	%	Est. % BF	%	Est. % BF	%	

FITNESS ASSEMENT		
Date:		
Cardiovascular Fitness	RHR:	RHR:
Protocol:	Time: HR:	Time: HR:
	Est. VO₂max:	Est. VO₂max:
	Rating:	Rating:
Muscular Fitness		
Modified Push-up Test	#: Rating:	#: Rating:
Partial Curl-up Test	#: Rating:	#: Rating:
Other:		
Other:		
Flexibility		
Sit and Reach Test	Inches: Rating:	Inches: Rating:
Shoulder Flexibility	Good Fair Poor	Good Fair Poor
Other:		
Other:		

Gloss-A-Dex

Abduction: movement of an extremity (i.e., arm, leg) away from the midline of the body. **pg. 55–56**

Action-Oriented Goal: a short-term goal that focuses on the specific steps or actions necessary to attain a desired outcome. Also called process goals or performance goals. **pg. 26**

Acute Injury: a single instantaneous incident of physical trauma to the body. **pg. 307**

Adduction: movement of an extremity (i.e., arm, leg) toward or across the midline of the body. **pg. 55–56**

Adenosine Triphosphate: the high-energy phosphagen molecule that supplies the energy necessary for all work (e.g., exercise) performed by the body. **pg. 84**

Aerobic Base: the point at which the body utilizes fat most efficiently as a substrate for energy production during oxygen-dependent (i.e., aerobic) physical activity or exercise. **pg. 199**

Aerobic Glycolysis: the bioenergetics system that supplies ATP during long duration, low-to-moderate-intensity exercise through the breakdown of carbohydrates (i.e., glucose). **pg. 85–86**

Agonist: the muscle or group of muscles which are primarily responsible for creating a particular joint action. Also known as the prime mover. **pg. 52**

All-or-None Principle: the contraction of all muscles within a given motor unit once the necessary threshold of central nervous system stimulation has been attained. **pg. 89**

Amino Acids: the structural components of protein including essential amino acids (i.e., those that must be ingested) and non-essential amino acids (i.e., those that can be manufactured by the body). **pg. 97**

Amotivation: a complete lack of motivation or lack of desire to engage in a certain behavior or an activity. **pg. 26**

Amphiarthrodial Joint: a slightly moveable joint often connected by fibrocartilaginous tissue. Also known as a cartilaginous joint. **pg. 46**

Anaerobic Glycolysis: the bioenergetics system that supplies ATP during short term, high-intensity exercise through the breakdown of glycogen (i.e., glucose). **pg. 85**

Anaerobic Threshold: the point during progressively intense exercise at which the muscles lose the ability to utilize oxygen to create energy (i.e., ATP) and blood lactate levels begin to sharply rise. **pg. 87**

Anatomical Position: standing in an tall position, feet hip-width apart with the toes pointing forward, the arms hanging to the sides of the body, palms of the hands facing forward, and the head and eyes looking straight ahead. **pg. 43**

Angular Momentum: the reluctance of a body segment or object to stop rotating around an axis of rotation as determined by the product of the object's mass, the distance from the axis of rotation, and the velocity of the object. **pg. 68**

Anorexia Nervosa: an eating disorder characterized by self-starvation, failure to maintain a minimally normal weight, an irrational fear of gaining weight or becoming fat, and a preoccupation with body shape. **pg. 130**

Antagonist: the muscle or group of muscles which oppose the agonist muscles. **pg. 62**

Anterior: a point or body part located on the front of the body. **pg. 43**

Anterior Pelvic Tilt: rotational movement of the pelvis such that the anterior superior iliac spine of the pelvis moves forward relative to the pubic bone. **pg. 156**

Appendicular Skeleton: the 126 bones that include the upper and lower extremities as well as the shoulder and pelvic girdles. **pg. 44**

Appreciative Inquiry: an approach to coaching behavioral change that focuses on exploring and amplifying an individual's strengths and that which is good. **pg. 34–35**

Arterial-Venous Oxygen Difference: the amount of oxygen removed from the arterial blood and taken into the mitochondria within the skeletal muscle. Also called oxygen extraction. **pg. 82**

Asthma: a chronic inflammatory disease that affects the lining of the airways within the lungs. **pg. 323**

Autogenic Inhibition: decreased muscle tension or relaxation of a muscle that is facilitated by stimulation of the Golgi tendon organs. **pg. 253**

Automated External Defibrillator: a small portable electronic device used to analyze the heart's rhythm and provide defibrillation of irregular heartbeats through the delivery of a small electrical shock. **pg. 317**

Axial Skeleton: the 80 bones that include the skull, spinal column, sternum, and ribs. **pg. 44**

Balance: the ability to control the position of the body against external forces. **pg. 73**

Ballistic Stretching: a method of flexibility training that utilizes rapid bouncing movements in an effort to lengthen and stretch the targeted muscle group. **pg. 254**

Basal Metabolic Rate: the minimum amount of energy needed to sustain basic life functions while lying at complete rest, in the morning, after sleep, and in a fasted state. **pg. 121**

Base of Support: the points of contact between the body and the ground or another surface or object. **pg. 73**

Beat: regular pulsation that creates an even rhythm within music. Also referred to as a count. **pg. 297**

Beats Per Minute: the number of beats of the heart per minute. **pg. 80.** Also refers to the number of beats that occur within one minute of music. **pg. 297**

Binge-Eating Disorder: an eating disorder characterized by recurrent episodes of eating significantly more food in a short period of time than most people would eat under similar circumstances, with episodes marked by feelings of lack of control. **pg. 131**

Blood Pressure: the pressure exerted by the circulating blood against the walls of the blood vessels, equal to the product of the cardiac output and the total peripheral vascular resistance. **pg. 81**

Body Composition: the relative amount of fat mass and lean body mass throughout the body, expressed as a percentage of body fat. **pg. 166, 191**

Body Mass Index: a calculation used to assess body weight relative to height such that BMI is equal to weight in kilograms divided by height in meters squared. **pg. 119, 150**

Bulimia Nervosa: an eating disorder characterized by frequent cycles of binge-eating and inappropriate compensatory purge behaviors intended to prevent weight gain. **pg. 130**

Calorie: a unit of energy defined as the amount of heat necessary to raise the temperature of one gram of water one degree Celsius. **pg. 98**

Carbohydrates: a macronutrient that serves as the body's preferred source of energy. **pg. 95**

Cardiac Muscle: the extremely efficient and fatigue-resistant muscle tissue that comprises the walls of the heart. **pg. 49**

Cardiac Output: the total amount of blood pumped or circulated by the heart per minute, equal to the product of the heart rate and the stroke volume. **pg. 81**

Cardiopulmonary Resuscitation: a life support method using chest compressions and rescue breathing intended to supply oxygen to the brain and other vital organs. **pg. 316–317**

Cardiorespiratory Endurance: the capacity of the circulatory and respiratory systems to deliver oxygen and nutrients to the working skeletal muscles to support continuous aerobic activity. **pg. 170, 191, 195**

Center of Gravity: the point at which the body's mass is concentrated and balanced between all three planes of motion. **pg. 73**

Cholesterol: a waxy, fat-like substance found in animal food products and produced by the liver of the body. **pg. 110–111**

Chondromalacia Patellae: a condition in which the cartilage lining the posterior surface of the patella becomes softened and swollen, progressing to fragmentation and flaking, and eventually to erosion of the cartilage down to the underlying bone. **pg. 309**

Chronic Injury: a state of injury that develops over an extended period of time as the result of cumulative stress to tissue within the body. **pg. 307**

Closed Kinetic Chain: an exercise during which the distal end (i.e., hand, foot) of the working body segment is in a fixed position and remains in constant contact with an immovable surface. **pg. 206**

Compressive Stress: a normal force that acts to shorten or compresses a tissue. **pg. 71**

Concentric: the phase of an isotonic muscle action during which the skeletal muscle shortens. **pg. 51**

Coordination: the ability to integrate several movements of the body simultaneously and sequentially to complete a complex task. **pg. 74**

DASH: an acronym representing the Dietary Approaches to Stop Hypertension. A dietary pattern characterized by high intake of fruit, vegetables, legumes, nuts; moderate intake of whole grains and low-fat or fat-free dairy products; and low in red meats, saturated fats, cholesterol, and sodium. **pg. 106**

Decisional Balance: the process of weighing the pros and cons related to behavioral change or the adoption of a new behavior. **pg. 23–24**

Deep: a point or a body part located further beneath (internal) or away from the surface of the body. **pg. 43**

Dehydration: fluid losses that exceed fluid replenishment (i.e., replacement). **pg. 101**

Delayed Onset Muscle Soreness: muscle soreness that typically begins about 24 hours after a new exposure to a physical overload (e.g., resistance training) and peaks about 48–72 hours post-exercise. **pg. 207**

Diabetes Mellitus: a group of metabolic diseases characterized by an inability to properly regulate blood glucose levels. **pg. 143, 325**

Diarthrodial Joint: a freely moveable joint containing a joint capsule, articular cartilage, and a synovial membrane producing synovial fluid. Also known as a synovial joint. **pg. 46**

Diastolic Blood Pressure: the pressure exerted by the circulating blood against the walls of the blood vessels during the relaxation phase of the cardiac cycle. **pg. 81, 149**

Dietary Guidelines for Americans: a set of dietary guidelines and key recommendations for the general public and 6 recommendations for special population groups published jointly by the Department of Agriculture and the Department of Health and Human Services. **pg. 105–111**

Disordered Eating: a broad range of maladaptive dietary behaviors, weight loss practices, and psychological disorders related to eating. **pg. 129**

Distal: a point on an extremity (e.g., arm or leg) located further away from the attached end of the limb or further from the center of the body. **pg. 43**

Dorsiflexion: the movement that brings the top (dorsal surface) of the foot toward the anterior aspect of the lower leg. **pg. 55–56**

Dynamic Stretching: a method of flexibility training that utilizes slow, controlled, and rhythmic movements to actively increase joint range of motion. **pg. 254**

Eating Disorders: four clinically diagnosable conditions including anorexia nervosa, bulimia nervosa, binge-eating disorder, and feeding or eating disorders not elsewhere classified. **pg. 129**

Eccentric: the phase of an isotonic muscle action during which the skeletal muscle lengthens. **pg. 51**

Elastic Deformation: the instantaneous return of a deformed object to its original shape once an external force is removed. **pg. 72**

Emergency Response Plan: a written plan outlining the policies and procedures related to emergency response within a fitness facility. **pg. 318**

Equilibrium: a state in which forces acting upon an object are equal. **pg. 68**

Eversion: the movement of the bottom of the foot outward, away from the midline of the body. **pg. 55–56**

Excess Post-Exercise Oxygen Consumption: the elevated consumption of oxygen after the cessation of an exercise session. Also known as the oxygen debt. **pg. 84**

Exercise: a subset of physical activity that includes planned, structured, and repetitive bodily movement performed to improve one or more components of physical fitness. **pg. 185**

Exertional Heat Cramps: painful involuntary muscle spasms, often affecting the lower extremities and abdomen, which may occur during or after prolonged strenuous exercise performed in hot and humid environments. **pg. 314**

Exertional Heatstroke: a life-threatening medical emergency characterized by dangerously high core body temperature, central nervous system dysfunction, and multiple organ system failure. **pg. 315**

Extension: a movement that increases the relative joint angle or moves two body segments further apart and back toward the anatomical position. **pg. 55–56**

External Rotation: a movement around the long axis of a bone or body segment away from the body. **pg. 55–56**

Extrinsic Motivation: motivation driven by or influenced by external factors or those outside of an individual. **pg. 26**

Fast Glycolytic Muscle Fibers: skeletal muscle fibers characterized by a fast speed of contraction, high force production, and energy production through anaerobic metabolism. Also labeled type IIb or IIx muscle fibers. **pg. 88**

Fast Oxidative Glycolytic Muscle Fibers: skeletal muscle fibers characterized by a fast speed of contraction, moderate-to-high force production, and energy production through anaerobic and aerobic metabolism. Also labeled type IIa muscle fibers. **pg. 88**

Fat: a macronutrient serving many important functions throughout the body including a source of energy during prolonged, low-intensity aerobic activity. **pg. 97**

Fatty Acid Oxidation: the bioenergetics system that supplies ATP during long duration, low-intensity exercise through the breakdown of fats (i.e., fatty acids). **pg. 86–87**

Female Athlete Triad: the interrelated combination of low energy availability, amenorrhea, and reduced bone mineral density sometimes seen among highly active females. **pg. 132**

First Class Lever: a lever system in which two opposing forces (e.g., muscle force, resistance force) are located on opposite sides of a fulcrum. **pg. 70**

FITT: an acronym representing frequency, intensity, time, and type of activity, which is applied to the design of cardiorespiratory training programs. **pg. 196–269**

Flexibility: the ability to move a joint through a full, pain-free range of motion. **pg. 178, 191, 253**

Flexion: a movement that decreases the relative joint angle or brings two body segments closer together. **pg. 55–56**

Force: an action upon an object causing acceleration, deceleration, or stabilization. **pg. 69**

Force Arm: in a lever system, the perpendicular distance of the muscle force from the axis of rotation. **pg. 69**

Frontal Plane: the anatomical plane that divides the body into the anterior and posterior sides. **pg. 44**

Fulcrum: the axis of rotation in a lever system. **pg. 69**

Functional: refers to an exercise that integrates multiple joints performing multi-planar, three-dimensional movement, which resembles activities of daily living or occupational activities. **pg. 73**

General Adaptation Syndrome: a concept proposed to explain the physiological response of the body to an imposed stress including the alarm stage, the resistance stage, and the exhaustion stage. **pg. 207**

Golgi Tendon Organs: sensory receptors located in the musculotendinous unit that are sensitive to changes in muscular tension and rate of tension change. **pg. 253**

Ground Reaction Force: the equal and opposite force applied against the body in response to the force applied by the body (e.g., foot) against the ground. **pg. 68**

GROW: a coaching model acronym which represents goal, reality, options, and what will you do. **pg. 35–36**

Health: a condition characterized by the absence of illness, disease, and injury as well as a state of optimal physical, social, and psychological well-being. **pg. 185**

Health Belief Model: a behavioral model that suggests an individual will modify their behavior to prevent a disease or an undesirable health condition if they believe they are susceptible to the disease or condition. **pg. 26**

Health-Related Physical Fitness: a set of attributes including cardiorespiratory endurance, muscular strength, muscular endurance, body composition, and flexibility. **pg. 189, 191**

Heart Rate: the number of beats or cardiac cycles of the heart per minute. **pg. 80, 149, 197**

Heart Rate Reserve: represents the difference between an individual's maximal heart rate and the resting heart rate. **pg. 198**

Heat Exhaustion: a common, yet potentially serious, heat illness often characterized by profuse sweating accompanied by cold, clammy skin. **pg. 315**

High-Density Lipoproteins: a lipoprotein that enables the transportation of lipids, cholesterol, and triglycerides through the bloodstream. Known as the 'good' cholesterol, HDLs are scavengers that gather and deliver cholesterol and lipids to the liver for breakdown and excretion. **pg. 110**

HIPAA: the Health Insurance Portability and Accountability Act of 1996. Regulates privacy of personal health information among health care providers and other covered entities. **pg. 347**

Horizontal Abduction: a movement of an extremity in the transverse plane (i.e., parallel to the ground) away from the midline of the body. **pg. 55–56**

Horizontal Adduction: a movement of an extremity in the transverse plane (i.e., parallel to the ground) toward or across the midline of the body. **pg. 55–56**

Hyperextension: the continuation of extension beyond the anatomical position. **pg. 55–56**

Hypertension: chronically elevated blood pressure defined as a systolic blood pressure greater than or equal to 140 mmHg or a diastolic blood pressure greater than or equal to 90 mmHg. **pg. 143, 326**

Hyponatremia: a condition in which the body's water-to-sodium ratio is severely elevated causing a decrease in plasma sodium concentration. **pg. 101**

Inferior: a point on the body located closer to the feet relative to another body part. **pg. 43**

Informed Consent: a document utilized to communicate the inherent risks and dangers associated with participation in exercise testing and training. **pg. 139, 348**

Intrinsic Motivation: motivation originating internally or within an individual such as performing a task for the inherent pleasure, satisfaction, or personal challenge derived from the task. **pg. 26**

Internal Rotation: a movement around the long axis of a bone or body segment toward the body. **pg. 55–56**

Interval Training: a method of exercise training which alternates short bouts of high-intensity exercise with short bouts of low-intensity active recovery for the purpose of increasing anaerobic threshold and exercise tolerance. **pg. 200**

Inversion: the movement of the bottom of the foot inward, toward the midline of the body. **pg. 55–56**

Isokinetic: a muscle action during which the skeletal muscle exerts a variable amount of force at a constant speed of movement modulated by the exercise equipment. **pg. 206**

Isometric: a muscle action during which force is produced, yet the muscle does not change length and no movement occurs. **pg. 51, 206**

Isotonic: a muscle action during which force is produced as the skeletal muscle shortens and lengthens to lift and lower a constant external load. **pg. 51, 205**

Karvonen Formula: a calculation based on heart rate reserve that is used to determine the target heart rate during cardiorespiratory exercise. **pg. 198, 270**

Kilocalorie: the amount of heat required to raise the temperature of one kilogram of water one degree Celsius. 1 kilocalorie is equal to 1,000 calories. **pg. 96, 120**

Kinetic Chain: the interconnected series of body segments and joints spanning from the feet to the head. **pg. 73, 155**

Kyphosis: an excessive posterior curvature or rounding of the thoracic spine. **pg. 156**

Lapse: a temporary departure from a desired behavior or a temporary return to an undesirable behavior. **pg. 21**

Lateral: a point on the body further away from the midline or the middle of the body. **pg. 43**

Law of Acceleration: states that a force applied to an object causes acceleration of the object in the direction of the force that is proportional to the force and inversely proportional to the mass of the object. **pg. 68**

Law of Action-Reaction: states that when an object applies a force to another object, there is an equal and opposite force applied back to the original object. **pg. 68**

Law of Inertia: states that an object at rest will stay at rest and an object in motion will stay in motion unless an external force acts upon the object. **pg. 68**

Liability Exposure: any situation that increases the risk of an injury, a medical emergency, or the severity of a medical emergency, as well as the risk of subsequent litigation. **pg. 340**

Ligament: fibrous connective tissue which connects bone to bone and provides passive stability to joints. **pg. 47, 308**

Lordosis: an excessive anterior curvature or arching of the lumbar spine. **pg. 156**

Low-Density Lipoproteins: a lipoprotein that transports fat molecules and cholesterol within the bloodstream. Known as the 'bad' cholesterol, LDLs contribute to the accumulation of plaque in the arteries causing atherosclerosis. **pg. 110**

Lower Cross Syndrome: a postural distortion pattern characterized by an anterior pelvic tilt, increased lumbar lordosis, internally rotated hips, adducted knees, and externally rotated feet. **pg. 160–161**

Maximal Oxygen Consumption: the highest amount of oxygen utilized by the body during maximal, exhaustive exercise, equal to the product of the maximal cardiac output and the maximal oxygen extraction. **pg. 83**

Measure: comprised of a series of downbeats and upbeats that are organized into a pattern within music. **pg. 297**

Medial: a point on the body located closer to the midline or the middle of the body. **pg. 43**

Median: a vertical line down the center of the body, which divides the body into the left and right halves. Also known as the midline. **pg. 43**

Metabolic Equivalent: a unit of measurement used to define the absolute energy expenditure or oxygen consumption of a specific level of activity. Also known as a MET. One MET is equivalent to 3.5 mL of oxygen consumed per kilogram of body weight per minute of activity. **pg. 83, 187**

Metabolism: the biochemical process of breaking down macronutrients to provide the energy necessary to sustain life and perform activity. **pg. 120**

Minerals: inorganic micronutrient elements essential for the maintenance of normal physiological processes throughout the body. **pg. 99–100**

Mitochondria: small organelles found throughout skeletal muscle within which ATP is produced aerobically. Known as the "powerhouse" of the muscle fiber (cell). **pg. 82**

Moment Arm: the perpendicular distance from the fulcrum to the applied force. **pg. 69**

Motivation: the degree of determination, drive, or desire with which an individual approaches or avoids a behavior. **pg. 26–28, 289**

Motivational Interviewing: a collaborative conversation style for strengthening a person's own motivation and commitment to change. **pg. 32–34, 123**

Motor Unit: the functional unit of the neuromuscular system including the nerve cell (i.e., motor neuron), the branches of the nerve cell (i.e., axon, dendrites), and the muscle fibers innervated by the nerve. **pg. 89**

Muscle Force: in a lever system, the internal force generated by the skeletal muscle(s). **pg. 69**

Muscle Spindles: sensory receptors within the skeletal muscle, which are sensitive to changes in length and rate of length change throughout the muscle. **pg. 253**

Muscular Endurance: the ability of a muscle or group of muscles to perform multiple repetitions against a submaximal external resistance. **pg. 175, 191, 205**

Muscular Strength: the ability of a muscle or group of muscles to exert maximal force against an external resistance. **pg. 174, 191, 205**

MyPlate: a graphic produced by the United States Department of Agriculture (USDA) intended to remind Americans of a well-balanced and healthy eating pattern. **pg. 111–113**

National Weight Control Registry: a large ongoing study seeking to identify and understand the strategies and behaviors of individuals successful at long-term maintenance of weight loss. **pg. 123**

Negligence: failure to act according to a generally accepted standard of care consistent with the manner in which a reasonable, prudent person would have acted under similar or identical circumstances. **pg. 339**

Neuroplasticity: the changes to or 're-wiring' of neural pathways within the brain resulting from exposure to new behaviors, environments, experiences, and neural processes. **pg. 21**

Non-Exercise Activity Thermogenesis: the energy expended during all bodily movement, which excludes sleeping, eating, structured exercise, and leisure-time physical activity. **pg. 121**

Normal Stress: a force that is applied perpendicular to an object's cross-section or parallel to the long axis of the object. **pg. 71**

Nutrient Dense Foods: those foods containing a high content of essential nutrients, yet a low caloric value. **pg. 106**

Nutrition Facts Label: an information panel required by the Food and Drug Administration (FDA) on all pre-packaged foods to provide the nutritional content within the food product. **pg. 112–116**

OARS: an acronym used to describe the core communication skills used during motivational interviewing. OARS stands for open-ended questions, affirmations, reflective listening, and summarizing. **pg. 33**

OMNI Scale of Perceived Exertion: a subjective scale ranging from zero to ten using both verbal and mode-specific pictorial descriptors distributed along an ascending slope from extremely easy to extremely hard, which is used to identify and monitor perceived exertion during various modes of physical activity and exercise. **pg. 198–199**

Open Kinetic Chain: an exercise during which the distal end (i.e., hand, foot) of the working body segment is 'open' to freely move through space. **pg. 207**

Osteoarthritis: a degenerative joint disease in which the cartilage that covers the ends of bones deteriorates, causing pain and loss of movement. **pg. 324**

Osteoporosis: a disease affecting the skeletal system in which low bone mineral density and changes in the microstructure of the bone increases the risk of fractures. **pg. 327**

Outcome-Oriented Goals: a long-term goal that is the result of the consistent performance of specific actions or behaviors. **pg. 29**

Overtraining: a chronic condition represented by decreased performance resulting from an imbalance between excessive training and inadequate recovery. **pg. 207, 312**

Oxygen Consumption: the amount of oxygen that is used by the body per minute, equal to the product of the cardiac output and the oxygen extraction. **pg. 83**

Oxygen Debt: the elevated consumption of oxygen after the cessation of an exercise session. Also known as the excess post-exercise oxygen consumption. **pg. 84**

Oxygen Deficit: the difference between the supply of and demand for oxygen during exercise, representing the oxygen that is missing relative to that which is needed to support the level of exercise. **pg. 83–84**

Oxygen Extraction: the amount of oxygen removed from the arterial blood and taken into the mitochondria within the skeletal muscle. Also called the arterial-venous oxygen difference. **pg. 81–82**

Patellofemoral Pain Syndrome: a condition characterized by complaints of pain behind and around the patella and through the anterior aspect of the knee. Also called runner's knee. **pg. 309**

Performance-Related Physical Fitness: a set of attributes including agility, coordination, balance, power, reaction time, and speed. Also known as the skill-related components of fitness. **pg. 189–191**

Periodization: the systematic manipulation of acute program variables intended to optimize fitness and performance gains while avoiding overuse, overtraining, and progression plateaus. **pg. 191, 211–213**

Phosphagen System: the bioenergetics system that supplies the immediate source of ATP during very short-term, high-intensity exercise. **pg. 84**

Phrase: a component of music consisting of 2 or more measures that can be combined to create an 8-count phrase (2 measures), a 16-count phrase (4 measures) or a 32-count phrase (8 measures). **pg. 297**

Physical Activity: any bodily movement produced by the use of the skeletal muscles that increases energy expenditure above resting levels. **pg. 185**

Physical Activity Guidelines for Americans: a set of physical activity recommendations, published by the U.S. Department of Health and Human Services, intended to guide Americans toward improved health through increased physical activity. **pg. 186–187**

Physical Activity Readiness Questionnaire: a popular preparticipation screening tool used by fitness professionals to identify those individuals at elevated risk, who should consult with their health care provider prior to beginning an exercise program. **pg. 140, 357**

Physical Fitness: a set of attributes possessed or attained by an individual that contribute to the ability to perform physical activity with vigor and without undue fatigue. **pg. 185**

Plane: a flat, level surface extending into space. **pg. 44**

Plantar Flexion: the movement of the bottom of the foot (plantar surface) toward the ground, pointing the toes away from the body. **pg. 55–56**

Plastic Deformation: the permanent change in shape of an object in response to an external force. **pg. 72**

Posterior: a point or body part located on the back of the body. **pg. 43**

Posterior Pelvic Tilt: rotational movement of the pelvis such that the anterior superior iliac spine of the pelvis moves backward relative to the pubic bone. **pg. 156**

Posture: the position of all body parts at any given time. **pg. 72, 155**

PRICE: an acronym representing protection, rest, ice, compression, and elevation, which indicates the immediate first aid and care recommended for many exercise-related injuries. **pg. 312**

Principle of Overload: refers to the application of a physiological or physical stress greater than that to which the body or targeted body system is normally subjected. **pg. 190**

Principle of Progression: indicates that as the body adapts and becomes accustomed to a specific level of overload, the training stimulus (i.e., overload) must be increased in order to stimulate additional changes and adaptations. **pg. 190**

Principle of Reversibility: refers to the gradual loss of conditioning (e.g., physiological and physical adaptations) in the absence of an appropriate training stimulus. Also known as detraining. **pg. 191**

Principle of Specificity: indicates that the training effect is specific to the training stimulus or stress applied to the body. Also known as the SAID principle: specific adaptations to imposed demands. **pg. 190**

Principle of Variation: refers to the strategic and meaningful manipulation of acute training variables necessary to promote a continuous training effect. **pg. 191**

Pronation: refers to the rotational movement turning the palms of the hand down or toward the posterior aspect of the body. Also refers to the combined movements of eversion and plantar flexion at the ankle. **pg. 55–56**

Proprioceptive Neuromuscular Facilitation: a method of flexibility training that alternates passive static stretches with muscle activation to facilitate increased joint range of motion. **pg. 254**

Protein: a macronutrient that serves as the building block for new tissue and tissue repair throughout the body. **pg. 96**

Protraction: movement of the scapula away from the midline of the body or the spinal column. **pg. 57**

Proximal: a point on an extremity (e.g., arm or leg) located closer to the attached end of the limb or closer to the center of the body. **pg. 43**

Pulmonary Ventilation: the amount of air inhaled and exhaled from the lungs per minute, equal to the product of the tidal volume and the respiratory rate. Also known as minute ventilation. **pg. 82**

Range of Motion: a measurement of flexibility often expressed in terms of the degrees of rotation around a joint or distance of linear movement of a body segment. **pg. 178**

Rate of Perceived Exertion: a subjective scale used to identify and monitor exercise intensity during cardiorespiratory exercise and physical activity. **pg. 198, 271**

Reciprocal Inhibition: the decreased neurological stimulation of a muscle group that corresponds to the activation of the opposing muscle group. **pg. 160, 253**

Recruitment: the simultaneous activation (i.e., contraction) of additional muscle fibers to produce greater force. **pg. 89**

Rehearsal Effect: the ability of the mind and muscles to recall repetitive activities. **pg. 280**

Rehearsal Moves: movements similar to those participants will perform in the class or during the chosen activity. **pg. 280**

Relapse: a long-term departure from a desired behavior or a return to an undesirable behavior, often accompanied by decreased motivation and desire to resume the desired behavior. **pg. 23**

Resistance Arm: in a lever system, the perpendicular distance of the resistance force from the axis of rotation. **pg. 69**

Resistance Force: in a lever system, the external force applied against a body segment. **pg. 69**

Respiratory Rate: the number of breaths taken per minute. **pg. 82**

Resting Metabolic Rate: the amount of energy expended in a resting and fasted state. **pg. 121–122**

Retraction: movement of the scapula toward the midline of the body or the spinal column. **pg. 57**

Rheumatoid Arthritis: an autoimmune disease in which the body's immune system mistakenly attacks the tissues of the joints. **pg. 324**

Risk Factors for Cardiovascular Disease: variables that have a strong association with the development of cardiovascular disease. **pg. 142–143**

Risk Management: a proactive administrative process intended to minimize liability exposures and subsequent liability losses for the fitness professional and the fitness facilities they represent. **pg. 341**

Rotation: a movement around the long axis of a bone or body segment. **pg. 55–56**

Rotational Inertia: refers to the reluctance of a body segment or object to rotate around an axis of rotation. **pg. 68**

Sagittal Plane: the anatomical plane that extends from the median, dividing the body into left and right sides. **pg. 44**

Sarcomere: the smallest functional unit within the skeletal muscle fiber designated by two Z-lines and containing the overlapping myofilaments: actin and myosin. **pg. 49, 51**

Scapulohumeral Rhythm: the synchronized movement of shoulder abduction and scapular upward rotation. **pg. 59**

Scope of Practice: defines the specific boundaries within which an individual may perform the tasks associated with their profession. **pg. 340**

Second Class Lever: a lever system in which the muscle force and the resistance force are located on the same side of the fulcrum, with the muscle force located further from the axis of rotation creating a force arm longer than the resistance arm. **pg. 70–71**

Self-Determination Theory: a behavioral theory suggesting that individuals seek to satisfy three primary psychosocial needs including a need for autonomy, a need to demonstrate competency, and a need for meaningful social interactions. **pg. 26**

Self-Efficacy: situation- or task-specific confidence held by an individual with regard to their ability to perform an activity or adopt a behavior. **pg. 23**

Self-Efficacy Theory: a theory related to behavioral change that describes how individuals form perceptions regarding their personal ability to perform an activity or to adopt a behavior. **pg. 24–25**

Self-Myofascial Release: a method of flexibility training during which an individual uses their own body weight to apply pressure to a targeted muscle using a foam roller or a similar device. **pg. 254**

Shear Stress: forces or loads that are applied in opposite directions, parallel to the cross-section of an object or perpendicular to the long axis. **pg. 71**

Shoulder Impingement Syndrome: a condition characterized by pain and reduced range of motion during abduction of the arm and overhead movements. **pg. 59, 310**

Size Principle: a neuromuscular principle indicating that muscle fibers are recruited in order of size beginning with smaller fibers (i.e., type I), progressing to larger fibers (i.e., type IIa), followed by the largest fibers (i.e., type IIb, type IIx). **pg. 89**

Skeletal Muscle: a voluntary muscle tissue that produces movement and stabilization of the skeletal system. Also known as striated muscle. **pg. 49–50**

Sliding Filament Theory: the widely-accepted theory describing the series of events involved in the contraction of a skeletal muscle. **pg. 51**

Slow Oxidative Muscle Fibers: skeletal muscle fibers characterized by a slow speed of contraction, low force production, and energy production through aerobic metabolism. Also labeled type I muscle fibers. **pg. 88**

SMART: a goal-setting acronym that represents specific, measureable, attainable, relevant, and time-bound. **pg. 26–27**

Smooth Muscle: an involuntary muscle tissue lining the internal organs and arterial blood vessel walls, which uses wave-like contractions to move substances through the body. **pg. 49**

SOAP Notes: an acronym representing subjective, objective, assessment, and plan, used as a method of documentation regarding participant progress with exercise sessions and programs. **pg. 349–350**

Social Cognitive Theory: a theory of behavioral change suggesting that new behaviors and learning are affected by three interdependent variables including personal characteristics, environmental factors, and behavioral attributes. **pg. 25**

Sprain: an overstretching or tearing of a ligament. **pg. 308**

Stability: the ease with which balance is maintained as influenced by the base of support, position of the center of gravity over the base of support, height of the center of gravity, and mass of the body. **pg. 73**

Standard of Care: represents the manner with which professional services should be delivered in order to provide reasonable assurance that the expected outcome is attained without unnecessary risk of harm. **pg. 339**

Static Stretching: a method of flexibility training in which a muscle is lengthened to a position of mild discomfort, but not pain, which is then held for an extended period of time. **pg. 253**

Steady State: a state of equilibrium during which the supply of oxygen is equal to the demand for oxygen to support a specific level of exercise. **pg. 80, 83, 199**

Strain: an overstretching or tearing of a muscle or tendon. **pg. 308**

Stroke Volume: the amount of blood pumped by the left ventricle of the heart per beat. **pg. 80**

Summation: the additive effect of multiple successive electrical stimuli delivered via the motor unit to the skeletal muscle fibers. **pg. 89**

Superficial: a point or a body part located closer to or on the surface of the body. **pg. 43**

Superior: a point on the body located closer to the head relative to another body part. **pg. 43**

Supination: refers to the rotational movement that turns the palms of the hand up or toward the anterior aspect of the body. Also refers to the combined movements of inversion and dorsiflexion at the ankle. **pg. 55–56**

Synarthrodial Joint: an immovable joint held together by tough, fibrous connective tissue. Also known as a fibrous joint. **pg. 46**

Synergist: a muscle or group of muscles that assist the prime mover to perform a specific joint action. **pg. 52**

Systolic Blood Pressure: the pressure exerted by the circulating blood against the walls of the blood vessels (i.e., arteries) during a left ventricular contraction of the heart. **pg. 81, 149**

Tempo: the rate of speed at which music is played. **pg. 298.** May also refer to the speed at which a resistance training exercise is performed. **pg. 208**

Tendon: a connective tissue that attaches the skeletal muscle to a bone. **pg. 51**

Tendonitis: an overuse injury characterized by inflammation and pain of a tendon. **pg. 310**

Tensile Stress: a normal force that acts to pull apart, elongate, or lengthen a tissue. **pg. 71**

Third Class Lever: a lever system in which the muscle force and the resistance force are located on the same side of the fulcrum, with the resistance force located further from the axis of rotation, creating a resistance arm longer than the force arm. **pg. 71**

Tidal Volume: the amount of air inhaled and exhaled by the lungs with each breath. **pg. 82**

Torque: the degree to which a force rotates an object around an axis of rotation, equal to the product of the force and the moment arm. **pg. 69**

Total Daily Energy Expenditure: the total amount of energy burned throughout the day. **pg. 121**

Total Peripheral Vascular Resistance: the systemic resistance to blood flow encountered or created throughout the arterial blood vessels. **pg. 81**

Training Effect: the physiological and physical adaptations resulting from regular exercise. **pg. 190**

Transtheoretical Model: describes the five stages of change that individuals move through when adopting a new behavior or making behavioral change. These stages include precontemplation, contemplation, preparation, action, and maintenance. **pg. 21–23, 289**

Transverse Plane: the anatomical plane extending parallel to the ground that divides the body into the upper and lower segments. Also called the horizontal plane. **pg. 44**

Twitch: a single electrical impulse delivered via the motor unit causing brief excitation of the muscle fibers followed immediately by relaxation. **pg. 89**

Upper Cross Syndrome: a postural distortion pattern characterized by a forward head position, protracted and elevated scapula, increased kyphosis, and forward-rounded shoulders. Also known as rounded shoulder syndrome. **pg. 160–161**

Valsalva Maneuver: characterized by holding one's breath while attempting to forcibly exhale against a closed glottis, thus preventing the air from escaping the lungs. **pg. 206, 208, 327**

Vertebral Column: the series of 33 interconnected bones including the cervical vertebrae, thoracic vertebrae, lumbar vertebrae, sacrum, and coccyx. **pg. 44, 46**

Viscoelastic: the ability of soft tissues within the body to display properties of both solids and fluids such that the tissue slowly returns to its original shape once an external force is removed. **pg. 72**

Vitamins: thirteen organic micronutrients essential for the maintenance of normal physiological processes throughout the body. **pg. 98–100**

Waist-to-Hip Ratio: a measurement used to assess an individual's regional fat distribution calculated by taking the waist circumference divided by the hip circumference. **pg. 151**

Answers to Chapter Review Questions

Chapter 1		Chapter 2		Chapter 3		Chapter 4		Chapter 5		Chapter 6		Chapter 7		Chapter 8		Chapter 9	
1.	B	1.	C	1.	B	1.	C	1.	C	1.	D	1.	C	1.	C	1.	A
2.	C	2.	B	2.	C	2.	B	2.	A	2.	B	2.	B	2.	B	2.	C
3.	D	3.	D	3.	D	3.	A	3.	C	3.	A	3.	B	3.	B	3.	B
4.	C	4.	B	4.	C	4.	D	4.	D	4.	D	4.	C	4.	C	4.	D
5.	A	5.	B	5.	B	5.	B	5.	B	5.	C	5.	B	5.	C	5.	C
6.	B	6.	A	6.	A	6.	A	6.	C	6.	C	6.	D	6.	B	6.	A

Chapter 10		Chapter 11		Chapter 12		Chapter 13		Chapter 14		Chapter 15		Chapter 16		Chapter 17		Chapter 18	
1.	C	1.	B	1.	C	1.	C	1.	C	1.	C	1.	B	1.	B	1.	D
2.	C	2.	C	2.	C	2.	C	2.	A	2.	D	2.	A	2.	C	2.	C
3.	D	3.	C	3.	B	3.	A	3.	C	3.	C	3.	D	3.	B	3.	B
4.	C	4.	C	4.	C	4.	D	4.	B	4.	C	4.	B	4.	A	4.	D
5.	C	5.	D	5.	D	5.	C	5.	A	5.	B	5.	A	5.	C	5.	C
6.	B	6.	C	6.	C	6.	D	6.	C	6.	D	6.	C	6.	A	6.	B

Chapter 19		Chapter 20		Chapter 21		Chapter 22		Chapter 23		Chapter 24		Chapter 25		Chapter 26		Chapter 27	
1.	B	1.	C	1.	D	1.	B	1.	D	1.	D	1.	C	1.	D	1.	A
2.	C	2.	C	2.	B	2.	A	2.	C	2.	B	2.	A	2.	A	2.	B
3.	D	3.	A	3.	D	3.	C	3.	B	3.	C	3.	B	3.	C	3.	D
4.	C	4.	D	4.	A	4.	D	4.	B	4.	B	4.	D	4.	D	4.	B
5.	B	5.	A	5.	A	5.	A	5.	C	5.	D	5.	D	5.	B	5.	D
6.	C	6.	B	6.	A	6.	B	6.	D	6.	B	6.	C	6.	A	6.	A

Notes

Notes

Notes

Notes